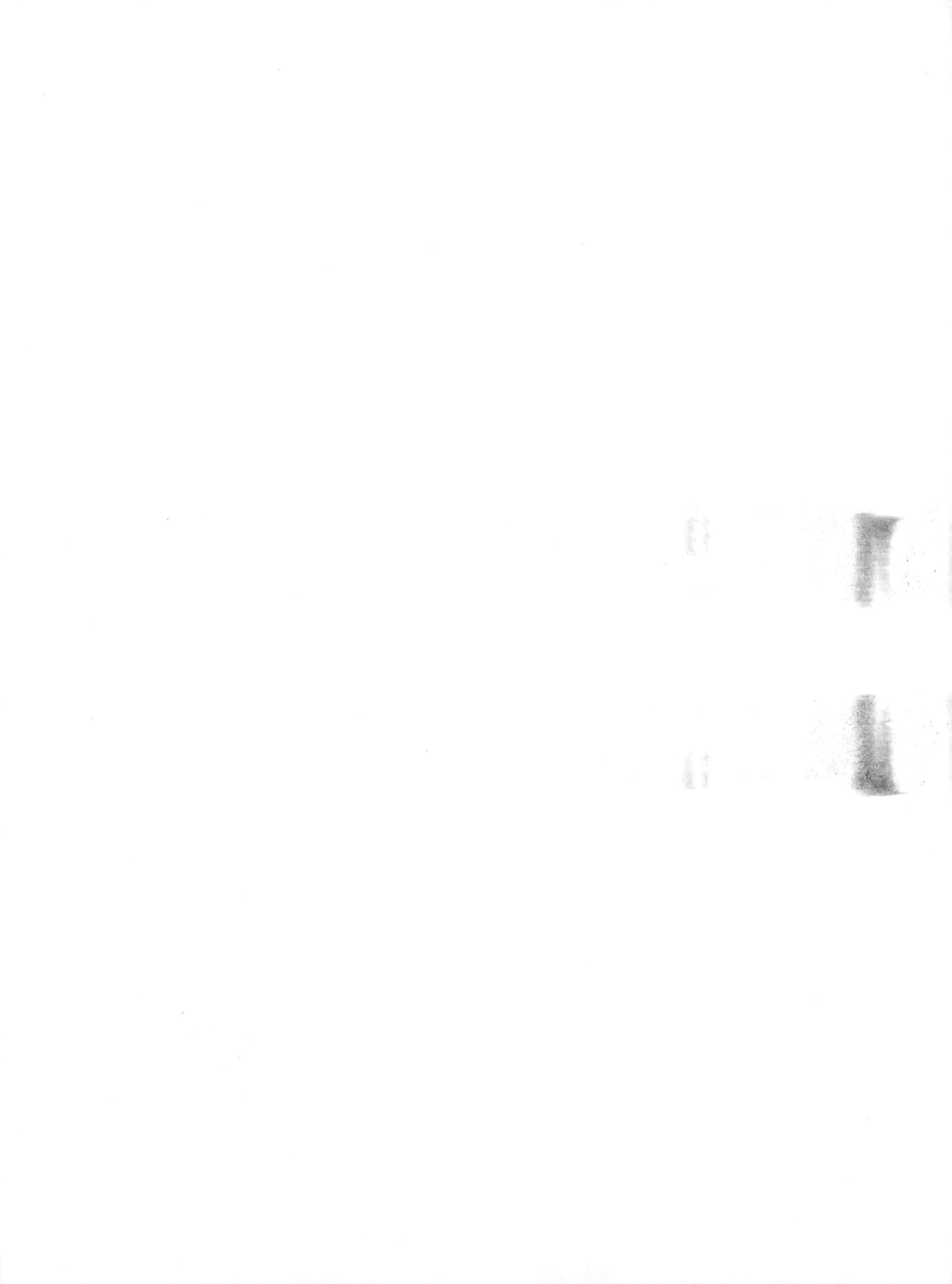

SALEM HEALTH
CANCER

SALEM HEALTH
CANCER

Second Edition

Volume I

Diseases, Symptoms and Conditions:
Achlorhydria – Ovarian epithelial cancer

Editors

Michael A. Buratovich, Ph.D.
Spring Arbor University

Laurie Jackson-Grusby, Ph.D.
Children's Hospital Boston, Harvard Medical School

Editor, first edition

Jeffrey A. Knight
Mount Holyoke College

SALEM PRESS
A Division of EBSCO Information Services, Inc.
Ipswich, Massachusetts

GREY HOUSE PUBLISHING

∞ The paper used in these volumes conforms to the American National Standard for Permanence of Paper for Printed Library Materials, Z39.48-1992 (R2009).

Note to Readers

The material presented in *Salem Health: Cancer* is intended for broad informational and educational purposes. Readers who suspect that they or someone whom they know or provide caregiving for suffers from cancer or any other physical or psychological disorder, disease, or condition described in this set should contact a physician without delay; this work should not be used as a substitute for professional medical diagnosis or staging. Readers who are undergoing or about to undergo any treatment or procedure described in this set should refer to their physicians and other health care team members for guidance concerning preparation and possible effects. This set is not to be considered definitive on the covered topics, and readers should remember that the field of health care is characterized by a diversity of medical opinions and constant expansion in knowledge and understanding.

Library of Congress Cataloging-in-Publication Data

Publisher's Cataloging-In-Publication Data
(Prepared by The Donohue Group, Inc.)

Names: Buratovich, Michael A., editor. | Jackson-Grusby, Laurie, editor.
Title: Cancer / editors, Michael A. Buratovich, Ph.D., Spring Arbor University, Laurie Jackson-Grusby, Ph.D., Children's Hospital Boston, Harvard Medical School.
Other Titles: Salem health (Pasadena, Calif.)
Description: Second edition. | Ipswich, Massachusetts: Salem Press, a division of EBSCO Information Services, Inc.; Amenia, NY: Grey House Publishing, [2016] | Editor, first edition, Jeffrey A. Knight, Mount Holyoke College. | Includes bibliographical references and index. | Volume I. Diseases, Symptoms and Conditions: Achlorhydria – Ovarian epithelial cancer – Volume II. Diseases, Symptoms and Conditions: Paget disease of bone – Zollinger-Ellison syndrome, Medical Specialties, Organizations, Social and Personal Issues – Volume III. Cancer Biology, Carcinogens and Suspected Carcinogens, Chemotherapy and Other Drugs, Complementary and Alternative Therapies, Lifestyle and Prevention – Volume IV. Procedures.
Identifiers: ISBN 978-1-61925-950-8 (set) | ISBN 978-1-68217-230-8 (vol. 1) | ISBN 978-1-68217-231-5 (vol. 2) | ISBN 978-1-68217-232-2 (vol. 3) | ISBN 978-1-68217-233-9 (vol. 4)
Subjects: LCSH: Cancer.
Classification: LCC RC265 .C336 2016 | DDC 616.99/4–dc23

First Printing

PRINTED IN THE UNITED STATES OF AMERICA

▶ Contents

▶ Publisher's Note

This second edition of *Salem Health: Cancer* includes 911 essays in 4 volumes on all aspects of cancer for all non-specialist interest groups—from those who have been diagnosed, to caregivers, family members, students, and readers with a general interest in health. The essays in this 4-volume set address diseases, conditions, symptoms, cancer-related syndromes, chemotherapy and other drugs, cancer centers, genetics, the biology of cancer, medical specialties, tests, procedures, complementary and alternative therapies, lifestyles, healthy and preventive strategies, and the many social and personal issues surrounding cancer, from cancer's impact on minority populations, finances, insurance, relationships, and emotional coping.

This comprehensive reference publication builds on the strength of the first, 2009 edition, with hundreds of updates and new topics. It will be of interest not only to public library patrons but also to premedical students and those building collections for the patient population.

Essays vary in length from 400 to 2,000 words, ranging from one to five pages. The material in this edition is arranged in ten categories:

- Cancer Biology
- Carcinogens & Suspected Carcinogens
- Chemotherapy & Other Drugs
- Complementary & Alternative Therapies
- Diseases, Symptoms & Conditions
- Lifestyle & Prevention
- Medical Specialties
- Organizations
- Procedures
- Social & Personal Issues

Each essay is written in one of six standard formats, all of which present a capsule definition of the topic, and all but the briefest essays list sources of further information from both print and online resources.

Specific formats are designed for readers for whom the information is compelling or urgent, fostering quick identification and retrieval of essential facts. For example, essays on diseases and conditions list "also known as" names and describe related conditions, risk factors, the disease process, incidence, symptoms, screening and diagnosis, treatment, and prognosis. Essays on carcinogens list "also known as" names for the chemical or substance, date it was identified by the government's report on carcinogens (RoC), cancers related to the carcinogen, exposure routes, principal places where the substance is found, populations at risk, symptoms to watch for, and a brief history of how we came to identify the substance as a carcinogen.

Essays on drugs list the Anatomical Therapeutic Chemical (ATC) classification system code if one exists; the types of cancer, or other condition for which the drug is indicated; the delivery routes (such as pill form or injection); the way the drug works; and side effects. Essays on procedures discuss why the procedure is performed, how to prepare, aftercare, risks, and the range of results. Essays on medical specialties identify not only the names of the specializations but also related subspecialists, the cancers they treat, how they are trained and certified, and the range of services and procedures they perform. Finally, a group of topics addressing social and personal issues, lifestyle choices, nutritional supplements, and complementary or alternative therapies are similarly formatted into subsections that call out key areas of interest for readers.

Special features of the set include tables throughout identifying the most important chemotherapeutic and other drugs and the symptoms and conditions they address, population statistics, survival rates, and other core information. Essays include "See also" cross-references to other essays in the set that are relevant to the topic. A fully cross-referenced "Complete List of Contents" at the beginning of every volume also assists readers in locating related topics of interest. Photographs identify typical instances of lesions, tumors, procedures, and anatomical cross-sections to locate areas of the body affected.

In addition, the following appendixes at the end of volume 4 provide information on the following:

- Drugs by Trade Name
- Associations and Agencies
- Cancer Centers and Hospitals
- Cancer Support Groups
- Carcinogens
- Glossary
- Bibliography

Salem Health: Cancer has benefited by the contributions of many experts—physicians, nurses, pharmacists, and professional medical writers—whose names are listed following this Publisher's Note. Salem Press thanks editors Michael A. Buratovich, Ph.D., Spring Arbor University and Laurie Jackson-Grusby, Ph.D., Children's Hospital Boston, Harvard Medical School.

▶ About the Editors

Michael Buratovich, Ph.D., is professor of biochemistry at Spring Arbor University in Spring Arbor, Michigan. He earned his BS in bacteriology and his MA in microbiology from UC Davis, and studied the function of tumor suppressor genes in the fruit fly, *Drosophila melanogaster*, in Dr. Peter Bryant's laboratory at UC Irvine. He also served as one of the editors for the 7th edition of the *Magill Medical Guide*, and has published over 100 articles in journals, encyclopedias, magazines, and books.

Laurie Jackson-Grusby, Ph.D., is an Assistant Professor in Pathology at Harvard Medical School, Children's Hospital Boston, and a faculty member of the Harvard Stem Cell Institute and Kirby Center for Neuroscience. She is a visiting instructor at the Harvard Extension school, where she teaches genetics. Her laboratory investigates the role of epigenetics in development of disease. She was awarded the Distinguished Scientist Award from the Sontag Foundation for her work on pediatric brain tumors.

▶ Contributors

Abbie L. Abboud, M.S., C.G.C.
Richard Adler, Ph.D.
Jane Adrian, M.P.H., Ed.M., M.T. (ASCP)
Paige E. Albert, B.S.,
Robert J. Amato, D.O.
Cathy Anderson, R.N., B.A.
Terry A. Anderson, B.S.
Wendell Anderson, B.A
Daruenie Andujar
Michele Arduengo, Ph.D., ELS
Bryan C. Auday, Ph.D
Bruce Baldwin, PhD
Tanja Bekhuis, Ph.D.
Paul F. Bell, Ph.D.
Raymond D. Benge, Jr., MS
Alvin K. Benson, Ph.D.
Anna Binda, Ph.D.
Robert Bockstiegel, B.S.
Scott A. Boerner, M.S.
Patricia Boone, Ph.D.
Andrea Bradford, M.A.
Wanda Todd Bradshaw, R.N.C., M.S.N.
Thomas L. Brown, Ph.D.
Suzette Buhr, R.T.R., C.D.A.
Amy Bull, D.S.N., A.P.N.
Michael A. Buratovich, Ph.D
Bharat Burman, B.A.
Jaime Stockslager Buss, M.S.P.H., ELS
Alex B. Cantrell, B.A.
Richard P. Capriccioso, M.D.
Mary Car-Blanchard, O.T.D., B.S.O.T.
Christine M. Carroll, R.N., B.S.N., M.B.A.
Kerry L. Cheesman, Ph.D.
Paul A. Clark, PhD
Wanda E. Clark, M.T. (ASCP)
Lisa M. Cockrell, B.S.
Pam Conboy, B.S.
Pamela S. Cooper, Ph.D.
Angela M. Costello, B.S.
Charlotte Crowder, M.P.H., ELS
Reyniel Cruz-Aguado, Ph.D.
D. Scott Cunningham, M.D., Ph.D.
Arun S. Dabholkar, Ph.D.
Helen Davidson, B.A.
Martiscia Davidson, A.M.
Tish Davidson, AM
Cynthia L. De Vine, B.A.
Jackie Dial, PhD
Jeremy W. Dugosh, PhD
Aldo C. Dumlao, M.D.
Patricia Stanfill Edens, R.N., Ph.D., LFACHE
Karen Nagel Edwards, PhD
Jill Ferguson, Ph.D.
Adi Ferrara, B.S.
Amber L. Fields, M.S.
K. Thomas Finley, Ph.D.
MaryAnn Foote, M.S., Ph.D.
Jo Gambosi, M.A., B.S.N.
James S. Godde, PhD
Zuri S.Goodman
Janet R. Green, M.S.P.H.
Katrina Green, R.N., B.S.N., O.C.N.
Silke Haidekker, PhD, ELS
Linda Hart, M.S., M.A.
Melanie Hawkins, B.S.N., R.N., O.C.N.
H. Bradford Hawley, MD
Peter B. Heller, Ph.D.
Collette Bishop Hendler, R.N., M.S.
Michelle L. Herdman, Ph.D.
Jennifer M. Hickin, B.S.
Carl W. Hoagstrom, Ph.D.
Christine G. Holzmueller, B.L.A.
Mary Hurd, M.A.
Bernard Jacobson, Ph.D.
Clair Kaplan, R.N., M.S.N., A.P.R.N. (WHNP),M.H.S., M.T. (ASCP)
Susan J. Karcher, PhD
Sarah Kasprowicz, M.D.
Michelle Kasprzak, R.N., B.S.N., O.C.N.
Keller Kaufman-Fox, B.A.
Debra B. Kessler, M.D., Ph.D.
Michael R. King, Ph.D.
Samuel V. A. Kisseadoo, Ph.D.
A. K. Khan, M.D., M.R.C.P.
M. A. Q. Khan, M.D., Ph.D.
Samreen F. Khan, M.S.
Samreen F. Khan, M.A.
Ing-Wei Khor, Ph.D.
Jeffrey A. Knight, Ph.D.
Marylane Wade Koch, MSN, RN
Robert Koch, DNSc, RN
Lalitha Krishnan, Ph.D.
Anita P. Kuan, Ph.D.
Steven A. Kuhl, Ph.D.
John S. Kuo, MD, PhD
Jeffrey P. Larson, P.T., B.S., A.T.C.
Jason F. Lee, MD, MPH
Magda Lenartowicz, MD, BA Hons (Gerontology)
Sara Levine
Lindsay Lewellyn, B.S.
Lisa M. Lines, M.P.H.
Marianne M. Madsen, M.S.
Judy Majewski, M.S.
Elizabeth A. Manning, Ph.D.

Amanda McQuade, Ph.D.

Kyle J. McQuade, Ph.D.

Ralph R. Meyer, Ph.D.

Vicki Miskovsky, B.S., R.D.

Paul Moglia, Ph.D.

Christina J. Moose, M.A.

Anita Nagypál, Ph.D.

Amy J. Neil, M.S., M.A.P.

Annette O'Connor, Ph.D.

David A. Olle, M.S.

Colm A. Ó'Moráin, M.A., M.D., M.Sc., D.Sc.

Ophelia Panganiban, B.S.

Jeannie V. Pasacreta, Ph.D., A.P.R.N.

Anna Perez, M.Sc.

Susan H. Peterman, M.P.H.

Jane Piland-Baker, MS

Diego Pineda, M.S.

Marcia Pinneau, R.N.

Nancy A. Piotrowski, Ph.D.

Victoria Price, Ph.D.

Christopher Pung, B.S., C.L.Sp. (CG)

Cynthia Racer, M.A., M.P.H.

Lillian Range, PhD

Bagirathy Ravishankar, Ph.D.

Pamela Richardson, M.S.

Alice C. Richer, R.D., M.B.A., L.D.

Gina Riley, PhD

Benjamin Noah Riley

Maria C. Rossi

Elizabeth D. Schafer, Ph.D.

Jason J. Schwartz, Ph.D., J.D.

Miriam E. Schwartz, M.D., M.A., Ph.D.

Banalata Sen, Phd, MPH

Terry J. Shackleford, Ph.D.

Nipa R. Shah, MD

Swati Sharma, MD

Martha A. Sherwood, PhD

Lisa J. Shientag, V.M.D.

R. Baird Shuman, Ph.D.

Vonne Sieve, M.A.

Dwight G. Smith, Ph.D.

Richard S. Spira, D.V.M.

Kelli Miller Stacy, ELS

Carol Ann Suda, B.S., M.T. (ASCP), S.Mt.

Shane B. Swing

Rena C. Tabata, M.Sc.

Dorothy P. Terry, R.N.

Susan E. Ullmann, M.T. (ASCP), M.A.

Oluseyi Adewale Vanderpuye, PhD

Nicole M. Van Hoey, Pharm.D.

Charles L. Vigue, Ph. D.

Linda August Vrooman, RN, MSN, OCN, CCRC, FNP-BC, NP-C

Catherine J. Walsh, Ph.D.

Stephanie Watson, B.S. Providence, RI

Marcia J. Weiss, J.D.

Bradley R. A. Wilson, Ph.D.

Nicola E. Wittekindt, Dr.Sc. (ETH Zürich)

Geetha Yadav, Ph.D.

Daniel L. Yazak, D.E.D.

John L. Zeller, M.D., Ph.D.

▶ Complete List of Contents

Volume 1

Volume 2

Diseases, Symptoms, and Conditions

Medical Specialties

Organizations

Social and Personal Issues

Volume 3

Cancer Biology

Carcinogens and Suspected Carcinogens

Chemotherapy and Other Drugs

Complementary and Alternative Therapies

Lifestyle and Prevention

VOLUME 4

Procedures

Appendixes

▶ Achlorhydria

Category: Diseases, Symptoms, and Conditions
Also known as: Profound hypochlorhydria

Related conditions: *Helicobacter pylori* infection, chronic atrophic gastritis, gastric adenocarcinoma, gastric carcinoid

Definition: Achlorhydria is the absence of acid secretion by the stomach caused by either atrophy of the acid-producing parietal cells or direct inactivation of the proton-pumping enzyme in parietal cells responsible for acid secretion.

Risk factors: The risk of achlorhydria increases with age and with long-term, untreated infection with the bacteria *Helicobacter pylori*. Patients with autoimmune conditions are also at increased risk. The condition has no predilection for sex or race.

Etiology and the disease process: Chronic inflammation of the stomach in response to untreated *H. pylori* infection lasting many years leads to the atrophy of stomach cells and a corresponding loss of acid-secreting capacity. Some patients may be more predisposed to achlorhydria in the presence of *H. pylori* because they respond to the infection by producing a specific inflammatory agent that is also a potent proton pump inhibitor. Autoimmune disease can also produce achlorhydria if the body makes antibodies that inactivate parietal cell proteins.

Achlorhydria is associated with the development of malignant cancer of the stomach. Over 60 percent of patients with gastric cancer have achlorhydria compared with 20 percent of healthy individuals. Acid normally acts as a disinfectant to prevent overgrowth of harmful bacteria; achlorhydria contributes to cancer development because the bacteria synthesize carcinogenic chemicals from nitrates present in food.

Achlorhydria is also associated with the formation of gastric carcinoid tumors. If acid output by the stomach is disrupted, the body overproduces the hormone gastrin, which stimulates overgrowth of enterochromaffin-like (ECL) cells in the stomach. This overgrowth may progress to carcinoid formation.

Incidence: Gastric carcinoids constitute 0.5 percent of gastric cancers. They are typically associated with autoimmune conditions and have a low risk of malignancy.

Symptoms: Achlorhydria itself causes no symptoms; rather, symptoms are secondary to the absence of acid. Lack of acid can cause vitamin B_{12} or calcium deficiency. Diarrhea may occur because of the overgrowth of bacteria.

Screening and diagnosis: Diagnosis is made by measuring the acidity of a stomach fluid sample after an intravenous injection of pentagastrin, which stimulates acid secretion in normal patients. Acidity will not increase in the stomach fluid of achlorhydric patients.

Treatment and therapy: Treatment focuses on addressing the underlying condition causing achlorhydria. Because vitamin B_{12} and calcium absorption are decreased, supplementation or injections of B_{12} may be necessary.

Prognosis, prevention, and outcomes: Restoration of normal acid production depends on prognosis and treatment for the underlying condition responsible for achlorhydria.

Pamela S. Cooper, Ph.D.

See also: Adenocarcinomas; Bacteria as causes of cancer; Gastric polyps; Gastrointestinal cancers; *Helicobacter pylori*; Hereditary diffuse gastric cancer; Premalignancies; Stomach cancers

▶ Acoustic neuromas

Category: Diseases, Symptoms, and Conditions
Also known as: Vestibular schwannomas

Related conditions: Neurofibromatosis type 2

Definition: Acoustic neuromas are benign (or nonmalignant) tumors that originate from Schwann cells surrounding the vestibular nerve (eighth cranial nerve) in the internal auditory canal. The term "neuroma" is somewhat misleading, as the tumors are not neuromas, nor do they arise from the acoustic or cochlear nerve. Acoustic neuroma typically occurs as unilateral (one-sided) sporadic tumors in 95 percent of all cases, but in rare cases tumors can be bilateral (two-sided) and are associated with an inherited syndrome called neurofibromatosis type 2 (NF2). Approximately 2 to 4 percent of patients diagnosed with acoustic neuromas have NF2 type, a prevalence of 1 in 50,000 in the general population.

Risk factors: Although high-dose ionizing radiation is a known risk factor of acoustic neuroma, environmental factors including noise exposure, radio frequency electromagnetic fields, and allergens have been reported as potential sources that may contribute to the formation of acoustic neuroma. One publication has reported the findings from an international multicenter case-control study that investigated the effects of these environmental factors in ninety-seven patients with acoustic neuroma and in age-matched control subjects. The study reported that increased risks were found for exposure to persistent noise and hay fever, but not for ionizing radiation or for regular mobile phone use.

Etiology and the disease process: Currently, the etiology of acoustic neuroma is not known. However, as an anomaly, it is rarely inherited. Nonetheless, neurofibromatosis type 2 should be suspected in young patients and those with family history. Neurofibromatosis is an autosomal dominant disease; thus patients who inherit a defective copy of the *NF2* tumor-suppressor gene have a 95 percent chance of developing bilateral tumors; however, half of the cases have no family history of NF2, which could indicate mutations in the germline that were not inherited.

Incidence: Sporadic acoustic tumors, the most common form of manifestation, occur in approximately 10 per 1 million persons per year—in other words the chance of an average person developing an acoustic neuroma in his or her lifetime is about 1 in 100,000. Neurofibromatosis is rarer, with only several thousand affected persons in the entire United States, corresponding to 1 in 40,000 individuals. However, a study has highlighted that the true incidence of acoustic neuroma may be higher than what has been envisaged, as 7 unsuspected schwannomas per 10,000 brain magnetic resonance imaging studies were identified, an equivalent of 0.07 percent. Acoustic neuromas, or schwannomas, occur largely in adults, typically in the fourth and fifth decades, with a mean presentation age of fifty years. They are uncommon in children; only thirty-nine cases had been reported as of 2007.

Symptoms: Acoustic neuromas are histologically benign; however, if large, they can cause hydrocephalus, brainstem compression, herniation, and eventually death. Hearing loss is the most prevalent symptom, occurring in more than 95 percent of patients, and the duration of hearing loss may extend to three or four years before clinical diagnosis is made—a majority of the patients experience one-sided, slowly progressing hearing impairment associated with high-frequency sounds. Alternative complaints or accompanying symptoms include tinnitus, dizziness, vertigo, and a sensation of fullness in the ear. With the progression of the tumor, patients may experience facial numbness, headaches, loss of coordination, and difficulty in swallowing. Vertigo is prevalent with smaller tumors, while unsteadiness, headache, and facial sensory disturbance are associated with large tumors.

Screening and diagnosis: Acoustic neuroma can be diagnosed by a number of screening methods. These include conventional audiometry, auditory brainstem response (ABR), and gadolinium-enhanced magnetic resonance imaging (MRI). Among these, gadolinium-enhanced MRI is the optimal diagnostic test. Typically, on MRI scans acoustic neuromas appear as dense and uniformly enhanced. Acoustic neuromas are staged according to their location and size. Small tumors are less than 1.5 centimeters (cm), moderate tumors between 1.5 and 3 cm, and large tumors greater than 3 cm in size. Based on the location, they are staged as intracanalicular (located in the internal auditory canal), cisternal (extending outside the internal auditory canal), compressive (having progressed to touch the cerebellum or brainstem), and hydrocephalus (having progressed to obstruct the drainage of cerebrospinal fluid in the fourth ventricle).

Treatment and therapy: The treatment options for acoustic neuroma include observation, microsurgery, stereotactic radiosurgery, and radiotherapy. Patients with advanced age or those deemed unfit for surgical intervention with small tumors at diagnosis are observed; treatment is withheld while tumor progression is monitored in serial imaging studies. However, treatment by observation has its own risks, as there is a greater risk of losing useful hearing.

If microsurgery is the choice for treatment, many factors need to be assessed when evaluating its primary and secondary outcomes. First, there are three standard surgical approaches, each with its own advantages and disadvantages: suboccipital, middle fossa, and translabyrinthine. In the suboccipital approach, the tumor is reached through the skull behind the ear. As the procedure involves the retraction of the cerebellum, the approach is intrinsically dangerous and prone to complications. Although the middle fossa method can preserve hearing in theory, this approach is also dangerous as it too requires the retraction of part of the brain. In the translabyrinthine approach, the tumor is accessed through the inner ear, and thus hearing loss is expected and inevitable. However, this method is unsuitable for large tumors. Second, microsurgery is technically challenging; therefore the rate of success is lower with a less experienced surgeon. Third, large tumors (greater than 3 cm) are difficult to resect without concomitant morbidity, such as facial palsy. Some of the complications that may arise from microsurgery are cerebrospinal fluid leak (12 percent of all cases), meningitis (5 percent), intracranial hemorrhage (2 percent), facial weakness with complete paralysis (31 percent), and delayed or partial paresis (50 percent).

Radiosurgery refers to the administration of a single fraction of radiotherapy using stereotactic techniques to localize the tumor and align the fields. Radiosurgery may be performed either with a Gamma Knife or a linear accelerator (linac) based system. Gamma Knife is an emerging treatment option for those who are at high risk during microsurgery. High-dose Gamma Knife procedures are less favored due to the possibility of radiation complications; thus low-dose radiation (for example, 13 gray, or Gy) therapies are advised because of safety and lower risk of facial weakness.

Radiotherapy refers to the administration of fractionated radiotherapy and includes stereotactic radiotherapy (radiation with other than gamma rays) and conventional radiotherapy techniques.

Complications of Gamma Knife radiosurgery include injury to facial and trigeminal nerves. However, with the current dosing regimen of 12.5 Gy, the risk of trigeminal or facial nerve injury has decreased significantly. Although the potential for complications is higher with microsurgical procedures than with radiotherapy or radiosurgery, an important issue that should be considered with irradiation therapies is the low risk of inducing malignancies within the radiation area. Current recommendations are to offer microsurgery and radiosurgery options for patients with definite treatment indications. While microsurgery is the treatment of choice for large tumors because of the low risk of radiation-induced malignancies, microsurgery is also considered for younger patients.

Prognosis, prevention, and outcomes: The microsurgical techniques for acoustic neuroma have improved the anatomical and functional preservation of the facial and cochlear nerves. These techniques, accompanied by continuous electrophysiological monitoring, have resulted in marked changes in the primary goals of management. In the past, the primary goal of acoustic neuroma management was to preserve the patient's life, whereas the objective today is to preserve the neurological function. Long-term follow-ups show negligible recurrence rates, suggesting that the preservation of neurological function does not restrict the tumor removal. Despite these advances, loss of nerve function and even deafness may occur postoperatively in some cases.

Bagirathy Ravishankar, Ph.D.

For Further Information

Battaglia, A., et al. "Comparisons of Growth Patterns of Acoustic Neuromas with and Without Radiosurgery." *Otology and Neurotology* 27 (2006): 705-712.

Mendenhall, W., et al. "Management of Acoustic Schwannoma." *American Journal of Otolaryngology* 25 (2004): 38-47.

Neff, B., et al. "The Molecular Biology of Vestibular Schwannomas: Dissecting the Pathogenic Process at the Molecular Level." *Otology and Neurotology* 27 (2006): 197-208.

Schlehofer, B., et al. "Environmental Risk Factors for Sporadic Acoustic Neuroma." *European Journal of Cancer* 43 (2007): 1741-1747.

Yohay, K. "Neurofibromatosis Types 1 and 2." *The Neurologist* 12 (2006): 86-93.

Other Resources

Acoustic Neuroma Association
http://anausa.org

American Cancer Society
http://www.cancer.org

See also: Ependymomas; Neurofibromatosis type 1 (NF1); Schwannoma tumors; Stereotactic Radiosurgery (SRS)

▶ Acute Lymphocytic Leukemia (ALL)

Category: Diseases, Symptoms, and Conditions
Also known as: Acute childhood leukemia, acute lymphoblastic leukemia, acute lymphoid leukemia

Related conditions: Acute myeloid leukemia, chronic lymphocytic leukemia, chronic myeloid leukemia

Definition: Acute lymphocytic leukemia (ALL) is a cancer of the white blood cells. A lymphocyte is a type of white blood cell made in the bone marrow that helps fight infection. In this fast-growing type of cancer, for unknown reasons, the bone marrow begins to make lymphocytes that develop abnormally. "Acute" means that the disease affects lymphocytes before they are fully formed and that it progresses rapidly if not treated.

Risk factors: Few risk factors exist for ALL. Receiving high doses of radiation, usually as treatment for another type of cancer, is one risk factor. Exposure to benzene may also be a factor. Risk increases in people with certain other diseases, such as Down syndrome, Fanconi anemia, Bloom syndrome, and some other genetic diseases. In about 25 percent of ALL cases, the patient has a chromosome mutation in which parts of chromosome 9 and chromosome 22 have changed places. Having a sibling, especially a twin, with ALL also increases the risk for this disease. Researchers are exploring lifestyle or environmental relationships, but it appears that many factors, including a combination of genetic and environmental factors, may be involved in developing ALL.

Etiology and the disease process: Through a genetic process that is not completely understood, cells in bone marrow begin to form abnormally. ALL can begin in two different types of lymphocytes, either B cells or T cells. As the abnormal lymphocytes quickly grow, they crowd out the red and white blood cells and platelets that the body needs and that are also created in the bone marrow. The symptoms of ALL come from the crowding out of these normal, healthy cells. These cells may then spread into the lining of the spine and brain.

Incidence: About 5,200 people in the United States were diagnosed with ALL in 2007. It is slightly more common in men than in women and slightly more common in white children than in children of other races. ALL occurs in people of all ages but has a peak incidence in children between the ages of two and five. After age five, risk decreases, then increases again in people over age fifty. It is the most common type of leukemia in children under the age of fifteen, accounting for about 80 percent of childhood leukemias. It occurs more often in developed countries and in people with higher socioeconomic status.

Symptoms: Symptoms of ALL include anemia, body aches, bone pain, bruises without any injury, enlarged lymph nodes, an enlarged spleen, excessive bleeding from minor injuries, fever with no illness or lasting low-grade fever, frequent infections, headaches, joint pain, nosebleeds, paleness, shortness of breath during activity, tiredness, vomiting, and unexplained weight loss.

Screening and diagnosis: There is no screening test for ALL. Blood and bone marrow tests are necessary to diagnose ALL. These tests look for abnormal lymphocyte cells. A bone marrow aspirate test (using a long needle to take marrow out of the bone) and a bone marrow biopsy (surgical removal of some bone marrow) are two possible tests. The bone marrow aspirate test looks for abnormal cells in the bone marrow and can also be used for other types of analysis. A bone marrow biopsy can show how much disease is already in the bone marrow. The results of these tests help determine which type of drug therapy to use and how long treatment should last.

If a patient has been diagnosed with ALL, a lumbar puncture may be performed to see if the abnormal cells have moved into the fluid surrounding the spine and brain. Chest X rays, ultrasounds, or additional blood tests may also be used to determine the spread of the disease.

Depending on where the cancer started and the results of testing, ALL may be categorized into early pre-B-cell ALL, common ALL, pre-B-cell ALL, mature B-cell ALL, pre-T-cell ALL, or mature T-cell ALL. The type of ALL helps determine which therapy to use and how long treatment should last. About 85 percent of ALL cases begin in B cells, and these cases are generally classified as lower risk.

ALL may also be classified or staged using the French-American-British (FAB) classification system. In this older system, ALL is classified according to the type of abnormal cells as follows:

- ALL-11: small, uniform abnormal cells
- ALL-12: large, varied abnormal cells
- ALL-13: large, varied, bubble-like cells

Age at Death for Acute Lymphocytic Leukemia, 2001-2005

Age Group	*Deaths (%)*
Under 20	21.4
20-34	15.9
35-44	9.7
45-54	11.2
55-64	11.7
65-74	12.7
75-84	11.5
85 and older	5.8

Source: Data from National Cancer Institute, Surveillance Epidemiology and End Results, Cancer Stat Fact Sheets, 2008

Note: The median age of death from 2001 to 2005 was forty-seven, with an age-adjusted death rate of 0.5 per 100,000 men and women.

Treatment and therapy: Patients diagnosed with ALL should start treatment immediately. The course and length of treatment chosen depend on the results of the patient's bone marrow tests, the patient's age, the number of ALL cells in the blood, whether certain chromosomal changes have already happened, whether ALL cells began in the B cells or the T cells, and whether ALL has spread to the brain covering or spinal cord. During therapy, bone marrow tests may be done again to make sure the treatment is destroying the cancer cells.

The first part of treatment for ALL is called induction therapy. This therapy helps kill ALL cells and get a patient's blood counts back to normal (remission). Some of the drugs used in induction therapy are given by mouth. Others are given in a vein, usually through the patient's chest. Most often, this chemotherapy for ALL involves combining drugs to improve the effects of the drugs. Often, ALL spreads into the lining of the spinal cord and the brain. To kill these ALL cells, drugs are injected directly into the spinal fluid. Radiation therapy may be used on the spine and brain either with or without the injected drugs.

Post-induction therapy, the second part of treatment for ALL, begins when a patient has reached remission. This type of therapy is needed because usually some ALL cells that cannot be detected by tests remain in the body. Post-induction therapy usually happens in two- or three-year cycles. The drugs used in post-induction therapy are usually different from those used in induction therapy, and the type of drugs used depends on how the patient responded to induction therapy and whether the patient has certain chromosome abnormalities. A patient may also need maintenance therapy after post-induction therapy to prevent the cells from regrowing.

T-cell ALL, infant ALL, and adult ALL are all forms of high-risk ALL. These types of ALL are usually treated with higher doses of drugs during both induction and post-induction therapy. Some patients with high-risk types of ALL may respond well to bone marrow or cord blood transplant therapy.

A bone marrow or cord blood transplant may be used when high doses of drugs are given to kill the ALL cells. These high doses of drugs may also kill healthy cells in the bone marrow. This transplant gives a patient healthy cells to replace the killed bone marrow cells. A transplant is a high-risk procedure and will probably not be used unless a patient does not have a good possibility of long-term remission with chemotherapy. High-risk ALL patients are more likely to have a transplant. The timing of a transplant is important; a patient has a better chance of a successful transplant when he or she is in remission at the time of transplant.

Prognosis, prevention, and outcomes: There is no known way to prevent ALL. Most children with ALL can be cured of this disease with proper treatment. The overall survival rate for children after chemotherapy is nearly 80 percent. Children with low-risk ALL have even higher survival rates.

Most adults also improve with treatment; the number of adults who have remissions has increased, and the length of adult remissions has improved. The overall survival rate for adults after chemotherapy is about 40 percent, and adults with low-risk ALL have even higher survival rates.

Marianne M. Madsen, M.S.

For Further Information

Abeloff, M. D., et al. *Clinical Oncology*. 3d ed. Orlando, Fla.: Churchill Livingstone, 2004.

Hoffman, R., et al. *Hematology: Basic Principles and Practice*. 4th ed. Orlando, Fla.: Churchill Livingstone, 2005.

Lichtman, M. A., et al., eds. *William's Hematology*. 7th ed. New York: McGraw-Hill, 2006.

Pui, C-H, ed. *Childhood Leukemias*. 2d ed. New York: Cambridge University Press, 2006.

Other Resources

Association of Cancer Online Resources
http://www.acor.org

CureSearch: National Childhood Cancer Foundation, Children's Oncology Group
http://www.curesearch.org

Leukemia and Lymphoma Society
http://www.leukemia-lymphoma.org

National Cancer Institute
http://www.cancer.gov/cancertopics/treatment/

See also: Acute Myelocytic Leukemia (AML); Aleukemia; Blood cancers; Childhood cancers; Chronic Lymphocytic Leukemia (CLL); Chronic Myeloid Leukemia (CML); Hemolytic anemia; Leukemias; Myelodysplastic syndromes; Myelofibrosis; Myeloproliferative disorders; Topoisomerase inhibitors

▶ Acute Myelocytic Leukemia (AML)

Category: Diseases, Symptoms, and Conditions

Also known as: Acute myeloid leukemia, acute myelogenous leukemia, acute myeloblastic leukemia, acute myelomonocytic leukemia, granulocytic leukemia, acute nonlymphocytic leukemia, acute promyelocytic leukemia

Related conditions: Acute lymphoblastic leukemia, myelodysplastic syndrome

Definition: Acute myelocytic leukemia (AML) describes a malignant proliferation in the bone marrow of an undifferentiated blood-forming cell of the myeloid line. AML begins with the genetic alteration of a single cell. That cell, called a blast cell, is the foundation from which the leukemia follows. The process of normal blood cell formation, or hematopoiesis, begins with undifferentiated cells, known as stem cells, inside the bone marrow. Stem cells differentiate into blasts, and these primitive blast cells give rise to red blood cells, platelets, and white blood cells. It is the accumulation of blast cells in the bone marrow and their failure to differentiate that has lethal consequences within just a few weeks or months if unchecked. Although the rate of success has improved, treatment is still associated with high mortality.

Risk factors: Certain genetic disorders have an associated AML risk, including Down syndrome, Fanconi anemia, and Shwachman-Diamond syndrome. Other risk factors include some forms of chemotherapy, radiation therapy, and exposure to tobacco smoke and benzene.

Etiology and the disease process: The process leading to acute myelocytic leukemia involves an interruption in progression of undifferentiated progenitor cells in the bone marrow that normally mature into red blood cells, white blood cells (neutrophils, eosinophils, basophils, and monocytes), or megakaryocytes. Megakaryocytes are bone marrow cells responsible for the production of platelets or thrombocytes necessary for blood clotting. Bone marrow is the soft interior of bones such as the skull, shoulder blades, ribs, pelvis, and backbones. It comes in two varieties: red marrow and yellow marrow. The red marrow, also called myeloid tissue, is the source of AML activity. Red blood cells, platelets, and most white blood cells arise from a parent cell in the red marrow. Many references limit discussion of AML to only the direct descendants of the myeloid line; these are the neutrophils, eosinophils, and basophils.

When blast cells do not mature properly, they accumulate in the bone marrow. It is the proliferation and the accumulation of this hematopoietic cell in the bone marrow that defines AML. Although research has not completely unraveled the process of this leukemic transformation, there is strong evidence of underlying chromosomal damage. For example, a variety of mutations are associated with AML, with damage to the gene for FMS-related tyrosine kinase (FLT3) being the most prominent. Normally, the receptor encoded by FLT3 signals undifferentiated blast cells in the bone marrow to proliferate when there is a need for additional circulating blood cells. The signal stops when the supply is sufficient, but in AML, the switch stays on, and unconstrained blast cell proliferation follows. Although AML begins with defective bone marrow cells, it generally moves quickly into the peripheral blood and may spread to other parts of the body, such as the liver, spleen, testes, brain, spinal cord, and lymph nodes.

Incidence: Because AML is associated with accumulating genetic defects, the incidence increases with age. AML ranges from 0.7 to 3.9 cases per 100,000 in people up through the age of sixty and increases to 6.7 to 19.2 cases per 100,000 in people who are over sixty. The median age of onset is more than sixty-seven years. Each year AML will strike about 13,400 adults and 650 children in the United States.

Symptoms: Clinical findings reflect the replacement of normal bone marrow elements with malignant blast cells. Probably the most consistent early complaints in AML are a history of increasing lethargy later followed by skin, soft-tissue, or respiratory infection. Some patients will have small red or purple spots on the body, called petechiae, resulting from broken blood vessels. Liver, spleen, and lymph node enlargement is common, as is weight loss. Some symptoms are nonspecific but quite common in AML patients. These include swollen gums; pale skin; black-and-blue marks; achiness in the knees, hips, or shoulder; mild fever; shortness of breath during even light exertion; and the slow healing of cuts.

Screening and diagnosis: The diagnostician must distinguish AML from other myeloproliferative disorders such as chronic myelogenous leukemia, and myelodysplastic syndrome. Although many supporting tests and symptoms point toward a diagnosis, the definitive finding of AML will require bone marrow aspirate and biopsy.

Short of biopsy examination, other indicators will raise suspicion. About one-third of AML patients will have an enlarged spleen and high levels of uric acid in the blood. The peripheral white blood cell count is not a good indicator, as it may be increased, decreased, or normal. However, there usually will be reduced numbers of granulocytes (neutrophils, basophils, and eosinophils) and platelets in the blood. Blast cells in the peripheral blood appear in only 15 percent of AML patients initially, but this number rises to half of those patients with decreased number of circulating white blood cells (leukopenia).

There is no standard staging system for AML. Generally, doctors describe the status of the condition as untreated, in remission, or recurrent. However, bone marrow examination more closely defines AML as belonging to one of eight cell subtypes. Doctors tailor the treatment to the subtype. The subtypes are as follows:

- M0: Myeloblastic, on special analysis
- M1: Myeloblastic, without maturation
- M2: Myeloblastic, with maturation
- M3: Promyeloctic
- M4: Myelomonocytic
- M5: Monocytic
- M6: Erythroleukemic
- M7: Megakaryocytic

Treatment and therapy: The goal of AML treatment is the destruction of the leukemic cells. However, this requires the suppression of bone marrow activity, which brings unfortunate side effects. With the bone marrow suppressed, fewer white cells are available to fight infection and fewer red cells and platelets are present to maintain a healthy oxygen exchange and clot formation. This almost always requires treatment with antibiotics and blood transfusions.

Initial treatment or induction therapy begins with a hospital stay of about a week using chemotherapy with a combination of drug types. Generally induction therapy requires more than one round of treatment, as it is likely that some AML cells will survive. Even if the induction therapy seems successful, the doctors assume that leukemic cells still exist though unrevealed on biopsy examination. In the unusual event that leukemia has spread to the brain or spinal cord, chemotherapy is also introduced into the cerebrospinal fluid.

At a later date, a follow-up round of less intensive treatments called consolidation therapy brings the patient back to the hospital to maintain remission status. Remission describes a normal peripheral blood profile, a normal bone marrow free of excess blasts, and a normal clinical status. Doctors generally reserve stem cell transplantation with more vigorous chemotherapy for those patients susceptible to relapse, although it is sometimes part of the consolidation regimen. However, there is some debate among doctors as to the risks and benefits of this treatment. For relapsed patients who are unable to undergo the rigors of stem cell transplantation, additional chemotherapy is generally not well tolerated or effective.

Doctors adapt specific chemotherapies to the subtype of the leukemia. Usually this will be some combination of an anthracycline-class agent with cytabrine. In some cases a third drug, 6-thioguanine, is added. Also factored into the treatment strategy are the patient's age, clinical status, and leukemia profile. Although quite variable, hospital stays for induction and consolidation therapies may require weeks or even months. Typically, chemotherapy will drive the patient's blood cell counts down to dangerously low levels. This will require drugs to elevate white blood cell counts as well as antibiotics and blood transfusions to protect against complications.

Prognosis, prevention, and outcomes: The prognosis of patients with AML largely depends on the patient's age. In part this is due to chemoresistance or the biological response of cells to survive the toxic stress of chemotherapy. Because chemoresistance tends to increase with age, important therapies are less effective in older patients. Also, the difference in the mechanisms of chromosome translocations in the young and older patients allows for a more favorable outcome in the younger patient.

In the absence of treatment, most people stricken with AML will die less than two months after the diagnosis. With therapy, between 20 and 40 percent of people survive for at least five years. The poorest prognoses are reserved for those patients older than sixty and for those developing AML following chemotherapy and radiation therapy for other cancers. In general, four years following consolidation therapy, approximately 40 percent of patients under sixty years of age will be free of any signs of leukemia, with that number dropping to 15 percent in older patients.

Richard S. Spira, D.V.M.
Updated by: Catherine J. Walsh

For Further Information

Dombret, H., & Gardin, C. (2016). An update of current treatments for adult acute myeloid leukemia. *Blood,*

127(1):53-61. Treatment guidelines for AML in adults patients.

Ezzone, Susan, & Schmit-Pokorny, Kim. (Eds.). (2007). *Blood and marrow stem cell transplantation: Principles, practices, and nursing insights*. Sudbury, MA: Jones and Bartlett. An encyclopedic treatment of stem cell transplants for blood-based cancers and diseases.

Hoffman, Ronald. (2005). *Hematology: Basic principles and practice* (4th ed.). St. Louis: Elsevier Churchill Livingstone. Useful hematology textbook that, though dated, remains very useful.

National Cancer Institute. 21st Century Adult Cancer Sourcebook: Adult Acute Myeloid Leukemia (AML), ANLL, Myelogenous or Myeloblastic Leukemia. (2011). Patient-directed, comprehensive information from cancer experts across the nation and includes signs, symptoms, treatment options, drugs, chemotherapy, staging, biology, prognosis, and survival.

O'Donnell, M. R., Abboud, C. N., Altman, J., Appelbaum, F. R., Arber, D. A., Attar, E., … Gregory, K. M. (2012). Acute myeloid leukemia. *Journal of the National Comprehensive Cancer Network*, 10(8):984-1021. Comprehensive and well-written review of AML.

Parker, James N. & Parker, Philip M. (Eds.). (2002). The official patient's sourcebook on adult acute myeloid leukemia: A revised and updated directory for the internet age. Icon Health Publications. A sourcebook for patients conducted independent internet-based research to complement their treatment, and provides information for patients to find information on topics related to acute myeloid leukemia.

Other Resources

Leukemia and Lymphoma Society

Acute Myeloid Leukemia.
www.lls.org/leukemia/acute-myeloid-leukemia

This website provides general overall of AML, causes, risk factors, treatment and other resources.
www.mayoclinic.org/diseases-conditions/acute-myelogenous-leukemia/basics/definition/con-20043431

Acute myelogenous leukemia (AML). A brief description of AML provided by staff at the Mayo Clinic, including Symptoms, risk factores, tests, and diagnoses, treatment. Includes additional resources for patients.

National Marrow Donor Program

Acute Myelogenous Leukemia.
http://www.marrow.org/PATIENT/Undrstnd_Disease_Treat/Lrn_about_Disease/AML/index.html

See also: Acute Lymphocytic Leukemia (ALL); Blood cancers; Childhood cancers; Chronic Lymphocytic Leukemia (CLL); Chronic Myeloid Leukemia (CML); Fanconi anemia; Genetics of cancer; Leukemias; Leukopenia; Myelodysplastic syndromes; Myeloproliferative disorders; Myelosuppression

▶ Adenocarcinomas

Category: Diseases, Symptoms, and Conditions
Also known as: Malignant adenomas, other names vary by type

Related conditions: Lung cancer, breast cancer, colon cancer, renal cell carcinomas

Definition: Adenocarcinoma is a type of cancer that develops in the epithelial tissue of glandular (secretory) organs. Although it is commonly associated with lung cancer (and is the most common form of lung cancer), adenocarcinoma can also develop in such organs as the breast, colon, kidney, liver, pancreas, prostate, and stomach. It is classified according to the kind of tissue from which it arose (such as lung or breast) or according to a particular product of the cells (such as mucinous adenocarcinoma). Adenocarcinoma can spread (metastasize) to other parts of the body and also destroy surrounding tissues.

Risk factors: Smoking increases the risk of almost every type of cancer. Other risk factors for adenocarcinoma vary by organ site. Age, race, family history, medication use, and lifestyle factors such as diet have been implicated in certain forms of adenocarcinoma.

Etiology and the disease process: Etiology of and the disease process for adenocarcinoma vary with the involved organ.

Incidence: Incidence of adenocarcinoma varies by type. Adenocarcinoma is the most common form of lung, pancreatic, prostate, and stomach cancer.

Symptoms: Symptoms of adenocarcinoma vary by type. Small adenocarcinomas may produce only mild symptoms that go undetected. Large adenocarcinomas produce more noticeable symptoms that vary with the site of

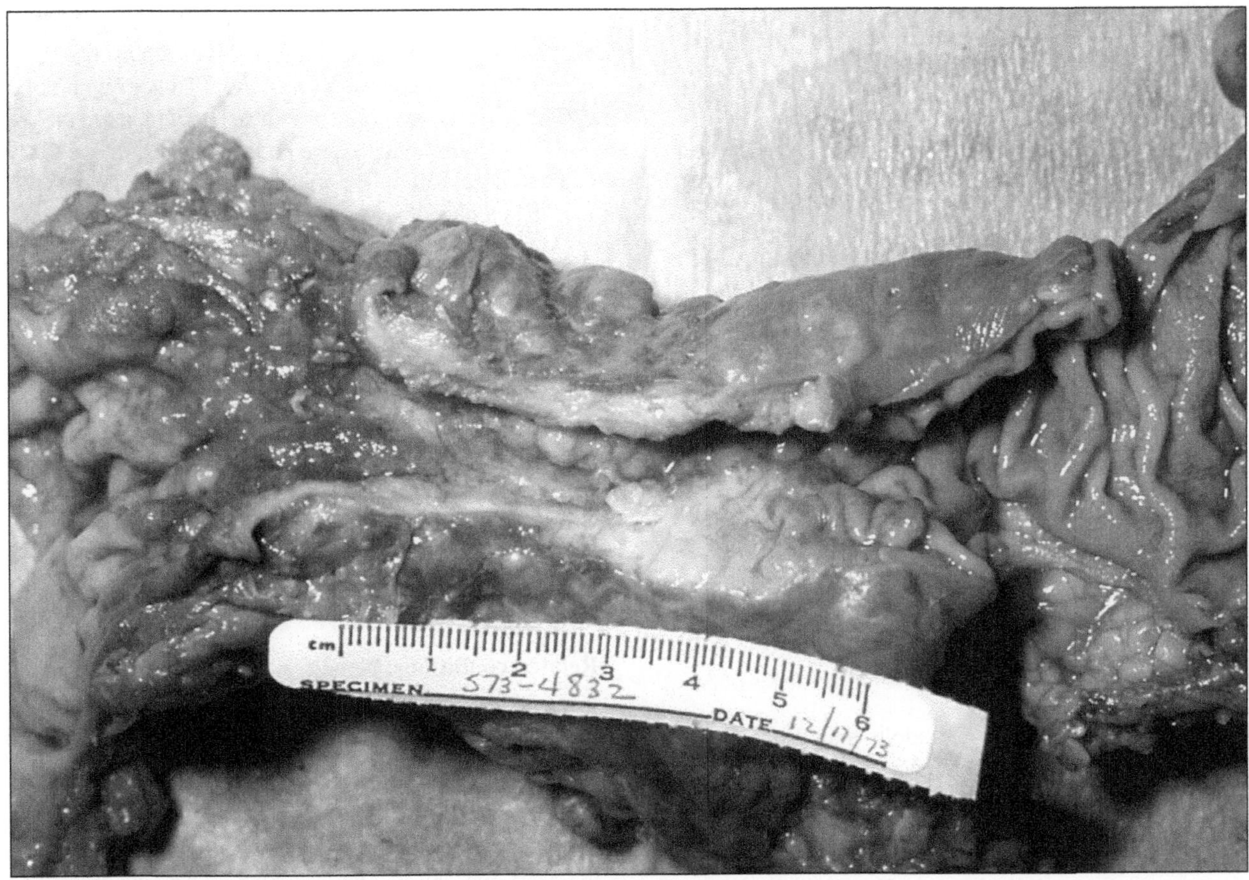

Asurgical specimen showing colonic adenocarcinoma. (Centers for Disease Control and Prevention)

involvement. The first signs of adenocarcinoma may be a noticeable lump and pain or discomfort.

Screening and diagnosis: Diagnosis of adenocarcinoma begins with a medical history and physical examination. Lumps are commonly biopsied, and specialized imaging techniques, such as X rays and computed tomography (CT) scans, are used to determine the extent of the disease (staging). Staging of adenocarcinoma varies by type.

Treatment and therapy: Specific treatment protocols vary by adenocarcinoma type and other factors, such as overall patient health and extent of the disease.

Conventional treatment options include surgery, chemotherapy, and radiation therapy. Early-stage, localized disease may be treated by surgery alone (surgical removal of the tumor and surrounding tissue) or surgery with adjuvant chemotherapy or radiation therapy. Advanced adenocarcinoma has no cure.

Newly emerging treatments for adenocarcinoma include hormone therapy and stem cell transplantation.

Prognosis, prevention, and outcomes: Without treatment, adenocarcinoma is fatal. Routine physical examinations and avoidance of risk factors, such as smoking, are keys to early detection and prevention.

Jaime Stockslager Buss, M.S.P.H., ELS

See also: Adenoid Cystic Carcinoma (ACC); Appendix cancer; Bile duct cancer; Breast cancer in children and adolescents; Bronchoalveolar lung cancer; Carcinomas; Duodenal carcinomas; Esophageal cancer; Fallopian tube cancer; Gallbladder cancer; Gastrointestinal cancers; Granulosa cell tumors; Head and neck cancers; *Helicobacter pylori*; Lung cancers; Mesothelioma; Mucinous carcinomas; Nasal cavity and paranasal sinus cancers; Oncogenic viruses; Pancreatic cancers; Prostate cancer; Rectal cancer; Salivary gland cancer; Small intestine cancer; Stomach cancers; Throat cancer; Urethral cancer; Urinary system cancers; Uterine cancer; Vaginal cancer; Vulvar cancer

▶ Adenoid Cystic Carcinoma (ACC)

Category: Diseases, Symptoms, and Conditions
Also known as: Adenocystic carcinoma, cribriform carcinoma, cylindroma, malignant cylindroma, AdCC

Related conditions: Adenoma, adenocarcinoma

Definition: Adenoid cystic carcinoma (ACC) is a rare malignant cancer of the secretory glands. Neoplasms usually originate in the major and minor salivary glands of the head and neck region but can also occur in places such as in the trachea, lacrimal glands, breast, skin, and vulva.

Risk factors: Environmental and genetic risk factors have not been identified.

Etiology and the disease process: There is little information available regarding pathogenesis except for some evidence suggesting that the *TP53* tumor-suppressor gene is inactivated in the most aggressive forms or stages of ACC.

Incidence: Both children and adults may develop ACC; however, most patients are diagnosed between the fourth and sixth decades of life. ACC affects more women than men at a ratio of approximately 3:2.

Symptoms: Signs and symptoms depend on the origin of the neoplasm.

Screening and diagnosis: Unfortunately, no screening tests exist because of a lack of serum markers. Diagnosis is made after histologic analysis obtained through biopsy or resection of a tumor. ACC is classified into three major groups according to distinctive histologic growth pattern: cribriform, tubular, and solid.

Treatment and therapy: The primary treatment option for adenoid cystic carcinoma is surgery. Postoperative radiotherapy or neutron beam therapy is sometimes recommended to help limit local failure. There is no effective chemotherapy for metastatic or unresectable ACC; however, several clinical trials are testing the effectiveness of new chemotherapeutic drugs (for example, paclitaxel and gemcitabine) when used alone or in combination with other drugs. Radiofrequency ablation and cryoablation are also being explored as treatment options.

Prognosis, prevention, and outcomes: ACC growth and disease progression tend to be slow but relentless. ACC is atypical of carcinomas and seldom metastasizes to regional lymph nodes. Distant metastasis is the predominant reason for treatment failure and occurs most frequently in the lung, followed by the liver. Tumors with solid growth patterns and perineural invasion of major nerves or positive margins tend to have poor prognosis. In one study that followed 160 ACC patients, disease-specific survival was 89 percent at five years and 40 percent at fifteen years.

Rena C. Tabata, M.Sc.

See also: Bronchial adenomas; Lacrimal gland tumors; Lung cancers; Nasal cavity and paranasal sinus cancers; Salivary gland cancer; Throat cancer

▶ Adenomatoid tumors

Category: Diseases, Symptoms, and Conditions
Also known as: Adenofibromyomas, Recklinghausen's tumors

Related conditions: None

Definition: An adenomatoid tumor is a small benign tumor of mesothelial origin usually occurring in the male epididymis or female Fallopian tube, ovary, or uterus. Rarely, these tumors can be seen within the testes and prostate. Extragenital adenomatoid tumors have also been identified in the heart, mesentery, pleura, lymph nodes, omentum, and adrenal glands. Because of its glandular appearance, it may be confused with an adenocarcinoma or metastatic carcinoma, especially signet ring cell carcinoma.

Risk factors: There are no known risk factors for adenomatoid tumors.

Etiology and the disease process: An adenomatoid tumor is a benign hamartoma that is a malformation resulting from faulty development in an organ and is made up of an abnormal mixture of tissue elements normally present at that site. Most adenomatoid tumors are composed of fibrous tissue separated by numerous slitlike pseudotubular spaces crossed by peculiar threadlike bridging strands, which are their typical morphologic feature. The most common benign tumor of the epididymis, adenomatoid tumors usually arise in the tail of the epididymis and may rarely invade adjacent testicular parenchyma. Although they may occur at any age, they are most commonly seen in patients between twenty and fifty years of age and are usually asymptomatic. Although usually under 5 centimeters (cm) in size, they can grow quite large under hormonal influence.

Incidence: In one study, the reported incidence of adenomatoid tumors is 1.2 percent, although the true incidence is probably greater, as most tumors are never biopsied because of their small size and similarity to leiomyomas of the uterus. When found in the male genital tract, these tumors are usually seen in an extratesticular location, usually involving the epididymis, representing approximately 30 percent of tumors arising in the paratesticular area.

Symptoms: Adenomatoid tumors usually are asymptomatic. However, when adenomatoid tumors occur in the genital tract, they can grow quite large and can be painful.

Screening and diagnosis: Often mistaken for uterine fibroids on magnetic resonance imaging, the radiologic appearance can vary from solid to cystic depending on the relative amounts of cystic spaces, smooth muscle, and fibrous tissue contained within the tumor. Ultrasound is useful in diagnosing adenomatoid tumors of epididymal origin. They usually appear as a round or oval, solitary, solid, well-circumscribed mass of variable echogenicity measuring between 5 millimeters (mm) and 5 cm. Occasionally they may appear cystic sonographically and rarely appear plaquelike and ill-defined.

Treatment and therapy: Surgical removal.

Prognosis, prevention, and outcomes: Excellent.

Debra B. Kessler, M.D., Ph.D.

See also: Endometrial cancer; Fallopian tube cancer; Fibrosarcomas, soft-tissue; Gynecologic cancers; Oophorectomy; Ovarian cancers; Ovarian cysts; Testicular cancer

▶ Adenomatous polyps

Category: Diseases, Symptoms, and Conditions
Also known as: Colorectal adenomas

Related conditions: Colon cancer, benign polyps, familial adenomatous polyposis (FAP)

Definition: Polyps are abnormal tissue growths stemming from the lining of mucous membranes. Colorectal adenomatous polyps are benign (noncancerous) polyps that project from the inner lining of the colon or rectum and protrude into the lumen of the intestines. Despite their benign characteristics, adenomatous polyps can become cancerous if not removed.

Risk factors: Adenomatous polyps are one of the most common types of colon polyp. Individuals over the age of fifty years are much more likely to develop these growths, as are those people with a family history of colon polyps. Additionally, having a mutation in the *APC* gene can cause a condition named familial adenomatous polyposis (FAP), a disorder that causes numerous polyps to grow in the intestines and almost always develop into tumors.

Etiology and the disease process: Adenomatous polyps are a collection of cells that display uncontrolled proliferation, forming a growth that stems from the inner lining of the colon.

Incidence: The prevalence of adenomatous polyps ranges from 10 to 25 percent of the population, depending on the type of screening procedure used.

Symptoms: Most adenomatous polyps are asymptomatic, and patients are unaware of their presence until they are identified through screening. When adenomatous polyps are not removed and continue to grow larger, they can eventually induce rectal bleeding, diarrhea, or constipation.

Screening and diagnosis: The most common screening method to detect adenomatous polyps is colonoscopy, a procedure by which a doctor inserts a viewing tube into the colon and removes any visually identified polyps. Other screening methods that may be used are flexible sigmoidoscopy and barium enema. Removed polyps are then biopsied to determine if they are benign or have developed into precancerous or cancerous lesions.

Treatment and therapy: When identified through screening, the general treatment is immediate removal of adenomatous polyps to prevent their possible development into cancer. Most doctors recommend that patients undergo subsequent colorectal screening on a regular basis for several years following the removal of adenomatous polyps.

Prognosis, prevention, and outcomes: When discovered and removed, adenomatous polyps do not significantly change a patient's quality of life. However, if left undetected, some of these polyps can develop into colon cancer, which has a higher mortality rate than any other cancer type in the United States. Some possible ways to prevent the development of adenomatous polyps is to maintain a diet that is high in fiber and low in fat, as well as refraining from smoking and excessive drinking.

Lisa M. Cockrell, B.S.

See also: Colon polyps; Colorectal cancer; Desmoid tumors; Duodenal carcinomas; Enterostomal therapy; Gardner syndrome; Gastric polyps; Genetics of cancer; Hereditary cancer syndromes; Hereditary polyposis syndromes; Polyps; Small intestine cancer; Stomach cancers; Turcot syndrome

▶ Adrenal gland cancers

Category: Diseases, Symptoms, and Conditions
Also known as: Pheochromocytoma, adrenal cortical cancer, adrenocortical cancer, neuroblastoma

Related conditions: Cushing syndrome, Conn syndrome, adrenogenital syndrome

Definition: The adrenal glands are hormone-producing endocrine glands located directly above the kidneys. The outer layer of each gland is called the adrenal cortex. Hormones produced in the adrenal cortex include cortisol (aids in regulating blood sugar level), aldosterone (aids in regulating fluid and electrolyte balance and blood pressure), and testosterone and estrogen (male and female sex hormones). A primary malignant tumor in the adrenal cortex—one that originates in that location—is called adrenocortical cancer. The inner area of each gland is called the adrenal medulla. Hormones produced in the medulla include epinephrine and norepinephrine, which help regulate the body's response to physical and emotional stress. A primary malignant tumor that originates in the medulla is called a pheochromocytoma. Another form of cancer that originates in the medulla is neuroblastoma, typically found in infants and children younger than age ten.

Adrenal tumors are commonly classified by their effect on hormone production in the affected area. Adrenal tumors that increase hormone production are called functioning tumors; those that do not produce hormones are called nonfunctioning tumors.

Risk factors: Although specific risk factors for adrenal cancers have not been identified, they have been associated with genetically linked familial syndromes, such as Li-Fraumeni syndrome, Beckwith-Wiedemann syndrome, and Carney complex.

Etiology and the disease process: The cause of adrenal cancer is unknown. Functioning tumors that secrete hormones produce changes in the body systems affected by those hormones. Nonfunctioning tumors typically grow large enough to produce pressure on other organs, causing discomfort or pain in the abdomen or flank.

Incidence: Primary adrenal gland cancers are rare, affecting only 1 or 2 persons per 1 million people. Approximately 60 to 80 percent of adrenal cancers are functional, secreting large amounts of adrenal hormones. Adrenocortical cancer is most common in men between the ages of forty and fifty; neuroblastoma most commonly affects children younger than age five; and pheochromocytoma is most common between ages thirty and forty.

Symptoms: A functioning adrenocortical cancer tumor typically produces excess amounts of cortisol and aldosterone, which can cause elevated blood pressure, weight gain, thirst, urinary frequency, facial swelling (moon face), cramping of the muscles in the arms and legs, and increased hair growth on the face, arms, and back. If the tumor produces sex hormones, men may develop a loss of sex drive, impotence, and enlarged breasts; women may develop a deeper voice, menstrual irregularities, and increased facial hair; and children may experience early puberty. A neuroblastoma can cause an unusual abdominal lump or fullness, weight loss, extreme tiredness, persistent diarrhea, flushing, sweating, elevated blood pressure, and behavior indicating the presence of abdominal pain. A pheochromocytoma can cause elevated blood pressure that is resistant to treatment, excessive sweating, severe headaches, tremors, rapid pulse, palpitations, and extreme anxiety.

A nonfunctioning adrenal cancer may not produce symptoms until the cancer is advanced or has metastasized. Typical symptoms are caused by the tumor pressing on other abdominal organs, causing pain or an abnormal feeling of fullness. Tiredness, fever, and weight loss may also be present.

Screening and diagnosis: There are no screening tests for adrenal cancer. Diagnosis begins with a thorough patient and family medical history and physical examination. If adrenal cancer is suspected, the patient's blood and urine are tested for elevated levels of adrenal hormones, and computed tomography scanning and magnetic resonance imaging are performed to identify tumors. The metaiodobenzylguanidine (MIBG) scan, during which images are taken after the injection of small amounts of radioactive materials, is used to detect the presence and location of a pheochromocytoma. Staging of adrenal cancer depends on the specific type of tumor.

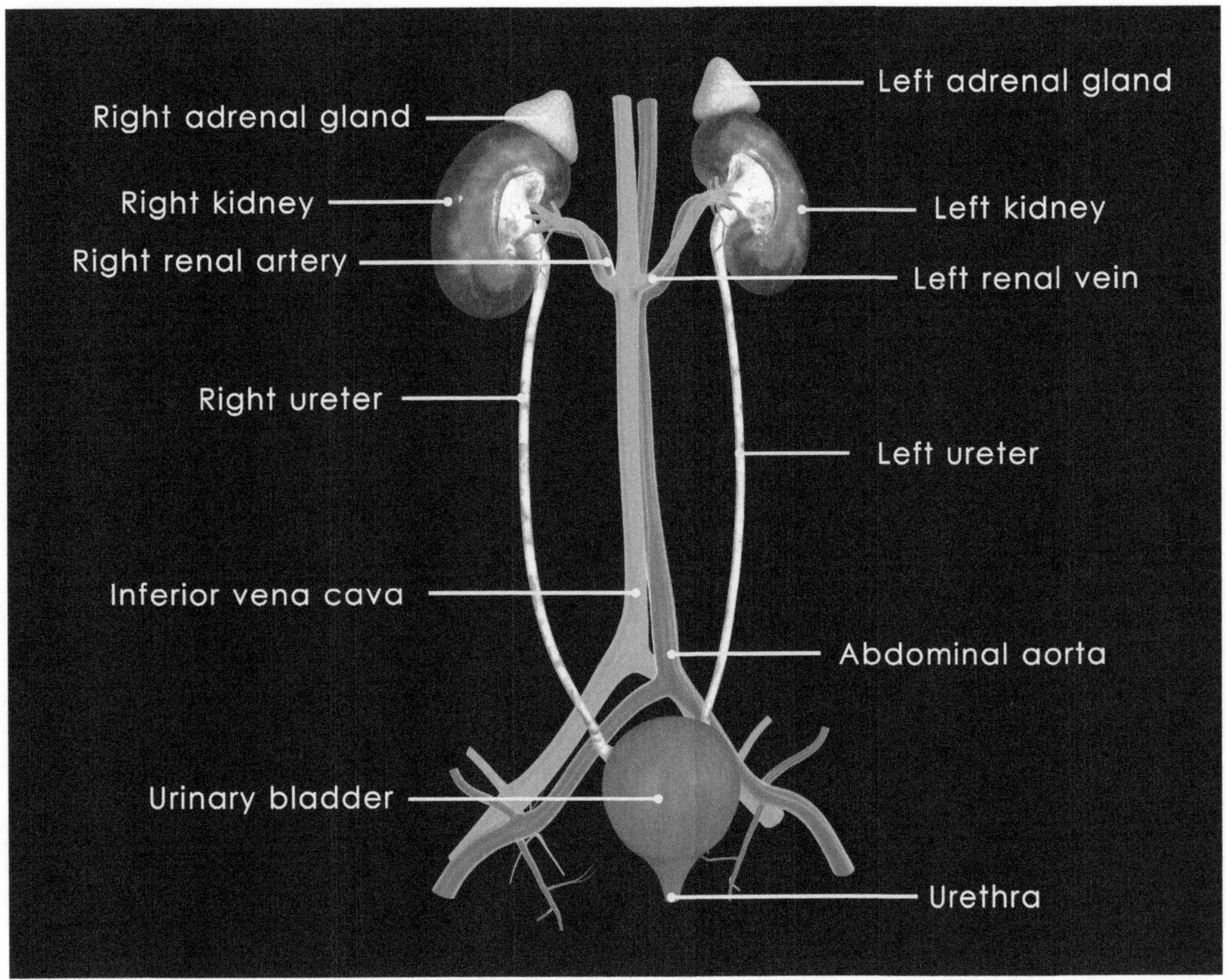

The adrenal glands are located on top of the kidneys. (iStock)

Treatment and therapy: Treatment for adrenal cancer usually includes surgery to remove the affected gland, followed by chemotherapy to destroy any remaining cancer cells. The type and combination of chemotherapeutic drugs used varies with the type of tumor.

Mitotane, most commonly used after surgery for adrenocortical cancer, blocks hormone production and destroys adrenal cancer cells. It is also used to treat inoperable, recurrent, and metastatic adrenocortical cancer. If the patient cannot tolerate mitotane therapy or it is ineffective, cisplatin is typically used, either alone or combined with cyclophosphamide and doxorubicin, fluorouracil and doxorubicin, or VP-16.

Following surgery, neuroblastoma may be treated with chemotherapy using carboplatin, doxorubicin, cyclophosphamide, and etoposide.

Surgery to remove a pheochromocytoma is typically preceded by the administration of medication to block the secretion of adrenalin, which can cause very high blood pressure and serious surgical complications. MIBG radiotherapy may be used after surgery or to treat metastatic pheochromocytoma.

Prognosis, prevention, and outcomes: There is no known prevention for adrenal cancer. The prognosis for adrenal cancer depends on the type of tumor and the stage of the disease. The five-year survival rate after surgery for adrenocortical cancer is approximately 10 to 35 percent; for localized pheochromocytomas it is about 95 percent. The prognosis for neuroblastoma varies widely depending on the child's risk grouping. The five-year survival rate ranges from about 95 percent for a low-risk child to about 30 percent for a high-risk child. Metastatic tumors of all types have a poor prognosis.

Dorothy P. Terry, R.N.

Relative Survival Rates for Adrenal Gland Cancers, 1988-2001

	Survival Rates (%)			
Cancer Type	*1-Year*	*3-Year*	*5-Year*	*10-Year*
Adrenal gland (all)	59.4	45.5	38.7	29.6
Adrenocorticol	66.0	48.5	41.2	31.3
Pheochromocytoma	84.5	73.0	64.8	44.0

Source: Data from L. A. G. Ries et al., eds., *Cancer Survival Among Adults: U.S. SEER Program, 1988-2001—Patient and Tumor Characteristics,* NIH Pub. No. 07-6215 (Bethesda, Md.: National Cancer Institute, 2007)

For Further Information

Bertagna, Xavier, ed. *Adrenal Cancer*. Montrouge, France: John Libbey Eurotext, 2006.

Souhami, Robert, and Jeffrey Tobias. *Cancer and Its Management*. Malden, Mass.: Blackwell, 2005.

Stern, Theodore A., and Mikkael A. Sekeres. *Facing Cancer: A Complete Guide for People with Cancer, Their Families, and Caregivers*. New York: McGraw-Hill, 2004.

Other Resources

American Cancer Society
http://www.cancer.org

Endocrine Web
http://www.endocrineweb.com

National Cancer Institute
http://www.nci.nih.gov/cancertopics

See also: Adrenocortical cancer; Computed Tomography (CT) scan; Cushing syndrome and cancer; Endocrine cancers; Endocrinology oncology; Hepatomegaly; Radiofrequency ablation

▶ Adrenocortical cancer

Category: Diseases, Symptoms, and Conditions
Also known as: Adrenal cortex carcinoma

Related conditions: Cushing syndrome, Conn syndrome, virilization

Definition: Adrenocortical cancer is an aggressive malignancy that occurs when a tumor develops in the tissue of the adrenal cortex, the outer layer of tissues that surround the adrenal gland and produce steroid hormones.

Risk factors: Certain hereditary diseases, including Li-Fraumeni syndrome, Beckwith-Wiedemann syndrome, and Carney complex, are the main known risk factors.

Etiology and the disease process: The cause of these tumors is unknown. An adrenocortical cancer tumor is either nonfunctioning or functioning, meaning that it overproduces certain hormones that the adrenal cortex normally produces. These hormones include cortisol, aldosterone, testosterone, and estrogen. Adrenocortical cancer commonly becomes malignant, spreading to the lung, liver, bone, and peritoneum (lining of the abdominal cavity).

Incidence: Adrenocortical cancer is relatively rare, affecting only 1 to 2 people out of 1 million every year. Although it generally occurs in adults between the ages of thirty and forty years, children can develop this cancer, usually under the age of six.

Symptoms: Nonfunctioning adrenocortical cancer tumors usually do not have symptoms. Functioning adrenocortical cancer tumors can generate many symptoms, owing to their overproduction of steroid hormones. Depending on the hormone, symptoms can include weight gain, high blood pressure, muscle weakness, acne, and changes in menstrual cycles.

Screening and diagnosis: Laboratory testing can be used to confirm changes in steroid hormone production. Abdominal radiological examination, such as computed tomography scanning and magnetic resonance imaging, can be used to determine the exact location and extent of the tumor. Adrenocortical cancer tumors are staged on a scale of I to IV, according to the size of the tumor and the degree of invasion, both locally and to distant sites.

Treatment and therapy: When discovered early, adrenocortical cancer can be cured through surgical removal of the tumor. However, because most tumors are not diagnosed until they are advanced, other treatment strategies such as radiation therapy and chemotherapy must be used. Most chemotherapy regimens to treat adrenocortical cancer include the drug mitotane, which is toxic to adrenal cortex cells, in addition to other chemotherapeutic agents such as cisplatin, doxorubicin, and etoposide.

Prognosis, prevention, and outcomes: The prognosis for patients diagnosed with adrenocortical cancer is generally very poor, and dependent on several factors. These include the ability of the tumor to be surgically removed, the stage of the cancer at diagnosis, the general health of the patient, and whether the tumor is recurrent.

Lisa M. Cockrell, B.S.

See also: Adrenal gland cancers

▶ Aleukemia

Category: Diseases, Symptoms, and Conditions
Also known as: Aleukemic myelosis, aleukemic leukemia

Related conditions: Acute and chronic myelogenous leukemia (AML and CML), acute and chronic lymphatic leukemia (ALL and CLL)

Definition: Aleukemia describes a condition in which a patient has a normal or reduced white blood cell count. Leukemia cells are present in the bone marrow. Leukemia cells may also be present in the blood. Aleukemia may be present in any of the four major types of leukemia: AML, CML, ALL, and CLL.

Risk factors: The risk factors are the same as those for leukemia. The risks include age, genetic diseases, prolonged exposure to some chemicals such as benzene, chemotherapies used to treat other forms of cancer, and exposure to high doses of radiation or tobacco smoke.

Etiology and the disease process: Aleukemias start when there is damage to the deoxyribonucleic acid (DNA) of blood cells. Normal cell development is interrupted, causing a decrease of mature cells and an increase in immature cells.

Incidence: Aleukemia is present at the start of about 25 to 30 percent of acute leukemias. It is more prevalent in hairy cell leukemia, which is a slow-growing subtype of CLL.

Symptoms: There may be no symptoms present. Patients may experience fatigue, weight loss, easy bruising, fever, and infections.

Screening and diagnosis: No specific screening test exists for aleukemia. A low white blood cell count found when a complete blood count (CBC) is done as part of a routine exam or in response to symptoms may lead to further testing and diagnosis. Diagnosis is made by the examination of blood smears and bone marrow for the presence of leukemia cells.

Staging is not done for any of the leukemias except CLL. The staging of CLL is based on imaging studies, blood tests, and bone marrow examination. The stages, ranging from Stage 0 to IV, are based on the involvement of lymph nodes, spleen, and liver, and decreasing numbers of red blood cells. The other forms of leukemia are classified by cell type.

Treatment and therapy: Treatment depends on the type of cell involved and the classification or staging level. In leukemias that progress slowly, treatment may not start until the disease is more advanced.

Prognosis, prevention, and outcomes: Prognosis depends on the type of cell involved and the rate of progression. No method of prevention exists. Treatment may slow the progress of the disease or cause complete remission. Some types of leukemia may not respond to treatment.

Wanda E. Clark, M.T. (ASCP)

See also: Acute Lymphocytic Leukemia (ALL); Acute Myelocytic Leukemia (AML); Anemia; Antiandrogens; Blood cancers; Chronic Lymphocytic Leukemia (CLL); Chronic Myeloid Leukemia (CML); Eosinophilic leukemia; Fanconi anemia; Leukemias

▶ Alopecia

Category: Diseases, Symptoms, and Conditions
Also known as: Alopecia disseminata, alopecia universalis, alopecia totalis, baldness, hair loss, acomia, pelade

Related conditions: Anagen effluvium, telogen effluvium

Definition: Alopecia is abnormal loss of hair, a common side effect of treatments for cancers, including chemotherapy and radiation therapy. There are many types of alopecia, with many causes, including certain skin cancers and other types of cancer that spread to the skin, although marked hair loss from skin cancer is extremely rare.

Risk factors: Chemotherapy for any cancer greatly increases the risk of alopecia, and radiation therapy increases the risk of hair loss from the irradiated area.

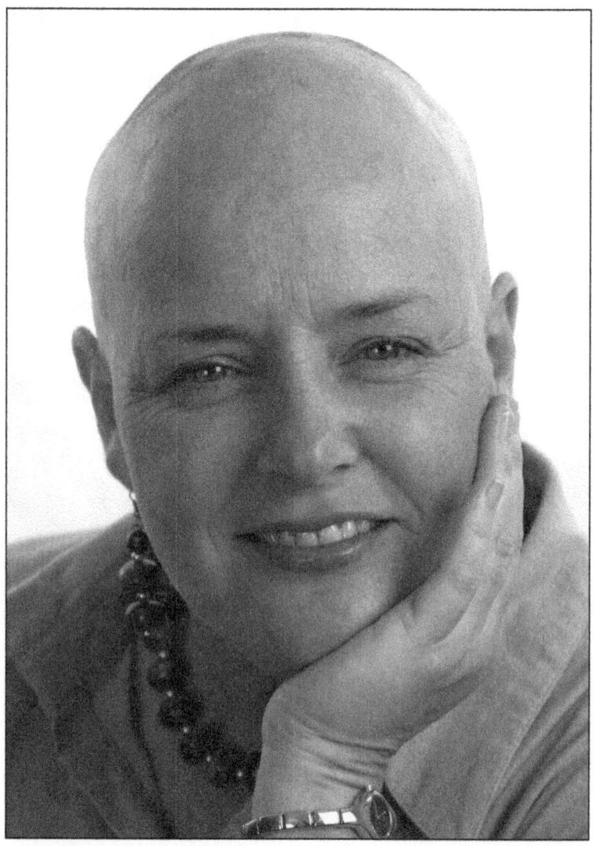

Chemotherapy has caused this woman to lose her hair. (iStock)

Etiology and the disease process: Each human hair grows from a hair follicle, an elongated pouch formed during fetal development by growth of the upper part of the skin, the epidermis, down into the lower part, the dermis. The lower part of the follicle, the hair bulb, contains the germinal matrix, the cells that form the hair. Each hair goes through a three-phase growth cycle: anagen, or active growth; catagen, or regression; and telogen, or resting. When the telogen phase for each hair is complete, a new anagen phase begins. Human hairs complete their recurring growth cycle, as old hairs are pushed out by new hairs, in random order. At any given time, about 85 percent of hairs are in the anagen, or active growth phase. Chemotherapeutic agents target rapidly reproducing cells, like cancer cells. Unfortunately, these agents do not know the difference between a cancer cell and the rapidly reproducing cells of the germinal matrix in a hair bulb. They stop cell division, or mitosis, in matrix cells, just as they do in cancer cells. The anagen phase comes to a stop, and in many cases, all the hair that is in the anagen phase is shed. Hair lost through chemotherapy almost always regrows, because the hair follicle is left intact. Radiation therapy also stops the reproduction of rapidly dividing cells, but in higher doses, radiation can damage the hair follicles it touches, preventing regrowth of hair.

Incidence: At least some degree of hair loss is likely with many forms of chemotherapy. Certain drugs or combinations of drugs are virtually certain to cause some degree of hair loss. A few drugs cause nearly complete hair loss.

Symptoms: Symptoms of alopecia related to cancer range from temporary thinning or breakage of a small patch of hair to loss of hair all over the body (alopecia disseminata, alopecia universalis, alopecia totalis), and hair loss can be temporary or permanent, depending on the cause.

Screening and diagnosis: Diagnosis of chemotherapy-related alopecia follows visible hair loss within days or weeks of administration of chemotherapeutic drugs.

Treatment and therapy: Therapies for alopecia caused by chemotherapy include administration of vitamins, minerals, or omega-3 and omega-6 fatty acids—substances that promote healthy hair. The benefit of these therapies on cancer-related hair loss is still being researched, and consumption of some vitamins and minerals may reduce the effectiveness of chemotherapy, so any treatment for hair loss during therapy should be approved by the treating physician. Treatment for cancer-caused alopecia includes treatment for the underlying cancer, which may include surgery or chemotherapy. Again, noticeable hair loss from cancer itself is extremely rare.

Prognosis, prevention, and outcomes: The prognosis for alopecia caused by chemotherapy depends on the chemicals used, the dosage, and the frequency of treatment. More intensive treatment is likely to cause more extensive hair loss. Whatever the amount or type of hair loss from chemotherapy, the prognosis is eventual regrowth of hair. Patchy regrowth may begin before chemotherapy is completed, an average of three to five months after initial hair loss from the first treatment. Because chemotherapy disrupts the matrix from which the hair is formed, including the melanocytes, or cells that give hair its color, regrown hair may differ in color or texture from the original hair. There has been some limited success in preventing scalp hair loss from chemotherapy through use of scalp cooling or a hairline tourniquet during administration of the chemotherapy. These, however, have been successful with only certain chemical agents. Their use has been questioned by some oncologists because, while they protect scalp follicles from damage, they also protect any cancer cells present in the scalp. Research trials are being conducted on other treatments that may reduce hair loss from chemotherapy. The prognosis for alopecia caused by radiation therapy depends on the dosage of radiation. High doses usually cause permanent hair loss to the irradiated area; low doses more often cause temporary, local hair loss.

Cathy Anderson, R.N., B.A.

For Further Information

Bleiker, T. O., N. Nicolaou, J. Traulsen, and P. E. Hutchinson. "'Atrophic Telogen Effluvium' from Cytotoxic Drugs and a Randomized Controlled Trial to Investigate the Possible Protective Effect of Pretreatment with a Topical Vitamin D_3 Analogue in Humans." *British Journal of Dermatology* 153, no. 1 (2005): 103-112.

Jothilakshmi, P. K., A. J. Watson, and E. Jude. "Acute Alopecia Due to Metformin Treatment for Polycystic Ovarian Syndrome." *Journal of Obstetrics and Gynaecology* 26, no. 6 (2006): 584-585.

Wang, J., Z. Lu, and J. L. Au. "Protection Against Chemotherapy-Induced Alopecia." *Pharmaceutical Research* 23, no. 11 (2006): 2505-2514.

Wyatt, A. J., G. D. Leonard, and D. L. Sachs. "Cutaneous Reactions to Chemotherapy and Their Management." *American Journal of Clinical Dermatology* 7, no. 1 (2006): 45-63.

Other Resources

Chemotherapy.com
http://www.chemotherapy.com

Healthline
http://www.healthline.com

WebMD
http://www.webmd.com

See also: Alkylating agents in chemotherapy; Chemotherapy; Cyclophosphamide; Paraneoplastic syndromes; Radiation therapies; Self-image and body image; Side effects

▶ Alveolar soft-part sarcomas

Category: Diseases, Symptoms, and Conditions
Also known as: Nonrhabdomyosarcoma soft-tissue sarcomas, ASPS

Related conditions: Soft-tissue sarcomas

Definition: Alveolar soft-part sarcoma is a slow-growing, malignant tumor that develops in deep soft tissues and muscles, most often in the thighs and buttocks. It is also found in the arm, chest, bladder, abdomen, and—in children—the head and neck. It gets its name from the way the tumor cells are clustered, resembling alveoli, or the air sacs of the lungs.

Risk factors: No risk factors are known, and alveolar soft-part sarcoma is nonhereditary.

Etiology and the disease process: The disease's etiology is murky. Early development of alveolar soft-part sarcoma appears to be linked to a genetic mutation involving the separation of a gene from chromosome 17 and its attachment to the X chromosome. A wealth of blood vessels allows tumor cells to enter the bloodstream and spread to other areas, usually the lungs and brain. Childhood alveolar soft-part sarcoma appears to have a different, and generally less aggressive, biology.

Incidence: Alveolar soft-part sarcoma is rare, with 40 to 80 new cases annually in the United States. About half of alveolar soft-part sarcoma patients are between the ages of fifteen and twenty-nine, and women generally outnumber men, especially among younger patients.

Symptoms: Common symptoms include a soft, painless lump, soreness, reduced range of motion, and numbness. Because alveolar soft-part sarcoma grows slowly in deep, elastic tissues, patients often do not notice symptoms until the cancer is advanced or has spread.

Screening and staging: Diagnostic procedures include laboratory tests and imaging studies such as computed tomography (CT) scans, magnetic resonance imaging (MRI), and bone scans. A biopsy is required, however, to confirm alveolar soft-part sarcoma. Tumors are staged based on size, grade, and degree of spread:

- Stage I: Low grade, with little potential for spreading
- Stages II and III: High grade, with increased potential for spreading
- Stage IV: Metastasis to distant organs

Other criteria are typically used for staging pediatric alveolar soft-part sarcoma.

Treatment and therapy: Surgical removal of the tumor and surrounding tissue is the primary treatment. Radiation therapy may be used before to shrink the tumor and after to kill any remaining cells, although it is used in children only if surgery alone is ineffective.

Chemotherapy is not generally beneficial. Other therapies are under study.

Prognosis, prevention, and outcomes: The five-year survival rate for patients with localized tumors is around 80 percent. If the disease has metastasized, the rate drops to 20 percent. However, long-term survival is possible even with spread because alveolar soft-part sarcoma grows slowly. The prognosis for children is considerably better, as their tumors are generally smaller and localized. Alveolar soft-part sarcoma can recur more than ten years after initial diagnosis, so long-term follow-up is recommended.

Judy Majewski, M.S.

See also: Dermatofibrosarcoma protuberans; Ewing sarcoma; Fibrosarcomas, soft-tissue; Hemangiosarcomas; Liposarcomas; Mesenchymomas, malignant; Rhabdomyosarcomas; Sarcomas, soft-tissue; Synovial sarcomas

▶ Amenorrhea

Category: Diseases, Symptoms, and Conditions
Also known as: Primary amenorrhea, secondary amenorrhea, absent periods, absent menses, absent menarche

Related conditions: Pregnancy, menopause, pituitary or gynecologic tumors

Definition: Amenorrhea is the absence of menstruation, whether temporary or permanent. Amenorrhea is normal prior to puberty, during pregnancy and lactation, and after menopause. Amenorrhea may also occur as the symptom of a variety of abnormal conditions, including pituitary or gynecologic tumors, and is an expected result of many chemotherapeutic cancer drugs.

Primary amenorrhea is the absence of menarche, the initial menstrual period, in women age sixteen and older. Menarche occurs normally in women between the eleventh and seventeenth year. The average age of menarche in the United States is 12.8 years.

Secondary amenorrhea is absence of menses for three months in a woman with previously normal menstruation and for nine months in a woman with oligomenorrhea, which is infrequent periods and fewer than the normal eleven to thirteen a year.

Risk factors: Both primary and secondary amenorrhea can be influenced by a host of other factors, some of which include immunodeficiency, anorexia nervosa, congenital abnormalities of the reproductive tract, obesity, diabetes, dietary restriction, starvation, metabolic disorders, drugs, and excessive physical exercise. Amenorrhea can also signal a pituitary or a gynecologic tumor, and it is a common and even expected result of chemotherapy or radiation treatment for cancer.

Etiology and the disease process: Amenorrhea is often due to the absence or change in hormones produced in the hypothalamus, the pituitary gland, or the ovaries (the triad that directs reproduction), and it can result from an abnormality in the outflow tract.

In primary amenorrhea, in the presence of secondary sex characteristics and a uterus, the most common cause is outflow tract obstruction with a transverse vaginal septum or imperforate hymen, both easily correctable. However, primary amenorrhea can also have a genetic cause.

The most common cause of secondary amenorrhea is pregnancy during a woman's reproductive years. Secondary amenorrhea may also be related to lifestyle choices. Athletes and ballet dancers who train vigorously often experience missed periods. Stress, obesity, and starvation can also result in secondary amenorrhea. In these cases, women stop menstruating because the ovaries do not produce enough estrogen in a cyclic manner to cause the uterine lining to thicken and shed normally.

If pregnancy is not the cause, the physician may test the patient's levels of hormones produced by the thyroid and the pituitary glands. When amenorrhea is accompanied by elevated levels of prolactin, galactorrhea, headaches, or visual disturbances, a pituitary tumor may be the cause. Adenomas are the most common cause of anterior pituitary dysfunction. Gynecological tumors such as ovarian cancer must also be ruled out in the presence of amenorrhea.

Cancer treatments such chemotherapy and radiation are often associated with amenorrhea. The greater the dose of the chemotherapeutic agent, the greater the chance of amenorrhea. Studies linking particular cancer treatments to the incidence of amenorrhea remain incomplete, but two drugs particularly linked to amenorrhea are doxorubicin and cyclophosphamide.

Incidence: In the United States, the incidence of primary amenorrhea is 2.5 percent. The incidence of secondary amenorrhea is between 1 and 4 percent.

Rarely, the cause of amenorrhea is a tumor of the pituitary. The true incidence of pituitary adenomas is difficult to know with certainty because they are often asymptomatic; autopsy estimates range from 2.7 to 27 percent.

Symptoms: The first sign of primary amenorrhea is the absence of menses. If the cause of absence of flow is an anomaly of the outflow tract of the blood, the patient may experience cramping and severe abdominal pain.

In the case of secondary amenorrhea, other that the absence of menstruation, symptoms may include:

- galactorrhea, in which case the breasts produce milk in a woman who is not pregnant or breastfeeding
- headache or reduced peripheral vision as a potential sign of an intracranial tumor
- hirsutism, or increased hair growth in a male pattern caused by excess androgen
- vaginal dryness, hot flashes, night sweats, or disordered sleep, suggesting ovarian insufficiency or premature ovarian failure (premature menopause)
- excessive weight gain or loss
- anxiety

Screening and diagnosis: With primary amenorrhea and the absence of secondary sex characteristics, the physician may order an ultrasound to determine if a uterus is present and measure the levels of two hormones produced by the anterior pituitary: the follicle stimulating hormone (FSH), which stimulates growth of the follicle in the ovary, and luteinizing hormone (LH), which triggers ovulation. Very low levels suggest that the gonads, or sex glands, have failed to develop or begin functioning.

Karyotyping to study the chromosome arrangement may reveal a genetic reason for the absence of menarche. An example is Turner syndrome, which is a congenital endocrine disorder caused by failure of the ovaries to respond to pituitary hormone stimulation. In addition to primary amenorrhea and failure of sexual maturation, the physical examination may note short stature. About one-third of the patients show webbing of the neck, marled cubitus valgus (a deformity of the arm in which the forearm deviates laterally), and developmental disabilities. Often genetic studies reveal the presence of only 45 chromosomes, the second X chromosome being absent.

Treatment and therapy: A thorough medical history often reveals the cause of amenorrhea, which can then be corrected by surgery, medication, or lifestyle changes. Secondary amenorrhea may be caused by some medications such as phenothiazines, some narcotics, and any condition related to pituitary insufficiency or thyroid dysfunction. For cases due to lifestyle choices, reducing the amount or intensity of exercise and maintaining a healthy weight should correct hormone levels and result in a return to regular periods.

If is determined to be a symptom of a pituitary or gyencologic tumor, the patient will undergo tests for malignancy and follow-up treatment and therapy indicated for the particular cancer diagnosed.

Prognosis, prevention, and outcomes: Most cases of amenorrhea are treatable, although some resulting from genetic conditions cannot be corrected. In women with low thyroid-stimulating hormone (TSH), or hypothyroidism, which is more often associated with hypermenorrhea or oligomenorrhea, the menstrual cycle is often returned to normal following hormone replacement therapy.

If a pituitary tumor is causing the amenorrhea, these tumors are rare and often asymptomatic, seldom resulting in death. They are typically slow growing and benign. However, the numerous hormones produced in the pituitary orchestrate many bodily functions, so patients with these tumors may face a lifetime of hormone replacement and long-term follow-up care.

Jane Adrian, M.P.H., Ed.M., M.T. (ASCP)

For Further Information

Bell, Ruth, et al. *Changing Bodies, Changing Lives: A Book for Teens on Sex and Relationships*. 3d ed. New York: Times Books, 1998.

Hobart, Julie A., and Douglas R. Smucker. "The Female Athlete Triad." *American Family Physician* 61, no. 11 (June 1, 2000).

Master-Hunter, Tarannum, and Diana L. Heiman. "Amenorrhea: Evaluation and Treatment. " *American Family Physician* 73, no. 8 (April 15, 2006).

Slap, Gail B. "Amenorrhea." In *The Gale Encyclopedia of Childhood and Adolescence*, edited by Jerome Kagan. Detroit: Gale, 1998.

Other Resources

American College of Obstetricians and Gynecologists
http://www.acog.org

American Society for Reproductive Medicine
http://www.asrm.org

See also: Alkylating agents in chemotherapy; Chemotherapy; Endometrial cancer; Infertility and cancer; Neuroendocrine tumors; Ovarian cysts; Sterility

▶ Anal cancer

Category: Diseases, Symptoms, and Conditions
Also known as: Cancer of the anus, anal canal cancer

Related conditions: Anorectum cancer, anal squamous intraepithelial lesions (ASIL), human papillomavirus (HPV), human immunodeficiency virus (HIV), acquired immunodeficiency syndrome (AIDS)

Definition: Anal cancer is a rare cancer that forms in the anus, which is at the end of the rectum. The anus is about 1.5 inches long and contains sphincter muscles that control bowel movements. Stool passes through the anus as it leaves the body.

Risk factors: There are several risk factors for anal cancer, including cigarette smoking and anal receptive sexual intercourse. Infection with the human papillomavirus (HPV16), the sexually transmitted disease that causes genital warts, can cause anal squamous intraepithelial lesions (ASIL), which may develop into anal cancer. People with a suppressed immune system from cancer, cancer treatments, organ transplantation, HIV, or AIDS have an increased risk of anal cancer. The number of people with both HIV and anal cancer is rising.

Etiology and the disease process: Researchers do not know the exact cause of the genetic changes that make healthy cells turn into anal cancer cells, although multiple risk factors have been identified. The anal cancer cells multiply and form masses or tumors.

Incidence: Anal cancer is a rare form of cancer; however, the number of new cases began to increase in the early 1980's. The incidence of anal cancer is 1 in 100,000 people. New cases in 2007 in the United States were estimated to reach 4,650. Anal cancer occurs more frequently in women than in men. Women are more likely to develop cancer in the anal canal. Men are more likely to develop cancer tumors on the outside of the anus. Anal cancer occurs most frequently in adults in their early sixties, at a median age of sixty-one years.

Symptoms: Anal cancer may not cause symptoms. Bleeding from the anus is a common early sign. This type of cancer may cause pain, itching, abnormal anal discharge, and changes in the diameter of stools. A mass or growth may develop in the anus. Nearby lymph nodes may be swollen. The anus may feel unusually full.

Screening and diagnosis: Screening tests for anal cancer are recommended for people with a high risk of anal cancer. Women should receive anal cancer screening as part of a yearly exam. Annual anal cancer screening is recommended for men after the age of fifty.

Stage at Diagnosis and Five-Year Relative Survival Rates for Cancer of the Anus, 1996-2004

Stage	*Individuals Diagnosed (%)*	*Survival Rate (%)*
Localizeda	49	81.7
Regionalb	32	61.1
Distantc	10	2.8
Unstaged	10	57.6

Source: Data from National Cancer Institute, Surveillance Epidemiology and End Results, Cancer Stat Fact Sheets, 2008
[a]Cancer still confined to primary site
[b]Cancer has spread to regional lymph nodes or directly beyond the primary site
[c]Cancer has metastasized

Anal cancer is diagnosed with a series of tests and procedures. A digital rectal exam (DRE) is used to check for lumps, masses, or growths in the anus. Endoscopy, using an anoscope or rigid protosigmoidoscopy, allows inspection of the interior anal canal. An anoscope is a thin tube with a viewing instrument and light that is inserted into the anus. A protosigmoidoscope is longer and allows sections of the colon to be viewed as well. Ultrasound, computed tomography (CT) scans, positron emission (PET) scans, and magnetic resonance imaging (MRI) scans are used to provide images of the anal structures and to help determine if the cancer has spread. Fine needle aspiration and sentinel lymph node biopsy are used to obtain cells for examination to confirm if cancer is present.

Staging is used to identify cancer growth and metastasis, plan treatment, and predict recovery. Fortunately, anal cancer rarely metastasizes.

- Stage I: Anal cancer is 2 centimeters (cm) or less.
- Stage II: Anal cancer is larger than 2 cm, is confined to the anus, and has not spread beyond the anus.
- Stage IIIA: Anal cancer is any size with spread to nearby lymph nodes or close areas, such as the bladder, urethra, or vagina.
- Stage IIIB: Anal cancer is any size with spread to nearby lymph nodes and close areas, or it has spread to lymph nodes in the pelvis.
- Stage IV: Anal cancer has spread to distant locations in the body.

Treatment and therapy: Chemoradiation is the treatment of choice for anal cancer. External radiation, brachytherapy, or both may be used. Chemotherapy 5-FU and Mutamycin (mitomycin) may be used in combination with radiation or surgery. Surgery is used for patients with residual anal cancer and includes local resection or abdominoperineal resection (APR).

Prognosis, prevention, and outcomes: Anal cancer screening, HPV testing, HIV testing, quitting smoking, knowing the STD status of sexual partners before intercourse, and not participating in anal sex may help prevent anal cancer. Condoms may reduce the risk of HPV and HIV, but they are not a guarantee. HPV vaccination is available for girls and women.

Many cases of anal cancer that are detected and treated early can be cured. However, anal cancer may recur even with treatment. It was estimated that 690 men and women with anal cancer would die in the United States in 2007, a rate of 0.2 per 100,000 people.

Mary Car-Blanchard, O.T.D., B.S.O.T.

For Further Information

Cranston, R. D., et al. "The Prevalence, and Predictive Value, of Abnormal Anal Cytology to Diagnose Anal Dysplasia in a Population of HIV-Positive Men Who Have Sex with Men." *International Journal of STD and AIDS* 18, no. 2 (February, 2007): 77-80.

Das, P., C. H. Crane, and J. A. Ajani. "Current Treatment for Localized Anal Carcinoma." *Current Opinions in Oncology* 19, no. 4 (July, 2007): 396-400.

Meyer, J., B. Czito, F. F. Yin, and C. Willett. "Advanced Radiation Therapy Technologies in the Treatment of Rectal and Anal Cancer: Intensity-Modulated Photon Therapy and Proton Therapy." *Clinical Colorectal Cancer* 6, no. 5 (January, 2007): 348-356.

Uronis, H. E., and J. C. Bendell. "Anal Cancer: An Overview." *Oncologist* 12, no. 5 (May, 2007): 524-534.

Other Resources

American Cancer Society

How Is Anal Cancer Diagnosed?

Http://www.cancer.org/docroot/CRI/content/CRI_2_4_3X_How_Is_Anal_Cancer_Diagnosed_47.asp

National Cancer Institute

Anal Cancer Treatment

http://www.cancer.gov/cancertopics/pdq/treatment/anal/patient

See also: Abdominoperineal Resection (APR); Anoscopy; Colostomy; Computed Tomography (CT) scan; Digital Rectal Exam (DRE); Endoscopy; Gastrointestinal cancers; Gastrointestinal oncology; Infectious cancers; Risks for cancer; Sexuality and cancer; Sigmoidoscopy

▶ Anemia

Category: Diseases, Symptoms, and Conditions

Also known as: Low red blood cell count, erythropenia, iron-poor blood

Related conditions: Cytopenia

Definition: Anemia is a low number of red blood cells, decreased volume of red blood cells, or a reduced concentration of hemoglobin.

Risk factors: For anemia of cancer, risk is associated with the type of cancer, stage of disease, and treatment regimen.

Etiology and the disease process: Anemia may be caused by deficiencies of vitamin B_{12}, folic acid, or iron; antibody formation; kidney failure; lead poisoning; bone-marrow dysfunction; chemotherapy; or radiation therapy. It can also result from infiltration of bone marrow by leukemia or lymphomas or from internal bleeding or excessive blood loss from repeated blood sampling.

Anemias caused by deficiencies in folic acid, vitamin B_{12}, and iron are generally known as nutritional anemias. In these forms of anemia, the endogenous hormone erythropoietin, responsible for red blood cell production, appears to be present in adequate amounts. Patients with cancer, however, can be anemic because of deficiencies in these nutrients.

The anemia of cancer, a subset of anemia of chronic disease, is marked by reduction in the amount of the hormone erythropoietin found in the circulation, suppression of bone marrow function, disturbances in iron metabolism, and activation of the inflammatory and immune systems in response to the insult of cancer that activates hormones, which in turn decrease the production of endogenous erythropoietin. Another form of anemia is aplastic anemia, which may be caused by chemotherapy, radiation therapy, or drugs.

In the normal state of health, endogenous erythropoietin is released by peritubular cells in the kidney cortex when specialized cells sense hypoxia (low oxygen

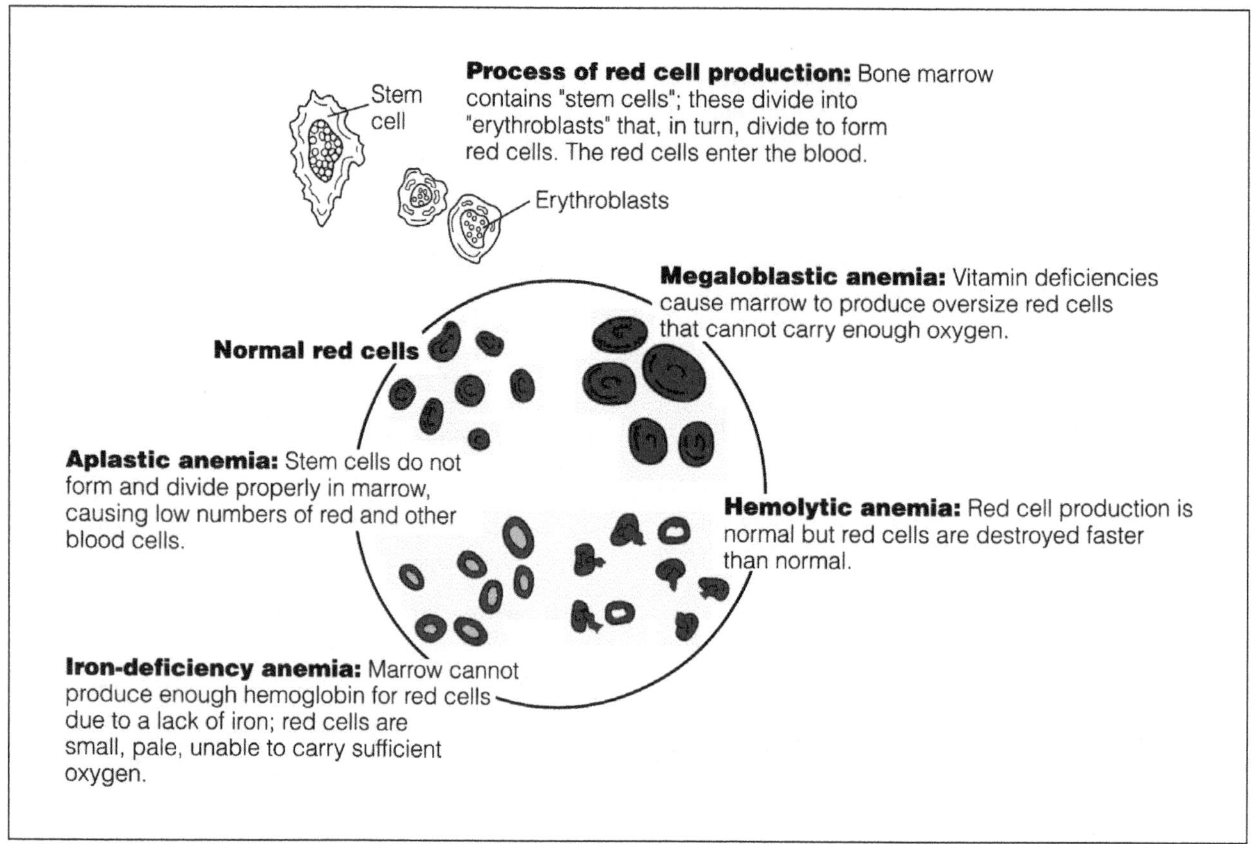

Numerous types of anemia exist.

content of the blood). In the bone marrow, erythropoietin stimulates the proliferation and differentiation of primitive cells (that is, progenitor cells) that will mature and differentiate into red blood cells. As the cells mature and differentiate, they synthesize hemoglobin, the iron-containing pigment that is responsible for carrying oxygen to all cells in the body and carrying carbon dioxide away from cells.

Incidence: It is estimated that the frequency of severe anemia, marked by a hemoglobin concentration less than 8 grams per deciliter (g/dl) across a broad range of cancers, is 5 to 20 percent, and that of mild anemia, marked by a hemoglobin concentration of 8 to 11 g/dl, is 25 to 45 percent.

Symptoms: Symptoms of anemia can include fatigue, pale skin (including nail beds and the lining of the eyelids), dizziness, chills, shortness of breath, rapid pulse, and chest pains.

Screening and diagnosis: A blood test can measure the hemoglobin concentration, or hematocrit; hemoglobin concentration is generally used, as it is more accurate than hematocrit. Other tests that are often done at the same time are red blood cell indices, which include red blood cell count, mean corpuscular volume (MCV), mean corpuscular hemoglobin concentration (MCHC), and mean corpuscular hemoglobin (MCH). Iron parameters, which include serum iron, total iron-binding capacity, percent transferrin saturation, and serum ferritin, are measured. A test for occult blood in the stool as a possible source of blood loss is often done, particularly in the setting of gastrointestinal cancers.

A normal red blood cell count is 3.5 to 5.0 × 10^{12}/liter for women and 4.3 to 5.9 × 10^{12}/liter for men. Hematocrit, the measure of the volume of red blood cells as a percentage of the total blood volume, is 37 to 47 percent for women and 45 to 57 percent for men. Normal concentration of hemoglobin is 14 to 17.5 g/dl for men and 12 to 16 g/dl for women.

Treatment and therapy: While anemia of cancer can be treated with transfusions of packed red blood cells, the standard of care at most cancer treatment centers is the use of recombinant human erythropoiesis-stimulating proteins such as epoietin alfa (Epogen or Procrit) or darbepoietin alfa (Aranesp). The recombinant human erythropoiesis-stimulating proteins are given as injections three times a week to once every three weeks depending on the patient's needs and type of recombinant protein used. The use of these recombinant proteins allows oncologists the option of not using red blood cell transfusions, with their small but inherent risks of autoimmunization and infection. The possibility of failure of bone marrow or stem cell transplantation increases with the number of previous transfusions. In cases of severe anemia, however, transfusions are routinely used because it takes several days for the erythropoiesis-stimulating proteins to increase red blood cell count and hemoglobin concentration.

Prognosis, prevention, and outcomes: The prognosis for anemia depends greatly on the type of anemia. For anemia of cancer, anemia may be directly related to prognosis and survival. Research suggests that it may be important to maintain hemoglobin concentration at a high level to decrease the effects of hypoxia, especially during treatment.

Because chemotherapy and radiation therapy target rapidly dividing cells, both cancer cells and bone marrow cells, it is difficult to prevent anemia due to treatment without reducing the efficacy of treatments. Also, the anemia of cancer involves endogenous inflammatory and immune functions, which cannot be prevented. Proper nutrition may be useful in preventing anemia caused by deficiencies in folic acid, iron, and vitamin B_{12}.

MaryAnn Foote, M.S., Ph.D.

For Further Information

Crawford, C., et al. "Relationship Between Changes in Hemoglobin Level and Quality of Life During Chemotherapy in Anemic Cancer Patients Receiving Erythropoietin Therapy." *Cancer* 95 (2002): 888-895.

Molineux, G., M. A. Foote, and S. G. Elliott, eds. *Erythropoietins and Erythropoiesis: Molecular, Cellular, Preclinical, and Clinical Biology*. Basel, Switzerland: Birkhäuser, 2003.

Other Resources

Anemia.com
http://www.anemia.com

MedlinePlus
Anemia
http://www.nlm.nih.gov/medlineplus/anemia.html

See also: Acute Lymphocytic Leukemia (ALL); Acute Myelocytic Leukemia (AML); Angiogenesis inhibitors; Antifungal therapies; Aplastic anemia; Blood cancers; Bone Marrow Transplantation (BMT); Chronic Lymphocytic Leukemia (CLL); Chronic Myeloid Leukemia (CML); Colony-Stimulating Factors (CSFs); Fanconi anemia; Hairy cell leukemia; Hematologic oncology; Hemolytic anemia; Stem cell transplantation; Thrombocytopenia; Transfusion therapy; Waldenström Macroglobulinemia (WM); Young adult cancers

▶ Angiosarcomas

Category: Diseases, Symptoms, and Conditions

Related conditions: Soft-tissue malignancy

Definition: Angiosarcomas are cancers that develop from blood vessels. Although the most common sites where they occur are the arms, legs, neck, and head, these tumors can occur anywhere on the body, most frequently on the skin or in the soft tissue. Angiosarcomas are made up of malignant cells that are rapidly proliferating and capable of extensive infiltration.

Risk factors: Some risk factors have been linked with the development of angiosarcoma. Primarily, these include previous exposure to radiation therapy or chemotherapy, as well as exposure to carcinogens such as certain polyester fibers or bone wax.

Etiology and the disease process: In many cases, angiosarcoma develops as a complication of a preexisting condition. For example, a radical mastectomy can lead to the development of an angiosarcoma in the soft tissue and skin of the breast. Additionally, foreign materials in the body, such as shrapnel, have resulted in angiosarcomas.

Incidence: Angiosarcoma is a very rare tumor type, occurring in only 2 to 3 patients out of 1 million individuals. Nearly half of all angiosarcomas develop in the head and neck regions, but they also can occur in the soft tissue of the lower and upper extremities. Least common of all angiosarcomas are those that occur in other areas of soft tissue, such as the breast, kidney, and liver.

Symptoms: Angiosarcomas in the soft tissues of the extremities may be identified as growing masses, while those that occur on the skin generally appear as blue or black nodules. Angiosarcomas that develop in other areas of soft tissue, especially within the abdominal cavity, are capable of growing quite large and often are not diagnosed until the size of the tumor begins to affect the surrounding tissues and organs.

Screening and diagnosis: Diagnosis occurs by recognizing the abnormal growths within the skin or extremities of the patient. Angiosarcomas within the abdominal cavity may remain undiagnosed until related symptoms become apparent, such as neuronal symptoms occurring from compression of the lumbar or pelvic nerves.

Treatment and therapy: Surgery and radiation therapy are common methods to treat angiosarcomas. Depending on the location, chemotherapy may also be used in combination with these other strategies. The most common chemotherapeutic agent to treat angiosarcoma is Adriamycin (doxorubicin).

Prognosis, prevention, and outcomes: Angiosarcomas are aggressive tumors that have a tendency to spread rapidly and frequently reoccur, even after treatment. The reported five-year survival rate for these patients is only 20 percent.

Lisa M. Cockrell, B.S.

See also: Accelerated Partial Breast Irradiation (APBI); Endotheliomas; Fibrosarcomas, soft-tissue; Hemangiosarcomas; Liver cancers; Lymphangiosarcomas; Sarcomas, soft-tissue; Veterinary oncology

▶ Aplastic anemia

Category: Diseases, Symptoms, and Conditions
Also known as: Bone marrow failure

Related conditions: Thrombocytopenia (low platelet count), neutropenia (low white count)

Definition: The bone marrow is responsible for producing all of the blood cells in the body. Aplastic anemia is a life-threatening condition caused when the bone marrow stops producing enough new cells to create new blood cells. The typical life span of red blood cells is 120 days, platelets about 6 days, and white blood cells about 1 day. The bone marrow needs to produce cells continuously to replace the dying cells. Aplastic anemia can be acquired or hereditary. The more common acquired aplastic anemia can be a temporary condition caused by exposure to toxic chemicals, pesticides, and benzenes. Common causes for the cancer patient are chemotherapy and radiation. Hereditary aplastic anemia is rare and can be associated with Fanconi anemia, Shwachman-Diamond syndrome, and dyskeratosis congenita.

Etiology and the disease process: Although the cause of most aplastic anemia is unknown, those cases induced by chemotherapy and radiation result from the therapy's suppression of bone marrow function. The bone marrow is not able to manufacture the cells that are needed to create red blood cells, platelets, and white blood cells.

Incidence: Aplastic anemia is a rare condition with only about 500 to 1,000 new cases each year in the United States. Of patients who are diagnosed with aplastic anemia, 20 percent have an inherited disorder as well.

Symptoms: The signs and symptoms of aplastic anemia may be seen immediately or can be slow to develop and be dependent on the blood counts themselves. Common symptoms include fatigue, dizziness, an irregular heart rate, fevers, frequent infections, frequent nose bleeds, oozing gums, blood in the stool, bruising, difficulty in stopping bleeding from a cut, and petechiae (similar to a red pinpoint rash, located on the arms, legs, and trunk). Patients may also complain of severe shortness of breath even while at rest.

Screening and diagnosis: Aplastic anemia is typically found when patients complain of fatigue to their physicians. The physical assessment includes looking for pale or yellow-tinted skin; listening to the heart, lungs, and breathing patterns; feeling the liver and spleen for enlargement; and checking for signs of bleeding. The physician may also assess the patient's environment to determine whether exposure to toxic chemicals or other triggers has occurred. Diagnostic testing includes analysis of blood, urine, and stool samples, and bone marrow aspiration and biopsy. The patient may also have images taken (X rays, computed tomography scans, and ultrasound) to look for enlarged organs. Once testing is complete, the aplastic anemia is staged according to how many cells are seen in the bone marrow. The three stages are moderate, severe, or very severe.

Treatment and therapy: The treatment for aplastic anemia depends on the severity and the patient's symptoms. The patient's overall health also determines what type of treatment can be tolerated. Moderate aplastic anemia is not treated, but the physician keeps a close eye on the blood counts and the patient's symptoms. If the aplastic anemia is caused by chemotherapy or radiation, the patient is treated with transfusions and growth factors.

Transfusions of red blood cells and platelets are the most common. Red blood cell transfusions help raise the hematocrit and hemoglobin, which improves the anemia symptoms. Epoietin alfa, a red blood cell growth factor, can be given to help the bone marrow release immature red blood cells from the bone marrow to mature and become functioning red cells.

Not all forms of aplastic anemia will respond to growth factors. Platelet transfusions will help the patient be able to form clots to stop bleeding. White blood cells are not typically transfused because of their short life span; however, they may be given to patients who have a severe infection. Patients with a low white blood cell count may receive filgrastim, a white blood cell growth factor, to stimulate the release of the immature white blood cells so that they can mature and fight off infections. Like the red cell growth factor, filgrastim may not be applicable for all forms of aplastic anemia.

Patients may receive medications such as antithymocyte globulin (ATG), cyclosporine, and methylprednisolone. Traditional therapy consists of the patient taking all three medications. It may take a few months before an improvement in blood counts is apparent. Patients may say that they are feeling better before their counts actually reflect an improvement. Antibiotics and antivirals may also be given to prevent infection.

Bone marrow transplants are more commonly used with younger patients to replace damaged bone marrow. Research is ongoing to develop additional treatments for aplastic anemia.

Prognosis, prevention, and outcomes: Historically aplastic anemia has had a poor prognosis. However, great strides have been made on the treatments available for aplastic anemia, and modern therapy has cured or managed the disease in many patients. Treatment can be effective but may take months before results are seen. Patients may also need to try different therapies to find one that works for them. Some forms of aplastic anemia can be prevented by avoiding exposure to toxins, radiation, and medication, but other forms cannot be prevented.

Katrina Green, R.N., B.S.N., O.C.N.

For Further Information

Klag, Michael J, ed. *Johns Hopkins Family Health Book.* New York: HarperCollins, 1999.

Schrezenmeier, Hubert, and Andrea Bacigalupo, eds. *Aplastic Anemia: Pathophysiology and Treatment.* New York: Cambridge University Press, 2000.

Other Resources

Aplastic Anemia & MDS International Foundation
http://www.aplastic.org

National Heart, Lung, and Blood Institute
http://www.nhlbi.nih.gov

See also: Anemia; Bone Marrow Transplantation (BMT); Fanconi anemia; Hairy cell leukemia; Hematologic oncology; Leukemias; Leukopenia; Myelodysplastic syndromes; Neutropenia; Transfusion therapy

▶ Appendix cancer

Category: Diseases, Symptoms, and Conditions
Also known as: Carcinoid tumor, colonic adenocarcinoma, mucinous cyst adenocarcinoma, signet-ring cell adenocarcinoma

Related conditions: Appendicitis, peritoneal carcinomatosis, disseminated peritoneal adenomucinosis

Definition: Appendix cancer is a cancerous tumor in the appendix, the pouchlike, thin tube with a closed end that is located in the lower right quadrant of the abdomen. The appendix, also called the vermiform appendix because its appearance is wormlike, is attached to the cecum, the first section of the large intestine, close to where it joins with the small intestine. It is not known to have a significant function in the body but may play a role in the immune system.

Cancerous tumors that originate in the appendix are part of the larger grouping of colorectal or gastrointestinal cancers. Types of appendix cancer include carcinoid tumor, mucinous cyst adenocarcinoma, colonic-type adenocarcinoma, and signet-ring cell adenocarcinoma.

Risk factors: Because appendix cancer is not common, no specific risk factors have been identified. However, risk factors for colorectal cancers in general include a diet high in red meat, lack of exercise, obesity, and cigarette smoking.

Stage at Diagnosis and Relative Survival Rates for Appendix Cancer, 1988-2001

	Survival Rates (%)		
Stage	*1-Year*	*5-Year*	*10-Year*
Stage I	97.4	89.9	83.2
Stage II	92.6	73.9	63.9
Stage III	87.2	48.3	37.0
Stage IV	65.9	25.4	16.2

Source: Data from L. A. G. Ries et al., eds., *Cancer Survival Among Adults: U.S. SEER Program, 1988-2001—Patient and Tumor Characteristics*, NIH Pub. No. 07-6215 (Bethesda, Md.: National Cancer Institute, 2007)

Etiology and the disease process: The cause of appendix cancer is unknown. It often goes undiagnosed until it causes appendicitis or the appendix ruptures. In a majority of patients, appendix tumors spread in a process called peritoneal seeding, in which multiple, initially small, tumors are produced throughout the abdominal cavity. Low-grade tumors grow more slowly and are generally less invasive, whereas high-grade tumors are faster growing and considerably more invasive.

Incidence: Cancer that starts in the appendix, or primary appendix cancer, is uncommon. Therefore, these cancers are usually included in the statistical data for colorectal cancer. and actual incidence rates are not available. One estimate is that about 1 percent of colorectal cancer cases in the United States are primary appendix cancer, with about 1,100 new cases diagnosed in 2007.

About 66 percent of appendix tumors are carcinoid tumors, 20 percent are mucinous cyst adenocarcinoma, and 10 percent are colonic-type adenocarcinoma. Signet-ring cell adenocarcinoma, which is very rare, is an aggressive cancer that is more difficult to treat than other adenocarcinomas.

Symptoms: People with appendix cancer may not experience symptoms until the disease is far advanced. The first reported symptoms are typically those of appendicitis, which include fever, pain in the lower right quadrant of the abdomen, nausea, and vomiting. Other symptoms may include bowel changes, abdominal bloating, pelvic pain, infertility, and an increase in waistline size, with possible navel protrusion. Some people experience no symptoms at all, and the cancer is found incidentally during surgery for another condition such as ovarian tumors.

Screening and diagnosis: There are no screening tests for appendix cancer. Most often it is found during surgery for another abdominal condition, either when a biopsy is performed on the tissue that has been removed or when the surgeon observes abnormalities or tumors in the abdomen. Computed tomography scanning, magnetic resonance imaging, and ultrasound can be performed if appendix cancer is suspected or to determine the extent of the cancer's spread. Radionuclide scanning is performed to determine the spread of a carcinoid tumor.

No standard staging system exists for appendix cancer. Instead, appendix tumors are usually classified by whether the cancer is confined to the appendix or has spread and how far: to distant organs or only to nearby tissues.

Treatment and therapy: The treatment of appendix cancer depends on the type of tumor, its size, and whether the cancer has spread. Surgery to remove the tumor along with nearby blood vessels, lymph nodes, and part of the large bowel is the most common treatment for tumors that are low grade and slow growing. Currently, the most effective treatment for higher-grade, more aggressive tumors and tumors that have seeded the abdomen is a procedure called cytoreductive or debulking surgery. During this procedure, the surgeon removes as much of the cancer in the abdomen as possible. When complete, it means that all visible tumors were removed; when incomplete, it means that some tumors could not be removed. This surgery is typically combined with intraoperative hyperthermic intraperitoneal chemotherapy; a high concentration of a chemotherapy solution is instilled in the abdomen during surgery. The solution, heated to just above normal body temperature, has been found to be effective because it destroys cancer cells and tumors that are too small to be seen and also because it can reach all surfaces in the abdomen. Postoperative intraperitoneal chemotherapy is also used in some cases.

Prognosis, prevention, and outcomes: The prognosis for appendix cancer varies greatly and depends on several factors, including the type of tumor, whether it has spread, and how it is treated. Complete cytoreductive surgery combined with intraoperative hyperthermic intraperitoneal chemotherapy has been found to be effective in increasing survival rates, especially with mucinous cyst adenocarcinoma. Appendix cancer has no known method of prevention.

Dorothy P. Terry, R.N.

For Further Information

Carmignani, C. P., and P. H. Sugarbaker. "Synchronous Extraperitoneal and Intraperitoneal Dissemination of Appendix Cancer." *European Journal of Surgical Oncology* 30, no. 8 (October, 2004): 864-868.

Holland, Jimmie C., and Sheldon Lewis. *The Human Side of Cancer*. New York: HarperCollins, 2000.

Sugarbaker, Paul H. "New Standard of Care for Appendiceal Epithelial Neoplasms and Pseudomyxoma Peritonei Syndrome?" *Lancet Oncology* 7, no. 1 (January, 2006): 69-76.

Other Resources

American Cancer Society
http://www.cancer.org

Appendix Cancer (Appendiceal Carcinoma) & Peritoneal Surface Malignancy
http://www.appendix-cancer.com

Cancer.Net
http://www.cancer.net/portal/site/patient

See also: Carcinoid tumors and carcinoid syndrome; Continuous Hyperthermic Peritoneal Perfusion (CHPP); Small intestine cancer; Stomach cancers

▶ Appetite loss

Category: Diseases, Symptoms, and Conditions
Also known as: Anorexia

Related conditions: Cachexia

Definition: Loss of appetite in cancer patients, referred to by medical professionals as anorexia, may result from either the cancer itself or the treatments used to combat the disease. Cancer-related anorexia is associated with weight loss and has been shown to correlate with a poorer outcome and a lower quality of life.

Risk factors: Those with cancer and undergoing chemotherapy for cancer are at risk.

Etiology and the disease process: Because many cancer treatments affect not only cancer cells but also healthy cells, several unwanted side effects may result. For instance, chemotherapy may reduce the turnover of taste receptor cells in the tongue, which may alter the flavor of food. Additional damage to other cell types in the mouth may result in sores, gum disease, dry mouth, and sore throat. Cells in the digestive tract may also be injured, resulting in abnormal gut motility and difficulty swallowing. Together, these effects may change the way food tastes and decrease the desire to eat.

Emotional side effects, such as fear and depression, as well as psychological effects, such as food aversion, can also contribute to the loss of appetite. Furthermore, many cancer patients with anorexia report early satiety, meaning that they feel full after eating only a small amount of food.

Biological causes for cancer-related anorexia also exist. Cytokines released by tumor cells or produced by immune cells in response to cancer may affect the central nervous system and the gastrointestinal tract to promote appetite loss. Specifically, the central nervous system is responsible for controlling food intake and energy homeostasis, while effects on the gastrointestinal tract can influence feelings of fullness. Examples of cytokines that may affect appetite include tumor necrosis factor-alpha (TNF-α), C-reactive protein, interleukin-1 beta (IL-1 beta), IL-6, and tumor-derived lipid mobilizing factor (LMF). However, there is some conflicting data as to whether blood levels of these cytokines correlate with, or are responsible for, the loss of appetite.

Incidence: In general, approximately 25 percent of cancer patients report loss of appetite. The incidence can be as high as 90 percent for patients with advanced cancers. However, different types of cancers tend to have different rates of anorexia. For example, approximately 60 to 80 percent of patients with cancers of the lung, stomach, pancreas, or esophagus have significant weight loss caused, in part, by anorexia. However, loss of appetite is not as frequent in patients with breast or prostate cancer.

Treatment and therapy: Cancer-related anorexia may be managed by either changing eating habits or taking medication. There are several dietary suggestions for cancer patients who struggle with loss of appetite. Liquid or powdered meal replacements as well as juice, soups, and milk-based drinks or shakes may be used in place of solid food to provide nutrients. Eating several small meals or snacks instead of three large meals per day may also be more feasible for patients with cancer-related anorexia. Additionally, drinking a glass of wine or exercising regularly may also stimulate the appetite. However, patients should consult with their doctors before consuming alcohol or beginning an exercise regimen.

The pharmacological treatment of cancer-related anorexia can be broadly divided into three groups: appetite stimulants, anticatabolic agents, and anabolic agents.

Examples of appetite stimulants include progestational agents (such as megestrol acetate and medroxyprogesterone), which can improve caloric intake. Corticosteroids (such as prednisolone and methylprednisolone) may improve appetite because of their inhibition of prostaglandin metabolism and IL-1 signaling. Cyproheptadine, an antihistamine, is also a serotonin antagonist, and its effects on this neurotransmitter in the brain can also promote an increase in appetite. A more controversial appetite stimulant is cannabis (marijuana), as it can stimulate CB1 receptors in the brain to enhance appetite.

Anticatabolic agents, which inhibit the production or activity of appetite-decreasing cytokines, are also important in combating cancer-related anorexia. Examples include thalidomide (a potent inhibitor of TNF-α production) and eicosapentaenoic acid (an inhibitor of adenylate cyclase activity and tumor-derived LMF activity).

Anabolic agents such as oxandrolone and fluoxymesterone have been studied as well, and they may build lean tissue mass by increasing muscle protein synthesis. The hormone androgen may also be useful in cancer patients (except for those with hormone-dependent tumors) as it can promote muscle growth and strength and may also induce the secretion of leptin, a hormone produced by adipose tissue to stimulate appetite.

Prognosis, prevention, and outcomes: Generally appetite loss resolves itself when its underlying cause is remedied. Although appetite loss can interfere with the healing process, it does not usually cause death in patients with early-stage cancers. However, cancer-related anorexia is often associated with cachexia, a wasting syndrome characterized by not only the loss of appetite but also weight loss, breakdown of muscle tissues, depletion of reserves within fat (adipose) tissue, fatigue, and weakness. In advanced-stage cancer, the cancer anorexia-cachexia syndrome is observed in about 80 percent of patients and is one of the most frequent causes of death.

Elizabeth A. Manning, Ph.D.

For Further Information

Behl, D., and A. Jatoi. "Pharmacological Options for Advanced Cancer Patients with Loss of Appetite and Weight." *Expert Opinion on Pharmacotherapy* 8, no. 8 (June, 2007): 1085-1090.

Perboni, S., and A. Inui. "Anorexia in Cancer: Role of Feeding-Regulatory Peptides." *Philosophical Transactions of the Royal Society B: Biolocial Sciences* 361, no. 1471 (July 29, 2006): 1281-1289.

Poole, K., and K. Froggatt. "Loss of Weight and Loss of Appetite in Advanced Cancer: A Problem for the Patient, the Carer, or the Health Professional?" *Palliative Medicine* 16, no. 6 (November, 2002): 499-506.

Rubin, H. "Cancer Cachexia: Its Correlations and Causes." *Proceedings of the National Academy of Sciences of the United States of America* 100, no. 9 (April 29, 2003): 5384-5389.

Other Resources

Cancer.Net
Appetite Loss
http://www.ascocancerfoundation.org/patient/Diagnosis+and+Treatment/Treating+Cancer/Managing+Side+Effects/Appetite+Loss

National Cancer Institute
Eating Hints for Cancer Patients: Before, During, and After Treatment
http://cancer.gov/cancertopics/eatinghints/page3

See also: Antidiarrheal agents; Cachexia; End-of-life care; Gastrointestinal cancers; Gerson therapy; Living with cancer; Medical marijuana; Pain management medications; Palliative treatment; Side effects; Taste alteration; Weight loss

▶ Ascites

Category: Diseases, Symptoms, and Conditions
Also known as: Peritoneal cavity fluid or peritoneal fluid excess, hydroperitoneum, abdominal dropsy, peritoneal carcinomatosis, malignant ascites

Related conditions: Late-stage cancer or liver disease, associated with ovarian, endometrial, breast, gastrointestinal (stomach, colon, pancreatic) cancer

Definition: Ascites is an abnormal accumulation of excess fluid in the abdominal (peritoneal) cavity that causes swelling or bloating. In late-stage cancer, tumor cells may be isolated from the fluid. Ascites can also occur with liver disease.

Risk factors: Ascites is not uncommon in cancer patients; 15 to 50 percent develop this condition at some time during their illness. Ascites is most common in patients with ovarian cancer but may also be present in patients with uterine, breast, colon, stomach, and pancreatic cancers. Liver involvement with cancer can increase the problem with ascites. Noncancerous conditions that can result in ascites include hepatitis, kidney failure, heart failure, and constrictive pericarditis (inflammation of the sac around the heart).

Etiology and the disease process: A lining of tissue, the peritoneum, supports the organs in the abdomen and covers the peritoneal cavity. Normally a small amount of body fluid lubricates this cavity and is kept in correct proportion by a pressure gradient. The liver stores blood and fluid depending on the pressure in the venous and arterial blood system. Under normal conditions, the lymphatic system drains 80 percent of the peritoneal fluid, so minimal accumulation occurs. When pathological or disease conditions occur, the fluid accumulates and edema settles in the peritoneal cavity.

In malignant ascites, a tumor may obstruct the lymphatic system so that drainage cannot occur. Liver involvement can cause a backup of fluid into the peritoneal cavity. In severe cases of ascites, gallons of liquid can fill the peritoneal cavity, pressing on the diaphragm (the muscles that separate the chest from the abdomen and allow a person to breathe).

Ascites is not actually a disease but a symptom of some pathological condition within the body. Some of the conditions that can result in ascites include cirrhosis of the liver (80 percent of ascites cases), pancreatic ascites, chylous ascites (a symptom of lymphoma), and cancer. Renal and endocrine ascites occur in rare instances.

Incidence: Approximately 10 percent of all cases of ascites occur in cancer patients. As many as half of all cancer patients will experience ascites. About 30 percent of all ovarian cancer patients have ascites, with as many as 60 percent presenting with ascites at death. Most cases result from disease that starts in the peritoneum or spreads from other body organs (metastasis).

Symptoms: Mild ascites may not be noticeable or present any symptoms. As the disease progresses, the abdomen can become more distended and swollen to the point of discomfort and pain. The patient may experience a feeling of heaviness. The patient may have trouble sitting, walking, or moving around. Fluid buildup may cause indigestion, nausea, or vomiting. The patient may experience diminished appetite with weight loss and general fatigue. When the fluid becomes excessive, the patient may have weight gain and shortness of breath. Some patients complain of swelling in the legs and ankles or experience hemorrhoids. Changes may occur in the navel as fluid collects. The severity of symptoms depends on the progression of the disease.

Screening and diagnosis: Diagnosis is confirmed using a physical exam and patient history along with X rays, ultrasound, computed tomography, or paracentesis with fluid analysis (removing fluid through a thin needle into the abdomen). Simple measuring of abdominal girth can provide a baseline for continued assessment.

Treatment and therapy: Treatment is targeted to the symptoms and to improve quality of life. One approach is to reduce sodium and fluid intake to decrease fluid buildup. Another is the use of diuretic drugs that promote removal of fluid through the kidneys as urination. Caution must be taken in the use of diuretics as the patient may experience hypovolemia (a drop in circulating blood volume through large loss of blood or fluid) with a severe drop in blood pressure or a potassium imbalance that can threaten the regular beat of the heart.

If discomfort is severe, a therapeutic paracentesis can be performed by the health care provider. This procedure drains fluid from the abdomen through a thin needle inserted into the peritoneal cavity. This procedure is generally performed with a local anesthesia. Rarely, surgery to shunt the fluid away from the abdominal cavity (peritoneovenous shunt) or specific chemotherapy may help. Repeated paracentesis as can be tolerated by the patient may be the only effective approach long term.

Few alternative or complementary approaches are effective for ascites. Diet can be modified to minimize sodium intake. The patient should consume potassium-rich foods such as low-fat yogurt, cantaloupe, or baked potatoes to assist with proper heart function.

Prognosis, prevention, and outcomes: The prognosis for ascites depends on the underlying cause and intensity of the problem. Generally, unless the cause is corrected, the fluid will return after draining with paracentesis. In fact, rapid reduction through the draining of fluid can result in rapid reaccumulation of fluid. Removing more than five liters at one time can result in hypotension, shock, and death.

Robert W. Koch, D.N.S., R.N.

For Further Information

Ginès, Pere, et al., eds. *Ascites and Renal Dysfunction in Liver Disease: Pathogenesis, Diagnosis, and Treatment.* 2d ed. Malden, Mass.: Blackwell Publishing, 2005.

Hawkins, Rebecca. "Clinical Focus: Ascites." *Clinical Journal of Oncology Nursing* 5, no. 1 (January/February, 2001).

Other Resources

Cancer.Net

Fluid in the Abdomen or Ascites

http://www.cancer.net/patient/Diagnosis+and+Treatment/Treating+Cancer/Managing+Side+Effects/Fluid+in+the+Abdomen+or+Ascites+-+ASCO+curriculum#mainContent idmainContent

MedlinePlus

Ascites

http://www.nlm.nih.gov/medlineplus/ency/article/000286.htm

See also: Cytology; Gallbladder cancer; Gastrointestinal cancers; Hepatomegaly; Krukenberg tumors; Mesothelioma; Paracentesis; Peritoneovenous shunts; Ultrasound tests

▶ Astrocytomas

Category: Diseases, Symptoms, and Conditions
Also known as: Gliomas

Related conditions: Primary brain tumors

Definition: Astrocytomas, the most common gliomas, are primary malignant brain tumors that can occur in most parts of the brain and occasionally in the spinal cord. As the name implies, astrocytomas are derived from astrocytes—nonneural support cells of the central nervous system. The types of astrocytomas based on clinical pathology include pilocytic astrocytoma, fibrillary astrocytoma, anaplastic astrocytoma, and glioblastoma multiforme. Because astrocytomas are primary brain tumors formed in the brain, they rarely spread to other parts of the body; however, they usually grow rapidly and invade surrounding normal brain tissue and therefore are life-threatening.

Risk factors: Brain tumors are caused by mutated or missing genes that result in abnormal cells. High-dose ionizing radiation used over time to treat brain tumors may on occasion cause secondary tumors. Exposure to certain chemicals such as pesticides, petrochemicals, and formaldehyde, and to electromagnetic fields over time increase the risk of developing astrocytomas.

Etiology and the disease process: Generally, malignant brain tumors are caused by changes in genetic structure due to inherited or environmental factors. It was thought that only 5 percent of primary brain tumors, including astrocytomas, are inherited; however, one study has shown that 80 percent of patients with grade IV astrocytoma (glioblastoma multiforme) had anomalous copies of chromosome 7. Familial clustering of gliomas is also associated with defined inherited tumor syndrome, including Li-Fraumeni syndrome, Turcot syndrome, and the neurofibromatosis I syndrome.

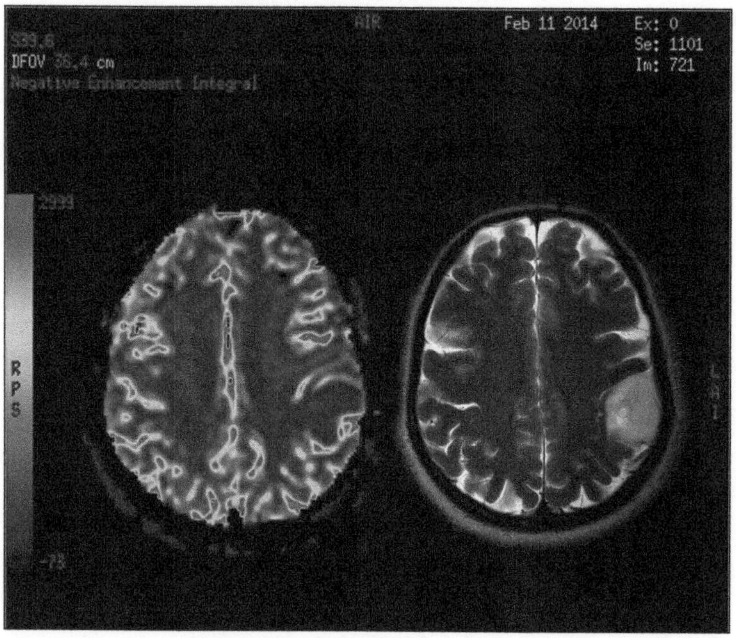

Incidence: Gliomas of both benign and malignant tumors account for 45 to 50 percent of all primary brain tumors; grade I and II astrocytomas account for 25 to 30 percent of all gliomas. Approximately 13,000 people in the United States die of malignant brain tumors every year, which represents about 2 percent of all cancer-related deaths.

Symptoms: Various symptoms may occur with astrocytomas, which depend largely on the location and size of the tumor. Seizure, focal neurologic deficits such as weakness or speech problems, and headaches are common symptoms. The headaches that are associated with brain tumors are typically worse in the morning and accompanied by vomiting. Sometimes increased pressure on the brain tissue can cause blurred, double, or even loss of vision. Behavioral changes may also follow with changes in mood and general state of well-being.

MRI scan of a brain tumor. (iStock)

Relative Survival Rates for Astrocytomas, 1988-2001

Years	*Survival Rate (%)*
1	62.3
2	48.4
3	42.7
5	35.8
8	30.7
10	27.8

Source: Data from L. A. G. Ries et al., eds., *Cancer Survival Among Adults: U.S. SEER Program, 1988-2001—Patient and Tumor Characteristics,* NIH Pub. No. 07-6215 (Bethesda, Md.: National Cancer Institute, 2007)

Screening and diagnosis: Methods of screening and diagnosing astrocytomas include computed tomography (CT) scans, magnetic resonance imaging (MRI), angiograms, X rays of the head and skull, and biopsies. Other brain scans, such as magnetic resonance spectroscopy (MRS), single-photon emission computed tomography (SPECT), or positron emission tomography (PET), provide a gauge of brain activity and blood flow. Brain tumors are graded based on the following criteria: mitotic index (growth rate), vascularity (blood supply), presence of necrotic center, invasive potential (border distinctness), and similarity to normal cells.

Accordingly, astrocytomas can be graded into four levels. Pilocytic astrocytoma are grade I tumors that are slow growing and do not invade the surrounding normal tissue, and are commonly diagnosed in children and young adults. Low-grade astrocytomas, including fibrillary or protoplasmic astrocytomas, are grade II tumors that grow slightly faster than grade I tumors and are invasive, with high incidence in the cerebrums of young adults and in the brain stems of children. Anaplastic astrocytomas are grade III, malignant and invasive tumors that occur in the same location as the low-grade astrocytomas and have a high recurrence rate. Glioblastomas multiforme are grade IV, a malignant type that is by far the most common glioma: Approximately 50 percent of astrocytomas are glioblastomas. The common sites of tumors are cerebral hemispheres in adults and the brain stem in children, and they typically contain more than one cell type.

Treatment and therapy: Treatment options differ according to size, grade, and location of the tumor. Tumors may be removed by craniotomy, an open-skull procedure. They may also be removed by ultrasonic aspiration, in which ultrasonic waves fragment the tumors, which are then aspirated. Alternatively, stereotactic radiosurgery may be performed with a Gamma Knife on benign, malignant, or metastatic tumors that are around 4 centimeters (cm) in size. Chemotherapy may be used as a primary therapy in young children or as an adjuvant after tumor removal with radiosurgery. For pilocytic and fibrillary astrocytomas, complete resection of the tumor is achieved; however, if excision is not possible because of the tumor's location, chemotherapy is indicated in young children and radiotherapy in adults. The treatment options for anaplastic astrocytoma and glioblastoma multiforme include total resection followed by radiotherapy and chemotherapy after surgery.

Prognosis, prevention, and outcomes: The prognosis and outcome of astrocytomas largely depend on the age of the patient, histological features of the tumor, and degree of neurologic or functional impairment. In low-grade astrocytomas, the mean survival time after surgery is six to eight years with the prognosis depending on whether the tumor undergoes progression to a malignant phenotype. Complete recovery is possible in pilocytic astrocytoma if total resection is achieved, while fibrillary astrocytomas show frequent recurrence. In patients with anaplastic astrocytomas and glioblastoma multiforme, the extent of resection is a prognostic factor; generally, younger patients below the age of forty-five have a better prognosis.

Bagirathy Ravishankar, Ph.D.

For Further Information

Arjona, D., et al. "Early Genetic Changes Involved in Low-Grade Astrocytic Tumor Development." *Current Molecular Medicine* 6 (September, 2006): 645-650.

Compostella, A., et al. "Prognostic Factors for Anaplastic Astrocytomas." *Journal of Neuro-Oncology* 81 (February, 2007): 295-303.

Miller, C. R., and A. Perry. "Glioblastoma." *Archives of Pathology and Laboratory Medicine* 131 (March, 2007): 397-406.

Robins, H. Ian, et al. "Therapeutic Advances for Glioblastoma Multiforme: Current Status and Future Prospects." *Current Oncology Reports* 9, no. 1 (2007): 66-70.

Szeifert, G., et al. "The Role of the Gamma Knife in the Management of Cerebral Astrocytomas." *Progress in Neurological Surgery* 20 (2007): 150-163.

Other Resources

Mayo Clinic
Gliomas
http://www.mayoclinic.org/glioma/astrocytomas.html

Neurosurgery Today
Astrocytoma Tumors
http://www.neurosurgerytoday.org/what/patient_e/tumors.asp

See also: Brain and central nervous system cancers; Cell phones; Craniotomy; Gamma Knife; Gliomas; Oligodendrogliomas; Spinal axis tumors

▶ Ataxia Telangiectasia (AT)

Category: Diseases, Symptoms, and Conditions
Also known as: A-T, Louis-Bar syndrome, Boder-Sedgwick syndrome

Related conditions: Nijmegen breakage syndrome

Definition: Ataxia telangiectasia (AT) is a rare primary immunodeficiency disease that causes ataxia (Greek for "lack of order"), or uncoordinated movements. Ataxia is caused by dysfunction of the central nervous system; in particular, the neural circuits that help coordinate movement. Telangiectasias are small, red spider veins caused by dilation of blood vessels. In AT these appear in the eyes, cheeks, and other skin surfaces.

Risk factors: AT is caused by mutations in the ATM gene (ataxia telangiectasia, mutated) located on chromosome 11q22-23, which codes for a 370kDa protein kinase. The ATM gene is 150kb with 66 exons. Individuals heterozygous for a mutated ATM gene have a two to three times increase risk of developing breast cancer and have an increase in radiation sensitivity.

Etiology and the disease process: The ATM protein kinase responds to double-stranded deoxyribonucleic acid (DNA) breaks by attaching phosphate groups to itself (a process known as "autophosphorylation"). ATM autophosphorylation converts this protein to its active form. This active ATM kinase is involved in the assembly of a multiprotein complex that helps the cell respond to DNA damage. ATM is also involved in triggering the accumulation of the tumor-suppressor protein p53, a master control switch to prevent cells from dividing. If the ATM protein is lacking, there is a delay in the accumulation of p53, so the cell continues to divide without DNA repair and increases the chances of mutations leading to cancer. Children with a mutated ATM gene generally have a poor prognosis with ataxia occurring around one year of age and progressive cerebellar atrophy beginning by age two.

The abnormal DNA repair due to mutations in the ATM gene does not explain the changes in non-dividing neurons. ATM may have a role in antioxidative defense, mitochondrial homeostasis, and DNA chromatin packing. The ATM gene codes for a sensor for reactive oxygen species which leads to the removal of nonfunctioning organelles.

Incidence: AT is a rare recessive genetic disease with an incidence of 1 in 40,000 to 1 in 100,000 live births.

Symptoms: There are several AT symptoms including 1) neurodegeneration, which causes uncoordinated movements; 2) immunodeficiency, such as a lack or reduced level of immunoglobulin A (IgA), immunoglobulin E (IgE), and immunoglobulin G2 (IgG2); 3) extreme sensitivity to ionizing radiation; and 4) an increased risk of cancer. Telangiectasias are not always present. Those with AT have frequent sinus and respiratory infections and can have recurring severe lung infections. The neurological problems result in delayed development of motor skills and poor balance, which are typically noted by two years of age. As the neurological degeneration continues, with progressive loss of muscle control, patients usually require a wheelchair for mobility in their teenage years. Slurred speech is generally present by age ten. AT patients also may have mild diabetes mellitus, premature gray hair, difficulty swallowing, and delayed physical and sexual development. Their intelligence quotient (IQ) is normal. People with AT have an increased risk of developing cancer, especially leukemia and lymphoma. Other cancers are also associated with AT, such as stomach, brain, ovary, skin, liver, larynx, and breast.

Screening and diagnosis: Ataxia, uncoordinated movements, is typically the symptom noted first. Telangiectasia may or may not be observed. Lab tests show a low lymphocyte count, especially of T and B lymphocytes. A screen of serum immunoglobulins may show low levels of IgA, IgG2, immunoglobulin G4 (IgG4), and IgE. Magnetic resonance imaging (MRI) and computed tomography (CT) scans may show cerebellar atrophy. AT patients also have elevated levels of alpha-fetoprotein and carcinoembryonic antigen in their sera. The size of the thymus may be examined by X-rays. A molecular diagnosis of AT includes sequencing of the ATM gene or examining closely linked markers if there is a family history of the disease. Also, a test of protein function or a cytogenetic test to look for specific breakpoints can be done.

Treatment and therapy: There is no specific treatment for AT; rather the specific symptoms are treated. Antibiotics are given to control infections and Gamma-globulin injections to help the dysfunctional immune system. Physical, occupational, and speech therapy can also be beneficial. Because of the sensitivity to ionizing radiation, AT patients with cancer should not receive radiation therapy or have unnecessary X rays for screening tests.

Prognosis, prevention, and outcomes: There is no cure for AT. Life expectancy varies, but often those with AT die in their twenties, although some live to their forties. Almost half of AT deaths are due to lung infections. If frequent infections can be controlled, then about 20 percent of those with AT die from cancer. About 28 percent of AT deaths are due to both pulmonary infections and malignancies. The parents of an AT child can have molecular diagnoses to assess their risk of having another child with AT. If both parents are carriers of a mutated ATM gene, there is a 25 percent risk of having a child with AT. Parents can have prenatal testing done to determine if the fetus has AT. Those who are carriers of a mutant ATM gene may be at a greater risk of developing cancers, especially leukemia and lymphoma, so more frequent cancer screenings may be beneficial to carriers. There is also evidence that ATM mutations are breast cancer susceptibility alleles. AT is a rare disease, but the study of the ATM gene has led to a better understanding of how the cell responds to double-stranded DNA damage.

Susan J. Karcher, PhD

For Further Information

Ahmed, M., & Rahman, N. (2006). ATM and breast cancer susceptibility. *Oncogene,* 25: 5906-5911.

Lavin, M. F., & Kozlov, S. (2007). ATM activation and DNA damage response. *Cell Cycle,* 6(8): 931-942.

Lee, Y., & McKinnon, P. J. (2007). Responding to DNA double-strand breaks in the nervous system. *Neuroscience,* 145: 1365-1374.

Lohmann, E., Krüger, S., Hauser, A-K., Hanagasi, H., Guven, G., Erginel-Unaltuna, N. … Gasser, T. (2015). Clinical variability in ataxia telangiectasia. *Journal of Neurology,* 262(7): 1724-1727.

Niida, H., & Nakanishi, M. (2006). DNA damage checkpoints in mammals. *Mutagenesis,* 21: 3-9.

Nissenkorn, A., & Ben-Zeev, B. (2015). Ataxia telangiectasia. *Handbook of Clinical Neurology,* 132: 199–214.

Perlman, S. L., Boder, E., Sedgewick, R. P. & Gatti, R. A. (2012). Ataxia–telangiectasia. *Handbook of Clinical Neurology,* 103: 307–332.

Shiloh, Y. (2006). The ATM-mediated DNA-damage response: Taking shape. *Trends in Biochemical Sciences,* 31: 402-410.

Other Resources

National Cancer Institute

Ataxia Telangiectasia: Fact Sheet.
http://www.cancer.gov/about-cancer/causes-prevention/genetics/ataxia-fact-sheet

National Institute of Neurological Disorders and Stroke

Ataxia Telangiectasia Information Page.
http://www.ninds.nih.gov/disorders/a_t/a-t.htm

See also: Family history and risk assessment; Genetic testing; Nijmegen breakage syndrome

▶ Barrett esophagus

Category: Diseases, Symptoms, and Conditions

Also known as: Barrett's esophagus, Barrett's metaplasia, Barrett's mucosa, Barrett's syndrome, columnar epithelium lined lower oesophagus (CELLO), columnar-lined esophagus

Related conditions: Esophageal adenocarcinoma, gastroesophageal reflux disease (GERD), hiatal hernia

Definition: Barrett esophagus is a condition in which some of the cells lining the esophagus (tube that carries food to the stomach) are replaced with a different type of cell similar to those lining the intestines, a process called intestinal metaplasia. Rarely, these cells develop into cancer of the esophagus (esophageal adenocarcinoma). This condition is named after Norman Barrett, who first described it in 1957.

Risk factors: Developing Barrett esophagus is linked to chronic heartburn and another common condition called gastroesophageal reflux disease (GERD). However, the chances of heartburn or GERD developing into Barrett esophagus are very small. Sometimes people who develop GERD have a part of the stomach that bulges through the diaphragm (hiatal hernia). This kind of hernia may trap acid in the esophagus and cause more damage, eventually leading to GERD and progressing into Barrett esophagus.

Etiology and the disease process: Normally, a round muscle (sphincter) near the bottom of the esophagus keeps stomach acid from washing back up into the esophagus. In people with GERD, some of the acid of the stomach leaks into the esophagus, possibly because of a weakness in the sphincter. In about 10 to 15 percent of these people, the acid changes the color and makeup of the cells lining the esophagus. These cells are much like cells in the intestines; they are darker than the normal esophagus tissue and more resistant to stomach acid. Rarely, Barrett esophagus cells develop into a precancerous state called dysplasia. Dysplasia, in some cases, then develops into esophageal cancer.

Incidence: About 700,000 adults in the United States have Barrett esophagus. It is very uncommon in children; the average age of diagnosis is sixty. It is twice as common in men as in women. Caucasians and Hispanics are more likely to develop this condition than those of other ethnic backgrounds.

Symptoms: Symptoms include chronic heartburn, chronic acid reflux, trouble swallowing or a feeling that something is stuck in the throat, weight loss, spitting up food, excessive burping, hoarseness, sore throat, and bleeding. Sometimes people with chronic heartburn will get some relief from their symptoms when they develop Barrett esophagus. The intestinal metaplasia may help protect the esophagus from the stomach acid because those cells are normally found in the intestines and are better able to withstand stomach acid.

Screening and diagnosis: Adults over the age of forty who have had chronic heartburn or acid reflux may be screened with an endoscopy to see whether they have Barrett esophagus. However, screening for this disease is not commonly recommended as an endoscopy is expensive and the rate of discovering the condition is very low. People who have no symptoms should not have an endoscopy just to see if they have this condition. Barrett esophagus can be diagnosed only by performing a biopsy on suspected tissue. There is no staging for Barrett esophagus.

Treatment and therapy: Treatment for Barrett esophagus involves avoiding further damage. Therapies that keep the acid in the stomach from moving up into the esophagus may include antacid-type medications or other medications that stop stomach acid production. Lifestyle changes, such as losing weight, stopping smoking, and avoiding certain foods, also help. Other ways to keep the acid in the stomach include eating smaller meals more often, wearing loose-fitting clothing, waiting two to three hours after eating before lying down, and elevating the head of the bed 8 to 10 inches. A type of surgery that reinforces the sphincter that keeps acid in the stomach may also help.

There is no cure for Barrett esophagus other than surgically removing the esophagus. This type of surgery is only performed on those who have already developed esophageal adenocarcinoma or are at very high risk for developing it. With this surgery, the affected part of the esophagus is removed, and the stomach is brought up and attached to the nonaffected part of the esophagus.

Possible treatments for removing Barrett esophagus cells are being investigated. These include various ways of destroying those cells with lasers or chemicals. However, removing the cells has not yet been proven to reduce the risk of Barrett esophagus recurring or developing into esophageal cancer. Removing the Barrett esophagus cells is usually recommended only when a patient has highly developed precancerous or already cancerous cells.

Prognosis, prevention, and outcomes: Barrett esophagus may not cause any problems or symptoms in those who have it. It is only significant because it is a precursor to esophageal adenocarcinoma, but even those who have Barrett esophagus have a less than 1 percent chance of developing this type of cancer. Those who have been diagnosed with Barrett esophagus should be screened regularly, every one to three years, to ensure that the cells are not developing into cancer.

Some ways of attempting to prevent further damage to the esophagus are to eat a diet low in fat and high in fruits, vegetables, and fiber. Avoiding smoking and maintaining a healthy weight may also help.

Marianne M. Madsen, M.S.

For Further Information

Parker, James, and Philip M. Parker, eds. *The Official Patient's Sourcebook on Barrett's Esophagus: A Revised and Updated Directory for the Internet Age*. San Diego, Calif.: Icon Health, 2004.

Shalauta, Saad R. "Barrett's Esophagus." *American Family Physician* 69, no. 9 (May 1, 2004): 2113-2118.

Sharma, Prateek, and Richard E. Sampliner, eds. *Barrett's Esophagus and Esophageal Adenocarcinoma*. 2d ed. Malden, Mass.: Blackwell, 2006.

Other Resources

Barrett's Oesophagus Foundation
http://www.barrettsfoundation.org.uk

MedicineNet.com
Barrett's Esophagus
http://www.medicinenet.com/barretts_esophagus/article.htm

National Digestive Diseases Information Clearinghouse
Barrett's Esophagus
http://digestive.niddk.nih.gov/ddiseases/pubs/barretts

See also: Esophageal cancer; Esophagectomy; Esophagitis; Histamine 2 antagonists; Premalignancies; Upper Gastrointestinal (GI) endoscopy

▶ Basal cell carcinomas

Category: Diseases, Symptoms, and Conditions
Also known as: Basal cell cancer, BCC

Related conditions: Basal cell epitheliomas

Definition: Basal cell carcinoma is a cancer in which the cancerous cells resemble the basal cells of the epidermis, the outer layer of the skin. It is the most common type of skin cancer.

Risk factors: Exposure to ultraviolet light is the primary risk factor. People with light skin and eyes are more susceptible because they have less melanin, the pigment that colors skin and blocks the sun's radiation. People who are exposed to more ultraviolet light because they work outdoors or use tanning booths are also at greater risk. Children are particularly susceptible to skin damage from the sun because they burn more readily. Arsenic exposure, usually from contaminated drinking water, is another risk factor.

Etiology and the disease process: Basal cell carcinomas are thought to begin in the upper part of the skin, the epidermis, or in a hair follicle. The basal cell layer forms the base of the epidermis. Basal cells continually divide to form new cells of skin, hair, or glands. They become cancerous when something disrupts their deoxyribonucleic acid (DNA) instructions for making normal new cells. The most common cause is ultraviolet radiation, probably UVB. These rays can hit the nuclei of skin cells and damage chromosomes or DNA. The body repairs most of the damage to chromosomes, but cells that are not repaired can begin to divide wildly and become cancer cells, which destroy surrounding cells or tissues. Basal cell carcinomas are slow growing and rarely spread to other parts of the body. If left untreated, however, they can do extensive damage to surrounding tissue.

Incidence: Basal cell carcinoma is the most common skin cancer in the United States, making up about 75 percent of skin cancers. Nearly a million new cases are reported each year, and about 90 percent of those are attributed to solar radiation, although some cases occur in skin rarely exposed to the sun. Men are at higher risk than women, probably because they have, in the past, worked outdoors more. Basal cell carcinoma is more common in adults than in children, and the elderly are the most likely candidates, as these cancers can take twenty to fifty years to manifest after radiation exposure.

Symptoms: The most common symptom of basal cell carcinoma is a skin lesion, which is a superficial growth or a sore that does not heal. There are many types of basal cell carcinoma and nearly as many types of lesions. Lesion size varies from a few millimeters to several centimeters, and some lesions are larger than they appear on the skin because they invade underlying tissues. The lesions are usually painless, though the surrounding skin can become irritated and tender. Some lesions are flat, reddish or crusty patches that can be mistaken for psoriasis or eczema. The color and appearance of lesions varies widely, from white or yellow and scarlike to pink, red, tan, brown, or black. Lesions are often waxy or translucent in appearance, and many are described as pearly. Some lesions are smooth and symmetrical, while others have irregular borders or a bumpy surface with superficial blood vessels. Other lesions have rolled edges with a crater in the middle. Many lesions bleed easily.

Screening and diagnosis: The U.S. Preventive Services Task Force evaluated routine screening for skin cancers in 2001 and did not find evidence to recommend whole-body skin examination for skin cancer, so health care providers look for skin cancers as circumstances allow or warrant. The diagnosis of basal cell carcinoma is made by histologic, or microscopic, examination of lesional cells from a sample of the lesion or from examination of the entire lesion. The type and variety of cancer are determined by the makeup and differentiation of cells.

Treatment and therapy: The most common treatment for basal cell carcinoma is surgical excision, or removal, of the lesion. Some normal tissue is taken all around the lesion so that the physician can be sure no cancer cells are left. Mohs surgery, which allows for better margin

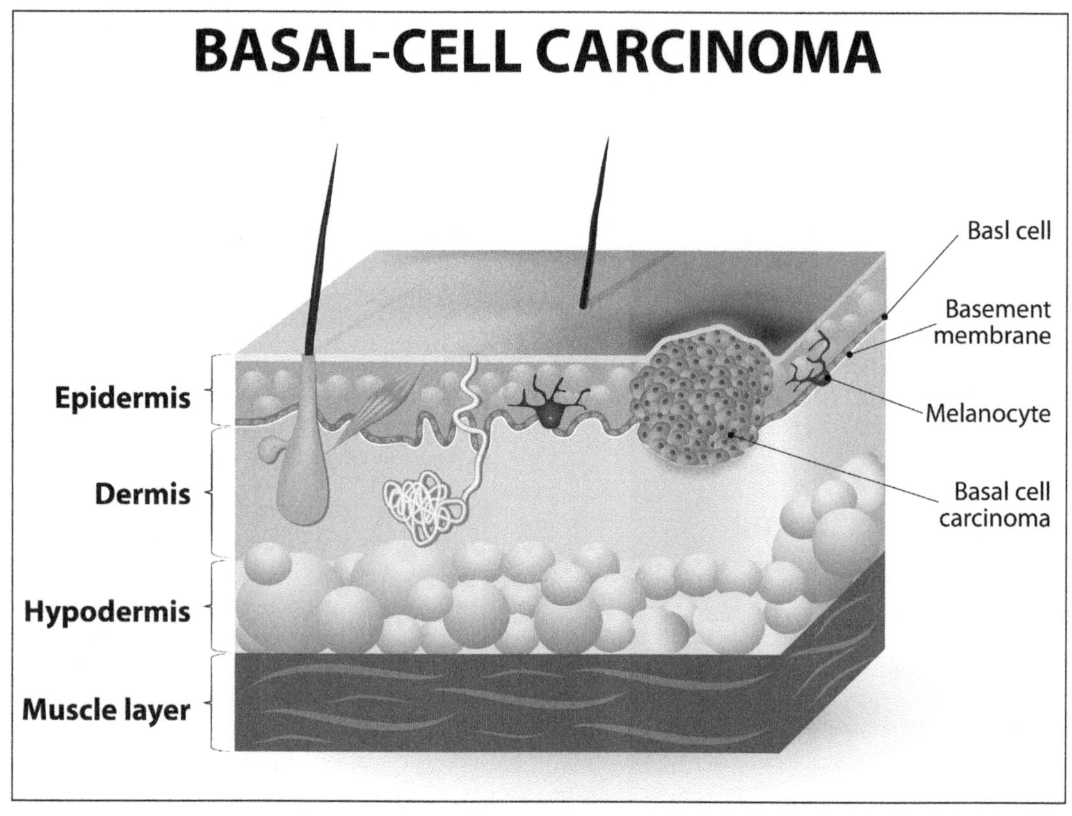

(iStock)

control, is the treatment of choice for sclerosing basal cell carcinoma. Other treatments include curettage and electrodesiccation, or scraping of the lesion and destroying the remaining tissue with electric current; cryosurgery, or freezing with liquid nitrogen; topical chemotherapy; radiation; laser surgery; and photodynamic therapy, in which a sensitizer is absorbed into the lesion, which is then exposed to a laser beam.

Prognosis, prevention, and outcomes: The cure rate is about 85 to 99 percent for primary tumors. One variant of basal cell carcinoma, called sclerosing, morpheaform, or infiltrating, is more likely to recur after treatment. This variant, which usually resembles a scar, is more difficult to treat because it grows in thin strands that may be missed in the tissue sample. Though death from basal cell carcinoma is extremely rare, untreated lesions can cause extensive damage and disfigurement, sometimes requiring skin grafts or reconstructive surgery. Early detection and treatment give the best outcomes. Basal cell carcinoma is also highly preventable through avoidance of excessive sun exposure, particularly in childhood. Childhood exposure to ultraviolet radiation can result in skin cancer that appears decades later. Limiting sun exposure, using sunscreen, and wearing sun-protective clothing and hats are useful methods of preventing damage to the skin from ultraviolet light.

Cathy Anderson, R.N., B.A.

For Further Information

Burns, C. A., and M. D. Brown. "Imiquimod for the Treatment of Skin Cancer." *Dermatology Clinics* 23, no. 1 (2005): 151-164.

Neale, R. E., et al. "Basal Cell Carcinoma on the Trunk Is Associated with Excessive Sun Exposure." *Journal of the American Academy of Dermatology* 56, no. 3 (2007): 380-386.

Noble, J. *Textbook of Primary Care Medicine*. 3d ed. St. Louis: Mosby, 2001.

Other Resources

Medem Medical Library
http://www.medem.com

Skin Cancer Foundation
http://www.skincancer.org

See also: Arsenic compounds; Bowen disease; Choriocarcinomas; Dermatology oncology; Electroporation therapy; Exenteration; Eye cancers; Eyelid cancer; Lip cancers; Medulloblastomas; Melanomas; Mohs surgery; Moles; Neuroectodermal tumors; Radical neck dissection; Skin cancers; Squamous cell carcinomas; Sunlamps; Turcot syndrome; Vulvar cancer

▶ Beckwith-Wiedemann Syndrome (BWS)

Category: Diseases, Symptoms, and Conditions
Also known as: Wiedemann-Beckwith syndrome, exomphalos-macroglossia-gigantism (EMG) syndrome

Related conditions: Hemihypertrophy (enlargement of one side of the body); hypoglycemia (low blood sugar); exomphalos (a protrusion of the umbilicus) or other abdominal wall defects such as umbilical hernia, omphalocele, and diastasis recti; visceromegaly (enlarged organs) or enlarged tongue or skeleton; adrenal gland abnormalities such as adrenocortical cytomegaly (enlarged cells of the adrenal cortex); dysplasia of the renal medulla; and embryonal cancerous tumors (tumors that arise from embryonic or fetal tissue) such as nephroblastoma (Wilms' tumor affecting the kidney, about 75 percent), hepatoblastoma (liver malignancy, about 1 to 11 percent), rhabdomyosarcoma (a soft-tissue tumor most commonly found in the head and neck, arms, and legs, and the renal and genital tracts, about 5 percent), and neuroblastoma (affecting primitive neuronal cells in the adrenal gland and behind the peritoneum, the serous tissue that lines the abdomen, about 4 percent)

Definition: Beckwith-Wiedemann syndrome (BWS) is a congenital overgrowth disorder caused by abnormalities in the 11p15.5 region of chromosome 11. The expression of the involved chromosome is variable and the penetrance (the degree to which features or characteristics resulting from the person's genetic makeup are seen by others) is incomplete. Penetrance is affected by either paternal or maternal transmission of information and gene control.

Risk factors: De novo mutations and inheritance through familial linkage are the primary risk factors. Analysis of the chromosomes is diagnostic in familial heritance, and all show transmission through the mother. Analysis of paternally derived BWS shows duplication or trisomy of the 11p15.5 region. These multiple copies result in a varying phenotype. Thus, different patterns of inheritance have been documented.

Etiology and the disease process: The overexpression of insulin-like growth factor-2 (IGF-2) is a key determinant of BWS. This overexpression occurs in the following manner. One set of chromosomes is inherited from the father, and the other is inherited from the mother. Each set of chromosomes contains a gene or a set of genes responsible for the characteristics of the new individual. Often, a gene on either the maternal or paternal chromosome is expressed, while the corresponding gene on the other parent's chromosome is silent. The expression of a gene on one parent's chromosome and the silence of the corresponding gene on the other parent's chromosome is termed imprinting. BWS develops when the normally expressed maternal gene is overactive. Deregulation of imprinted growth regulatory genes on chromosome 11, region 11p15.5, results in an imbalance between maternal and paternal allele expression. This region contains the genes for insulin and insulin-like growth factor-2 (IGF-2), both potent stimulators of fetal growth. This genetic aberration triggers exaggerated growth in the fetus, both in overall size as well as the enlargement of various structures and organs. Other tissues sensitive to abnormal growth factors respond by producing a high incidence of embryonal tumors and other anomalies. The loss of IGF-2 imprinting results in an overexpression of IGF-2 and leads to an enlarged body, organs, and overstimulation of embryonic tissues, which are the basis for various tumors affecting the kidneys, liver, and adrenal glands.

Incidence: BWS occurs in approximately 1 in 14,000 live births in the regular population in the United States. The incidence is higher with in vitro births (assisted reproductive technology). Because of phenotypic variation, many individuals with BWS may go undiagnosed, especially if the penetrance is mild or subtle.

Symptoms: Major symptoms include macroglossia (large tongue), pre- or postnatal growth greater than the ninetieth percentile, and abdominal wall defects. Minor symptoms include hypoglycemia, ear creases or helical indentations, facial nevus flammeus (port-wine stain), a large placenta at birth, and polyhydramnios (excessive amniotic fluid). Abnormalities in all body systems have been reported in association with BWS.

Screening and diagnosis: Because of the high incidence of embryonal tumor formation, abdominal ultrasonographic examinations are necessary every three months, especially in the first six years of life (the period when most embryonal tumors manifest). Wilms' tumor is rapidly progressive, and even individuals who have been examined every six months have been found to have late-stage disease. Diagnosis is by imaging studies (ultrasound, magnetic resonance imaging, computed tomography, bone scans), biopsy, laboratory tests (complete blood count, blood smear, alpha-fetoprotein, tests to evaluate functioning of the involved organs).

Staging is a process to determine whether the cancer has spread (metastasized) to other sites. Classification includes:

- Stage I: The cancer can be completely removed by surgery.
- Stage II: A majority of the cancer is removed by surgery with a small amount remaining at the primary site.
- Stage III: The cancer has spread to the lymph nodes.
- Stage IV: The cancer has spread to distant sites in the body.
- Recurrent: The cancer has returned after it has been treated.

Treatment and therapy: Hypoglycemia must be prevented and, if present, rapidly treated to prevent central nervous system abnormalities, especially mental retardation. Embryonic tumors require treatment (surgery, radiation, chemotherapeutic drug administration). Macroglossia is treated with surgery to ensure a patent (open) airway and normal mouth and speech development. Other anomalies are given standard treatment for the problem.

Prognosis, prevention, and outcomes: Prevention requires a decision by affected individuals not to reproduce. Prenatal genetic testing is currently not available. Prenatal ultrasound examination may lead to early detection of an affected fetus. If the pregnancy is continued, medical personnel can be alerted, thus allowing prompt attention to the infant at birth to detect problems and intervene in a timely manner, hopefully preventing some complications. Prognosis depends on the range of morbidities and their management.

Wanda Todd Bradshaw, R.N.C., M.S.N.

For Further Information

Cohen, M. Michael. "Beckwith-Wiedemann Syndrome: Historical, Clinicopathological, and Etiopathogenetic Perspectives." *Pediatric and Developmental Pathology* 8 (2005): 287-304.

Smith, Adam C., Sanaa Choufani, José C. Ferreira, and Rosanna Weksberg. "Growth Regulation, Imprinted Genes, and Chromosome 11p15.5." *Pediatric Research* 61, no. 5 (2007): 43R-47R.

Weksberg, Rosanna, Cheryl Shuman, and Adam C. Smith. "Beckwith-Wiedemann Syndrome." *American Journal of Medical Genetics, Part C* 137C (2005): 12-23.

Other Resources

Beckwith-Wiedemann Syndrome Family Forum
http://www.beckwith-wiedemann.info

Online Mendelian Inheritance in Man
http://www.ncbi.nlm.nih.gov/sites/entrez?db=OMIM

See also: Adrenal gland cancers; Adrenocortical cancer; Nephroblastomas; Rhabdomyosarcomas; Wilms' tumor

▶ Benign Prostatic Hyperplasia (BPH)

Category: Diseases, Symptoms, and Conditions
Also known as: Benign enlargement of the prostate (BEP), lower urinary tract symptoms (LUTS)

Related conditions: Prostate cancer, urinary retention

Definition: Benign prostatic hyperplasia (BPH) refers to an enlarged prostate gland. The prostate is a reproductive gland in men that produces semen, the fluid that nourishes and transports sperm. It is about the size and shape of a walnut and is located below the bladder. The gland surrounds the urethra, the tube that carries urine outside the body. The prostate grows in size in most men as they age.

Risk factors: Increasing age and a family history of BPH contribute to the risk of developing this condition.

Etiology and the disease process: The exact cause of BPH is unknown. It is not cancerous, nor does it increase the risk of developing prostate cancer.

Incidence: Approximately 50 percent of men between the ages of fifty-one and sixty and 90 percent over age eighty develop BPH. About half of all men diagnosed with BPH have moderate to severe symptoms.

Symptoms: The enlarged prostate presses down on the urethra and irritates or obstructs the bladder. Common symptoms include frequent urination two or more times per night, a sudden urge to urinate, a weak urine stream, dribbling after urinating, straining to urinate, the inability to prevent urine leakage, or the sensation that the bladder is not empty even after urinating. In extreme cases, urinary retention, the complete inability to urinate, is a problem.

Screening and diagnosis: The evaluation typically consists of a complete medical history, a digital rectal exam to feel the size of the prostate, a urinalysis to check for blood or infection in the urine, a prostate-specific antigen (PSA) blood test to screen for prostate cancer, and questions to assess the severity of symptoms. Additionally, urine flow rate, a post-void residual urine test, a pressure-flow study, an X ray of the urinary tract, or cystoscopy (a test using a scope inserted into the urethra and bladder) may be recommended.

Treatment and therapy: Depending on the severity of symptoms, treatment can include lifestyle modifications, such as decreasing the intake of fluid before bedtime and limiting the consumption of alcohol and caffeine, or medication to increase urine flow. In extreme cases, surgery to remove part of the prostate may be recommended.

Prognosis, prevention, and outcomes: Many men with BPH have only minor symptoms and are able to manage their discomfort with lifestyle modifications. A yearly exam is recommended to monitor symptoms and the impact of BPH on daily life.

Vonne Sieve, M.A.

See also: Digital Rectal Exam (DRE); Prostate cancer; Prostate-Specific Antigen (PSA) test; Prostatectomy; Prostatitis; Saw palmetto; Transrectal ultrasound; Urologic oncology

▶ Benign tumors

Category: Diseases, Symptoms, and Conditions
Also known as: Mass, benign neoplasm, noncancerous tumor

Related conditions: Lipoma, chondroma, adenoma, hemangioma

Definition: A benign tumor is a noncancerous growth that does not invade nearby tissue or spread to other parts of the body. Benign tumors are caused by cell overgrowth and are thus distinct from other tissue formations, such as cysts or abscesses. A tumor is a mass of tissue that serves no useful purpose and exists at the expense of healthy tissues. Benign tumors do not exhibit any of the three characteristics of malignant tumors: Benign tumors do not invade nearby tissues, do not metastasize, and do not grow in an unlimited, accelerated manner.

Risk factors: The specific risk factors for benign tumors vary depending on the location of the tumor and the tissue type. For example, risk factors for benign breast tumors include such factors as body mass index, height, and breast size. Problems with the body's immune system can cause tumors, both malignant and benign. Certain viruses can also play a role in tumor formation, as in cervical cancer and hepatocellular carcinoma. Exposure to loud sounds or music can increase the risk of developing benign tumors in the ears, as can repeated exposure to cold water. Smoking can cause benign tumors to appear in the lower lip.

Etiology and the disease process: The source of most benign tumors is a discrete population of cells that have been altered through acquired genetic defects. Such abnormal tissue masses are termed benign neoplasms. Benign tumors are usually encapsulated, meaning that they are confined to a specific, localized area and surrounded by a thin layer of tissue. This limits the growth rate and invasive potential of the tumor. In the liver, the most common benign tumors are hemangiomas. These tumors are made of abnormal blood vessels, most likely present at birth but only detected later when they cause symptoms or are identified on an ultrasound or computed tomography (CT) image obtained for another reason. Hemangiomas occur more frequently in women. Infections can cause benign tumors to appear in the larynx, which can be detected by symptoms of hoarseness.

Incidence: Benign tumors are common and usually not life-threatening. However, benign tumors cause more than 13,000 deaths annually, compared with more than 500,000 annual deaths due to malignant tumors. Benign tumors can cause serious injury or death by pressing on vital organs (such as the brain), tissues, or nerves in the vicinity of the growth. Benign tumors in the kidneys can range in size from 1 millimeter to several centimeters without causing any symptoms or requiring treatment. Benign tumors in the lungs are relatively rare, making up only 7 to 10 percent of all tumors in the lungs. Benign tumors in the stomach account for 5 to 10 percent of all stomach tumors, afflicting many people between the ages of forty and fifty. Men are two to four times more likely to develop benign stomach tumors compared with women.

Symptoms: Benign tumors may be asymptomatic or may cause one or more of the following symptoms depending on their location and their specific tissue type: itching, obstruction of the intestines, bleeding or occult blood loss resulting in anemia, cosmetic changes, hormonal syndromes caused by hormones secreted by the tumor, compression of the blood vessels or vital organs, and pain or dysfunction induced by pressure. Benign tumors in the nose have the following symptoms: hard breathing, bleeding, headache, or severe eye pain and blurring.

Screening and diagnosis: When a tumor is found, a biopsy is performed to determine whether the tumor is benign or malignant. Although usually not life-threatening, once diagnosed, benign tumors should be monitored regularly, as a benign tumor may progress and become a malignant tumor. For instance, a colon polyp is a type of benign tumor, but most incidences of colon cancer develop from colon polyps. The most common benign tumors of the ear occur behind the ear. They can also occur within the ear canal or on the scalp and can be discovered during a routine ear examination, which includes audiometry (hearing tests) and tympanometry (middle ear testing). When looking into the ear, the doctor may observe cysts or benign tumors within the ear canal.

Treatment and therapy: Often a benign tumor will require no treatment if it is located in a low-risk area where it will not cause symptoms or disturb proper function of an organ. If causing symptoms, benign tumors are usually treated by surgery. Benign tumors may also be removed for cosmetic reasons. The incidence of recurrence after surgery is typically low. Chemotherapy and radiation therapy are usually ineffective in the treatment of benign tumors. Benign tumors of the brain may be surgically removed to prevent harmful effects on the surrounding normal brain tissue.

Prognosis, prevention, and outcomes: Benign tumors tend to grow more slowly than malignant tumors and are less likely to threaten health. If a tumor is benign, the prognosis is generally very good. The situation can be more serious if the tumor is located in the brain.

Michael R. King, Ph.D.

For Further Information

Black, Peter McL. *Living with a Brain Tumor: Dr. Peter Black's Guide to Taking Control of Your Treatment.* New York: Henry Holt, 2006.

DeMonte, Franco, et al., eds. *Tumors of the Brain and Spine*. New York: Springer, 2007.

Moore, Stephen W. *Griffith's Instructions for Patients.* 7th ed. Philadelphia: Elsevier Saunders, 2005.

Other Resources

Genetics Home Reference
Benign Tumors
http://ghr.nlm.nih.gov/conditionGroup=benigntumors

Medline Plus
Benign Tumors
http://www.nlm.nih.gov/medlineplus/benigntumors.html

See also: Acoustic neuromas; Adenomatoid tumors; Birt-Hogg-Dubé Syndrome (BHDS); Brachytherapy; *BRAF* gene; Carcinogens, known; Carney complex; Castleman disease; Chemoprevention; Cowden syndrome; Craniopharyngiomas; Endotheliomas; Fibroadenomas; Gastrointestinal Stromal Tumors (GISTs); Gestational Trophoblastic Tumors (GTTs); Glomus tumors; Hemangioblastomas; Hystero-oophorectomy; Lacrimal gland tumors; Leiomyomas; Metastasis; Multiple endocrine neoplasia type 1 (MEN 1); Multiple endocrine neoplasia type 2 (MEN 2); Phyllodes tumors; Pineoblastomas; Radical neck dissection; Sertoli cell tumors; Tuberous sclerosis

▶ Bile duct cancer

Category: Diseases, Symptoms, and Conditions
Also known as: Intrahepatic cholangiocarcinoma, extrahepatic cholangiocarcinoma, perihilar cancer, Klatskin tumors

Related conditions: Sclerosing cholangitis, liver cancer

Definition: Bile is a fluid produced by the liver that aids in the digestion of fats. Bile is transported from the liver through a series of tubes, called bile ducts, to either the gallbladder, which stores and concentrates the bile, or directly to the small intestine. Bile duct cancer forms in the inner layer of these ducts. It can develop in the smaller ducts within the liver, where it is called intrahepatic cholangiocarcinoma, or in ducts outside the liver, where it is called extrahepatic cholangiocarcinoma. Extrahepatic cholangiocarcinoma is divided into two types, depending on where the cancer originates. Perihilar cancer develops in the bile duct close to its exit point from the liver. Distal bile duct cancer develops close to where the bile duct empties into the small intestine. Approximately 95 percent of cholangiocarcinomas are adenocarcinomas.

Risk factors: Conditions that irritate the bile ducts have been linked to an increased risk of developing cholangiocarcinoma. These disorders include bile duct stones, congenital bile duct cysts, viral hepatitis, sclerosing cholangitis (especially in people who smoke), and nonviral cirrhosis. Other risk factors include ulcerative colitis, liver flukes (parasites found in Asian countries), and obesity. Exposure to some chemicals, including polychlorinated biphenyls, dioxin, and Thorotrast (previously used in X-ray diagnosis), also increase the risk of developing this cancer.

Etiology and the disease process: The exact cause of most cholangiocarcinomas is unknown. Patients with no known risk factors often develop this cancer. Cholangiocarcinoma is a slow-growing cancer that can remain undetected until it has reached an advanced stage. It originates in the mucosal cells that line the ducts and spreads throughout the layers of the ducts. Eventually, the ducts become blocked, preventing the flow of bile. When the cancer grows through the walls of the ducts, it can invade the liver, gallbladder, small and large intestines, and blood vessels that serve the liver.

Incidence: Primary cholangiocarcinoma is a rare disease that is most common in Asian countries because of its association with liver flukes. Approximately 90 percent of cholangiocarcinomas are extrahepatic, with about 65 percent perihilar tumors and 25 percent distal cancers. About 4,000 people in the United States develop this cancer each year, most of whom are men, and about 70 percent of them are older than age sixty-five. The American Cancer Society has noted an increase in the incidence of intrahepatic cholangiocarcinoma, possibly because of improved diagnostic testing.

Symptoms: Most cholangiocarcinomas do not produce symptoms until they are in the advanced stages. Jaundiced and itchy skin, dark urine, and pale bowel movements may occur if the ducts become blocked and bilirubin, a chemical in bile, is forced into the blood vessels. Other symptoms include fever, bloating, loss of appetite, weight loss, and fatigue.

Screening and diagnosis: There are no screening tests for cholangiocarcinoma. Diagnosis typically is made during surgery for a gallbladder disorder or during diagnostic tests for other conditions. Blood chemistry and liver function tests, though not specific for this cancer, may show abnormal results. Tumor-marker studies may show the presence of carcinoembryonic antigen and cancer antigen 19-9 (CA 19-9). Ultrasound, computed tomography scanning, magnetic resonance imaging, endoscopic retrograde cholangiopancreatography, positron emission tomography, and percutaneous transhepatic cholangiography are imaging studies used to diagnose cholangiocarcinoma, determine treatment options, and assess the spread of the disease. Biopsy and biliary brushing may be performed to obtain cells for differential testing. Staging is based on the number of tumors present and the extent of their spread to other organs.

Relative Survival Rates for Bile Duct Cancer, 1988-2001

	Survival Rates (%)	
Years	*Intrahepatic*	*Extrahepatic*
1	27.9	43.7
2	19.5	25.4
3	8.5	17.5
5	4.8	12.8
8	3.4	9.8
10	3.2	9.7

Source: Data from L. A. G. Ries et al., eds., *Cancer Survival Among Adults: U.S. SEER Program, 1988-2001—Patient and Tumor Characteristics,* NIH Pub. No. 07-6215 (Bethesda, Md.: National Cancer Institute, 2007)

Note: The median survival time for bile duct cancer is 5.6 months, for extrahepatic bile duct cancer, 9.4 months.

Treatment and therapy: Traditional treatment for cholangiocarcinoma includes surgery, chemotherapy, and radiation therapy. Surgery for intrahepatic cholangiocarcinoma always involves the removal of part of the liver and is a difficult procedure. In many cases, the cancer is too far advanced at the time of diagnosis for surgery to be successful or safe for the patient. Surgery for extrahepatic cholangiocarcinoma usually involves the removal of the bile duct, gallbladder, and parts of the liver and small intestine. It may also include the resection of part or all of the pancreas. When the cancer cannot be removed, symptoms may be relieved by creating a bypass around the tumor blocking the bile duct or inserting a biliary drain.

Chemotherapy and radiation therapy may be used before surgery to shrink a tumor, in place of surgery when the tumor is inoperable, and after surgery to destroy cells that may have spread. Common chemotherapeutic agents used include fluorouracil, cisplatin, doxorubicin, and gemcitabine. Radiation is commonly administered in the form of tiny seeds that are implanted into the duct, delivering high-dose radiation directly to the tumor.

Other forms of treatment that are being tested include using a person's own immune system to fight the cancer, introducing viruses that seek out and destroy cancer cells, and photodynamic therapy, in which a special light is used to activate a drug that has been administered for the purpose of destroying cancer cells.

Prognosis, prevention, and outcomes: The overall survival rate for cholangiocarcinoma is poor, with fewer than 20 percent surviving five years after diagnosis. Although there is no definitive way to prevent this disease, reducing exposure to its risk factors may prevent its development.

Dorothy P. Terry, R.N.

For Further Information

Holland, Jimmie C., and Sheldon Lewis. *The Human Side of Cancer*. New York: HarperCollins, 2000.

Souhami, Robert, and Jeffrey Tobias. *Cancer and Its Management*. Malden, Mass.: Blackwell, 2005.

Stern, Theodore A., and Mikkael A. Sekeres. *Facing Cancer: A Complete Guide for People with Cancer, Their Families, and Caregivers*. New York: McGraw-Hill, 2004.

Other Resources

American Cancer Society
http://www.cancer.org

Cancer.Net
http://www.cancer.net/portal/site/patient

See also: Afterloading radiation therapy; Alkaline Phosphatase Test (ALP); Carcinoid tumors and carcinoid syndrome; Cholecystectomy; Computed Tomography (CT) scan; Endoscopic Retrograde Cholangiopancreatography (ERCP); Endoscopy; Gallbladder cancer; Gastrointestinal cancers; Infection and sepsis; Infectious cancers; Iridium seeds; Klinefelter syndrome and cancer; Liver cancers; Pancreatectomy; Pancreatic cancers; Percutaneous Transhepatic Cholangiography (PTHC)

▶ Birt-Hogg-Dubé Syndrome (BHDS)

Category: Diseases, Symptoms, and Conditions
Related conditions: Renal cell carcinoma, pulmonary cysts

Definition: Birt-Hogg-Dubé syndrome (BHDS) is a rare, genetically linked syndrome named after the three Canadian doctors who first identified it as a skin disorder. It consists of three types of benign skin growths: fibrofolliculomas, white or flesh-colored tumors that occur in hair follicles; trichodiscomas, overgrowths of tissues in hair disks; and acrochordons, commonly called skin tags. These growths are typically found on the face, neck, chest, and scalp.

Since the identification of BHDS in 1977, further study of patients with the syndrome has revealed additional abnormalities that characteristically develop in affected individuals. The most common of these conditions include benign and cancerous kidney tumors, lung cysts, and spontaneous pneumothorax.

Risk factors: BHDS is genetically linked, meaning that it is associated with a defect in one or more genes. Although, in most cases, the gene responsible for BHDS has been passed through families, evidence of genetic mutation in people with no familial link has also been identified. Patients with a defective gene who also smoke have a higher risk of developing kidney cancer.

Etiology and the disease process: BHDS is caused by a mutation in the gene encoding the protein folliculin, which functions as a tumor suppressor that regulates cell proliferation. When folliculin is absent or not functioning properly, it cannot control cellular growth and division, which leads to tissue overgrowth and the formation of tumors. Folliculin is present in many types of tissues but is primarily found in skin, lung, and kidney cells.

The folliculin gene (FCLN) is located on chromosome 17p11.2. BHDS is an autosomal dominant trait that would have a probability of 50% if either parent is affected. FLCN has been shown to interact with two other folliculin-interacting proteins produced by FNIP1 and FNIP2. Studies in knockout mice have shown that dysfunction of these three genes causes metabolic changes that lead to kidney tumors. Researchers hope these latest findings lead to new treatments for kidney cancers.

BHDS usually begins with the formation of skin growths. As the disease progresses, these growths increase in number and size. Slow-growing kidney tumors can develop as single or multiple tumors in one or both kidneys. Several types of tumors have been associated with BHDS, including benign tumors such as renal oncocytomas, and cancerous tumors such as chromophobe renal carcinoma, and clear cell carcinoma. Benign tumors often become cancerous as the disease progresses.

Incidence: BHDS is very rare; it is estimated to be present in about six hundred families worldwide. A precise incidence rate is unknown because people are not routinely tested for the presence of the FCLN gene. There is no indication that race or gender influences a person's risk of having the gene or developing the disease. The typical age at which a person begins to display signs of BHDS is between the late twenties and early forties. The incidence of kidney cancer in people with BHDS may be as low as 30 percent; however, the incidence of lung cysts is estimated to be about 90 percent.

Symptoms: Although some people with BHDS have no noticeable symptoms of the disease, the development of fibrofolliculomas or acrochordons is usually the first indication that the person is affected. Initially looking like small, white pimples, fibrofolliculomas typically become larger and more prolific as time passes. The development of polyps in the mouth or colon may also indicate BHDS and should be investigated further. Lung cysts, which usually do not cause respiratory problems or lung cancer, may be detected during routine examinations or testing for other conditions. Multiple or bilateral kidney tumors are often the first indication of BHDS.

Screening and diagnosis: Several recurrent tests are recommended for people with BHDS and those with family members who have BHDS. Recommendations include an annual kidney ultrasound and chest X-ray, computed tomography (CT) scanning or magnetic resonance imaging (MRI) every two years, and biopsies of suspicious skin growths. Deoxyribonucleic acid (DNA) testing to check for genetic alterations should be considered for individuals who have family members with the disease. Genetic counseling should precede any such testing.

The disease is typically diagnosed after skin lesion biopsies are positive for fibrofolliculomas or when multiple kidney tumors and lung cysts are identified.

Treatment and therapy: There is no specific medical treatment recommended for the skin tumors associated with BHDS. Surgical removal, electrodesiccation, and dermabrasion have been used without long-term success. A relatively new procedure for BHDS-related skin tumors is laser skin resurfacing, which has been successful in several cases; however, the long-term results are unknown.

Both benign and cancerous kidney tumors are removed surgically. However, new tumors often form in place of the ones removed. When possible, only part of the kidney is removed to prolong the patient's kidney function. Experimental treatments to destroy the cancer cells may be used on recurrent tumors. These include cryoablation (freezing the tumor) and radio frequency ablation (killing the tumor with heat). In cancers that are not controllable with surgery, or in which the cancer has metastasized, angiogenesis or mTOR inhibitors are an option.

Prognosis, prevention, and outcomes: The prognosis for BHDS depends on whether kidney cancer develops and the success of its treatment. BHDS cannot be prevented. Birt-Hogg-Dubé syndrome (BHDS)

Dorothy P. Terry, R.N.
Updated by: Annette O'Connor, Ph.D.

For Further Information

Hasumi, H., Baba, M., Hasumi, Y., Furuya, M. & Yao, M. (2015), Birt–Hogg–Dubé syndrome: Clinical and molecular aspects of recently identified kidney cancer syndrome. *International Journal of Urology,* 23(3), 204-210. doi: 10.1111/iju.13015

Lindor, N. M., Hand, J., Burch, P. A. & Gibson, L. E. (2001). Birt-Hogg-Dubé syndrome: An autosomal dominant disorder with predisposition to cancers of the kidney, fibrofolliculomas, and focal cutaneous mucinosis. *International Journal of Dermatology,* 40(10), 653-656.

Pavlovich, C. P., Grubb, R. L., Hurley, K., Glenn, G. M., Toro, J., Schmidt, L. S., … Linehan, W. M. (2005). Evaluation and management of renal tumors in the Birt-Hogg-Dubé syndrome. *American Journal of Surgical Pathology,* 173(5), 1482-1486.

Pomery, Chris. (2004). *DNA and family history.* Toronto: Dundurn Press.

Other Resources

BHD Foundation:
http://www.birthoggdube.org/id1.html

The BHD Foundation website deals with all aspects of the disease and has information for families and health care providers. It includes information from the International BHD Symposia

Genetics Home Reference.
https://ghr.nlm.nih.gov/condition/birt-hogg-dube-syndrome

This website provides information on various genetic conditions that impact health. It has an extensive bibliography for both medical professionals and patients.

See also: Hereditary Leiomyomatosis and Renal Cell Cancer (HLRCC); Kidney cancer; Urinary system cancers

▶ Bladder cancer

Category: Diseases, Symptoms, and Conditions
Also known as: Transitional cell carcinoma

Related conditions: Kidney cancer

Definition: Bladder cancer is a cancer that forms in the inner lining of the bladder.

Risk factors: Researchers do not completely understand the causes of bladder cancer; however, several carcinogens, family history, and prior diagnosis of bladder cancer remain the chief causes. Smokers are at greatest risk for developing bladder cancer as well as people with exposure to certain chemical dyes in the rubber- and leather-processing, textile, and printing industries.

Etiology and the disease process: The wall of the bladder is lined with cells called transitional cells and squamous cells. More than 90 percent of bladder cancers begin in the transitional cells and are called transitional cell carcinomas. About 8 percent of bladder cancer patients have squamous cell carcinomas. Cancer that is only in cells in the lining of the bladder is called superficial bladder cancer and often recurs after treatment.

Cancer that begins as a superficial tumor may grow through the lining and into the muscular wall of the bladder. This invasive cancer may extend through the bladder wall into a nearby organ such as the uterus, vagina, or prostate gland or into nearby lymph nodes, in which case cancer cells may have spread to other lymph nodes or other organs such as the lungs and liver or to the bones.

Incidence: Primarily occurring in men and women over the age of forty, bladder cancer is diagnosed in 38,000 men and 15,000 women each year in the United States. According to the National Cancer Institute, this is the fourth most common type of cancer in men, and the eighth most common in women. Caucasians get bladder cancer twice as often as African Americans and Hispanics. People with family members who have bladder cancer as well as people who have previously had bladder cancer are more likely to get the disease.

Symptoms: Bladder cancer often causes no symptoms until it reaches an advanced state that is difficult to cure. The most common symptom of bladder cancer is blood in the urine (hematuria). Some patients experience pain or burning during urination, or a change in urinary habits, such as a frequent urge to urinate.

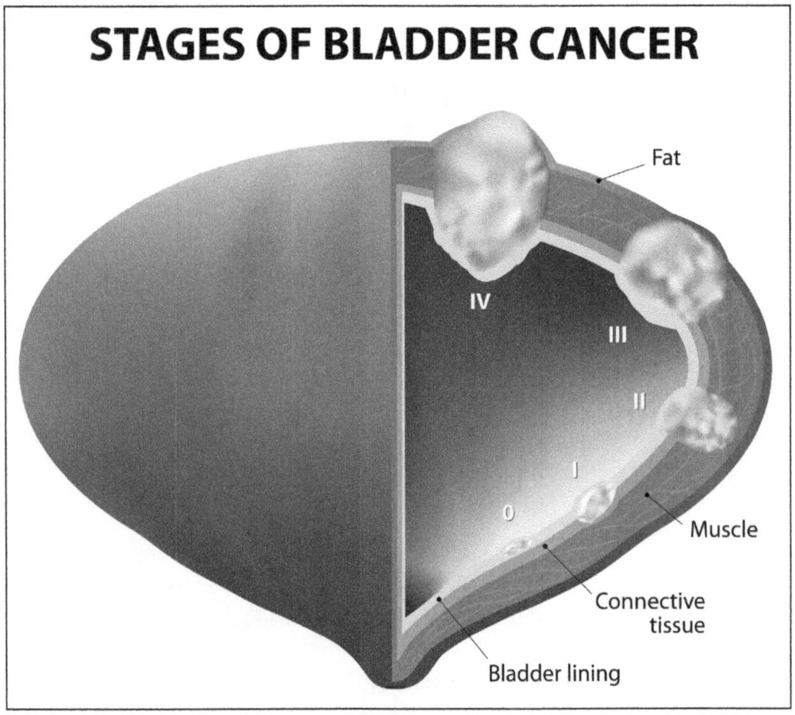

(iStock)

Screening and diagnosis: Screening tests include a medical interview, a physical examination, urinalysis, urine cytology, and cystoscopy. The urinalysis determines if the urine contains abnormalities such as blood, protein, sugar, and solids. Urine cytology is a microscopic examination of urine to detect any abnormal cells that have sloughed off the bladder wall and have been released in the urine. If necessary, cytoscopy is performed with a very narrow tube with a light and camera inserted through the urethra to examine the inside of the bladder. If bladder cancer is suspected, a physician may order a computed tomography (CT) scan, pyelography, or biopsy. The CT scan is helpful for a three-dimensional view of the bladder and urinary tract to determine if any masses or tumors exist in the bladder or if the cancer has spread to other organs. Pyelography involves injecting a special dye into a vein or the urethra and examining a series of

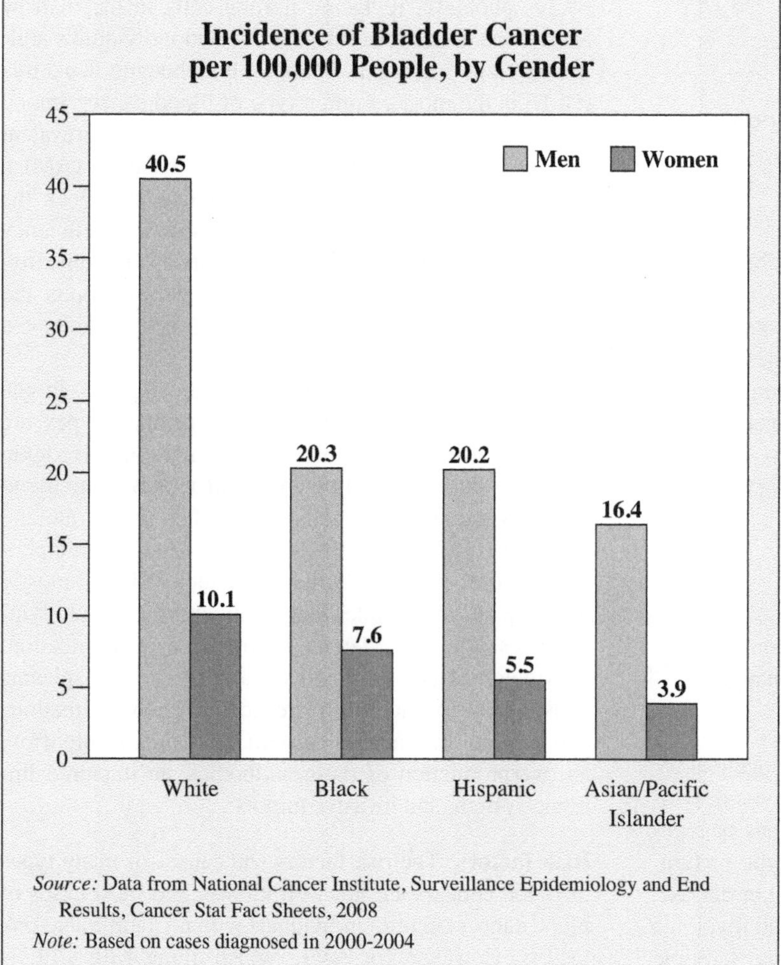

Source: Data from National Cancer Institute, Surveillance Epidemiology and End Results, Cancer Stat Fact Sheets, 2008

Note: Based on cases diagnosed in 2000-2004

timed-interval X rays of the urinary system to determine if abnormalities exist. The biopsy is typically performed during cytoscopy, and abnormal cells can be detected with a microscope.

Staging refers to the size of the cancer and the extent to which it has invaded the bladder wall and spread to other parts of the body. High-grade tumors are significantly more aggressive and life-threatening than low-grade tumors. Approximately 10 percent of bladder cancer is found to be superficial bladder cancer in situ, which is a highly aggressive, early manifestation of bladder cancer.

Treatment and therapy: The physician may treat superficial bladder cancer with transurethral resection (TUR) by inserting a cystoscope into the bladder through the urethra and using a tool with a small wire loop on the end to remove the cancer and to burn away any remaining cancer cells with an electric current. For invasive bladder cancer or cancer involving a large portion of the bladder, surgery is performed to remove the entire bladder, nearby lymph nodes, part of the urethra, and the nearby organs that may contain cancer cells. In some cases of low-grade cancer, only part of the bladder is removed in a procedure called segmental cystectomy.

Radiation therapy uses high-energy rays to kill localized cancer cells to shrink the tumor before surgery or if surgery is not an option. Chemotherapy uses one drug or a combination of drugs to kill cancer cells. Superficial bladder cancer can be treated with local chemotherapy; once per week for several weeks, a catheter is inserted through the urethra and remains in the bladder for several hours. If the cancer has deeply invaded the bladder or spread to lymph nodes or other organs, chemotherapy may be used to treat the entire body.

Biological therapy, or immunotherapy, uses the body's natural immune system to fight cancer by inserting a catheter with a solution containing live, weakened bacteria to kill cancer cells in the bladder.

Prognosis, prevention, and outcomes: Bladder cancer has one of the highest recurrence rates of all cancers. If treated once, patients must continue a course of follow-up screenings. The five-year survival rate for patients with early-stage bladder cancer is 85 percent. Most patients with bladder cancer (up to 80 percent) will be diagnosed with a superficial tumor. Patients with tumors invading the bladder wall have a five-year survival rate of 60 to 75 percent.

Robert J. Amato, D.O.

For Further Information

Dunetz, Gary N. *Bladder Cancer: A Resource Guide for Patients and Their Families.* Bloomington, Ind.: AuthorHouse, 2006.

Ellsworth, Pamela. *One Hundred Questions and Answers About Bladder Cancer.* Sudbury, Mass.: Jones & Bartlett, 2005.

Schoenberg, Mark P., et al. *The Guide to Living with Bladder Cancer.* Baltimore: Johns Hopkins University Press, 2000.

Other Resources

Mayo Clinic
Bladder Cancer
http://www.mayoclinic.com/health/bladder-cancer/DS00177

National Cancer Institute
Bladder Cancer
http://www.nci.nih.gov/cancertopics/types/bladder

See also: 4-Aminobiphenyl; Bacillus Calmette Guérin (BCG); Cystography; Cystoscopy; Gastrointestinal oncology; Kidney cancer; Squamous cell carcinomas; Transitional cell carcinomas; Urethral cancer; Urinary system cancers; Urography; Urostomy

▶ Blood cancers

Category: Diseases, Symptoms, and Conditions
Also known as: Hematopoietic neoplasms, malignant neoplasms, bone marrow diseases

Related conditions: Leukemia (acute myelogenous or myelocitic leukemia, or AML; acute lymphocytic or lymphoid leukemia, or ALL; chronic myelogenous or myelocitic leukemia, or CML; chronic lymphocytic or lymphoid leukemia, or CLL), lymphoma (Hodgkin disease, or HD; non-Hodgkin lymphoma, or NHL), and myeloma (plasma cell dyscrasia, plasma cell myeloma, multiple myeloma, myelomatosis)

Definition: Blood cancers are those that arise from an abnormality in the production of any of the mature blood cells or their precursor stem cells. Not all bone marrow disorders, such as anemia, are cancers. The three main types of blood cancer are leukemia, lymphoma, and myeloma.

Leukemia is a cancer of any of the five dominant types of white blood cells. It occurs when the bone marrow produces abnormal white blood cells, which replicate, limiting the ability of healthy cells to function. Chronic leukemia develops slowly, while acute leukemia develops quickly. Of the four subtypes of leukemia, the acute forms exhibit immature blood-forming cells or blasts, and the chronic forms exhibit few or no blast cells but changes in the presentation of marrow cells. Acute lymphocytic leukemia (ALL), also known as acute lymphoid leukemia, is the most common type of blood cancer among those under nineteen years of age. ALL is characterized by lymphoblasts replacing normal cells in the marrow and lymph nodes lowering the affected individual's ability to fight infection. Chronic lymphocytic leukemia (CLL) is the most common type of blood cancer among those fifty years of age and older and the most prevalent type of leukemia. Acute myelogenous leukemia (AML), in which leukemic blast cells proliferate and block the production of normal marrow cells, results in a deficiency of red blood cells, white cells, and platelets. Chronic myelogenous leukemia (CML) is seen mostly in adults and begins with a change in a single stem cell, a future red cell, white cell, or platelet.

Lymphomas originate in malignant changes in the lymphatic or immune system. The primary types are Hodgkin disease and non-Hodgkin lymphoma. Hodgkin disease is characterized by abnormal T or B white blood cells. As the abnormal cells divide, they proliferate and can spread throughout the body. Non-Hodgkin lymphoma is a cancer of the lymphoid tissue, which is mostly made up of lymph nodes that manufacture and store lymphocytes, white blood cells that protect against infection.

Myelomas are progressive blood cancers of plasma cells, which produce antibodies to fight against infections and regulate the immune system. Myeloma results from an overproduction of these antibodies, an impaired immune system, and invasive tumors.

Risk factors: The risk factors and causes of many types of blood cancers are not well known, and most cases of blood cancer occur in individuals with no identifiable risk factors. However, for AML, which along with CLL is among the most common types of blood cancer seen in adults, these specific risk factors have been found: Down syndrome and other genetic disorders, chronic exposure to ionizing radiation and chemicals such as benzene in the workplace, high doses of radiation therapy and the chemotherapies used to treat lymphoma or other types of cancer, and tobacco smoke. Those who are immunosuppressed with certain human retroviruses and bacteria, such as the Epstein-Barr virus (EBV) in Africa; those with human immunodeficiency virus (HIV); and those with human T-cell leukemia virus (HTLV) are at greater risk of developing lymphomas. Familial clustering also has been associated with the development of lymphomas.

Etiology and the disease process: Cancer develops as a result of a variety of factors and over a number of years. Blood cancers differ widely by group and within each subtype in their progression, causes, and molecular presentation. The leukemias begin in two types of white blood cells: neutrophils and monocytes, which are germ-ingesting cells, and lymphocytes, which are immune-defense cells. Abnormal white blood cells in the bone marrow multiply and enter the bloodstream, crowding out normal cells. Lymphomas develop when these immune-defense cells multiply and cause tumors in the lymph nodes or other parts of the immune system. Development of blood cells through the hematopoietic process is arrested, and abnormal blood cells proliferate. Every stage of hematopoietic development can result in a particular type of cancer. Non-Hodgkin lymphoma (NHL) is manifested by well-differentiated cells with slow progression, while other forms are more aggressive with lymphocytes of limited differentiation. Tumors of the bone marrow are characteristic of myelomas. In myeloma, cells that are to become immune cells develop in the bone marrow from stem cells, as will all blood cells. A major type of white blood cells, B lymphocytes, which typically develop into plasma cells, undergo multiple genetic changes as they change into plasma cells, causing malignant plasma cells to develop. These myeloma cells travel throughout the bloodstream, reside in the bone marrow, and damage healthy tissue. The myeloma interferes with the plasma cell's production of protective proteins called immunoglobulins or antibodies by producing M proteins or abnormal immunoglobulin, making those affected susceptible to infection.

Incidence: The most common forms of leukemia seen in adults aged fifty and over are chronic lymphocytic leukemia (CLL) and acute myelogenous leukemia (AML). The incidence of acute lymphocytic leukemia (ALL) increases in those over sixty years of age. In 2007, new cases of CLL were estimated at 15,340 and new cases of AML at 13,410. The National Cancer Institute (NCI) reports that between 2000 and 2004, the average median age at diagnosis for leukemia was sixty-seven, with 23.7 percent between the ages of seventy-five and eighty-four. Based on cases diagnosed during this period, the age-adjusted incidence rate for leukemia was 12.3 per 100,000 men and women per year. Chronic leukemias accounted for 7 percent more cases than acute leukemias.

It was estimated that 71,380 cases of lymphoma would be diagnosed in the United States in 2007. The majority of these cases, 63,190, were projected to be of the non-Hodgkin type. Incidence rates of Hodgkin lymphoma tend to be higher among men than women. Non-Hodgkin lymphoma also is more commonly diagnosed among men, particularly those aged sixty to sixty-four (52.3 in every 100,000 men in this age group). According to the NCI's cancer surveillance data, the median age for diagnosis of lymphoma was sixty-four, with the majority of cases, 21.3 percent, diagnosed between the ages of seventy-five and eighty-four. Non-Hodgkin lymphoma is the fifth most common cancer among men and women.

It was estimated that 19,900 new cases of myeloma would be diagnosed in the United States in 2007. NCI data indicated that the median age for diagnosis of myeloma was seventy, with the majority, 28.1 percent, between the ages of seventy-five and eighty-four. Incidence rates for all types of leukemia are higher among men than women and higher among African Americans than those of European descent. New cases of multiple myeloma are estimated to be diagnosed at a rate of 5 to 6 per 100,000 people each year. The incidence rate of myeloma is higher for men than women across racial and ethnic groups.

Symptoms: Signs and symptoms of blood cancers vary widely and may be similar to those of other, less severe illnesses. Symptoms vary based on the category and subtype of blood cancer; for example, symptoms of acute leukemia may include pallor, shortness of breath with exertion, lack of energy, night sweats or a mild fever, slow healing of cuts and bruises, unexplained weight loss, tiny red spots under the skin, bone and joint aches and pains, and low white blood cell count (especially neutrophils and monocytes). Although specific bone marrow and blood tests are needed to diagnose any type of blood cancer, some of those affected with certain subtypes of leukemia may have enlarged lymph nodes in the neck, groin, or armpit, and they may suffer from frequent infections.

Often individuals who have Hodgkin disease or non-Hodgkin lymphoma experience painless, swollen lymph nodes, loss of appetite, vomiting, bloating, abdominal pain, fullness (due to enlargement of the liver, spleen or abdominal lymph nodes), pain in the lower back, bone pain, constant coughing, and unexplained lethargy.

Early symptoms of myeloma are bone pain, particularly with movement, and infections involving the skin, the urinary tract, the bronchial tract, or lungs. These symptoms may also be accompanied by pallor resulting from anemia, weakness, and exaggerated fatigue.

Screening and diagnosis: Blood tests and specific bone marrow tests are needed to diagnose blood cancer; however, individuals in early stages of the disease may not have symptoms suggesting cancer. Current evidence does not suggest that routine blood screening before the onset of symptoms will detect cases of blood cancer and lead to improved medical outcomes or be cost effective in those at average risk of developing cancer according to their medical, family, and occupational history. The first

Estimated New Blood Cancer Cases and Deaths by Gender, 2007

	New Cases			Deaths		
Blood Cancer Type	*Men*	*Women*	*Total*	*Men*	*Women*	*Total*
Leukemias (all)	24,800	19,440	44,240	12,320	9,470	21,790
Acute myeloid leukemia	7,060	6,350	13,410	5,020	3,970	8,990
Chronic myeloid leukemia	2,570	2,000	4,570	240	250	490
Acute lymphocytic leukemia	3,060	2,140	5,200	820	600	1,420
Chronic lymphocytic leukemia	8,960	6,380	15,340	2,560	1,940	4,500
Other leukemias	3,150	2,570	5,720	3,680	2,710	6,390
Lymphomas (all)	38,670	32,710	71,380	10,370	9,360	19,730
Hodgkin disease	4,470	3,720	8,190	770	300	1,070
Non-Hodgkin lymphoma	34,200	28,990	63,190	9,600	9,060	18,660
Multiple myeloma	10,960	8,940	19,900	5,550	5,240	10,790

Source: Data from American Cancer Society, *Cancer Facts and Figures 2007* (Atlanta: Author, 2007)

indication that a person has blood cancer may be the results of a blood test performed as part of an annual physical. The blood sample may reveal anemia or changes in white blood cells, a possible indicator of leukemia. If an individual has symptoms that suggest blood cancer, the physician will take a medical history and check for swelling of the liver, spleen, or lymph nodes in the armpits, groin, or neck. Urinalysis will also be performed to detect substances or cellular material in the urine. Other tests include a blood test to assess blood cell count, a cytogenetic exam to analyze the number and shape of chromosomes to check for genetic abnormalities, a bone marrow aspirate to check for cancerous cells in liquid bone marrow, and a bone marrow biopsy to check for cancerous cells in the bone specimen. If cancerous cells are present, additional tests may be ordered to ascertain if the disease has spread and to organs or systems. These tests include tumor-marker tests (immunophenotyping, based on the type of antigen or marker on the surface of the cell), a spinal tap or lumbar puncture to obtain a sample of cerebrospinal fluid, chest X rays (for signs of infection or lymph node involvement), or ultrasound scans.

Staging is used to assess the extent or severity of the disease, to plan treatment, and to predict the outcome or prognosis. Classification of each type of blood cancer into stages is based on the site that is affected, the progression of the disease, and the appearance of the affected cells. For example, CLL is staged according to the risk-based Rai classification system using symptoms such as blood lymphocyte count, presence of enlarged lymph nodes or organs, platelet count, and anemia. Other forms of leukemia, such as acute leukemia, are not staged because of acute onset, which typically means the cancer has spread to other organs at the time of diagnosis.

Although leukemic cancerous cells circulate in the blood and bone marrow, in lymphomas cells form tumors in lymphatic tissue. The Ann Arbor staging system is used for staging both Hodgkin disease and non-Hodgkin lymphomas on the basis of specificity of site of lymph node involvement. The TNM (tumor/lymph node/metastasis) system may be used to stage the size of a tumor, lymph node involvement, and existence or extent of spread through other parts of the body. The International Staging System (ISS) is used for staging multiple myelomas based on blood tests for two proteins, albumin and beta-microglobulin, which are markers for the disease.

Treatment and therapy: Blood cancers are typically treated with one or more of the following: chemotherapy, radiation therapy, stem cell transplantation, and immunotherapy. A treatment plan is created using an anticancer agent such as chemotherapy, sometimes in combination with radiation therapy. The goal of chemotherapy, drugs given in combination and via different methods of delivery, is to destroy cancerous cells or to stop them from growing and multiplying, producing long-term remission or a cure. Radiation may be used to treat localized cancers such as lymphomas and certain types of leukemia, or it may be used to relieve symptoms when cancerous growths cause pain or pressure on bones, nerves, or organs. However, chemotherapy and radiation therapy can cause long-term or late effects, affecting fertility or growth and causing learning disabilities or illnesses secondary to the primary cancer such as leukemia.

Chemotherapy doses considered tolerable by most patients may not be sufficient to arrest, cause remission in, or cure acute leukemia, myeloma, or lymphoma. In patients who may be at high risk of relapse, who relapse after a successful course of treatment, or who do not respond as expected to conventional treatment, stem cell transplantation (transplanting cells from which blood cells and immune cells arise) can enable production of normal blood cells such that intensive chemotherapy can bring about recovery. Immune treatments (using antibodies from the patient or a donor) may be used alone or in combination with other therapies to attack cells that remain after chemotherapy and that may attach to antigens on the malignant cells. They also are used as vaccines to suppress malignant cells that remain in the body following therapy. New chemotherapies, immunotherapies, vaccines, gene therapies, and types of bone marrow transplants to suppress the growth of cancerous cells and affect the course of the disease are always being developed and tested. Patients need to be reminded that pain and uncomfortable symptoms arising from the toxic effects of cancer treatments can be managed by consulting with their physicians. Supportive care to improve functioning and quality of life, transfusions, antibiotics to protect against infection, and a healthy diet and lifestyle are critical for those undergoing cancer treatment.

Prognosis, prevention, and outcomes: Many factors affect the outcome of a patient's blood cancer, including the type, location, and stage of disease as well as individual and demographic factors such as the person's general health, age, and response to treatment. A cancer survivor will undergo follow-up care, which includes frequent monitoring of blood counts, X rays, urine tests, imaging tests such as computed tomography (CT) or positron emission tomograph (PET) scans. Those whose remission lasts five years are considered cured. Survival rates for those with blood cancer have been rising since 1975 and the advent of more effective cancer treatments, according to the NCI's *Cancer Trend Report 2005 Update*. No specific guidelines for preventing blood cancer exist, as its causes are not known and many types are relatively rare. Limiting exposure to environmental toxins and leading healthy lifestyles may help prevent blood cancers in those of average risk. The relative overall five-year survival rate of leukemia between 1996 and 2003 was nearly 50 percent, a survival rate that has more than tripled in patients diagnosed with leukemia since 1947. Relative survival rates vary by age of diagnosis, race, gender, and type of leukemia. Of all types of leukemia, those with CLL had the highest relative survival rate during this period, with 75.8 percent surviving.

Hodgkin disease is considered one of the most curable cancers, with many patients cured after their initial treatment. The five-year survival rate has increased dramatically since the 1960's, reaching 86 percent of patients of all races who were diagnosed with the disease between 1996 and 2003. Similarly, due to advances in treatment of non-Hodgkin lymphoma, the mortality rate has declined considerably since the 1980's.

Susan H. Peterman, M.P.H.

For Further Information

Adler, Elizabeth M. *Living with Lymphoma: A Patient's Guide*. Baltimore: Johns Hopkins University Press, 2005.

Hoffman, Barbara, ed. *A Cancer Survivor's Almanac: Charting Your Journey*. Minneapolis: National Coalition for Cancer Survivorship, 1996.

Mauch, Peter M., et al., eds. *Hodgkin's Disease*. Philadelphia: Lippincott Williams & Wilkins, 1999.

Wiernik, Peter Harris, ed. *Neoplastic Diseases of the Blood*. 4th ed. New York: Cambridge University Press, 2003.

Other Resources

American Cancer Society
http://www.cancer.org

International Myeloma Foundation
http://www.myeloma.org

The Leukemia and Lymphoma Society
http://www.leukemia-lymphoma.org

Memorial Sloan-Kettering Cancer Center
http://www.mskcc.org

National Cancer Institute
http://www.cancer.gov

See also: Acute Lymphocytic Leukemia (ALL); Acute Myelocytic Leukemia (AML); Aleukemia; Amyloidosis; Anemia; Aplastic anemia; Bone marrow aspiration and biopsy; Bone Marrow Transplantation (BMT); Burkitt lymphoma; Chronic Lymphocytic Leukemia (CLL); Chronic Myeloid Leukemia (CML); Cutaneous T-Cell Lymphoma (CTCL); Disseminated Intravascular Coagulation (DIC); Down syndrome and leukemia; Eosinophilic leukemia; Fanconi anemia; 5Q minus syndrome; Hairy cell leukemia; Hemolytic anemia; Hodgkin disease; Human T-Cell Leukemia

Virus (HTLV); Hypercalcemia; Leukemias; Leukopenia; Leukoplakia; Lymphocytosis; Lymphomas; Multiple myeloma; Myelodysplastic syndromes; Myelofibrosis; Myeloma; Myeloproliferative disorders; Myelosuppression; Neutropenia; Pheresis; Polycythemia vera; Richter syndrome; Sézary syndrome; Stem cell transplantation; Superior vena cava syndrome; Thrombocytopenia; Thymomas; Thymus cancer; Transfusion therapy; Umbilical cord blood transplantation; Waldenström Macroglobulinemia (WM)

▶ Bone cancers

Category: Diseases, Symptoms, and Conditions
Also known as: Osteosarcoma, osteogenic sarcoma, bone tumor

Related conditions: Li-Fraumeni syndrome, Gardner syndrome, retinoblastoma, leukemia, human immunodeficiency virus (HIV) infection

Definition: Bone cancers are malignant, unregulated proliferation of neoplasia (new tissue growth) in bone cells. The most common type of bone cancer is osteosarcoma, a highly malignant tumor composed of cells derived from growing connective tissue cells of bone. Osteochondromas are the most common cancerous primary bone tumors, with giant cell tumors developing in the thighbone near the knee. Ewing sarcoma is the second most common form of childhood bone cancer and is found mostly in the extremities. Chondrosarcomas are cancerous bone tumors that appear in the cartilage of bone in middle age. Other rare sarcomas are parosteal osteosarcomas involving both the bone and membranous covering, fibrosarcomas originating in the ends of bones in the arm or leg and then spreading to soft tissue, and chordomas that develop on the skull or spinal cord. Multiple myeloma is a hematologic cancer that frequently causes bone tumors.

Risk factors: The exact cause of osteosarcoma is not known, but inherited or acquired deoxyribonucleic acid (DNA) mutations are the suggested causes. Risk factors include the presence of a benign bone disease; previous treatment with radiation for another cancer, especially at a young age; teenage growth spurts; and disproportionate tallness with age. Certain rare, inherited cancers are also risk factors, such as Gardner syndrome, Li-Fraumeni syndrome (a rare family predisposition to multiple types of cancers caused by a mutation in a cancer-suppressing gene), and retinoblastoma (a malignant tumor of the retina that usually occurs in children younger than five years old). Studies suggest that occupational exposure to wood preservatives and certain herbicides increases the risk of developing soft-tissue sarcomas.

Suggested risk factors for myeloma bone disease include age (it rarely occurs under the age of forty), family history, smoking, exposure to petroleum and other chemicals, and exposure to high amounts of radiation. Atomic radiation from nuclear explosions and high-dose exposure to ionizing radiation are known to be risk factors for bone cancer but on a small scale. Virus infections make relatively minor contributions to human bone cancer, except the human immunodeficiency virus (HIV), which causes sarcoma.

Etiology and the disease process: Bone cancers are among the class of mesenchymal cancers that originate from the mesenchyme (bone and other tissues derived from embryonic mesoderm). Abnormal or partially differentiated cells develop in the bone marrow and can enter the general circulation and ultimately cause leukemia. (Leukemia can also result from blocked hemopoietic cell differentiation that causes abnormal cells to accumulate in bone marrow.) Initial mutation in a gene linked to DNA repair will cause other mutations to arise and spread more rapidly. Bone cancers usually develop rapidly and metastasize through the lymph channels of the body. Metastatic tumors frequently involve the axial more than the appendicular skeleton.

Malignant primary bone tumors originate in hard bone, in the soft tissue of blood vessels and nerves, or in tissues containing muscles, fat, or fiber. Osteosarcomas can grow quickly along the edge or end of a fast-growing long bone of the arms or legs, sometimes affecting the pelvis, shoulder, and skull. Osteosarcoma may metastasize into nearby tissues of the foot, tendons, and muscles, or spread through the bloodstream to other organs or bones in the body.

Ewing sarcoma originates from immature nerve tissue in the bone marrow of the leg, hips, ribs, and arms, but it is mostly found in the extremities, rapidly infiltrating the lungs and metastasizing to other bones, kidneys, heart, adrenal glands, and other soft tissues.

Chondrosarcomas usually originate in cartilage in ribs, legs, or hip bones. These grow slowly and take years to spread to other parts of the body.

Incidence: In the United States, about 2,400 cases of cancers of bones and joints are reported annually. The American Cancer Society in 2004 reported incidence rates in the United States to be approximately 1 in 113,333 people, or 2,400 people. In 2005, 2,570 new cases of bone and joint cancer were reported, along with 1,210 deaths.

Osteosarcoma and Ewing sarcoma occur mostly in children, adolescents, and young adults, accounting for 10 to 15 percent of all childhood bone cancers but constituting only 1 percent of all cancers. Most other types of bone cancers are usually found only in adults.

Osteosarcoma occurs slightly more often in male than female children and youths, usually between the ages of ten and twenty, and represents one-fifth of all bone tumors. Approximately 900 new cases of osteosarcoma are reported each year in the United States.

Ewing sarcoma occurs in 0.6 in one million people in the United States, more often in male than female children and youths between the ages of ten and twenty, and accounts for 16 percent of bone cancers.

Chronic leukemia, resulting from bone marrow cancer, is the most common form of leukemia and is twice as common in men as in women. It is ten times more common in adults than in children but accounts for 75 percent of childhood leukemias, with a five-year survival rate of 80 percent.

Genetic association crops up with bone cancer but scarcely accounts for more than 10 percent of cancers.

Symptoms: Pain is the most common symptom of bone cancer, associated with weakened bones and fractures. Symptoms may include swelling around the affected site, increased pain with activity or lifting, limping, and decreased movement of the affected limb. The soft bone tissues grow very large and push aside normal tissue. The initial symptom is usually a painless lump or swelling, which later becomes sore and painful as it presses against nearby nerves and tissues.

Symptoms of Ewing sarcoma include pain, swelling and redness around the site of the tumor, typical small round blue cells, fatigue, fever, paralysis and incontinence (if the tumor is in the spinal region), numbness, tingling, weight loss, and decreased appetite.

The symptoms for myeloma bone disease are pain, constipation, nausea, vomiting, fractures in bones, weakness or numbness in legs, weight loss, weakness, fatigue, repeated infections, and problems with urination.

Screening and diagnosis: In addition to a complete medical history and physical examination, diagnostic procedures for bone cancers such as osteosarcoma and Ewing sarcoma may include multiple imaging studies, such as X rays, of the tumor and sites of possible metastasis. Osteosarcomas are classified according to subtypes and grades determined by X rays and histological analysis:

- Low grade: intraosseous low grade, parosteal
- Intermediate grade: periosteal
- High grade: conventional, telangiectatic, central, small cell, high-grade surface

Age at Death for Cancer of the Bones and Joints, 2001-2005

Age Group	*Deaths (%)*
Under 20	14.8
20-34	14.3
35-44	7.1
45-54	9.5
55-64	11.5
65-74	13.7
75-84	18.3
85 and older	10.7

Source: Data from National Cancer Institute, Surveillance Epidemiology and End Results, Cancer Stat Fact Sheets, 2008

Note: The median age at death from 2001 to 2005 was fiftyeight, with an age-adjusted death rate of 0.4 per 100,000 men and women.

A radionuclide bone scan is used to determine the cause of pain or inflammation to rule out any infection or fractures. Magnetic resonance imaging (MRI) is done to rule out any associated abnormalities of the spinal cord and nerves. A computed tomography (CT) scan provides more detailed images than general X rays. A complete blood count (CBC) measures the size, number, and maturity of different blood cells in a specific volume of blood, and urine and blood tests (including blood chemistries) are also used for diagnosis.

A biopsy is performed on a tissue specimen to determine if cancer or other abnormal cells are present and to determine other courses of action. Myeloma bone disease is additionally diagnosed with aspiration (an examination of a small amount of bone marrow fluid). Cell sorting devices can identify the number of proliferation cells or ploidy status of the nuclear DNA. Chemical proteins (serving as antigens) detected by specific antibodies provide information on the state of cancer cells. Polymerase chain reaction (PCR) kits, which amplify and detect altered DNA base sequences in minute samples of cells, provide additional tumor markers. They make it possible to diagnose cancer types that are difficult to categorize by conventional pathology. Screening of serum sample glycoprotein antigens in the general circulation reveals undetected cancer, and monitors established cancer.

Treatment and therapy: Treatment of bone tumors depends on the type of tumor. Treatment is more likely to succeed if fewer cancer cells exist at the beginning of treatment. If the cancer has metastasized, chemotherapy or radiotherapy is used. Chemotherapy is used as a primary therapy or as an addition to other types of treatment and is the main method for treating advanced bone cancer. Typical drugs used are ifosfamide, cisplatin, methotrexate, and doxorubicin, plus some natural products. Drugs are more effective when used in combination.

Treatment of osteosarcoma and Ewing sarcoma may include surgery (biopsy, bone/skin grafts, reconstructions, resections, limb salvage procedures), amputation, prosthesis fitting and training, rehabilitation including physical and occupational therapy, psychosocial adapting, supportive care (for the side effects of treatment), antibiotics (to prevent and treat infections), and continued follow-up care (to determine response to treatment, detect recurrent disease, and manage the side effects of treatment).

Treatment of osteosarcoma depends on the subtype and grade of the tumor. Low-grade tumors are surgically removed and usually not treated with chemotherapy. Intermediate-grade tumors are treated with both surgery and chemotherapy. High-grade tumors consist of immature cells, which require aggressive chemotherapy. Most osteosarcomas do not respond to radiation therapy.

Treatment of myeloma bone disease includes radiation therapy and medications (to control pain), chemotherapy, fracture treatment, bone marrow transplantation, and alpha interferon for immunotherapy.

The most common treatment for soft-tissue sarcomas is surgical removal of the tumor, followed by radiation, chemotherapy, or both. Photodynamic therapy involves laser activation of sensitive compounds that generate free radicals.

Dietary adjustments, massage, reflexology, acupuncture, and relaxation techniques can relieve pain, anxiety, tension, and depression. Regular exercise provides physical strength and also reduces mental and emotional stress.

Prognosis, prevention, and outcomes: Prognosis for bone cancers involves predictions of the rate of growth, the likelihood of the cancer to metastasize, the most effective drug or treatment procedure, and the patient's needs. Prognosis for osteogenic, Ewing, and other sarcomas greatly depends on the extent of the disease; the size and location of the tumor; presence or absence of metastasis; the tumor's response to therapy; the patient's age, overall health, and tolerance of specific medications, procedures, and therapies; and continuous follow-up care for the side effects of radiation and chemotherapy as well as secondary malignancies that could occur.

Prompt medical attention and aggressive therapy are important for the best prognosis. Five-year event-free survival is expected for 85 percent of patients whose low-grade osteosarcoma tumors are surgically removed without chemotherapy and for 75 percent of patients with high-grade tumors requiring aggressive chemotherapy. About 50 percent of patients without metastatic Ewing sarcoma may have long-term disease-free survival.

The five-year survival rate for sarcomas is about 90 percent if the cancer is discovered before spreading and less than 30 percent for sarcomas that have already metastasized at the time of diagnosis. Since sarcomas arise from chemical reactions within cells, chemoprevention (with minimal side effects) would presumably curb cancer. New legal requirements for carcinogen testing minimize the hazards associated with industrial products; carcinogens cause less than 1 percent of cancers in developed countries. Nevertheless, cancer is still the second highest cause of death in the Western world, suggesting the need for more research and effective controls.

Lifestyle modifications for bone cancer prevention include diet management, control of food additive use, tobacco avoidance, regulation of reproductive factors such as contraception, reduction of alcohol consumption, screening for early detection of cancer, and appropriate use and disposal of industrial products.

Samuel V. A. Kisseadoo, Ph.D.

For Further Information

Beers, Mark H., ed. *The Merck Manual of Medical Information.* 2d ed. Whitehouse Station, N. J.: Merck Publishing, 2003.

King, Roger J. B., and Mike W. Robins. *Cancer Biology.* 3d ed. New York: Pearson/Prentice Hall, 2006.

O'Neill, Catherine E., ed. *New Developments in Bone Cancer Research.* New York: Nova Biomedical Books, 2006.

Pappo, A. S., ed. *Pediatric Bone and Soft Tissue Sarcomas.* New York: Springer, 2005.

Singh, Gurmit, and Shafaat A. Rabbani, eds. *Bone Metastasis.* Totowa, N.J.: Humana, 2005.

Other Resources

American Cancer Society
http://www.cancer.org

Free Health Encyclopedia
Bone Cancers
http://www.faqs.org/health/topics/75/Bone-cancers.html

Spectrum Health
http://www.spectrum-health.org

See also: Amputation; Bone scan; Childhood cancers; Ewing sarcoma; Fibrosarcomas, soft-tissue; Giant Cell Tumors (GCTs); Laryngeal cancer; Li-Fraumeni Syndrome (LFS); Limb salvage; Metastasis; Nasal cavity and paranasal sinus cancers; Nuclear medicine scan; Orthopedic surgery; Paget disease of bone; Rothmund-Thomson syndrome; Sarcomas, soft-tissue; Simian virus 40; Spinal axis tumors; Uterine cancer; Veterinary oncology; Young adult cancers

▶ Bone pain

Category: Diseases, Symptoms, and Conditions
Also known as: Skeletal pain

Related conditions: Bone metastasis, fracture

Definition: Bone pain is an uncomfortable response to disease, infection, inflammation, or trauma to bone.

Risk factors: Those at greatest risk for bone pain not caused by fracture or other trauma are those with bone disease, including bone cancers.

Etiology and the disease process: Bone pain in cancer may be caused by tumors in or near bones or conditions that cause damage within the bone, such as multiple myeloma. Cancer that spreads, or metastasizes, to bone from another part of the body can result in bone pain. Medications given to stimulate the production of blood cells in the bone marrow may cause temporary bone pain.

Incidence: Bone pain is experienced in more than half the cases of bone metastasis. There is a higher incidence in patients with advanced disease, particularly in those with breast and prostate cancers.

Symptoms: Symptoms include limited mobility, swelling in the area of pain, fatigue, and lack of appetite. Loss of height is associated with bone compression in the vertebrae. Burning or tingling sensations may indicate nerve involvement. Fracture, a late sign of advanced disease, is another source of pain.

Screening and diagnosis: Bone lesions are detected on X rays, positron emission tomography (PET) and computed tomography (CT) scans, and magnetic resonance imaging (MRI). A biopsy is necessary to determine if cancer has spread to the bone. The level of pain is assessed using a variety of scales. A commonly used scale uses a zero to ten rating, where zero correlates with no pain and ten with the worst possible pain. Other evaluations are employed to describe the type and quality of pain.

Treatment and therapy: Chemotherapy and radiation alleviate or diminish pain by reducing tumor size. Bone pain is managed with medications, including nonsteroidal anti-inflammatory drugs (NSAIDs), steroids, muscle relaxants, opioids, antidepressants, and antianxiety drugs. Nonpharmaceutical interventions used alone or in conjunction with medication can be effective. Examples include physical therapy, exercise, acupuncture, aromatherapy, biofeedback, breathing exercises, hypnosis, massage, and nerve stimulation. Surgery may be necessary to stabilize weakened bones with rods or special cements.

Prognosis, prevention, and outcomes: Prognosis depends on the ability to treat the underlying cause of the pain. An increase in bone pain may indicate disease progression that can lead to serious injury, including fracture, loss of bladder and bowel control, and paralysis. Chronic bone pain can be effectively managed to maximize functionality and quality of life in cases in which it cannot be completely eradicated.

Linda August Vrooman, R.N., B.S.N., O.C.N.

See also: Acute Lymphocytic Leukemia (ALL); Amputation; Blood cancers; Bone cancers; Bone scan; Chronic Lymphocytic Leukemia (CLL); Chronic Myeloid leukemia (CML); Limb salvage; Multiple myeloma; Myelofibrosis; Myeloma; Neuroblastomas; Neuroectodermal tumors; Orthopedic surgery; Paget disease of bone; Pain management medications; Radiopharmaceuticals; Waldenström Macroglobulinemia (WM); Young adult cancers

▶ Bowen disease

Category: Diseases, Symptoms, and Conditions
Also known as: Bowen's disease, squamous cell carcinoma in situ

Related conditions: Squamous cell carcinoma (SCC), Bowenoid papulosis, erythroplasia of Queyrat

Definition: Bowen disease refers to a type of skin cancer considered squamous cell in situ, named after John Bowen, who documented it in 1912. It may arise anywhere on the skin or the mucous membranes. Bowen disease of the glans penis is called erythroplasia of Queyrat. Unlike other premalignant cancers, Bowen disease possesses a low potential for progression to invasive SCC (less than 5 percent) and an even lower potential for metastasis. Another characteristic feature of Bowen disease is its greater propensity to spread over skin than to invade deeper skin layers. Although its malignant potential is low, extensive skin damage can result from delays in treatment.

Risk factors: Repeated exposure to the sun and exposure to the human papillomavirus (HPV), particularly HPV 16, and to arsenic have been implicated as risk factors for Bowen disease. However, more often than not, no risk factor can account for disease development.

Etiology and the disease process: Bowen disease originates from the overproliferation of squamous cells, the flat superficial cells that make up the upper layer of the skin (epidermis). The entire epidermal layer is involved in Bowen disease. Triggers of this overproliferation include ultraviolet light from chronic sun exposure and exposure to HPV 16. Both can damage or alter cellular deoxyribonucleic acid (DNA) and the cellular controls regulating cell division. The *TP53* gene is particularly susceptible to ultraviolet light damage and has been implicated as one of many possible mechanisms of cancer proliferation apart from Bowen disease. Arsenic has been hypothesized to enhance the carcinogenic properties of ultraviolet irradiation, as it has a propensity to accumulate in the skin as well as the lungs, bladder, kidney and liver.

Incidence: The incidence of Bowen disease has been estimated to range from 14 to 142 cases per 100,000. There is also a predilection for whites as well as older adults.

Symptoms: Bowen disease manifests in an insidious manner and often mimics other diseases before being diagnosed. It often appears as a reddish, nonpigmented, raised, and scaly lesion that gradually enlarges. The lesion is easily identifiable as it is well demarcated from surrounding normal skin. The most common sites are the head, neck, and extremities, although any part of the skin or mucous membrane may be affected. As the lesion enlarges, it thickens and starts to exhibit crusting, fissures, or ulcers. These lesions are usually solitary unless malignancy is present. Nonetheless, a full skin examination is warranted.

Screening and diagnosis: Bowen disease can easily be mistaken for other skin cancers such as invasive SCC and basal cell carcinoma. Therefore, a punch or shave biopsy of the lesion is essential to initiate appropriate treatment irrespective of location. The sample must include the full thickness of the epidermis and, as much as possible, hair structures in deeper layers. Staging of Bowen disease as a squamous cell carcinoma is not applicable unless invasion of the underlying dermis is seen during microscopic examination. Apart from routine skin examinations as part of a regular physical examination, there are no formal screening tests for Bowen disease.

Treatment and therapy: Medical and surgical treatments are available, although the latter are preferred. Medical treatment consists of topical treatment with either 5-fluorouracil (5-FU) or imiquimod 5 percent cream. 5-FU is used on the lesion after keratolytic therapy (controlled chemical breakdown) or cryotherapy (freezing). Iontophoresis can also be used to deliver the drug by inducing a drug "gradient" within the lesion. In women, 5-FU must not be taken during pregnancy. Radiotherapy using X rays or grenz rays is reserved for patients who cannot undergo surgery or those with multiple lesions. Lesions may also be treated with photodynamic therapy, in which a chemical agent increases photosensitivity only within tumor cells. This microenvironment is then exposed to a specific wavelength of light, which causes local toxin and oxygen radical release and immune system activation, leading to tumor cell death.

There are many surgical options including excision of both the lesion and a small margin (4 millimeters) of normal tissue, Mohs micrographic surgery, curettage and electrodesiccation, cryotherapy, and carbon dioxide laser ablation. Simple excision is preferred for small lesions in nonproblematic areas where deformities can be easily corrected. Mohs micrographic surgery, which is a very precise procedure also used in removing other skin cancers, is more suited to removing larger or recurring lesions and in areas where skin conservation is required for cosmetic reasons or functional preservation (for example, the face or joints). Curettage and electrodesiccation, cryotherapy, and carbon dioxide laser ablation are also effective treatments but do not provide pathologic specimens to confirm tumor eradication, particularly with deeper-lying lesions.

Prognosis, prevention, and outcomes: The overall prognosis of patients after treatment is excellent. Recurrence is often associated with inadequate removal of the lesion or malignant transformation and spread. Some of the sequelae of treatment include skin deformity, scarring, infection, and underlying damage to blood vessels and nerves.

Prevention is aimed at decreasing unnecessary ultraviolet light exposure. This includes patient education regarding sun exposure and measures such as wearing protective clothing and sunscreen with an SPF of at least 15 and avoiding exposure to the sun between 10 A.M. and 4 P.M.

Aldo C. Dumlao, M.D.

For Further Information

Fossel, Michael B. *Cells, Aging, and Human Disease.* Oxford, England: Oxford University Press, 2004.

Gupta, Renu. *Skin-Care.* Delhi, India: Diamond Pocket Books, 2000.

McCally, Michael. *Life Support: The Environment and Human Health.* Cambridge, Mass.: MIT Press, 2003.

Other Resources

American Cancer Society

Treating Bowen Disease

http://www.cancer.org/docroot/CRI/content/CRI_2_4_4X_Treatment_of_bowens_disease_51.asp

American Osteopathic College of Dermatology

Bowen's Disease

http://www.aocd.org/skin/dermatologic_diseases/bowens_disease.html

See also: Complementary and alternative therapies; Penile cancer; Premalignancies; Skin cancers; Vulvar cancer

▶ Brain and central nervous system cancers

Category: Diseases, Symptoms, and Conditions

Also known as: Brain tumors, central nervous system (CNS) tumors, gliomas, glioblastomas, astrocytomas, meningiomas, neuromas

Related conditions: Seizures, psychiatric symptoms (including abnormal personality and behavioral characteristics), loss of memory and cognition

Definition: Brain and central nervous system cancers are masses of abnormal cells (malignant tumors) in the brain and central nervous system that grow rapidly and can invade surrounding normal tissue. Brain tumors are named for both the type of cell from which they arose and their location in the brain. For example, schwannomas are named after the Schwann cells, astrocytomas after astrocytes, oligodendrogliomas after oligodendrocytes, meningiomas after the meninges or brain membranes, and pinealoblastomas after the pineal gland. Exceptions are medulloblastomas, which are undifferentiated neuroectodermal tumors of the cerebellum, and central neuroblastomas, which affect the brain cortex. The naming system for pediatric brain tumors is still evolving and remains controversial.

Risk factors: Chemicals such as vinyl chlorides, aromatic hydrocarbons, and N-nitroso compounds in cigarettes; ionizing radiation; electromagnetic fields; and viral infections have been suggested as possible environmental risk factors. Some brain cancers appear to be more common in people working with radiation and chemicals, such as employees of nuclear plants and oil refineries. However, none of these environmental factors have been conclusively shown to cause brain cancer. Genetic risk factors include inherited diseases such as tuberous sclerosis and von Hippel-Lindau disease.

Etiology and the disease process: The causes of brain and central nervous system cancers are still unproven. Environmental, genetic, medical, and lifestyle factors may all play a role in causing these cancers. Brain tumors can be primary or secondary. Primary tumors originate in the brain and are rarer than secondary brain tumors, accounting for around one-fourth of all brain tumors. Once they occur, primary brain tumors rarely metastasize to other tissues beyond the spinal cord. Examples of primary brain tumors are schwannomas, astrocytomas, medulloblastomas, meningiomas, and oligodendrogliomas. Secondary or metastatic tumors originate elsewhere in the body and migrate or metastasize to the brain. The types of cancer most likely to metastasize to the brain are breast cancer, lung cancer, melanoma, and colon cancer. Nasopharyngeal cancer can also metastasize to the brain via the cranial nerve or through openings in the bone at the base of the skull called foramina.

Incidence: The annual incidence of primary invasive central nervous system tumors in the United States is 6.6 per 100,000 people, with an estimated 4.7 deaths per 100,000 people annually. Approximately 20,500 new cases of brain and central nervous system cancers occurred in the United States in 2007, as well as an estimated 12,740 deaths from these cancers. Brain tumors account for 85 to 90 percent of all primary central nervous system tumors. Primary brain tumors have a higher incidence in whites than in blacks and are more common in men than in women, with three out of five sufferers being men. Brain tumors usually arise in early or middle adult life and are most common in people older than sixty-five. However, brain cancer can occur at any age.

Primary brain tumors are rarer than secondary brain tumors, with a ratio of 1 primary brain tumor to every 3 secondary brain tumors. Some experts put this ratio at closer to 1:10, attributing the increased detection of secondary tumors to more sensitive imaging methods. The most common primary brain tumors are astrocytomas, glioblastomas, meningiomas, and other mesenchymal tumors, which make up around 65 percent of all primary brain tumors. The most common primary spinal tumors are schwannomas, meningiomas, and ependymomas, accounting for 79 percent of primary spinal tumors.

Secondary or metastatic brain tumors occur in 20 to 40 percent of brain cancer patients. About 80 percent of secondary tumors occur in the cerebral hemispheres, 15 percent in the cerebellum, and 5 percent in the brain stem. Multiple metastases to the brain are more common than solitary metastases, occurring in more than 70 percent of cases.

Symptoms: Symptoms of brain tumors include persistent headaches that become more intense and frequent, seizures, problems walking and speaking, vision problems (including blurred vision, double vision, or loss of peripheral vision), loss of memory and cognition, personality or behavioral changes, abnormal breathing rates, dizziness, nausea or vomiting, loss of hearing, and hormonal disorders.

In one study of brain tumors and seizures, seizures were observed in more than 38 percent of patients with primary brain tumors and in 20 percent of patients with cerebral metastases. Oligodendrogliomas are more likely than other types of central nervous system tumors to be associated with seizures.

Screening and diagnosis: The first step of brain tumor screening involves a neurological exam to test vision, hearing, balance, coordination, and reflexes. If the neurological exam results warrant further testing, the doctor may order brain imaging scans, such as computed tomography (CT) and magnetic resonance imaging (MRI) scans, which produce pictures of the brain in which tumors can be distinguished by means of dyes or magnetic fields. Computed tomography is better at detecting bone calcification and skull lesions. Magnetic resonance imaging is better for detecting soft-tissue and spinal cord tumors. Other tests include an angiogram, in which a dye is injected into the blood to highlight the blood vessels in and around the brain, X-ray scans of the head and skull to reveal changes to skull bones and calcium deposits associated with brain tumors, and positron emission tomography (PET), which identifies areas of abnormal brain metabolism. The discovery of genetic mutations (changes in specific genes) that are linked to different types of cancers has opened the door to future genetic screening for at-risk individuals. A genetic screen involves taking a blood sample and analyzing the deoxyribonucleic acid (DNA) in the sample for genetic mutations that are known to cause a specific type of cancer.

When a tumor is detected on a brain scan, a biopsy is usually performed to make a diagnosis. A biopsy involves taking a sample of the tumor; this can be done in a separate procedure or during surgery to remove the tumor. The tumor can be biopsied by open craniotomy, in which the cranium or skull is opened to expose the brain, allowing a sample of the tumor to be surgically removed. Hard-to-reach tumors can be sampled by means of a needle biopsy. A small hole, known as the "burr" hole, is drilled in the cranium, and tumor cells are extracted with a narrow-bore needle. The tumor sample is frozen and cut into very thin slices, which are then examined under a microscope. This allows the medical team to confirm the presence of a tumor and determine the specific type of tumor. Additional tests may also be performed to help pinpoint the tumor type.

There is no standard method for staging brain tumors. Along with the tumor grade, the type of cell from which the tumor originated and the location in the central nervous system are used for classifying the tumor. Grade I tumors grow slowly and rarely spread to other tissues. The following types of brain tumors are classified as Grade I: pilocytic astrocytomas, Grade I meningiomas, and Grade I ependymomas. Grade II tumors typically grow slowly but may spread to other tissues. Grade II tumors include diffuse astrocytomas, Grade II meningiomas, oligodendrogliomas, Grade II ependymomas, oligoastrocytomas (made up of a mixture of oligodendrogliomal and astrocytomal cells), pinealcytomas, and craniopharyngiomas. Grade III tumors contain fast-growing cells that often spread to other tissues. Grade III tumors include anaplastic astrocytomas, anaplastic oligodendrogliomas, anaplastic ependymomas, anaplastic oligoastrocytomas, and pinealoblastomas. Grade IV tumors grow rapidly, spread aggressively, and contain cells that appear very different from normal cells. Grade IV tumors include gliobastomas and medulloblastomas, which usually occur in children and adults aged twenty-one to forty.

Treatment and therapy: The most common treatment for brain and central nervous system cancers involves surgery to remove as much of the tumor as possible without disrupting neurological function. Surgery usually does

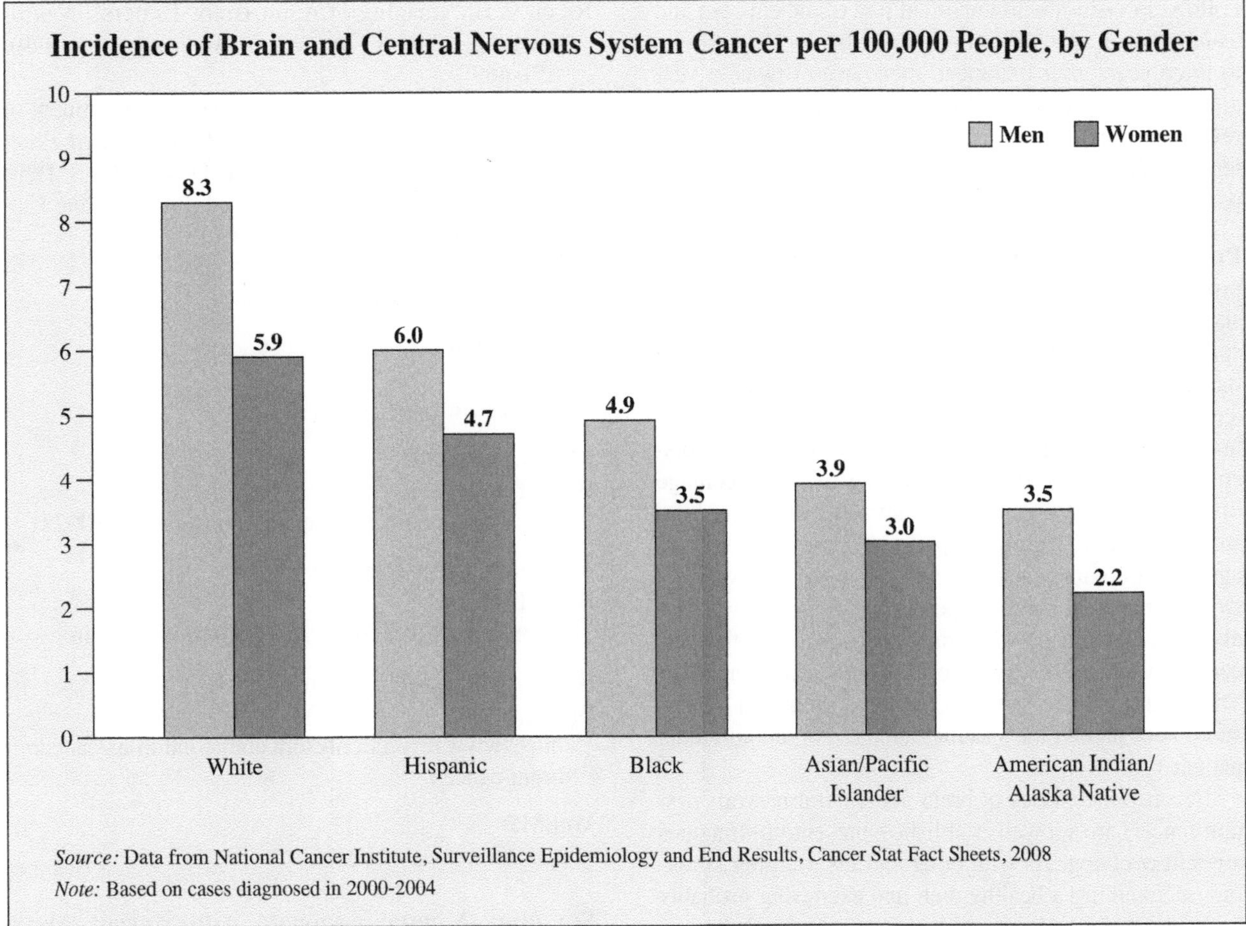

Source: Data from National Cancer Institute, Surveillance Epidemiology and End Results, Cancer Stat Fact Sheets, 2008
Note: Based on cases diagnosed in 2000-2004

not result in the removal of all tumor tissue. In addition, some tumors are located deep in the brain and cannot be reached without considerable damage to the surrounding tissue. These tumors are sometimes diagnosed without conducting a biopsy and treated by nonsurgical means. Radiation treatment and chemotherapy can be used to remove cancer cells remaining after surgery and to treat deep-seated tumors that are not amenable to surgical removal. Radiation therapy is effective for a wider range of brain and spinal cord tumors than chemotherapy. Radiation can enhance the cure rate and prolong disease-free survival. A common type of radiation treatment is external beam radiation therapy (EBRT). Chemotherapy has been shown to prolong disease-free survival in patients with gliomas, medulloblastomas, and some germ-cell tumors. Chemotherapy includes the use of dexamethasone, mannitol, furosemide, and nitrosourea. Anticonvulsants are also used to treat cancer patients with seizures.

The majority of brain tumors are accompanied by multiple metastases. These can be treated with a combination of surgery or radiosurgery and whole-brain radiation therapy (WBRT). Radiosurgery is useful for lesions that have a diameter smaller than 3 centimeters. Corticosteroids and anticonvulsants can also be used as needed. Chemotherapy is not as widely used for metastatic brain tumors but may be effective for brain metastases from chemosensitive primary tumors.

New therapies that are currently being tested include the use of tyrosine kinase receptor inhibitors, farnesyl transferase inhibitors, viral-based gene therapy, and oncolytic viruses. Patients with tumors that do not respond well to the commonly used treatments can look into clinical trials using combinations of novel therapies with EBRT.

Surgery to remove brain tumors can sometimes result in the damage of normal brain tissue. This can cause partial paralysis, changes in sensation, muscle weakness, and defects in thinking and language function. These patients may be referred for physical and speech therapy to regain muscle and language functions, respectively.

Follow-up visits are an important part of patient care and usually occur every three to four months for the first two to three years after treatment, then once or twice a year after that. The doctor will discuss treatment side effects, review medical history, and conduct various tests to determine if the cancer has recurred or metastasized to other parts of the body.

Prognosis, prevention, and outcomes: A cancer patient's prognosis depends on age (whether younger or older than sixty), the number and location of tumors in the brain and spinal cord, the rate of tumor growth and metastasis, and the tumor's response to treatment. The prognosis is better for brain metastases from breast cancer and worse for brain metastases from colon cancer. When doctors discuss survival rates, they are referring to the percentage of people with a specific type and stage of cancer who survive for a predetermined period of time after their diagnosis. A common statistic is the five-year survival rate. Doctors may talk about the percentage of people who are alive, the percentage who are symptom-free, or the percentage who are disease-free five years after diagnosis. These numbers are averages for large groups of people and do not predict the specific outcome for an individual patient.

Because the causes of brain and central nervous system cancers are not well established, prevention strategies are still evolving. As with other cancers, quitting smoking, maintaining a healthy diet, and exercising probably have beneficial and preventive effects. A novel therapy that has been approved in Switzerland under the brand name DCVax-Brain involves vaccination with dendritic cells that recognize molecules on an individual patient's tumor cells.

When examining outcomes for brain cancer survivors, it is important to also consider their quality of life. A survivor's quality of life has been directly linked to cognitive impairment, especially defects in speech and language.

Ing-Wei Khor, Ph.D.

For Further Information

Connelly, J. M., and M. G. Malkin. "Environmental Risk Factors for Brain Tumors." *Current Neurology and Neuroscience Reports* 7 (2007): 208-214.

Hutter, A., et al. "Brain Neoplasms: Epidemiology, Diagnosis, and Prospects for Cost-Effective Imaging." *Neuroimaging Clinics of North America* 13 (2003): 237-250.

Ricci, P. E. "Imaging of Adult Brain Tumors." *Neuroimaging Clinics of North America* 9 (1999): 651-669.

Wen, P. Y., P. M. Black, and J. S. Loeffler. "Treatment of Metastatic Cancer." In *Cancer: Principles and Practice of Oncology*, edited by V. T. DeVita, Jr., S. Hellman, and S. A. Rosenberg. 6th ed. Philadelphia: Lippincott Williams & Wilkins, 2001.

Other Resources

Cedars-Sinai
Brain Tumors
http://www.csmc.edu/5192.html

MayoClinic.com
Brain Tumor
http://mayoclinic.com/health/brain-tumor/DS00281

National Cancer Institute
Brain Tumor
http://www.cancer.gov/cancertopics/types/brain

Revolution Health
Brain Cancer
http://www.revolutionhealth.com/conditions/cancer/brain-cancer/

WebMD
http://www.webmd.com

See also: Acoustic neuromas; Astrocytomas; Ataxia Telangiectasia (AT); Carcinomatous meningitis; Cell phones; Cognitive effects of cancer and chemotherapy; Craniotomy; Gliomas; Leptomeningeal carcinomas; Meningeal carcinomatosis; Meningiomas; Neuroblastomas; Neuroectodermal tumors; Neuroendocrine tumors; Neurofibromatosis type 1 (NF1); Neurologic oncology; Oligodendrogliomas; Orbit tumors; Pheochromocytomas; Primary central nervous system lymphomas; Schwannoma tumors; Spinal axis tumors; Spinal cord compression; Turcot syndrome; Von Hippel-Lindau (VHL) disease; Wilms' tumor Aniridia-Genitourinary anomalies-mental Retardation (WAGR) syndrome and cancer

▶ Breakthrough pain

Category: Diseases, Symptoms, and Conditions
Also known as: Episodic or incident pain

Related conditions: Breakthrough pain may be related to tumor progression or nerve compression as a result of cancer. It may also be a result of a treatment, including surgery, or a variety of painful disorders, such as arthritis.

Definition: Breakthrough pain is a transient and intermittent flare of severe pain that "breaks through" analgesic medications.

Risk factors: Anyone undergoing treatment for trauma, illness, and other painful conditions is at risk for breakthrough pain. Cancer patients—particularly those with advanced disease—are at high risk for breakthrough pain.

Etiology and the disease process: Breakthrough pain generally is the result of whatever is causing a patient's baseline persistent pain.

Incidence: Approximately one-half to two-thirds of cancer patients and up to 86 percent of people taking pain-reducing medication for chronic pain experience breakthrough pain. The frequency of breakthrough pain varies among individuals; most patients with cancer-related pain have several episodes daily. Often, breakthrough pain flares up just before the patient is to take the next dose of pain medication; this is termed end-of-dose failure.

Symptoms: The severity, duration, and cause of breakthrough cancer pain vary among patients. Typically, breakthrough pain happens fast. The average duration is approximately thirty minutes, but it may last from seconds to hours. Breakthrough pain is often unpredictable; it may occur spontaneously or it may be triggered by an activity, such as coughing or moving. It may manifest as an intensified or all-over dull sensation, or it may be a localized sharp pain.

Screening and diagnosis: There is no independently validated measurement available for the evaluation of breakthrough pain.

Treatment and therapy: Breakthrough pain medications are generally short-acting and work rapidly to control sudden flares of pain. Breakthrough pain medications may be administered in several ways: orally, by injection, intravenously, under the tongue (sublingually), rectally, or transmucosally. Traditionally, opioid derivatives, such as morphine, administered intravenously, have been one of the fastest ways to alleviate breakthrough pain. A patient-controlled analgesia device (PCA) allows for convenient intravenous administration of pain medication. One drug that specifically treats breakthrough pain is oral transmucosal fentanyl citrate. Fentanyl citrate dissolves rapidly (within five to ten minutes) via the mucous membranes. Cognitive techniques (including relaxation training, hypnosis, imagery, and distraction) and touch and music therapy may also help relieve breakthrough pain.

Prognosis, prevention, and outcomes: Breakthrough pain medications are often called rescue medicines and are taken only at the time of an episode. It is important to take rescue medications at the earliest signs of breakthrough pain, as it is harder to control pain when it is allowed to build up.

Anita Nagypál, Ph.D.

See also: Antinausea medications; Brief Pain Inventory (BPI); Pain management medications

▶ Breast cancers

Category: Diseases, Symptoms, and Conditions
Also known as: Metastatic breast cancer (MBC), ductal carcinoma in situ (DCIS), lobular carcinoma in situ (LCIS)

Related conditions: Intraductal papillomas, noncancerous adenomas (growths) of the breast tissue, cysts

Definition: Breast cancer is the occurrence of a malignant tumor in the breast tissue. The most commonly diagnosed breast tumors are ductal carcinoma in situ (DCIS) and lobular carcinoma in situ (LCIS). When discovered early, these tumors are easily treated. However, if gone undetected, the tumors can eventually metastasize, meaning that some of the cancer cells detach from the tumor and spread throughout the body, acting as "seeds" to trigger the further development of malignancy in distant body parts. Once metastatic breast cancer (MBC) forms, the cancer becomes much more difficult to treat.

Risk factors: Some risk factors have been established as very important for determining patients who would benefit from more careful preventative care and observation. However, the presence of one or more risk factors does not necessarily mean that the patient will actually develop a breast tumor. Conversely, up to 70 percent of women who develop breast cancer did not have any known risk factors before diagnosis.

Women who previously had a breast tumor in one breast have a significantly increased risk of developing cancer in the other breast. The cancer in the second breast

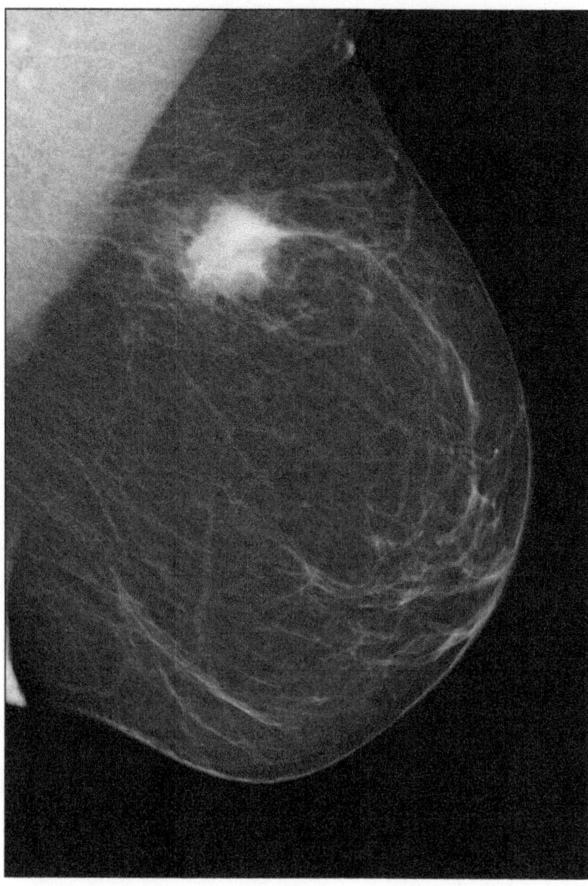

A mammogram showing a breast tumor. (iStock)

is considered unrelated and not a recurrence of the cancer in the first breast. Several factors are considered to moderately increase the risk of breast cancer in some women. As women age, they develop an increasing risk of developing breast cancer. For example, women between the ages of forty and forty-nine have a 1 in 68 risk of developing breast cancer; this risk nearly doubles to 1 in 37 for women between the ages of fifty and fifty-nine. Nearly half of women diagnosed with breast cancer are over sixty-five and postmenopausal. Mutations in two key genes, *BRCA1* and *BRCA2*, have also been associated with an increased risk of developing breast cancer. These genes are considered tumor suppressors, and mutations can lead to their dysfunction. These mutations seem to be inherited, and having a direct family relative with breast cancer also increases the risk of developing breast cancer. This is most true for first-degree relatives, such as a mother, sister, or daughter. One first-degree relative with breast cancer can nearly double the risk for an individual to develop breast cancer; two first-degree relatives with breast cancer causes the individual to be up to five times as likely to develop breast cancer.

Other factors have been shown to only slightly increase the risk of developing breast cancer. These include obesity and increased alcohol intake. Further, women who began to menstruate early (prior to age twelve), who enter into menopause late (after age fifty-five), or who never have children have a small increase in the chance of developing breast cancer. This is thought to be due to the increased exposure these women have to estrogen, a hormone that can increase breast cancer development.

Etiology and the disease process: One of the most commonly accepted models of breast cancer formation stems from the development of genetic aberrations in breast cells. Activated mutations in oncogenes, genes responsible for the growth and proliferation of cells, and inhibitory mutations in tumor-suppressor genes that negatively regulate cell growth play an instrumental role in cellular transformation. Cell transformation is the process by which a normal cell changes into a tumorigenic cell, capable of growing into a malignant mass. A breast tumor begins when one or more tumorigenic cells form within the epithelial layer, the internal tissue lining of the breast. As the tumor grows, it spreads past the epithelium, invading into the deeper tissues of the breast. If left untreated, the breast tumor will eventually metastasize, as the tumor cells break away from the primary tumor and are dispersed throughout the body via the circulatory system.

Breast cancers are primarily differentiated as hormone-receptor-positive or -negative. These receptors are the estrogen receptor (ER), progesterone receptor (PR), or both. The distinctions among these tumors are critical, as they are a major determinant in choosing the proper therapy. Both hormone receptors have a similar action: After either hormone binds to its respective receptor inside the cell, it subsequently transports into the nucleus, where it plays a major role in regulating gene expression.

Incidence: Breast cancer is one of the most frequently diagnosed cancers in women in the United States, with an estimated more than 175,000 new cases per year. Breast cancer development seems to be affected by race, with a higher incidence occurring in white and African American women compared with Hispanic, American Indian, and Asian American women. Breast cancer is second only to lung cancer in inducing cancer-related deaths in women, but it is the primary cause of cancer-related mortality in younger women, ages twenty to fifty-nine. Since the early 1990's, the incidence of breast cancer-related deaths has steadily decreased, a reduction most dramatically seen in younger white and African American women. The cause of this reduction is attributed to both improved anticancer therapy and earlier diagnostic abilities. The risk of a woman developing breast cancer at some point in her lifetime is nearly 1 in 8, or 13 percent. Although breast cancer most often occurs in women, it can rarely occur in men.

Symptoms: Early breast cancer is usually free of symptoms. The first sign of breast cancer is most often a persistent lump in the breast. As the tumor develops, the individual may begin to experience other symptoms, including swelling of the armpit or breast and thickening of the breast tissue. Patients may also notice slight pain or tenderness in the breast. Changes in how the nipple looks is also frequently observed with breast cancer.

Screening and diagnosis: A clinical breast exam is a common method to detect lumps or abnormal changes in the breast tissue. If a lump is detected, the clinician will assess the characteristics of the lump. Lumps that are soft, smooth, and round and move about easily are more likely to be benign, compared to hard, nonsymmetrical lumps that are tightly attached to the breast tissue, which are more likely to be cancerous. It is also recommended that women perform monthly breast self-examinations at home to detect changes between checkups. Subtle changes that may not register as a lump by touch can often be detected by mammograms, X-ray images taken of the breast. Further, many clinicians use mammograms to provide a more detailed look at lumps identified during an examination. Ultrasound and magnetic resonance imaging (MRI) can be used to directly image breast abnormalities. If a clinician feels that a certain breast abnormality warrants further investigation, a biopsy is performed to remove tissue that a pathologist can use to determine if any cancer is present.

At the time of first diagnosis, most patients are diagnosed either with early, localized breast cancer or regional breast cancer. Only a small minority of patients receive a primary diagnosis of metastatic breast cancer (MBC). Recurrent breast cancer is a malignancy that has returned after previously being treated to the point of not being detected. Recurrence may occur locally in or near the breast or in distant parts of the body, such as the bone, liver, or lungs.

Once a diagnosis is made, the stage of the breast cancer is determined. This is necessary for the physician to determine the extent of the disease and to prescribe the appropriate treatment. Stage 0 is described as in situ carcinoma. In situ carcinoma is noninvasive, meaning the cancer cells have not begun to spread beyond the epithelium, or tissue surface. The most common breast cancer of this stage is ductal carcinoma in situ (DCIS), in which cancerous cells develop within the milk ducts. Stage I is the earliest form of invasive breast cancer. At this point, the tumor is smaller than 2 centimeters (cm) in diameter and is confined to the breast. In Stage II, the tumor is either between 2 and 5 cm and has spread to the lymph nodes under the arm or is larger than 5 cm but has not spread outside the breast. Stage III is characterized by larger tumors that may have spread to lymph nodes and areas beyond the underarm, such as behind the breastbone or near the collarbone. Stage IV is the most advanced stage. At this point, the cancer is classified as distant metastatic cancer.

Stage at Diagnosis and Five-Year Relative Survival Rates for Women with Breast Cancer, 1996-2004

Stage	*Women Diagnosed (%)*	*Survival Rate (%)*
Localized[a]	61	98.0
Regional[b]	31	83.5
Distant[c]	6	26.7
Unstaged	2	56.9

Source: Data from National Cancer Institute, Surveillance Epidemiology and End Results, Cancer Stat Fact Sheets, 2008

[a]Cancer still confined to primary site

[b]Cancer has spread to regional lymph nodes or directly beyond the primary site

[c]Cancer has metastasized

Treatment and therapy: The main goals of breast cancer therapy are to eradicate the tumor and prevent its recurrence. Treatments can be categorized as either local or systemic, and the use of either or both is determined by the extent and stage of disease. Local therapies include surgery and radiation therapy. Surgery can be either minimal, such as a lumpectomy in which only the lump is removed, or more drastic, such as a mastectomy in which the majority of the breast is removed. If the breast cancer has spread to local lymph nodes, these also may be removed at the time of surgery. Surgery is often used in conjunction with other therapies, including radiation therapy and systemic drug therapy. Once the breast cancer has metastasized and become MBC, surgery is not a viable therapeutic option. For MBC, systemic therapy is generally the standard treatment and consists of three main categories: chemotherapy, endocrine therapy, and biological therapy.

The most effective chemotherapeutic agents for breast cancer are taxanes and anthracyclines, although other drug classes can be used. Despite the benefit these drugs can offer in lengthening patient survival, the accompanying toxic side effects can dramatically decrease the patient's quality of life. Endocrine therapy is the standard of care for hormone-receptor-positive breast cancer. The most common type of endocrine therapy is the selective estrogen receptor modulator (SERM) tamoxifen, which can reduce the proliferative effect that estrogens have in the breast tumor cells. Although tamoxifen is generally tolerated better than chemotherapies, there is a high risk for developing resistance, after which the drug loses its benefit. The newest addition to the breast cancer therapy arsenal is targeted biological therapy. The prototypical example of this in breast cancer is trastuzumab, an antibody that recognizes and inhibits the human epidermal growth factor receptor (HER2) present on the surface of the breast cancer cell. HER2 is an effective breast cancer target because it is often overactivated in breast cancer, increasing the proliferative signaling downstream of its activation.

Prognosis, prevention, and outcomes: The improvement of screening and diagnostic techniques has been instrumental in increasing the discovery of breast cancer early in development, when it is most easily treated. Additionally, the development of novel drugs and therapies has caused a significant increase in extending survival of breast cancer patients. Clinicians measure disease outcome by measuring survival rates; a disease-free survival of at least five years is generally considered to be a cure. Currently, the five-year survival rate for patients diagnosed with local breast cancer that has not spread beyond the breast is 98 percent. This survival rate is lowered to 83.5 percent in patients with regional metastasis. Patients with Stage IV metastatic breast cancer have a five-year survival rate of only 26.7 percent.

Much effort has gone into determining methods of preventing breast cancer. Because many breast tumors depend on estrogen for growth and survival, decreasing unnecessary estrogen exposure may help prevent breast cancer. Some women with an especially high risk of breast cancer may elect to have an oophorectomy, surgery to remove both ovaries, the primary source of estrogen in premenopausal women. Additionally, regular exercise may reduce the amount of estrogen naturally produced by the body, decreasing the amount of estrogen to which the breast is exposed. An extreme preventative measure in women with a high risk for developing breast cancer is prophylactic mastectomy, a surgical procedure to remove the breast before any signs of cancer.

Lisa M. Cockrell, B.S.

For Further Information

Bowcock, Anne M, ed. *Breast Cancer: Molecular Genetics, Pathogenesis, and Therapeutics*. Totowa, N.J.: Humana Press, 1999.

Craig, Jordan V., and Barrington J. A. Furr, eds. *Hormone Therapy in Breast and Prostate Cancer*. Totowa, N.J.: Humana Press, 1999.

Grobstein, Ruth H. *The Breast Cancer Book: What You Need to Know to Make Informed Decisions*. New Haven, Conn.: Yale University Press, 2005.

Kufe, Donald W., et al., eds. *Holland Frei Cancer Medicine 7*. 7th ed. Hamilton, Ont.: B. C. Decker, 2006.

Manni, Andrea, ed. *Endocrinology of Breast Cancer*. Totowa, N.J.: Humana Press, 1999.

Other Resources

American Cancer Society
http://www.cancer.org

National Breast Cancer Foundation
http://www.nationalbreastcancer.org

National Cancer Institute
Breast Cancer
http://www.cancer.gov/cancertopics/types/breast

Susan G. Komen for the Cure
http://www.komen.org

See also: Accelerated Partial Breast Irradiation (APBI); Adenocarcinomas; Aging and cancer; Antiestrogens; Antiperspirants and breast cancer; Birth control pills and cancer; Breast cancer in children and adolescents; Breast cancer in men; Breast cancer in pregnant women; Breast implants; Breast reconstruction; Breast ultrasound; Calcifications of the breast; Childbirth and cancer; Clinical Breast Exam (CBE); Cutaneous breast cancer; Diethylstilbestrol (DES); Duct ectasia; Ductal Carcinoma In Situ (DCIS); Ductal lavage; Ductogram; Estrogen-receptor-sensitive breast cancer; Fertility drugs and cancer; Fibroadenomas; Fibrocystic breast changes; Genetic counseling; Genetic testing; Hormone receptor tests; Hormone Replacement Therapy (HRT); Invasive ductal carcinomas; Invasive lobular carcinomas; Lobular

Carcinoma In Situ (LCIS); Lumpectomy; Lumps; Lymphadenectomy; Lymphangiography; Lymphangiosarcomas; Lymphedema; Mammography; Mastectomy; Medullary carcinoma of the breast; Metastasis; Microcalcifications; Needle localization; Obesity-associated cancers; Phyllodes tumors; Pregnancy and cancer; Premalignancies; Progesterone receptor assay; Tubular carcinomas; Wire localization

▶ Breast cancer in children and adolescents

Category: Diseases, Symptoms, and Conditions
Also known as: Phyllodes tumors

Related conditions: Adenocarcinoma

Definition: Breast cancer is a malignant tumor that originates from breast cells. Most breast masses in children and adolescents are benign rather than cancerous in nature. One study noted fewer than fifty documented cases of breast cancer in girls between the ages of three and nineteen. Of these cases, juvenile secretory carcinoma was the most common and responsible for more than 80 percent of cases. The second most common form of breast cancer was intraductal carcinoma.

Breast tumors called phyllodes tumors, although usually seen in women around forty-five years old, may occur in adolescents and have been reported in girls as young as ten years. These tumors may be benign, intermediate, or malignant. Another form of breast cancer in adolescents is primary breast carcinoma, which has been reported in girls between the ages of three and nineteen. However, in adolescents, most malignant breast masses are metastases from other cancers, such as Hodgkin disease, non-Hodgkin lymphoma, primary hepatocellular carcinoma, neuroblastoma, and rhabdomyosarcoma.

Average Incidence of Breast Cancer, 1975-2000

Age Group	*Incidence (per million people)*
15-19	1.3
20-24	12.1
25-29	81.1

Source: Data from A. Bleyer, M. O'Leary, R. Barr, and L. A. G. Ries, eds., *Cancer Epidemiology in Older Adolescents and Young Adults Fifteen to Twenty-Nine Years of Age, Including SEER Incidence and Survival: 1975-2000,* NIH Pub. No. 06-5767 (Bethesda, Md.: National Cancer Institute, 2006)

Risk factors: Risk factors for breast cancer in adolescents include having received chest-wall radiation and having a family history of breast cancer. If a child or adolescent receives radiation therapy to treat cancer of the chest area, the person's risk for developing breast cancer later in life is significantly higher. The younger radiation was initiated, the higher the risk. This is especially the case when radiation is given to girls whose breasts are developing.

Etiology and the disease process: Breast masses in children before and during puberty usually are breast buds. The development of breast buds in children is usually the first sign of puberty. The development of breast buds in children who are too young for puberty may indicate premature thelarche, or precocious puberty. Biopsy is warranted for cystic lesions that do not resolve with aspiration and for suspicious solid lesions.

Some cancers start in glandular tissue that basically produces and secretes a substance. The ducts and lobules of the breast are glandular tissue, and the cancers starting in these areas are sometimes called adenocarcinomas.

Incidence: Breast cancer in children and adolescents is rare. Generally, the lifetime probability of developing breast cancer is 1 in 6 overall, and 1 in 8 for invasive breast cancer. Globally, and in terms of all ages, breast cancer incidence rates are highest in North America and northern Europe, and lowest in Asia and Africa.

Symptoms: The most common finding with breast cancer in adolescents is a hard irregular mass and usually one that does not cause symptoms. As the cancer grows, symptoms may include a change of shape, size, and feel of the breast. Another symptom is bloody, yellow, or green, puslike drainage from the nipple. Advanced symptoms include bone or breast pain, swelling of the arm on the same side of the body as the breast with cancer, and weight loss. If metastasis occurs, other symptoms can include difficulty breathing, skin rash that is generalized, limb swelling, and back pain.

Screening and diagnosis: Because a mass may not produce symptoms in the initial stages, all adolescents, especially girls with a family history of breast cancer or other malignancies, should have their breasts clinically examined regularly and should conduct monthly self-examination. Ultrasonography is the preferred imaging modality for breast masses in adolescents because of the increased density of the adolescent breast. Also the large amount of fibroglandular tissue makes mammography difficult to interpret. The accuracy of ultrasonography in differentiating solid from cystic lesions is 96 to 100 percent. Research suggests that an evaluation is warranted if no breast development occurs by the age of thirteen.

The stage of breast cancer is based on tumor size; involvement of the skin, chest wall, or local lymph nodes; and whether the cancer has spread to other organs (metastasis). Stage I and Stage II are referred to as early stage or localized breast cancer. In Stage I the tumor size is less than 2 centimeters (cm) with no lymph node involvement. Stage II can exhibit lymph node involvement, but the nodes are small. The primary tumor size is larger than 2 cm but not larger than 5 cm. A tumor that is larger than 5 cm must be node-negative to be considered early stage.

Stage III breast cancers are referred to as locally advanced breast cancer. In this stage, the tumors are large and greater than 5 cm across. There can be extensive axillary nodal involvement or nodal involvement of the soft tissues above or below the collarbone. A tumor is also designated Stage III if it extends to underlying muscles of the chest wall or the overlying skin. In Stage III, the breast may be undergoing the inflammatory process and appear red and swollen.

Stage IV breast cancer, also known as metastatic breast cancer, consists of tumors that have spread to areas such as the brain, bones, skin, and even other organs. There may be any number of affected lymph nodes, and the primary tumor may be any size.

Treatment and therapy: The subsequent management of the adolescent with a breast mass depends on the type of mass. Surgical resection (excisional biopsy) may be necessary for cystic lesions that do not resolve with aspiration, when aspiration is not productive or not feasible, and for suspicious solid lesions. Although uncommon, more advanced forms of breast cancer have the potential to be treated similarly to the condition found in adults.

Prognosis, prevention, and outcomes: The five-year survival rate refers to the number of patients who live at least five years after their cancer is found. According to the American Cancer Society (ACS), the five-year survival rates for persons with breast cancer that is appropriately treated are 100 percent for Stage I, 81 to 92 percent for Stage II, 54 to 67 percent for Stage III, and 20 percent for Stage IV.

Jeffrey P. Larson, P.T., B.S., A.T.C.

For Further Information

American Joint Committee on Cancer. *AJCC Cancer Staging Manual.* 5th ed. Philadelphia: Lippincott-Raven, 1997.

Barry, Joanne. "Reaching Out to Educate." *Canadian Nurse* 103, no. 8 (October, 2007): 34-35.

Mandrell, B. N. "Secondary Breast Cancer in a Woman Treated for Hodgkin Lymphoma as a Child." *Oncology* 21 (October, 2007): 27-29.

Twombly, R. "Childhood Cancer Survivor Study Doubles to Examine Late Effects of New Treatments." *Journal of the National Cancer Institute* 99, no. 21 (November 7, 2007): 1574-1576.

Other Resources

National Cancer Institute
Breast Cancer
http://www.cancer.gov/cancertopics/types/breast

UpToDate
Overview of Breast Masses in Children and Adolescents
http://patients.uptodate.com/topic.asp?file=adol_med/11491

See also: Adenocarcinomas; Breast cancers; Breast Self-Examination (BSE); Calcifications of the breast; Childhood cancers; Clinical Breast Exam (CBE); Cutaneous breast cancer; Phyllodes tumors; Young adult cancers

▶ Breast cancer in men

Category: Diseases, Symptoms, and Conditions
Also known as: Infiltrating or invasive ductal carcinoma, ductal carcinoma in situ, inflammatory breast cancer, Paget disease of the nipple

Related conditions: Gynecomastia, fibroadenomas, papillomas

Definition: Breast cancer occurs in men when malignant (cancerous) cells develop in the breast tissue of the male breast. The cancer can then spread into other tissues.

Risk factors: Advanced age is a risk factor for men, just as it is for women. The median age of diagnosis for male breast cancer is sixty-eight. Men who have a close female relative with breast cancer are at risk and may be evaluated for the presence of a mutation in the *BRCA2* gene. This mutation is responsible for 15 percent of breast cancers in men, and men with the mutation have a 6 percent lifetime risk for breast cancer. Other risks include radiation exposure (which may be occupational but is more often a result of treatment of other cancers) and liver disease, such as cirrhosis, which causes an increase in estrogen and a decrease in androgen hormones. Obesity and cigarette smoking may also play a role as risk factors.

Many male breast cancers are estrogen-receptor-positive, which means that estrogen will increase the risk of development or accelerated growth of the cancer. Estrogen is given to some men to slow the growth of prostate cancer and is used by some men who are undergoing gender transformation. One risk specific to men for the development of breast cancer is Klinefelter syndrome, a genetic mutation involving at least one extra X chromosome, a condition that affects 1 in 850 men. These men have higher levels of estrogen and lower levels of androgens and therefore are at particular increased risk.

Etiology and the disease process: There are a number of risk factors for male breast cancer, but none of the known causes can be eliminated. Most male breast cancers are invasive, infiltrating ductal carcinomas and are far more treatable in early localized stages. Therefore, efforts should be concentrated on early identification and treatment by increasing awareness of risk factors, heightening surveillance of those with nonmodifiable risks, and attempting to change those risks that can be modified.

Incidence: Both men and women have breast tissue, and breast cancer occurs in men but is much rarer in men than in women, comprising only 1 percent of all cancers in men. The American Cancer Society states that in the United States in 2005 more than 1,500 cases of male breast cancer were diagnosed and almost 500 deaths occurred.

Symptoms: Symptoms of breast cancer in men include breast lumps as well as nipple and skin changes. The cancer is most often diagnosed when a man goes to his doctor after finding a mass below the nipple in one breast.

Nipple changes can include redness or patchy scaling of the skin, nipple retraction (pulling inward), and nipple discharge. Skin changes may include puckering and dimpling as well as redness and scaling; however, chest hair may obscure subtle skin changes, and men are not accustomed to examining their breasts in a way that would help them find early lumps. Even when men find early symptoms, they may be misinformed about male breast cancer or embarrassed and delay seeking medical care.

Screening and diagnosis: Providing information that male breast cancer does occur and describing early symptoms may be the best screening tools to offer. Screening for male breast cancer is not common among primary care providers, but if a lump is detected or brought to the provider's attention by the patient, the first step is a mammography done with spot compression or magnification and possibly ultrasound, followed by a biopsy. A biopsy is the only definitive way to diagnose breast cancer.

Staging assesses the size, location, lymph node involvement, and degree of metastasis of the cancer, ranging from Stage 0, which is the earliest stage, to Stage IV, which is the most advanced.

Treatment and therapy: Treatment usually involves surgery to remove the breast tissue and often lymph nodes and some of the chest muscles as well. Sentinel lymph node biopsy can be used to attempt to avoid more radical removal of lymph nodes. Radiation therapy and chemotherapy may be employed.

If the cancer is determined to be estrogen-receptor-positive, the antiestrogen drug tamoxifen can be used to slow the growth and reproduction of cells that require estrogen. Another drug used in treatment is megace, an antiandrogen drug that blocks the effects of androgen in the breast.

Prognosis, prevention, and outcomes: Prognosis is similar for male and female breast cancer when cancers of the same stage are compared; however, male breast cancer often is not discovered as early as is female breast cancer. Early detection is especially important because men have less breast tissue than women, and therefore their cancers can more easily reach and invade the chest muscles. Age at diagnosis and general health

Stage at Diagnosis and Five-Year Relative Survival Rates for Invasive Male Breast Cancer, 1988-2001

Stage	*Survival Rate (%)*
Localized[a]	96.9
Regional[b]	78.1
Distant[c]	23.0
Unstaged	64.2

Source: Data from L. A. G. Ries et al., eds., *Cancer Survival Among Adults: U.S. SEER Program, 1988-2001—Patient and Tumor Characteristics,* NIH Pub. No. 07-6215 (Bethesda, Md.: National Cancer Institute, 2007)

[a]Cancer still confined to primary site

[b]Cancer has spread to regional lymph nodes or directly beyond the primary site

[c]Cancer has metastasized

influence outcomes. With advanced medical care, five-year survival rates now vary from close to 100 percent for cancers caught in Stage 0 to 25 percent for cancers that have progressed to Stage IV. Prevention efforts center on screening for risk factors that may heighten surveillance for disease and on patient education about early self-detection of changes in the male breast. Outcome also depends on prevention of recurrence, and increased screening as well as adjuvant chemotherapy may improve long term outcomes.

Clair Kaplan, R.N., M.S.N., A.P.R.N. (WHNP), M.H.S., M.T. (ASCP)

For Further Information

Berek, J. S., and N. F. Hacker. *Practical Gynecologic Oncology*. Philadelphia: Lippincott Williams & Wilkins, 2005.

DeVita, V. T., S. Hellman, and S. A. Rosenberg. *Cancer: Principles and Practice of Oncology*. 7th ed. Philadelphia: Lippincott Williams & Wilkins, 2005.

Estala, E. M. "Proposed Screening Recommendations for Male Breast Cancer." *The Nurse Practitioner* 31, no. 2 (2006): 62-63.

Other Resources

American Cancer Society
http://www.cancer.org

National Cancer Institute
Male Breast Cancer Treatment
http://www.cancer.gov/cancertopics/pdq/treatment/malebreast/

See also: Breast cancers; Breast Self-Examination (BSE); Clinical Breast Exam (CBE); Cutaneous breast cancer; Ductal Carcinoma In Situ (DCIS); Invasive ductal carcinomas

▶ Breast cancer in pregnant women

Category: Diseases, Symptoms, and Conditions
Also known as: Gestational breast cancer, lactational breast cancer, postpartum breast cancer

Related conditions: Lactating adenoma, fibroadenoma, cystic disease, lobular hyperplasia, milk retention cyst (galactocele), abscess, lipoma, hamartoma, leukemia, lymphoma, sarcoma, neuroma, tuberculosis

Definition: Gestational breast cancer is defined as breast cancer that occurs during pregnancy or up to one year thereafter.

Risk factors: It is generally believed that breast cancer is years in the making; thus, pregnancy itself can be an aggravating risk factor for breast cancer because the physiologic changes that occur in the breast during pregnancy may mask an occult or nonpalpable mass. Further, there is often denial on the part of the physician or patient that breast cancer can occur during pregnancy, further aggravating the underlying risk. Moreover, the elevated levels of estrogen (hundredfold increase) and progesterone (thousandfold increase) during pregnancy may also stimulate cancer growth. Other traditional risk factors for breast cancer include a history of benign breast disease, menarche (onset of menstrual activity) before the age of twelve, drinking three or more alcohol-containing drinks daily, increased bone density, a sedentary lifestyle, nulliparity (no previous live births), first birth after the age of thirty, a first-degree relative (mother or sister) with breast cancer, upper socioeconomic status, a history of endometrial or ovarian cancer, chest irradiation, increased breast density, a history of breast cancer, dietary fat intake (especially saturated fat), and obesity.

Etiology and the disease process: Like all cancers, breast cancer arises when an oncogene (cancer-causing gene) is activated or the tumor-suppressor gene controlling the oncogene is silenced. Regardless of the precipitating risk factor, breast cancer appears to reflect the cumulative exposure to estrogen and progesterone.

Incidence: Of all women diagnosed with breast cancer, only 12.7 percent will be between the ages of twenty and forty-four; of these women, only 10 percent will be pregnant at the time of diagnosis. Based on several analyses, the actual incidence of breast cancer during pregnancy has been estimated to fall between 1/3000 and 1/10,000 of all pregnant women. Breast cancer during pregnancy is second only to cervical cancer as the most common malignancy occurring during pregnancy. Of concern is that the incidence will most likely increase as women delay childbearing. In fact, women who have their first term pregnancy after the age of thirty have a twofold to threefold increased risk of breast cancer compared with women who have their first term pregnancy before the age of twenty.

Symptoms: Most often, women with breast cancer during pregnancy complain of a painless mass in the breast or a nipple discharge; a bloody nipple discharge is particularly concerning.

Screening and diagnosis: All pregnant women should undergo a complete physical examination at the time they register for prenatal care, including a thorough breast examination. All new breast masses or nipple discharges should be evaluated promptly and not delayed until the pregnancy has been completed. The mean age at diagnosis of breast cancer during pregnancy is thirty-two to thirty-four years. In most cases, the disease is advanced at the time of diagnosis. In general, the number of positive lymph nodes is greater, the tumors are larger, the steroid hormone status is more often negative, the number of cells synthesizing deoxyribonucleic acid (DNA) is greater, the number of mutations involving *BRCA1* and *BRCA2* is greater, and the tumor suppressor p53 is more often downregulated. Although the usefulness of mammography has been questioned in women less than thirty-five years of age because of higher breast density, mammography during pregnancy (in which breast density is increased) has been shown to be 90 percent sensitive in detecting malignancies. The irradiation exposure to the fetus is negligible and should not be a deterrent. Ultrasound, which carries no fetal irradiation risk, has been shown to be 100 percent sensitive in detecting a malignancy when the breast mass is palpable. The diagnosis rests, however, with pathologic confirmation, which can be obtained with a fine needle biopsy, a core needle biopsy, or an excisional biopsy. Staging is performed to determine if metastasis has occurred.

Treatment and therapy: The management of breast cancer during pregnancy has the same goal as in patients who are not pregnant. Termination of pregnancy is not indicated. Surgery is generally delayed until the second trimester, and for nonmetastatic diseases, a modified radical mastectomy is considered the standard conservative procedure. Similarly, even though all chemotherapeutic agents are category D (teratogenic), they have accumulated a favorable safety profile when used in the second and third trimesters. Fetal malformations range from 19 percent in the first trimester to 1.3 percent in the second and third trimesters based on nearly 100 pregnant women treated with 5-fluorouracil, doxorubicin, and cyclophosphamide (a standard chemotherapeutic regimen).

Prognosis, prevention, and outcomes: Women who are diagnosed with breast cancer during pregnancy are often diagnosed at a later stage, because breast changes during pregnancy, including increased breast size and changes in breast texture, make small, early-stage tumors harder to detect and diagnose. Roughly half of new cases are found in a late stage (III or IV), as compared with just over a quarter of cases that are diagnosed at Stage I and another quarter or so at Stage II. The five-year survival rate for women with negative lymph nodes is 82 percent; however, lymph node metastasis occurs in 65 percent of women with breast cancer during pregnancy. The overall survival for breast cancer during pregnancy is 70 percent.

D. Scott Cunningham, M.D., Ph.D.

For Further Information

Barnes, D. M., and L. A. Newman. "Pregnancy-Associated Breast Cancer: A Literature Review." *Surgical Clinics of North America* 87 (2007): 417-430.

Leslie, K. K., and C. A. Lange. "Breast Cancer and Pregnancy." *Obstetrics & Gynecology Clinics of North America* 32 (2005): 547-558.

Other Resources

National Breast Cancer Foundation
http://www.nationalbreastcancer.org/about-breast-cancer/

National Cancer Institute
http://www.cancer.gov

Susan G. Komen for the Cure
http://cms.komen.org/komen/AboutBreastCancer/index.htm

See also: Adenocarcinomas; Breast cancers; Breast Self-Examination (BSE); Calcifications of the breast; Childbirth and cancer; Clinical Breast Exam (CBE); Cutaneous breast cancer; Duct ectasia; Ductal Carcinoma In Situ (DCIS); Ductal lavage; Ductogram; Estrogen-receptor-sensitive breast cancer; Pregnancy and cancer

▶ Bronchial adenomas

Category: Diseases, Symptoms, and Conditions
Also known as: Bronchial gland tumors, mucous gland adenomas, bronchial carcinoid tumors, cylindromas

Related conditions: Carcinoid syndrome

Definition: A bronchial adenoma is a slow-growing tumor in the windpipe (trachea) or in the large air passages (bronchi) leading from the windpipe to the lungs.

Risk factors: The cause and risk factors for bronchial adenomas are not known.

Etiology and the disease process: A bronchial adenoma can be one of several types of tumors that begin in the mucous glands; the main types of tumors are carcinoids and adenoid cystic carcinoma (also called cylindroma). The tumors are usually small and slow growing and therefore may not be diagnosed for years. Symptoms of bronchial adenoma may be confused with those of bronchial asthma or chronic bronchitis.

Incidence: Approximately 1 to 3 percent of pulmonary (relating to the lungs) tumors are bronchial adenomas. Bronchial adenomas can be found in individuals of all ages but usually are found in people between the ages of thirty and fifty; the incidence is equal for men and women.

Symptoms: Some of the symptoms of bronchial adenomas are difficulty breathing, hoarseness, a persistent cough, coughing up blood (hemoptysis), wheezing sounds, or pneumonia that recurs or is slow to end.

Screening and diagnosis: A chest X ray, computed tomography (CT) scan, or magnetic resonance imaging (MRI) can be used to detect a tumor. Often physicians will use a bronchoscopy, a procedure in which a thin, flexible tube with a very small camera is used to look at the trachea and bronchi and to take a sample of cells (biopsy) for testing. This test can distinguish a bronchial adenoma from other types of tissue growths. Sometimes it may be necessary to insert a needle through the chest wall, between the ribs, to take the biopsy for determination of the type of tumor.

Treatment and therapy: Treatment of bronchial adenoma is by surgical removal of the tumor. Surgery may be bronchoscopic surgery (during a bronchoscopy) if the tumor is small or open-lung surgery. There is a small chance of recurrence of a bronchial adenoma and a very small chance of metastases. Laser ablation (removal) of a bronchial adenoma may be done through a bronchoscope, especially for tumors that have recurred.

Prognosis, prevention, and outcomes: Following removal of the tumor there is an excellent long-term prognosis for individuals with a bronchial adenoma.

Vicki Miskovsky, B.S., R.D

See also: Adenocarcinomas; Adenoid Cystic Carcinoma (ACC); Bronchoalveolar lung cancer; Bronchography; Bronchoscopy; 1,4-Butanediol dimethanesulfonate; Carcinoid tumors and carcinoid syndrome; Coughing; Laryngeal cancer; Lung cancers; Pneumonia

▶ Bronchoalveolar lung cancer

Category: Diseases, Symptoms, and Conditions
Also known as: Non-small-cell lung cancer (NSCLC), bronchioloalveolar lung cancer, lung adenocarcinoma

Related conditions: Pleural effusion, pneumonia

Definition: Bronchoalveolar lung cancer is a type of NSCLC that arises in the alveoli (air sacs of the lung). It can begin as either a single site or multiple sites, or spread rapidly as a pneumonic form. Bronchoalveolar lung cancer is less likely than other types of NSCLC to spread beyond the lungs.

Risk factors: The most common cause of lung cancer is smoking cigarettes. Another major cause is exposure to secondhand smoke. Other risk factors include exposure to radon gas or asbestos, environmental pollution, tuberculosis, lung disease, and an inherited predisposition to lung cancer.

Etiology and the disease process: With bronchoalveolar lung cancer, cells in the alveoli begin to grow wildly. As they grow, they progress along the alveolar walls. Multiple sites may develop and then converge to consolidate some areas of the lungs. An obstructed area of the lung may become pneumonic.

Incidence: NSCLCs account for about 75 percent of all lung cancers. Bronchoalveolar lung cancer makes up about 2 to 3 percent of this group. Although 10 percent of patients with lung cancer in the United States are nonsmokers, 25 to 30 percent of patients with bronchoalveolar lung cancer are nonsmokers. It is more common in women.

Symptoms: The symptoms of bronchoalveolar cancer are coughing, shortness of breath, wheezing, chest pain, large amounts of watery sputum, and hemoptysis (coughing up blood). On physical examination, the lungs are dull to percussion (tapping on the chest wall), and breath sounds may be weak or absent on auscultation (listening with a stethoscope). If the tumor is pressing on a nerve, it can cause shoulder pain or hoarseness.

Screening and diagnosis: Currently, there is no accurate, inexpensive screening test for bronchoalveolar lung cancer. Researchers are working to develop such a test by looking at a marker in the blood and also at breath analysis.

To diagnose lung cancer, pulmonary function tests and a chest X ray may be performed. Chest X rays can demonstrate most lung cancers, except the very small.

More sensitive tests are computed tomography (CT) scans, magnetic resonance imaging (MRI), and positron emission tomography (PET) scans.

To differentiate between the types of lung cancer, a biopsy of the tumor must be performed. Bronchoscopy, thoracoscopy, or mediastinoscopy may be performed to examine pulmonary secretions and the lymph nodes of the lung. If the cancer exists on the periphery of the lung, it may be necessary to perform a needle biopsy through the chest wall. If none of these procedures is effective in determining the type of lung cancer, a surgical procedure called a thoracotomy (opening the chest) can be performed.

The actual diagnosis of bronchoalveolar lung cancer is made by the pathologist, who examines the tumor cells under a microscope. The pathologist identifies the type of lung cancer and stages the cancer. All NSCLCs are staged in the same way, using a combination of numeric tumor grading and the TNM (tumor/lymph node/metastasis) stages. The stages are as follows:

- Stage IA, T1 N0 M0: The tumor is less than 3 centimeters (cm) and there is no lymph node involvement or metastases.
- Stage IB, T2 N0 M0: The tumor is greater than 3 cm, but it has not spread beyond the lung.
- Stage IIA, T1 N1 M0: The tumor is less than 3 cm, and there is spread to local lymph nodes.
- Stage IIB, T2 N1 M0, or T3 N0 M0: Either the tumor is greater than 3 cm, or it has spread into the outside of the lungs, the chest cavity, or the pericardium (sac around the heart).
- Stage IIIA, T 1-3 N2 M0, or T3 N1 M0: Either the cancer has spread to distant lymph nodes but has not metastasized, or the cancer has spread into adjacent tissues and muscles and has spread to local lymph nodes.
- Stage IIIB, T4 N3 M0: Either the cancer has spread to nearby organs or it has spread to distant lymph nodes but has not metastasized.
- Stage IV, M1: The cancer has metastasized to distant organs.

Treatment and therapy: Treatment of lung cancer can include surgery, chemotherapy, and radiation. To remove a bronchoalveolar tumor, the surgeon can perform a wedge resection, a lobectomy, or a pneumonectomy. Chemotherapy for lung cancers is effective only 35 percent of the time. The most commonly used drugs are combinations of cisplatin (Platinol), carboplatin (Paraplatin), vinorelbine (Navelbine), vincristine (Oncovin), vinblastine (Velban), paclitaxel (Taxol), docetaxel (Taxotere), and gemcitabine (Gemzar). Newer chemotherapy drugs that interfere with cell growth and reproduction as well as angiogenesis (formation of new blood vessels) are being used. They are gefitinib (Iressa), erlotinib (Tarceva), and bevacizumab (Avastin).

Radiation therapy for bronchoalveolar lung cancer is not effective as a cure, so it is reserved for treatment when surgery is not possible.

Prognosis, prevention, and outcomes: Patients with lower stage cancers survive longer than those with high-stage cancers. Research has shown that patients who have never smoked respond better to treatments for bronchoalveolar cancer. The best way to avoid lung cancer is by not smoking and by avoiding exposure to secondhand smoke.

Christine M. Carroll, R.N., B.S.N., M.B.A.

For Further Information

Houlihan, Nancy G. *Lung Cancer*. Pittsburgh: Oncology Nursing Society, 2004.

Hunt, Ian, Martin Muers, and Tom Treasure. *ABC of Lung Cancer*. Malden, Mass.: Blackwell, 2008.

Roth, Jack A., James D. Cox, and Waun Ki Hong, eds. *Lung Cancer*. 3d ed. Malden, Mass.: Blackwell, 2008.

Other Resources

LungCancer.org
http://www.lungcancer.org/

MayoClinic.com
Lung Cancer
http://www.mayoclinic.com/health/lung-cancer/DS00038

National Cancer Institute
Lung Cancer
http://www.cancer.gov/cancertopics/types/lung

See also: Adenocarcinomas; Adenoid Cystic Carcinoma (ACC); Bronchial adenomas; Bronchography; Bronchoscopy; 1,4-Butanediol dimethanesulfonate; Carcinoid tumors and carcinoid syndrome; Coughing; Laryngeal cancer; Lung cancers; Pneumonia

▶ Burkitt lymphoma

Category: Diseases, Symptoms, and Conditions
Also known as: B-cell lymphoma, small noncleaved cell lymphoma

Related conditions: Non-Hodgkin lymphoma

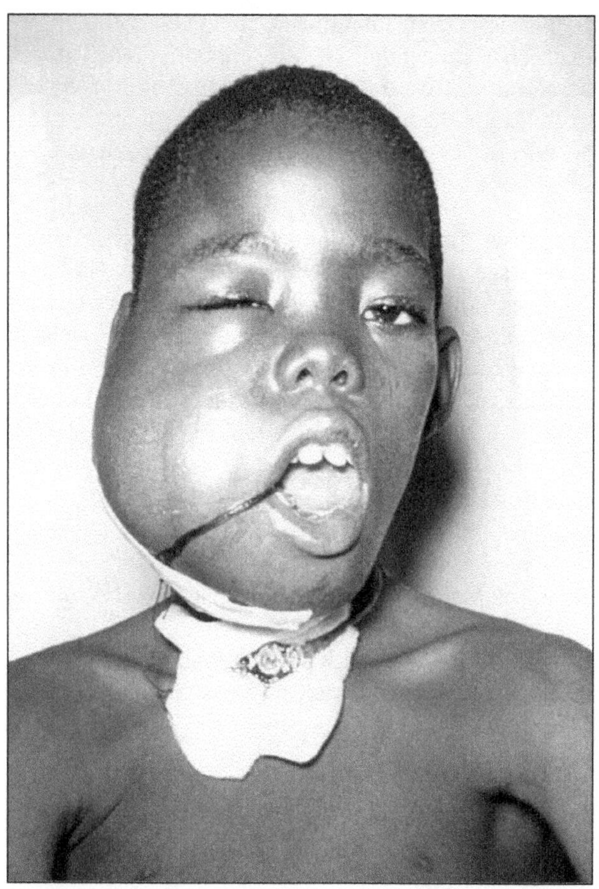

A child with a large facial tumor caused by Burkitt lymphoma. (Centers for Disease Control and Prevention)

Definition: Burkitt lymphoma, first described by Denis Parsons Burkitt in 1956, is an aggressive type of non-Hodgkin lymphoma (NHL) that develops from B lymphocytes, the cells that produce antibodies and fight infections. NHL is the most common cancer of the lymphatic system.

Risk factors: Most people who develop Burkitt lymphoma have no identifiable risk factors, however, there are several factors that may lead to its development. These include age, sex, exposure to chemicals that damage deoxyribonucleic acid (DNA), infections such as the Epstein-Barr virus (EBV), and a weakened immune system—especially in HIV/AIDS patients.

Etiology and the disease process: In North America, most cases of Burkitt lymphoma are sporadic and caused by a chromosomal rearrangement. Of these rearrangements, 85 percent involve a translocation between chromosomes 8 and 14 [t(8;14)(q24;q32)] which moves the *MYC* gene from its normal location on chromosome 8 to the vicinity of the gene producing immunoglobulin G (IgG) on chromosome 14. In 10 percent of Burkitt lymphoma cases, *MYC* has been translocated to the vicinity of antibody-producing genes on either chromosome 2 or chromosome 22.

In its new chromosomal location, *MYC* is overactive and results in uncontrolled cell growth. The *MYC* gene encodes for a transcription factor that activates other genes. One activated gene is *HMG-I/Y*, which transforms normal B lymphocytes into rapidly growing tumor cells with its protein product.

Burkitt lymphoma is endemic in equatorial Africa. It is associated with not only chromosomal translocations but also the Epstein-Barr virus (EBV), which also causes infectious mononucleosis and other cancers. About 30 percent of Burkitt lymphoma patients in the United States harbor EBV.

In children, the disease usually begins in the abdomen, develops rapidly, and metastasizes quickly. Abdominal swelling, fluid retention, and vomiting often occur. In adults, the disease often begins with a painless enlargement of a lymph gland or abdominal swelling. Depending on the location of the affected lymph node, a variety of conditions may develop. Occasionally, Burkitt lymphoma affects the blood and may result in anemia, increased bleeding, and susceptibility to infections. The B cells may invade other tissues, causing a variety of symptoms.

Because the cancer is one of the most rapidly growing human tumors, most cases are in either Stage III or Stage IV at the time of diagnosis.

Incidence: Burkitt lymphoma is common in central Africa, where it accounts for as much as 50 percent of cancer deaths in children. The disease is relatively rare in the United States, but when it does occur, the average age at diagnosis is seven years, and the disease accounts for about 3 percent of the total cancer deaths in people under twenty years old. The disease is also three times as likely to occur in boys as in girls and is more common in Caucasian children than children of other races. Also, it is 1,000 times more likely to occur in AIDS patients.

Symptoms: Although most cases in the United States develop in the abdomen, the first symptom is usually a painless swelling of an axillary, neck, or groin lymph node. The affected lymph node or nodes will grow rapidly and may form lumps. Depending on where the disease develops, other symptoms may occur. In Africa, where Burkitt lymphoma is endemic, the disease often affects the face and jaw, causing extensive swelling.

Screening and diagnosis: Diagnosis is by biopsy of the affected tissue followed by histological and immunochemical histological examination. Other methods used to diagnose the disease include: spinal fluid analysis, blood cell and platelet counts, X rays, computed tomography (CT) scans, gallium scans, tumor cell DNA electrophoresis, and positron emission tomography (PET) scans. The St. Jude's Children's Research Hospital system is commonly used to stage the disease in children.

- Stage I: Lymphoma is localized to a single site.
- Stage II: Lymphomas involve more than one site but are localized to one side of the body.
- Stage III: Lymphomas involve multiple sites on both sides of the body but do not involve bone marrow or the nervous system.
- Stage IV: Lymphomas involve the bone marrow or the nervous system.
- The Ann Arbor system is used for adults with the disease.
- Stage I: Lymphoma is limited to one lymph node either above or below the diaphragm or is limited to one organ.
- Stage II: Lymphomas are either in two or more lymph nodes on the same side of the diaphragm or are limited to one organ and the lymph nodes near that organ.
- Stage III: Lymphomas have spread to lymph nodes on both sides of the diaphragm and may involve an organ.
- Stage IV: Lymphomas have metastasized throughout one or more organs and may involve lymph nodes.

Treatment and Therapy: Burkitt lymphoma is treated with intensive chemotherapy involving a combination of chemotherapeutic agents such as the EPOCH (etoposide, prednisolone, oncovin, cyclophosphamide, hydroxydaunorubicin) combination regimen often supplemented with rituximab (R-EPOCH). Other combinations of chemotherapeutic agents such as CODOX-M/IVAC (cyclophosphamide, doxorubicin, vincristine, methotrexate/ifosfamide, etoposide, high dose cytarabine) are also used—often in combination with rituximab. If large tumors are involved, radiation therapy may be indicated. In some cases, surgery may be required to remove affected tissues. Stem cell therapy, bone marrow transplants, and monoclonal antibodies also have been used to treat the disease.

Prognosis, prevention, and outcomes: If the disease is relatively localized and has not spread, aggressive chemotherapy can cure up to 80 percent of the cases. If the central nervous system or the bone marrow has become involved, the effectiveness of treatment is significantly less.

Charles L. Vigue, Ph.D.

For Further Information

Evans, A., & Blum, Kristie A. (Eds.). (2015). *Non-Hodgkin Lymphoma: Pathology, Imaging, and Current Therapy* (Cancer Treatment and Research). New York: Springer.

Marcus, R., Sweetenham, J. W., & Williams, M. E. (Eds.). (2014). *Lymphoma: Pathology, Diagnosis, and Treatment* (Cambridge Medicine). New York: Cambridge University Press.

Robertson, Erle. (Ed.). (2012). *Burkitt's Lymphoma* (Current Cancer Research) (2013th Edition). New York: Springer Science-Business Media.

Mauch, P.M., Armitage, J.O., Coiffier, B., Dalla-Favera, R., Harris, N. L, (Eds.). (2004). *Non-Hodgkin's Lymphomas.* Philadelphia, PA: Lippincott Williams & Wilkins.

Other Resources

Leukemia and Lymphoma Society.
http://www.leukemia-lymphoma.org/hm_lls

Lymphoma Information Network.
Burkitt's Lymphoma/Leukemia.
http://www.lymphomainfo.net/nhl/types/burkitts.html

National Cancer Institute.
Non-Hodgkin Lymphoma.
http://www.cancer.gov/cancertopics/types/non-hodgkins-lymphoma

Lymphoma Research Foundation.
Non-Hodgkin Lymphoma.
http://www.lymphoma.org/site/pp.asp?c=bkLTKaOQLmK8E&b=6300139&gclid=CNWqst2928kCFYIaHwodvycP-g#burkitts

See also: Childhood cancers; Epstein-Barr Virus; Genetics of cancer; Hepatitis C virus (HCV); Hodgkin disease; Infectious cancers; Lymphomas; Molecular oncology; MYC oncogene; Non-Hodgkin lymphoma; Oncogenic viruses; Proto-oncogenes and carcinogenesis; Viral oncology; Virus-related cancers; Young adult cancers

▶ Cachexia

Category: Diseases, Symptoms, and Conditions
Also known as: Wasting syndrome, anorexia-cachexia syndrome

Related conditions: Anorexia

Definition: Cachexia is a complex syndrome in which changes in the way the body uses food—particularly fat and carbohydrates—lead to loss of muscle and fat. Anorexia (loss of appetite) is sometimes, but not always, associated with cachexia.

Risk factors: Certain cancers such as lung cancer or any cancer of the digestive tract—particularly of the esophagus, stomach, and pancreas—are more likely to be accompanied by cachexia. It is also common in advanced cancer, although infrequently it occurs in early cancers, sometimes even before diagnosis. Cachexia can also occur with acquired immunodeficiency syndrome (AIDS).

Etiology and the disease process: In cancer-related cachexia, it is thought that the tumor releases chemicals that change food metabolism. Patients with cachexia tend to have poor appetites. Even with nutritional supplementation, the wasting cannot be reversed while the cancer remains.

Incidence: When diagnosed, about 80 percent of patients with cancers in the upper gastrointestinal tract and 60 percent of patients with cancers of the lung have already lost considerable weight. More than 80 percent of patients who die from any cancer or from AIDS have cachexia. Patients with any solid tumor except breast cancer are generally more prone to cachexia, and it is also more common and more pronounced as the disease progresses in children and in the elderly.

Symptoms: Cachexia is one of the most overwhelming symptoms of cancer, demolishing quality of life with numbing fatigue, loss of appetite or changes to taste, and severe weight loss of 10 percent or more of body weight.

Screening and diagnosis: When a person experiences unexplained weight or appetite loss or fatigue, medical practitioners without more specific clues might perform such general screens as a complete blood count and a chest X ray. When the source of the problem is suspected, tests are more specific.

With a known cancer, cachexia diagnosis is based on clinical history, substantial weight loss, and physical examination. The concentration of plasma albumin in blood will usually be low. Extensive diagnostics are not normally required.

Treatment and therapy: The best course of action for cachexia is treatment of the underlying disease. After successful treatment, patients regain lost muscle and fat mass.

Prognosis, prevention, and outcomes: Prognosis is very poor with cachexia in advanced disease. When cachexia occurs in the early stages of cancer, the cancer that causes it is often responsive to treatment, and successful treatment removes the source of changes to metabolism.

Jackie Dial, Ph.D.

See also: Antinausea medications; Appetite loss; Nutrition and cancer treatment

▶ Calcifications of the breast

Category: Diseases, Symptoms, and Conditions
Also known as: Microcalcifications, macrocalcifications

Related conditions: Hyperplasia, precancer of the duct, fibroadenoma

Definition: Calcifications are calcium deposits in breast tissue, not detectable by touch but visible on mammograms as white spots. Macrocalcifications are large deposits, not indicative of cancer. Microcalcifications appear as tiny white specks on mammograms. Scattered throughout a mammogram, they are usually not cause for concern. They may indicate possible precancer when they appear in irregular patterns or are concentrated in one area of the breast.

Risk factors: Macrocalcifications and 80 percent of microcalcifications are harmless. Women in their childbearing years are prone to microcalcifications.

Etiology and the disease process: Macrocalcifications are related to changes in the breast due to inflammation, injury, or aging. Microcalcifications may appear in areas of rapidly dividing cells and therefore can indicate precancer.

Incidence: Macrocalcifications occur in about half of women over age fifty and in about 1 in 10 women under the age of fifty. Microcalcifications are usually evident in women only during their childbearing years.

Symptoms: No symptoms are associated with calcifications of either kind.

Screening and diagnosis: Calcifications are visible only on radiologic images. Macrocalcifications are harmless and require no further attention. Doctors may order special magnified mammographic views of microcalcifications in clusters or in odd patterns. Generally a biopsy is not needed at the first appearance of suspect patterns. Doctors typically have the patient repeat the mammogram three to six months later. If the repeat mammogram does not exhibit any obvious changes in the pattern or number of microcalcifications, a regular schedule of mammograms is adequate to monitor further changes. If microcalcifications appear particularly suspect on first appearance or if changes are noted in the repeat mammogram, a core needle biopsy or a surgical biopsy can be done to rule out precancer.

Treatment and therapy: If a patient has microcalcifications removed for biopsy that prove to be precancerous, she should be followed closely with regular mammograms to identify any future occurrences.

Prognosis, prevention, and outcomes: Macrocalcifications and the majority of microcalcifications (80 percent) have no relation to cancer. If a precancerous area is identified in microcalcifications, it can be removed completely many years before it has a chance to develop into actual cancer, and the patient's prognosis is excellent. Any other suspect microcalcifications should be removed fully and analyzed. Patients should be closely followed for the occurrence of new microcalcifications. After menopause, microcalcifications generally no longer occur.

Charlotte Crowder, M.P.H., ELS

See also: Breast ultrasound; Ductogram; Fibroadenomas; Hormone Replacement Therapy (HRT); Lobular Carcinoma In Situ (LCIS); Microcalcifications; Tubular carcinomas; Wire localization

▶ Cancer syndromes resulting from DNA repair defects

Category: Diseases, Symptoms and Conditions
Also known as: DeSanctis-Cacchion syndrome, Lynch syndrome

Related conditions: Ataxia telangiectasia, Bloom syndrome, Fanconi anemia, Hereditary Non-polyposis colorectal cancer (HNPCC), Xeroderma pigmentosum

Definition: Damage to DNA generally takes one of several forms. It may involve cross-linking of nucleotides, often the result of exposure to ultraviolet light, but also the result of oxygen radicals generated during metabolism, mismatching of nucleotide pairs, or double-stranded breakage. Several signaling mechanisms have evolved to detect DNA damage, either activating repair mechanisms, or blocking movement through the cell cycle and inducing cell death (apoptosis). Any defects in repair mechanisms may predispose the cell into becoming malignant.

Etiology and the disease process: DNA damage may result either from external or environmental sources such as ultraviolet light originating from sunlight (or tanning parlors), or endogenous errors during DNA replication in S phase of the cell cycle. Either may result in mutations to regulatory factors (tumor suppressors, cyclins or cyclin-dependent kinases). Other internal factors which may play a role in mutations include reactive oxygen metabolites, and even some therapeutic drugs. The most critical of these mutations produce breaks in one or both strands of DNA, destroying the integrity of the molecule. Some 150 gene products, termed DNA damage response proteins (DDR), are known to be involved in repair mechanisms. Mutations in any of these genes may result in a malignant transformation of the cell.

A significant proportion of DDR proteins are kinases, enzymes which regulate through phosphorylation of substrates. Two networks in particular play critical roles in regulating repair: the ataxia-telangiectasia mutated (ATM) kinases, and ATM-Rad3-related (ATR) kinases. The *BRCA1* gene, known to be associated with genetically-related breast cancer, is known to activate either kinase network. Each kinase system functions in activating checkpoints – largely involving the p53 protein – which prevent the replicating cell from proceeding past the G_1/S or G_2/M phases of the cell cycle.

DNA repair of single nucleotide errors may involve enzymes, encoded by the nucleotide excision repair (*NER*) genes, which excise the incorrect bases, creating a gap which is repaired by DNA Polymerase ⊠; the strand is rejoined using a DNA ligase. Single or double-stranded breaks are more problematic. Rejoining of broken ends utilizes a DNA-dependent kinase (DNA-PK) bringing ends together for joining by the ligase.

A second method of rejoining DNA breaks involves homologous recombination; the broken ends rejoin through a recombination procedure mediated by the *BRCA1* and *BRCA2* gene products.

Breast cancers associated with *BRCA1* and *BRCA2* genes: Mutations in the breast cancer genes *BRCA1* and *BRCA2* account for approximately 25% of hereditary breast cancers, and some 10% of all breast cancers, approximately 20,000 of the nearly 200,000 total diagnosed cases per year in the United States. Nearly two-thirds of women who inherit a mutated form of *BRCA1* will develop breast cancer by age 70, though often much earlier in life, while approximately half the women who inherit a mutated *BRCA2* gene will develop breast cancer by age 70.

In addition, mutations in these genes have been linked with increased risk of ovarian cancers. The normal products of these genes are associated with DNA repair mechanisms in the cell. The mutation may be inherited from either the mother or father, a single copy of which is sufficient to put the individual at greater risk.

Women at greater risk, such as those of Ashkenazi (Eastern European) Jewish ancestry, or women with a sibling who developed early breast cancer (prior to age 40), may undergo genetic testing for the mutated gene. If the test is positive for the mutation, some women choose to undergo double mastectomy to eliminate the breast cancer risk entirely.

Hereditary Non-polyposis Colorectal Cancer: HNPCC represents two forms of colorectal cancers associated with inherited dominant forms of mutated mismatch DNA repair genes (MMR) such as the *MLH1* and *MSH2*. Mutations in one or both of these genes are found in 45-50% of the approximately 8000 cases of HNPCC diagnosed in the United States each year, accounting for 5% of the total cases of colorectal cancers. Diagnosis of HNPCC is primarily on histological findings, difficult because only small differences appear from those in other forms of colorectal cancer. The presence of multiple neoplasms in the colon may be indicative of the disease. In addition, increased incidence of the disease in close family members, accounting for between 5-15% of the colorectal cases, is also indicative of the hereditary nature of the disease. As with most forms of treatment of colorectal cancer, surgical removal is the primary form of treatment.

Xeroderma pigmentosum: XP represents a group of rare genetic disorders, with an incidence approximately one per one million persons, and characterized by extreme sensitivity to ultraviolet light, generally that originating from sunlight. Characteristic symptoms such as reddening or blistering of the skin, especially after several minutes of exposure to sunlight, usually appear shortly after birth, and increase in intensity as the child becomes older. Unless the individual completely avoids exposure to sunlight, skin cancers, especially melanomas, often appear by the first decade of life. The eyes are particularly sensitive to sunlight, which may take the form of blistering, cataracts and even cancer.

At least eight forms of XP have been described, with varying degrees of severity. Most result from inborne mutations of NER genes which function in the excision and replacement of nucleotide errors. The primary risk factors are exposure to sunlight, or use of therapeutic drugs which could potentially damage DNA. There is no specific treatment beyond that of treatment or removal of cancerous lesions.

Richard Adler, Ph.D.

For Further Information

Curtin, Nicola. "DNA repair dysregulation from cancer driver to therapeutic target." *Nature Reviews/Cancer* 12 (December 2012): 801-818.

Friedberg, Errol, et al. *DNA Repair and Mutagenesis.* Washington, DC: ASM Press, 2006.

Friedenson Bernard. "The BRCA1/2 pathway prevents hematologic cancers in addition to breast and ovarian cancers." *BMC Cancer.* 2007;7:152. doi:10.1186/1471-2407-7-152.

Kelley, Mark (ed.). *DNA Repair in Cancer Therapy.* Waltham, MA: Elsevier Inc., 2012.

Pelengaris, Stella and Michael Khan (eds.) *The Molecular Biology of Cancer.* Malden, MA: Blackwell Publishing, 2006.

Other Resources

American Cancer Society
http://www.cancer.org/cancer/cancercauses/geneticsandcancer/heredity-and-cancer

Breast Cancer Gene Test
http://www.webmd.com/breast-cancer/breast-cancer-brca-gene-test

National Cancer Institute
http://www.cancer.gov/about-cancer/causes-prevention/genetics

Xeroderma Pigmentosum Society, Inc.
http://www.xps.org/

See also: Cell cycle regulation, Cell death, Chromatin, DNA repair, Hereditary Non-polyposis

▶ Candidiasis

Category: Diseases, Symptoms, and Conditions
Also known as: Thrush, yeast infection, fungal infection

Related conditions: Fever, infections, and sepsis in cancer treatment

Definition: *Candida* species are fungi that are found as part of the normal flora in humans and are also major human pathogens. The diseases caused by *Candida* species are termed candidiasis.

Risk factors: Candida colonization increases after antibiotic (antibacterial) therapy, and the broader the spectrum of antibacterial therapy, the greater the growth. Cancer surgery, particularly if it involves the gastrointestinal (including oral) or female genital tract, can allow candida present in the normal flora of these areas to enter into the previously protected underlying tissues. Cancer chemotherapy can impair the immune system by decreasing the production of white blood cells by the bone marrow. When corticosteroids are used as part of the cancer chemotherapy, both neutrophil and lymphocyte function is impaired. Radiation can damage mucous membranes and, in some cases, the bone marrow as well. Vascular catheters used to administer cancer chemotherapy and other drugs are frequently ports of entry for candida. Urinary and gastrointestinal catheters can also assist invading organisms. Leukemias, lymphomas, and bone marrow metastases can result in diminished numbers of the normally functioning neutrophils and lymphocytes essential to fight invading organisms.

Etiology and the disease process: *Candida* species are commensal organisms and are found as part of the normal human flora because of their ability to adhere to and persist on mucosal surfaces. It is only when this natural balance is upset that these opportunistic pathogens cause disease. Candidal organisms possess a number of virulence factors. Production of hydrolytic enzymes (proteinases and lipases) can alter protective mucous membranes, allowing penetration into the tissues beneath. The cell wall of *Candida* species is made up of beta-glucans, mannoproteins, and chitins (carbohydrates). Different growth conditions can result in changes in cell-wall components that drastically alter the morphology. Outside the body and on mucosal surfaces, *Candida* species exist as yeasts (round or oval, single-celled organisms). When tissues are invaded, the amount of cell-wall chitin is increased, and mycelia (long filaments) are formed rather than yeasts. This phenomenon is called dimorphism and may make the organism more challenging for the immune system. Formation of finger-like projections from yeast cells (pseudohyphae) seems to be important in penetration into host cells. These and other candida virulence factors are important contributors to disease causation, but it is the impaired immune system of the host that usually tips the balance.

Incidence: Autopsies of leukemia patients reveal disseminated candidiasis involving major organs in 20 to 33 percent of cases. Bloodstream invasion has been documented in more than 10 percent of patients with leukemia and about 1 percent of patients with lymphoma. The incidence is lower in patients with solid tumors and in children.

Symptoms: Symptoms can be quite varied, as many different areas of the body and organs can be infected. Oral discomfort and swallowing pain and difficulty may accompany oral and esophageal candidiasis. Abdominal pain can occur with stomach and intestinal ulcerations caused by candida in cancer patients. Vaginal discharge and itching is often associated with candida vaginitis. Endophthalmitis can cause blurred vision. Infected peripheral and central intravascular catheters may have minimal symptoms heralding the underlying suppurative thrombophlebitis. However, the most common symptom or sign of candidiasis, especially disseminated, is fever.

Screening and diagnosis: The diagnosis of candidiasis may be presumptively made by physical examination of the cancer patient. Examination of the skin and oral cavity for plaques, ulcers, and erythema may be revealing. Candida endophthalmitis, resulting from bloodstream infection, is strongly suspected when characteristic cotton-wool lesions are observed on ophthalmoscopic examination of the retina. A new heart murmur may be the result of candida endocarditis associated with vascular catheter infection. Rales and decreased breath sounds may be present during candida pneumonia. Intraluminal urine seen in indwelling urinary catheters is frequently cloudy with white fluffy debris when urinary candida infection occurs. Intravascular catheter sites may reveal erythema, induration, or purulent drainage, but these signs can be subtle or absent in the neutropenic patient.

Endoscopic examination can be helpful with gastrointestinal candidiasis, particularly esophagitis. Computed tomography (CT) and magnetic resonance imaging (MRI) scans of the abdomen can demonstrate abscesses.

Blood tests for candida antigens, beta-glucan, and polymerase chain reaction (PCR) may provide a specific diagnosis. Microscopic examination of urine and tissue biopsies is also helpful. Culture of blood, urine, tissue biopsies, and the like provides specific diagnostic information, and the cultured *Candida* can be speciated and tested for susceptibility to antifungal agents.

Treatment and therapy: The relatively nontoxic azole and echinocandin antifungals are most often used to treat candidiasis. Amphotericin B has long been standard therapy for invasive candidiasis, but the comparatively high toxicities have limited its use to refractory or resistant cases. If candida has been cultured, then fungal susceptibilities can be used to guide therapy. It is important to begin therapy as early as possible to achieve the best outcome, and this mandates that therapy be commenced in high-risk cancer patients before the availability of diagnostic studies if candidiasis is suspected. Adjunctive measures are also important. Vascular, gastrointestinal, or urinary catheters should be removed if possible. Immune function must be optimized. Colony-stimulating factors can increase neutrophil numbers in the neutropenic cancer patient.

Prognosis, prevention, and outcomes: Disseminated candidiasis with candidemia in cancer patients has a crude mortality rate of 70 to 75 percent with an excess mortality rate of about 40 percent. Without treatment survival rates are less than 5 percent.

Prevention is best accomplished by reducing the risk factors for infection. Removing catheters promptly, treating neutropenia, and using antibacterials only when absolutely necessary are all beneficial. Antifungal prophylaxis has been shown to reduce the incidence of candidiasis in cancer patients with neutropenia and also in patients for whom treatment has included bone marrow or solid organ transplantation.

H. Bradford Hawley, M.D.

For Further Information

Bodey, Gerald P., ed. *Candidiasis*. 2d ed. New York: Raven Press, 1993.

Ostrosky-Zeichner, Luis, et al. "Deeply Invasive Candidiasis." *Infectious Disease Clinics of North America* 16 (2002): 821-835.

Pappas, Peter G., et al. "Guidelines for Treatment of Candidiasis." *Clinical Infectious Diseases* 38 (2004): 161-189.

Other Resources

Centers for Disease Control and Prevention
Candidiasis
http://www.cdc.gov/nczved/dfbmd/disease_listing/candidiasis_gi.html

Mycology Online
Candidiasis
http://www.mycology.adelaide.edu.au/Mycoses/Cutaneous/Candidiasis/

See also: Antifungal therapies; Fever; Gastrointestinal complications of cancer treatment; Taste alteration

▶ Carcinoid tumors and carcinoid syndrome

Category: Diseases, Symptoms, and Conditions
Also known as: Gastrointestinal tract tumors, adenocarcinoid tumors

Related conditions: Colon cancer, small bowel lymphoma

Definition: A carcinoid tumor arises from hormone-producing cells that line the small intestine, appendix, bronchi, colon, pancreas, ovaries, testes, bile ducts, gallbladder, stomach, and liver. Carcinoid syndrome is a group of symptoms caused by the release of hormones from a carcinoid tumor.

Risk factors: No risk factors for carcinoid syndrome or carcinoid tumors have been identified, although they are thought to be related to a genetic mutation that is either inherited or spontaneous.

Etiology and the disease process: Carcinoid tumors are slow-growing tumors that develop from enterochromaffin cells. These cells secrete hormones such as serotonin, histamine, prostaglandins, polypeptides, and tachykinins. Some 65 percent of carcinoid tumors occur in the gastrointestinal tract, and 25 percent are found in the lungs. The remaining 10 percent arise from other organs, or the primary site is unknown. Benign carcinoid tumors are small and have a low rate of recurrence. Malignant carcinoid tumors tend to be larger than 2 centimeters (cm) and are more likely to metastasize (spread to other organs). They also can invade adjacent tissue.

The hormones secreted by gastrointestinal carcinoid tumors are broken down in the liver, so patients with these types of tumors do not experience carcinoid syndrome. However, if there are liver metastases, carcinoid syndrome can develop. Carcinoid tumors of the lungs, ovaries, and testes are more likely to cause carcinoid syndrome.

Incidence: Research suggests a rate of from 1.5 to 8 cases per 100,000 people. Carcinoid syndrome is rare.

Symptoms: Large gastrointestinal tumors may cause abdominal pain, abdominal mass, bleeding, nausea and vomiting, obstruction, and diarrhea.

Carcinoid tumors of the lungs cause coughing, chest pain, wheezing, blood-tinged sputum, and pneumonia. Lung carcinoid tumors cause the carcinoid syndrome about 20 percent of the time.

The most common symptom of the carcinoid syndrome is facial flushing that can last from hours to days. Other common symptoms are diarrhea, abdominal pain, wheezing, valvular heart disease, sweating, rapid heart rate, weight gain, weakness, secondary diabetes, and increased body and facial hair. These symptoms are caused by the high levels of hormones released by the tumor.

Screening and diagnosis: There is no routine screening for carcinoid tumors. Larger carcinoid tumors can be diagnosed by computed tomography (CT) scans or magnetic resonance imaging (MRI). If the CT scan shows abnormal lymph nodes or a liver tumor, a needle biopsy can be performed.

Carcinoid tumors can also be found by somatostatin (a hormone) receptor scintography, a nuclear imaging scan. This scan uses indium 111 octreotide as a radioactive dye. Octreotide has an affinity for hormone-producing cells. This test is quite accurate, but it can miss very small tumors and tumors that do not have somatostatin receptors.

Two other nuclear imaging procedures are used. They are positron emission tomography (PET) and metaiodobenzylguanidine (MIBG) scans. The PET scan picks up areas of the body with higher than normal metabolism. Like octreotide, MIBG is attracted to carcinoid tumors.

The only way to verify that a tumor is a carcinoid tumor is to biopsy it. Biopsy may be done by endoscopy, bronchoscopy, or needle biopsy.

Diagnosis of carcinoid syndrome can be done by performing a twenty-four hour urine test for 5-hydroxyindolacetic acid (5-HIAA). The normal rate of urinary excretion of 5-HIAA is 8 milligrams (mg). Persons with carcinoid syndrome can excrete between 100 and 2,000 mg of 5-HIAA.

The staging for carcinoid tumors is based on the primary site.

Treatment and therapy: If a carcinoid tumor is less than 2 centimeters (cm) in size, it can be removed by surgery. If the carcinoid tumor is larger than 2 cm, there are multiple tumors, or there are metastases, a cure is less likely. Surgery may be performed to ease the symptoms from the tumor or the carcinoid syndrome.

Sometimes the goal of surgery is debulking (decreasing the size of the tumor). This is done to decrease symptoms of carcinoid syndrome or in preparation for chemotherapy or radiation therapy. Debulking can be performed by surgical resection, cryoablation (freezing), radiofrequency ablation (radiation), or hepatic artery embolization (blocking the blood supply to the liver).

Chemotherapy may be used to treat carcinoid tumors. The chemotherapeutic drugs most frequently used are 5-fluorouracil (Adrucil), cyclophosphamide (Cytoxan), streptozocin (Zanosar), and doxorubicin (Adriamycin). Interferon, an immune system stimulator, may be used with chemotherapy. Chemotherapy is effective in about 30 percent of cases, and its effects are short term.

External radiation therapy can be administered to decrease tumor size and to decrease the symptoms that the patient is experiencing. Radiation is not effective against liver metastases.

Medications can be used to treat carcinoid syndrome. Octreotide has been effective in reducing the size of some carcinoid tumors. Imodium, lomotil, ondansetran (Zofran), and cyproheptadine (Periactin) may eliminate the diarrhea. Tamoxifen (nolvadex), phenothiazides, gastric histamine receptor antagonists, phentolamine alpha blockers, and corticosteroids may decrease the flushing.

Patients with carcinoid syndrome must take a niacin supplement and ingest adequate protein. Carcinoid tumors use nicotinic acid (a niacin breakdown product) and tryptophan to create serotonin and can deplete the body's stores of niacin.

Prognosis, prevention, and outcomes: With appropriate treatment, a person with carcinoid cancer or carcinoid syndrome can live for ten to fifteen years with a fairly good quality of life. There is no way to prevent carcinoid tumors.

Christine M. Carroll, R.N., B.S.N., M.B.A.

For Further Information

Babovic-Vuksanovic, Dusica, et al. "Familiar Occurrence of Carcinoid Tumors and Association with Other Malignant Neoplasms." *Cancer Epidemiology Biomarkers and Prevention* 8 (August, 1999): 715-719.

Wilander, Erik, Monalill Lundqvist, and Kjell Öberg. *Gastrointestinal Carcinoid Tumors*. New York: Fischer, 1989.

Zuetenhorst, Johanna M., and Babs G. Taal. "Metastatic Carcinoid Tumors: A Clinical Review." *The Oncologist* 10, no. 2 (February, 2005): 123-131.

Other Resources

American Cancer Society

Detail Guide: Gastrointestinal Carcinoid Tumors
http://www.cancer.org/docroot/CRI/CRI_2_3x.asp?dt=14

Medicinenet

Carcinoid Syndrome (Carcinoid Tumor)
http://www.medicinenet.com/carcinoid_syndrome/article.htm

See also: Achlorhydria; Antidiarrheal agents; Appendix cancer; Barium swallow; Bronchial adenomas; Duodenal carcinomas; Endocrine cancers; Gastric polyps; Gastrointestinal oncology; Grading of tumors; 5-Hydroxyindoleacetic Acid (5HIAA) test; Imaging tests; Interferon; Neuroendocrine tumors; Nuclear medicine scan; Small intestine cancer; Stomach cancers; Surgical biopsies; Thymomas; Thymus cancer

▶ Carcinoma of Unknown Primary origin (CUP)

Category: Diseases, Symptoms, and Conditions

Related conditions: Skin cancer, lung cancer, prostate cancer, breast cancer, lung cancer, recurrent carcinoma

Definition: Carcinoma of unknown primary origin (CUP) is an abnormal growth of cells, resulting in malignant (metastasized) cancer with no known origin. Carcinoma represents the most common cancers, including the common forms of skin, breast, prostate, lung, and colon cancer.

Risk factors: Malignant transformation can be caused by exposure to toxic carcinogens such as such as radiation, tobacco smoke, and certain chemicals. Some viruses have been linked to cancer: Epstein-Barr virus and lymphoma, human papillomavirus and cervical cancer, hepatitis B virus and liver cancer, and Kaposi sarcoma-associated virus and Kaposi sarcoma. Additionally, many carcinomas are the result of a random genetic mutation, resulting in abnormally formed cells that can be cancerous. There are strong hereditary factors involved in carcinoma, so that having a family history of cancer can mean being predisposed to developing cancer.

Etiology and the disease process: The origin of carcinoma is in the cells of the epithelium, which lines both the outside (skin) and the inside cavities and lumen of tissues and organs. In normal tissue, cells multiply to form new cells, and the old or damaged cells self-destruct by apoptosis, or cell suicide. However, when cells undergo malignant transformation (genetic mutations that lead to cancer), they divide and grow at a rapid rate, and tumors form and grow. Tumors can grow quickly if the cells are dividing at a high rate, while slow-growing tumors result from slowly dividing cells. As more and more of these dividing cells accumulate, the normal tissue becomes diseased. The cancer can spread to other regions of the body.

Incidence: Over 80 percent of all diagnosed cancers are a result of carcinoma. Of those, 2 to 4 percent are carcinomas of unknown origin, in that they have metastasized from an unknown location.

Symptoms: Symptoms of carcinoma of unknown primary origin include local symptoms, metastasis symptoms, and systemic systems. Local symptoms include unusual bumps, nodes, cysts, or swelling; bleeding (usually found internally or in urine tests); and pain from compression of the tissues surrounding the area of a tumor growth. Metastasis symptoms include enlarged lymph nodes, neurological symptoms, an enlarged liver, and occasionally coughing or broken bones. Systemic symptoms refer to symptoms that affect the entire body, such as weight loss, excessive sweating, hormonal changes, or lack of iron in the bloodstream.

Screening and diagnosis: Cancer is usually classified according to the tissue from which the cancerous cells originate, as well as the normal cell type they most resemble. Sometimes, however, although cancerous cells are present, their origin is unknown.

Depending on symptoms present, a patient may undergo several tests including blood, urine, stool tests, and X rays. If carcinoma is suspected, the physician will usually order a biopsy to examine a small piece of the cancerous tissue under a microscope. Cancer is determined to be carcinoma of unknown primary origin when there is no evidence to determine the origin of the cancerous cells.

By examining the pattern of spreading for the cancer, the physician may derive more information about where it originated. In cancers that appear above the diaphragm, lung cancer is usually the cause. Research has shown that over half of patients with carcinoma of unknown primary origin have cancer that originated in the lung or pancreas.

According to the National Cancer Institute, physicians classify carcinoma of unknown primary origin into one of the following categories:

- Poorly differentiated carcinomas: The cancer cells look very different from normal cells.
- Metastatic melanoma to a single nodal site: Cancer of the cells that color the skin (melanocytes) has spread to lymph nodes in only one part of the body.
- Cancer in the cervical lymph nodes: Cancer is in the small, bean-shaped organs that make and store infection-fighting cells (lymph nodes) in the neck area.
- Isolated axillary metastasis: Cancer has spread only to lymph nodes in the area of the armpits.
- Inguinal node metastasis: Cancer has spread to lymph nodes in the groin area.
- Multiple involvement: Cancer has spread to several different areas of the body.

Treatment and therapy: Treatment of carcinoma of unknown primary origin depends on the suspected origin of the cancer, the microscopic analysis of the cancer cells, and other factors.

Surgery is a common treatment for carcinoma of unknown primary origin; the cancer and a small portion of the healthy tissue surrounding it are removed. Various surgical procedures are used, depending on the location of the cancer.

Radiation therapy is often used before surgery to shrink tumors or after surgery to kill remaining cancer cells; it can also be used as a therapy without surgery.

Chemotherapy is a systemic treatment that uses drugs to kill cancerous cells. Once the drugs enter the body and travel through the bloodstream, they kill cancerous cells throughout the body. Drugs can be administered orally or by injection into the veins or muscles. Occasionally chemotherapy is administered after surgery has removed all cancer cells as a preventive measure to ensure that new cancer cells do not develop (adjuvant therapy).

Hormone therapy has shown success in halting the production of hormones that assist in the growth of cancerous cells. Synthetic hormones or other drugs block the body's natural hormones, or hormone-producing glands are removed by surgery.

If carcinoma of unknown primary origin has been categorized, the treatment is more specific. If the cancer is classified as poorly differentiated cells or discovered within the abdomen, the most common treatment is chemotherapy. If the cancer is found in the neck area, treatment may include removal of the lymph nodes and tonsils, radiation therapy, or neck surgery. A lymph node dissection may be performed if the cancer has spread to the lymph nodes. When cancer is found in lymph nodes near the armpit, surgery is performed to remove the nodes and often the breast tissue, along with radiation and chemotherapy. If the cancer is found in the lymph nodes near the groin area, surgery is performed to remove the lymph nodes and some groin tissue. If the cancer is found in several areas of the body, usually a systemic therapy such as chemotherapy or hormone therapy will be used to deliver treatment to the entire body.

Prognosis, prevention, and outcomes: The prognosis for patients with carcinoma of unknown primary origin is poor. The average survival is approximately three to five months; 25 percent of patients survive one year, and only 10 percent of patients survive five years. Studies have shown that cancer found in the lymph nodes has a longer survival rate. Colonoscopies, mammograms, and prostate cancer screenings can lead to early detection and possibly longer survival times.

Robert J. Amato, D.O.

For Further Information

Fizazi, Karim, ed. *Carcinoma of an Unknown Primary Site*. New York: Taylor & Francis, 2006.

Icon Health. *The Official Patient's Sourcebook on Carcinoma of Unknown Primary: A Revised and Updated Directory for the Internet Age*. San Diego, Calif.: Author, 2002.

Other Resources

American Cancer Society

Detailed Guide: Cancer of Unknown Primary
http://www.cancer.org/docroot/CRI/CRI_2_3x.asp?rnav=cridg&dt=58

National Cancer Institute

Cancer of Unknown Primary
http://www.nci.nih.gov/cancertopics/types/unknownprimary/

See also: Breast cancers; Carcinogens, known; Carcinogens, reasonably anticipated; Carcinomas; Carcinosarcomas; Lung cancers; Metastasis; Prostate cancer; Skin cancers; Survival rates

▶ Carcinomas

Category: Diseases, Symptoms, and Conditions
Also known as: Epithelial cell cancer

Related conditions: Dysplasia, metaplasia

Definition: Carcinoma refers to any type of cancer that arises from epithelial cells. Carcinomas are distinguished from cancers of connective tissue (sarcomas), from cancers of blood-forming cells (leukemias and lymphomas), and from germ-cell tumors (teratomas). Carcinomas arising from stratified squamous epithelium are termed squamous cell carcinomas; those arising from glandular epithelium are termed adenocarcinomas.

Risk factors: Risk factors fall into two categories: environmental and hereditary. Environmental risk factors include exposure to carcinogenic chemicals or ionizing radiation, or infection with oncogenic viruses. Thousands of carcinogenic chemicals are known, and many are subject to strict regulations regarding exposure. Exposure to ionizing radiation, the most important source of which is the ultraviolet portion of sunlight, is another risk factor. Other important risk factors are inborn genetic variations that predispose individuals to particular cancers and immune system dysfunction.

Etiology and the disease process: Epithelial cells are more prone to malignant transformation than other types of cells because they are routinely exposed to the outside environment. Therefore, carcinoma is far more prevalent than sarcoma, leukemia, or other forms of cancer. The etiology of carcinoma hinges on cellular alterations that confer several key traits on the cell: unregulated growth, stimulation of new blood vessel formation, tissue invasion, and metastatic potential. Infection by oncogenic viruses causes carcinoma by introduction of foreign genes into the cell; these oncogenic genes (oncogenes) can confer the attributes of malignancy to the infected cells. Gene disruption can cause carcinoma via abnormal activation of oncogenes or, alternatively, by abnormal inactivation of tumor-suppressor genes.

Incidence: Carcinoma is by far the most prevalent form of cancer, accounting for more than 90 percent of new cancer cases and cancer deaths. In 2005, there were approximately 1.2 million new cases and 500,000 deaths from carcinoma in the United States.

Symptoms: Symptoms of early carcinoma vary widely according to the epithelial cells affected and their growth pattern. Advanced or terminal carcinoma symptoms include cachexia, pain, fatigue, and depression.

Screening and diagnosis: Carcinoma screening consists of careful inspection of epithelial cells at risk as well as blood tests for circulating tumor markers. Inspection for skin cancer may be as straightforward as looking for suspicious changes on the skin, whereas screening for cervical cancer involves scraping or brushing cells from the uterine cervix followed by staining and microscopic examination (a Pap smear). Blood tests can also be used to screen for carcinoma based on shedding of tumor-specific molecules into the circulation. A blood test for prostate-specific antigen (PSA) is used to screen men at risk for prostate cancer; those with high levels are then candidates for diagnostic biopsy. Diagnosis of carcinoma is usually done by pathologists based on microscopic examination of biopsied tissue. Features of carcinoma include cellular traits such as abnormally large nuclei, loss of multicellular organization, and disruption of the basement membrane. Staging of carcinoma is based on searches for malignant cells in adjacent structures and lymph nodes. Carcinoma staging uses the International Union Against Cancer (UICC) and American Joint Committee on Cancer (AJCC) system that describes the tumor itself, lymph node involvement, and metastatic lesions; however, other staging systems are also used, such as Dukes' classification of colon cancer.

Treatment and therapy: Treatment options for carcinoma include surgery, chemotherapy, radiotherapy, immunotherapy, monoclonal antibody therapy, and other, less common approaches. Treatment plans are made based on the disease grade and stage and the functional status of the patient. Surgical therapy (mechanical removal of the tumor) reliably reduces the tumor burden and offers complete resection as the best outcome. Examples include surgical removal of the breast (mastectomy) or prostate (prostatectomy). Chemotherapy (systemic administration of anticarcinoma drugs) can damage tumor cells anywhere in the body, usually by interfering with deoxyribonucleic acid (DNA) replication. Many chemotherapy regimens harm healthy tissue as a dose-limiting toxicity. Radiotherapy is the use of high-energy electromagnetic radiation (X rays or gamma rays) to damage or kill cancer cells; radiation can be delivered from the outside or by implantation of radioactive pellets (brachytherapy). Immunotherapy refers to attempts to attack carcinoma cells with the patient's own immune cells. Monoclonal antibody therapy depends on knowledge of signal transduction pathways and uses antibodies to block or disrupt the malignant cells' growth. An example includes the use of monoclonal antibodies against human epidermal growth factor receptor 2 (HER2) such as trastuzumab to interfere with signals generated by the HER2 receptor in breast cancer.

Prognosis, prevention, and outcomes: Although some types of carcinoma are quite deadly, many forms are indolent and manageable. Prognosis depends mostly on the type of carcinoma, the histologic grade, and the anatomic stage. Prevention efforts can reduce the incidence of carcinomas within populations and take the form of avoidance of or reduction of exposure to carcinogens. Examples include smoking-cessation campaigns to prevent some cases of lung cancer and promotion of sunscreen use to prevent some cases of melanoma. Individuals may further reduce their risk of cancer by losing weight and being physically active. Outcomes continue to improve because of the integration of treatments and supportive care.

John B. Welsh, M.D., Ph.D.

For Further Information

Hanahan D., and R. A. Weinberg. "The Hallmarks of Cancer." *Cell* 100 (2000): 57-70.

Kufe, D. W., et al., eds. *Holland Frei Cancer Medicine*. 7th ed. Hamilton, Ont.: BC Decker, 2006.

Ruddon, R. W. *Cancer Biology*. 4th ed. New York: Oxford University Press, 2007.

Schottenfeld, D., and J. F. Fraumeni, Jr., eds. *Cancer Epidemiology and Prevention*. New York: Oxford University Press, 2006.

Weinberg, R. A. *The Biology of Cancer*. New York: Garland Science, 2007.

Other Resources

American Cancer Society
http://www. cancer.org

National Cancer Institute
http://www.cancer.gov

See also: Adenocarcinomas; Adenoid Cystic Carcinoma (ACC); Adrenocortical cancer; Appendix cancer; Ascites; Basal cell carcinomas; Bile duct cancer; Birt-Hogg-Dubé Syndrome (BHDS); Bladder cancer; Bowen disease; Breast cancer in men; Breast cancers; Bronchoalveolar lung cancer; Carcinoma of Unknown Primary origin (CUP); Carcinomatosis; Carcinomatous meningitis; Carcinosarcomas; Cervical cancer; Chordomas; Choriocarcinomas; Comedo carcinomas; Ductal Carcinoma In Situ (DCIS); Duodenal carcinomas; Endocrine cancers; Epidermoid cancers of mucous membranes; Ethnicity and cancer; Fallopian tube cancer; Gallbladder cancer; Granulosa cell tumors; Hereditary Leiomyomatosis and Renal Cell Cancer (HLRCC); Hereditary mixed polyposis syndrome; Hereditary non-VHL clear cell renal cell carcinomas; Hereditary papillary renal cell carcinomas; Invasive ductal carcinomas; Invasive lobular carcinomas; Leptomeningeal carcinomas; Liver cancers; Lobular Carcinoma In Situ (LCIS); Lung cancers; Medullary carcinoma of the breast; Meningeal carcinomatosis; Merkel Cell Carcinomas (MCC); Metastatic squamous neck cancer with occult primary; Mucinous carcinomas; Multiple endocrine neoplasia type 2 (MEN 2); Ovarian epithelial cancer; Pancreatic cancers; Parathyroid cancer; Penile cancer; Pituitary tumors; Prostate cancer; *SCLC1* gene; Skin cancers; Small intestine cancer; Squamous cell carcinomas; Stomach cancers; Teratocarcinomas; Thymus cancer; Transitional cell carcinomas; Trichilemmal carcinomas; Tubular carcinomas; Urethral cancer; Urinary system cancers; Uterine cancer; Vaginal cancer; Virus-related cancers; Vulvar cancer; Yolk sac carcinomas

▶ Carcinomatosis

Category: Diseases, Symptoms, and Conditions
Also known as: Carcinosis

Related condition: Metastasis

Definition: Carcinomatosis is a condition in which a malignant tumor (or carcinoma), originating in the epithelial cells lining the internal and external surfaces or passageways that run through all organs, has spread via the bloodstream or lymphatic system through a process called metastasis. This is in contrast to carcinoma in situ, in which the cancer has not spread to neighboring tissues and involves only the cells where it originated. Although strictly speaking carcinomatosis should be used only for epithelial cancers, or carcinomas, it is sometimes employed to describe other types such as sarcomas—cancers of connective tissues such as bone, cartilage, or fat—that have spread widely throughout the body. Carcinomatosis is also used to describe a cancer in a relatively large region of the body.

Risk factors: Cancer risk increases as a function of smoking; consuming a high-fat diet; being overweight or obese; unprotected exposure to the sun's ultraviolet rays;

increasing age; gender (often men have a higher risk); race (which race has an increased risk depends on the cancer); poverty and thus access to health care, screening, and early diagnosis; genetics (sometimes tied to ethnicity or religion); or environment (exposure to pollution, toxins, and ionizing radiation). However, every cancer has distinct risk factors.

Etiology and the disease process: Just as every cancer has distinct risk factors, every cancer also has distinct, organ-specific causes. However, what is common among cancers is the out-of-control growth and accumulation of abnormal cancer cells. Carcinogens—substances that cause gene mutation—may be chemical, irradiative, viral, immunological, or hereditary.

Incidence: In the United States the incidence of cancer among men is as follows: prostate, 33 percent; lung, 13 percent; colorectal, 10 percent; bladder, 7 percent; non-Hodgkin lymphoma, 6 percent; and skin melanoma, 5 percent. Among women the rates were breast, 32 percent; lung, 12 percent; colorectal, 11 percent; endometrial, 6 percent; and non-Hodgkin lymphoma, 4 percent.

Symptoms: Most cancers develop from a single aberrant cell. This cell then proliferates to generate a clinically detectable tumor, which may be benign or malignant. In some cases, multiple primary tumors may occur; this may or may not be followed by metastasis. The symptoms may evidence the progression from normal cell through premalignant lesions to fully malignant cancers capable of moving to distant sites.

Screening and diagnosis: Screening may be general through blood tests, X rays, computed tomography (CT scans), and endoscopy. However, for some cancers, there are specific screening tests. For example, for prostate cancer, screenings include digital rectal examinations to detect irregularities of the prostate gland and blood tests to detect levels of prostate specific antigen (PSA), but prostate biopsies are more definitive. Similarly, colonoscopies (colorectal examinations) help identify precancerous or cancerous polyps or tumors that may also be confirmed by biopsies, and Pap smears test for abnormal cells that might signal the start of cervical cancer.

Most types of cancer are categorized in Stages I, II, III, and IV. These stages of cancer are based on the extent of spread and whether the cancer has moved to lymph nodes or other organs. Each stage classification is slightly different for every type of cancer, ranging from the least extensive spread (Stage I) to the most extensive (Stage IV), where the cancer has spread through the bloodstream beyond the primary site; that is, it has metastasized. The condition of carcinomatosis usually refers to cancers in Stage III or IV.

Treatment and therapy: Treatment options include surgery, radiation therapy, chemotherapy, and hormone therapy. Radiation therapy uses X rays or other high-energy rays to kill cancer cells or shrink tumors. Radiation may be used alone, or before or after surgery. Chemotherapy uses drugs (singly or in combination) to kill cancer cells. Alternative therapies include dietary formulas, homeopathy, or hypnotherapy. Complementary therapies consist of such procedures as massage or even music, often to reduce the anxiety that often accompanies a cancer diagnosis.

Prognosis, prevention, and outcomes: Thanks to the increasing numbers of diagnostic tools and treatment options, the prognosis for specific forms of cancer has improved even though predicting the outcome of any individual treatment is very difficult.

As for prevention, avoidance of smoking drastically reduces the incidence of lung cancer, while reducing the body mass index to below twenty-five cuts down the risk of colon, kidney, pancreatic, esophageal, uterine, and breast cancer. Reducing the intake of processed meats and to a lesser extent red meat diminishes the likelihood of colorectal cancer. Limiting direct exposure to the sun reduces malignant skin melanomas. Modifying not only lifestyle risk factors but also occupational factors such as avoiding the inhalation of asbestos fibers at the workplace also helps cancer prevention. The use of specific drugs may also be preventive, as is testing for such genes as *BRCA1* and *BRCA2*, which cause breast cancer. Various forms of screening such as Pap smears, colonoscopies, and PSA tests have also been found to be effective preventive measures.

As for outcomes, mortality rates for the most common forms of cancer among men were as follows: lung cancer, 31 percent; prostate, 10 percent; colorectal, 10 percent; pancreatic, 5 percent; and blood leukemia, 4 percent. Among women, the corresponding figures were lung, 27 percent; breast, 15 percent; colorectal, 10 percent; ovarian, 6 percent; and pancreatic, 6 percent.

Peter B. Heller, Ph.D.

For Further Information

Eyre, Harmon J., et al., eds. *Informed Decisions: The Complete Book of Cancer Diagnosis, Treatment, and*

Recovery. 2d ed. Atlanta, Ga.: American Cancer Society, 2002.
"Facts About Cancer." In *American Medical Association Family Medical Guide*. 4th ed. Hoboken, N.J.: John Wiley, 2004.
Kleinsmith, L. J. *Principles of Cancer Biology*. San Francisco: Pearson Benjamin Cummings, 2006.
Tannock, I. F., et al., eds. *The Basic Science of Oncology*. 4th ed. New York: McGraw Hill, 2005.
Turkington, Carol A., and William LiPera, eds. *The Encyclopedia of Cancer*. New York: Facts on File, 2005.

Other Resources

American Cancer Society
http://www.cancer.org

National Cancer Institute
http://www.cancer.gov

See also: Appendix cancer; Ascites; Carcinomatous meningitis; Carcinosarcomas; Fallopian tube cancer; Gynecologic cancers; Hyperthermic perfusion; Leptomeningeal carcinomas; Lumbar puncture; Meningeal carcinomatosis

▶ Carcinomatous meningitis

Category: Diseases, Symptoms, and Conditions
Also known as: Meningeal carcinomatosis, leptomeningeal carcinomatosis, leptomeningeal metastasis

Related conditions: Almost any type of cancer can be associated with this condition, but it is generally seen with melanoma and breast and lung cancers.

Definition: Carcinomatous meningitis is the spread or infiltration of tumor cells from a primary central nervous system (CNS) source, such as a brain tumor, or from a distant or secondary source, such as a lung or breast tumor, via the blood to the subarachnoid space, where it spreads via the fluid covering the brain, called the cerebral spinal fluid (CSF), to involve the coverings of the brain, known as the leptomeninges. The leptomeninges are further subdivided into the pia mater and the arachnoid. The space between the two is called the subarachnoid space, and this space acts as the conduit for the spread of tumor cells as it contains the CSF fluid.

Risk factors: In adults, primary brain tumors such as oligodendroglioma or secondary tumors, also called metastases, from lung, breast, melanoma, lymphoma, ovarian, or gastric cancer can spread to the brain surfaces. In children, primary brain tumors such as ependymoma, pineal tumors, meduloblastoma, germinoma, or glioblastoma can spread to the leptomeninges.

Etiology and the disease process: The leptomeninges are the coverings of the brain. The leptomeninges can be further subdivided into the pia mater, a thin translucent sheet or membrane that adheres to the surfaces of the brain and spinal cord, and the arachnoid, a delicate weblike membrane between the dura and pia mater. The space between the two is called the subarachnoid space and is filled with fluid called cerebral spinal fluid, which nourishes the brain and cushions it.

When tumor cells invade the subarachnoid space between the pia mater and the arachnoid, that invasion is called carcinomatous meningitis. Unlike other forms of meningitis, where the invading organism is a bacteria, fungus, or virus, the invaders in carcinomatous meningitis are cancer cells, and therefore it is not an infection.

Tumor growth in carcinomatous meningitis is along the CSF and can involve the dura, pia-arachnoid, or rarely the spinal cord itself. In adults, tumor growth usually results from spread of a primary brain tumor (a cancer that starts in the brain) such as oligodendroglioma or of secondary cancers from lymphoma, melanoma, or lung, breast, or gastric tumors. A secondary cancer occurs when cancer cells leave the primary site (usually the breast in carcinomatous meningitis) and spread to another organ or different parts of the body (metastasize). These secondary cancer cells can stay inactive for many years, so even when a cancer appears to have been successfully treated, it can recur. No one knows what triggers the cancer cells to become active again. It is estimated that between 3 and 5 out of every 100 patients with cancer will develop carcinomatous meningitis, and it can occur with any type of cancer but most commonly occurs in breast cancer.

Incidence: The incidence of carcinomatous meningitis is increasing because cancer patients are surviving longer. It is seen in about 3 to 5 percent of patients who have cancer.

Symptoms: Patients usually complain of nonspecific symptoms such as headache or back pain, or focal neurologic deficits such as weakness in an extremity.

Screening and diagnosis: Carcinomatous meningitis can be diagnosed by magnetic resonance imaging (MRI) or myelography together with computed tomography (CT). A cerebral spinal fluid (CSF) or spinal tap (also called a lumbar puncture), whereby a needle is inserted into the spinal fluid within the subarachnoid space and the CSF fluid is sampled, is the usual form of diagnosis, although CSF cytology is negative in 10 percent of cases. On non-contrast CT, there is obliteration of basal cisterns or sulci with hydrocephalus as an indirect sign. Contrast-enhanced MRI is more sensitive than CT and typically shows enhancement of the basilar cisterns or sulci with focal subarachnoid masses less common. It should be noted that up to 30 percent of confirmed cases of meningeal metastases will have a negative MRI.

Treatment and therapy: This disease is difficult to cure, and the treatment aim is usually to ameliorate symptoms, usually by chemotherapy injected into the spinal fluid via lumbar puncture (intrathecal methotrexate) or by radiotherapy to the brain.

Prognosis, prevention, and outcomes: Some patients respond to treatment; however, the prognosis is generally poor, with death occurring within one month if the disease is untreated. Treatment can extend median survival to three to six months. New treatment options involving new chemotherapy regimens are being tested.

Debra B. Kessler, M.D., Ph.D.

For Further Information

Carpenter, Malcolm B. *Core Text of Neuroanatomy*. 2d ed. Baltimore: Williams & Wilkins, 1981.

Grossman, Robert I., and David M. Yousem. *Neuroradiology: The Requisites*. St. Louis: Mosby-Year Book, 1994.

Osborn, Anne G. *Diagnostic Neuroradiology*. St. Louis: Mosby-Year Book, 1994.

Robbins Pathologic Basis of Disease. 5th ed. Philadelphia: W. B. Saunders, 1994.

Watanabe, M., R. Tanaka, and N. Takeda. "Correlation of MRI and Clinical Features in Meningeal Carcinomatosis." *Neuroradiology* 35 (1993): 512-515.

Other Resources

American Cancer Society
http://www.cancer.org

National Cancer Institute
http://www.cancer.gov

See also: Acoustic neuromas; Carcinosarcomas; Craniotomy; Infection and sepsis; Leptomeningeal carcinomas; Lumbar puncture; Meningeal carcinomatosis

▶ Carcinosarcomas

Category: Diseases, Symptoms, and Conditions
Also known as: Mixed epithelial-stromal carcinomas, mixed epithelial-nonepithelial malignant tumors, collision tumors, malignant mixed mullerian tumors, sarcocarcinomas

Related conditions: Carcinoma, carcinoma in situ, carcinoma of unknown primary, carcinomatosis, carcinomatous meningitis

Definition: Carcinosarcomas are malignant tumors (abnormal masses of tissue that can invade and destroy local tissue and spread to other regions) that are a combination of carcinoma (cancer of epithelial tissue, which is skin or tissue that lines organs) and sarcoma (cancer of connective tissue, such as bone) that occur throughout the body. The stromal (connective tissue) component is usually high grade (contains abnormal cells that will most likely grow and spread quickly). The mesenchymal (the mass of tissue that develops mainly from the mesoderm, the middle layer of the trilaminar germ disc during development) component is classified into two groups: the homologous form composed of cell types that are normally found and the heterologous form composed of cell types that are not normally found.

Risk factors: Tamoxifen (a nonsteroidal triphenylethyl compound), widely used as adjuvant therapy in the treatment of breast cancer, has been positively correlated with the development of uterine carcinosarcoma. Radiation and chemical exposure also have been associated with carcinosarcomas.

Etiology and the disease process: The cause of carcinosarcomas is poorly defined. For malignant mixed mullerian tumors (carcinoma of the endometrium), based on histological staining preparations, the epithelial and stromal components are presumed to originate from the same cell.

Incidence: Incidence depends on the type of carcinosarcoma. Uterine carcinosarcoma is estimated at 33.4 and 17.0 per million in black and white women respectively.

Symptoms: Carcinosarcomas can occur anywhere in the body. They often produce no signs and symptoms in their early stages. They may grow and produce a lump or swell. A tumor may cause pain if it impinges on nerves or muscles. The tumor may cause blockage, bleeding, or other pathological features depending on the location.

Screening and diagnosis: Carcinosarcomas, like many cancers, are staged according to their size and location, their spread to lymph nodes, their spread to other regions in the body, and their grade. Magnetic resonance imaging (MRI), computed tomography (CT), and ultrasound are frequently used for diagnosis. Biopsies are conducted to determine the malignancy and the grade (aggressiveness) of the tumor.

Treatment and therapy: Treatment options for carcinosarcomas, as with other cancers, depends on size, type, location, and stage.

Prognosis, prevention, and outcomes: Prognosis and outcome are determined primarily by depth of invasion and stage.

Rena C. Tabata, M.Sc.

See also: Carcinoma of Unknown Primary origin (CUP); Carcinomatosis; Carcinomatous meningitis; Meningeal carcinomatosis; Metastatic squamous neck cancer with occult primary; Uterine cancer

▶ Cardiomyopathy in cancer patients

Category: Diseases, Symptoms, and Conditions
Also known as: Doxorubicin-induced cardiomyopathy, secondary cardiomyopathy, bleomycin-induced cardiomyopathy, radiation-induced cardiomyopathy

Related conditions: Breast cancer, esophageal cancer, lymphoma, metastases from primary cancers

Definition: Cardiomyopathy is a disease in which the heart muscle is abnormally enlarged, thickened, or stiffened, decreasing its ability to pump blood. According to the World Health Organization, cardiomyopathies can be divided into three types: dilated, restrictive, and hypertrophic, both primary (or idiopathic) and secondary. Cardiomyopathy in cancer patients involves the secondary type of cardiomyopathy, due to a specific cause, usually chemotherapeutic agents such as doxorubicin as well as radiation, which is often employed for lymphoma or cancer of the breast or esophagus. In addition, metastases to the heart muscle from a cancer found elsewhere in the body can result in a restrictive form of cardiomyopathy.

Risk factors: Risk factors for cardiomyopathy in cancer patients include radiation and chemotherapy.

Some Common Symptoms of Cardiomyopathy

- Tiredness
- Weakness
- Abnormal heart rhythm (rapid or pounding)
- Heart murmur
- Swelling of legs, ankles, and feet
- Bloating of the abdomen
- Shortness of breath while at rest or after exercise
- Dizziness, fainting, or light-headedness during exercise

Source: National Heart, Lung, and Blood Institute

Etiology and the disease process: Both doxorubicin and bleomycin cause a dilated type of cardiomyopathy in which both the left and right ventricles are enlarged. The drugs most frequently associated with cardiotoxicity are doxorubicin (Adriamycin) and daunorubicin, which are anthracyclines. The total dose of anthracyclines a person receives determines the probability of developing chronic cardiomyopathy. Other chemotherapeutic drugs that can cause dilated cardiomyopathy include mitoxantrone, interferon, aldesleukin, trastuzumab (a monoclonal antibody), bleomycin, cyclophosphamide, 5-fluorouracil, vincristine, vinblastine, busulfan, mitomycin C, cisplatin, amsacrine, paclitaxel, and docetaxel. In dilated cardiomyopathy due to chemotherapeutic agents, the left ventricle typically demonstrates global hypokinesis, whereas the right ventricle has a less severe abnormality of contractility. Because of the ventricular dilatation, both mitral and tricuspid regurgitation are common, and patients with this condition also exhibit reduced ejection fractions. Decreased cardiac output, decreased stroke volume, and decreased systolic function are seen as well. Mural thrombi may also be present due to akinesis of the cardiac apex.

Radiation to the chest can cause a restrictive form of cardiomyopathy. In this condition the normal heart muscle is replaced by abnormal tissue. This abnormal tissue restricts the diastolic relaxation of the heart muscle so that the heart has normal ventricular size and contractility but aberrant diastolic relaxation leading to elevation of end diastolic pressures of the ventricles.

Incidence: The incidence of congestive heart failure secondary to cardiomyopathy from epirubicin is 0.7 percent. Doxorubicin is more cardiotoxic than epirubicin, and the incidence of congestive heart failure ranges from 3 to 4 percent.

Symptoms: In restrictive cardiomyopathy, the signs and symptoms are related to congestive failure and arrhythmias. In dilated cardiomyopathy due to chemotherapeutic agents, occasionally these agents will cause an acute cardiotoxic effect, with symptoms such as abnormal heart rhythms and electrocardiogram changes.

Screening and diagnosis: Chest X ray demonstrates the paradox of a huge heart with clear lungs in dilated cardiomyopathy. In the restrictive form of cardiomyopathy, the chest X ray often shows a normal-size heart with pulmonary congestion. Because the resultant abnormal physiology of restrictive cardiomyopathy is similar to that of constrictive pericarditis, distinction between these two entities is difficult. Magnetic resonance imaging (MRI), like computed tomography (CT), demonstrates a pericardial thickness greater than 4 millimeters in all patients with constrictive pericarditis, but this is rarely seen in restrictive cardiomyopathy.

In restrictive cardiomyopathy, the electrocardiogram shows low voltage in the late stages, and echocardiography shows decreased diastolic function with normal to decreased ejection fractions. In dilated cardiomyopathy, echocardiography always demonstrates a decreased ejection fraction because of an enlarged left ventricle with global hypokinesis. Systolic function is normal in restrictive cardiomyopathy, whereas it is always decreased in dilated cardiomyopathy. The reverse is true with diastolic function, where it is normal in dilated cardiomyopathy but decreased in restrictive cardiomyopathy. Gated myocardial scintigraphy shows decreased left ventricular ejection fraction, shortened ventricular ejection time, and decreased rate of ejection in dilated cardiomyopathy. Because marked focal wall abnormalities are usually absent in dilated cardiomyopathy, this may help distinguish it from end-stage coronary artery disease, which can manifest with focal-wall motion abnormalities.

Treatment and therapy: Nuclear medicine techniques have become important in monitoring left and right ventricular function in patients receiving chemotherapeutic agents that are cardiotoxic, including anthracyclines such as doxorubicin and daunorubicin. Gated myocardial scintigraphy is reproducible, allowing for serial assessment of ejection fractions and the selection of patients who may best tolerate the medication. Gated myocardial scintigraphy is especially important in monitoring patients to determine the onset of cardiac toxicity. Many clinicians allow the ejection fraction to fall to 0.45 in patients receiving doxorubicin before discontinuing therapy. Newer forms of anthracyclines called liposome encapsulates have been shown to be less toxic to the heart and still effective against cancer.

Prognosis, prevention, and outcomes: Lifestyle changes can reduce symptoms of heart failure from cardiomyopathy. Reducing salt and fluid intake and avoiding alcohol are beneficial as well as a judicious exercise plan to increase stamina without overtaxing a failing heart. Some patients whose cardiomyopathy progresses despite medication may be candidates for cardiac transplant.

Debra B. Kessler, M.D., Ph.D.

For Further Information

Brandenberg, R. O., et al. "Report of the WHO/ISFC Task Force on Definition and Classification of Cardiomyopathies." *Circulation* 64 (1981): 437A.

Brant, William E., and Clyde A. Helms. *Fundamentals of Diagnostic Radiology*. Baltimore: Williams and Wilkins, 1994.

Mettler, Fred A., and Milton J. Guiberteau. *Essentials of Nuclear Medicine Imaging*. 3d ed. Philadelphia: W. B. Saunders, 1991.

Other Resources

American Heart Association
Cardiomyopathy
http://www.americanheart.org/presenter.jhtml?identifier=4468

The Cardiomyopathy Association
http://www.cardiomyopathy.org/

See also: Nuclear medicine scan; Radionuclide scan

▶ Carney complex

Category: Diseases, Symptoms, and Conditions
Also known as: Nevi, atrial myxoma, myxoid neurofibroma, and ephelides (NAME) syndrome; lentigine, atrial myxoma, mucocutaneous myxoma, blue nevi (LAMB) syndrome

Related conditions: Cushing syndrome, multiple thyroid nodules, benign tumors

Definition: Discovered in 1985 by J. Alden Carney, Carney complex is a very rare, inherited genetic condition that can cause a variety of symptoms, ranging from skin pigmentation to tumor growth throughout the body. It primarily involves the endocrine system and, depending on the severity of its symptoms, can lead to cancer or heart failure.

Risk factors: Because Carney complex is an inherited condition, risk factors include family members with Carney complex. Genetic testing or screening is advised for patients with family members who have been previously diagnosed with Carney complex.

Etiology and the disease process: The genes *PRKAR1A* and *CNC2* have been identified in causing Carney complex. It is thought that additional genes are also involved.

Incidence: Carney complex is a rare condition with only 400 cases being documented worldwide.

Symptoms: Onset of Carney complex usually begins in a person's twenties, and symptoms can include spotted pigmentation of the skin on the eyes, lips, mouth, and genitals, as well as heart-related conditions, such as tumors in the chambers of the heart, which, while typically benign, can lead to stroke or heart failure. These tumors can also be found in the thyroid, adrenal gland, breast, brain, and testes. Symptoms of these tumors can include rash, fever, and joint pain.

Screening and diagnosis: Although no standard screening guidelines exist for Carney complex, it is recommended that people suspected of having the disease receive an echocardiogram and blood tests (particularly for prolactin, cortisol, and insulin-like growth factor 1, or IGF-1) once a year, as well as frequent skin, thyroid, and genital exams. If a diagnosis of Carney complex is made, patients should be referred to an oncologist, as there is an increased risk in the development of cancer in patients with Carney complex.

Treatment and therapy: Treatment and therapy are based on the symptoms exhibited by the patient.

Prognosis, prevention, and outcomes: As Carney complex has been diagnosed in less than 400 people throughout the world, with approximately 50 to 75 percent of those cases due to genetic inheritance, prevention is limited to repetitive screening and genetic testing. The outcome of Carney complex is determined by the severity of the symptoms and the speed of diagnosis.

Anna Perez, M.Sc.

See also: Adrenal gland cancers; Adrenocortical cancer; Cushing syndrome and cancer; Endocrine cancers; Genetic counseling; Genetic testing

▶ Castleman disease

Category: Diseases, Symptoms, and Conditions
Also known as: Angiofollicular lymph node hyperplasia, angiomatous lymphoid, Castleman tumor, giant benign lymphoma, Castleman's disease

Related conditions: Angiocentric immunoproliferative lesion, lymphomatoid papulosis

Definition: Castleman disease is a rare disorder of the lymphatic system that causes the growth of benign tumors. Two localized forms often appear in the mediastinum: hyaline-vascular, accounting for almost 90 percent of the cases, and plasma cell. The multicentric type involves several different areas of the body.

Risk factors: Human immunodeficiency virus (HIV) infection is the only known risk factor. It is much more common in HIV patients, particularly in those who have developed acquired immunodeficiency syndrome (AIDS).

Etiology and the disease process: The etiology of this disease remains unknown. Increased production of interleukin-6 (IL-6) in the lymph nodes may play a role in the development of the disease. Human herpesvirus 8 (HHV-8) also plays a role in the development of the multicentric type.

Incidence: Although the number of patients diagnosed annually is unknown, Castleman disease is a very rare condition. Two leading cancer centers in the United States each see about two cases per year. The number of cases has been rising over the past twenty years, however, as the incidence of HIV infection has increased.

Symptoms: Most patients who have the hyaline-vascular type are asymptomatic. Those who have the plasma cell type may have excessive sweating, fatigue, fever, skin rash, or weight loss. Those who have the multicentric type may have a variety of symptoms depending on the areas affected—a common finding is enlarged liver or spleen.

Screening and diagnosis: There is no screening method. Diagnosis is suggested by the appearance of benign lymphatic tumors on imaging studies and the presence of elevated IL-6 levels. Definitive diagnosis can be made only by removal or biopsy of the tumor for histologic examination.

Treatment and therapy: Therapy is usually symptomatic. For localized types, the most common treatment is surgical removal of the tumor. Corticosteroids are used to treat specific symptoms associated with plasma cell and multicentric types, and the multicentric type is sometimes treated with chemotherapeutic agents.

Prognosis, prevention, and outcomes: Prognosis for the localized types is good following complete surgical removal of the tumor. Prognosis is poor, however, for the multicentric type, with an overall mortality rate of 50 percent and median survival of twenty-six months.

Jeremy W. Dugosh, Ph.D.

See also: Benign tumors; Cutaneous T-Cell Lymphoma (CTCL); Lymphomas; Mycosis fungoides

▶ Cervical cancer

Category: Diseases, Symptoms, and Conditions
Also known as: Cervical squamous cell/adenocarcinoma, cervical intraepithelial neoplasm (CIN)

Related conditions: Squamous intraepithelial lesion (SIL), dysplasia, human papillomavirus (HPV) infection

Definition: Cervical cancer is a slow-growing cancer of the female reproductive organs. The two primary types of cervical cancer are squamous cell carcinoma and adenocarcinoma. Classified by microscopic examination, squamous cell carcinoma accounts for 90 percent of diagnosed cases. The majority of the remaining cases are classified as adenocarcinoma, a cancer that develops from the mucus-producing gland cells in the endocervix. Additionally, a very small minority of cervical cancer cases demonstrate characteristics of both types and are therefore classified as adenosquamous or mixed carcinomas.

Risk factors: The most significant risk factor for developing cervical cancer is infection with high-risk types of human papillomavirus (HPV). HPV is sexually transmitted, and certain sexual behaviors can increase the risk of infection: sex at an early age, multiple sexual partners (directly or indirectly through a partner who has multiple sexual partners), and sex with an uncircumcised partner. Although use of condoms does not eliminate the potential for HPV infection because any skin-to-skin contact can be sufficient to transmit the virus, condoms nonetheless do provide limited protection. Studies have identified the following additional risk factors:

- Obesity/low-fiber diet
- Smoking
- Concomitant infection with another sexually transmitted disease such as human immunodeficiency virus (HIV), herpes simplex virus (HSV), or chlamydia
- Long-term oral contraceptive use
- Multiple full-term pregnancies
- In utero exposure to diethylstilbestrol (DES, a hormone prescribed from 1940 to 1971 for some pregnant patients considered at high risk for miscarriage)
- Family history of cervical cancer

Etiology and the disease process: Human papillomavirus (HPV) is a group of more than one hundred distinct viruses, with approximately forty strains capable of infecting the genital tract. Researchers have classified fifteen HPV types as high risk for cancer development, with a nearly two-thirds prevalence of types 16 and 18 in cervical cancer samples. In the vast majority of cases, HPV infection is spontaneously cleared by a healthy immune system. In a minority of cases, however, the virus can remain latent for years before eventually converting normal cervical cells to cancerous ones. Because only a small percentage of women infected with HPV progress to cervical cancer, lifestyle and immune system competence are believed to play a vital role in the progression of the disease.

Incidence: Cancer of the cervix is second only to breast cancer in prevalence among women worldwide. Nearly 500,000 new cases are diagnosed each year, with a greater than 80 percent occurrence in developing countries.

Age-standardized incidence rates fall in the 15 per 100,000 range for most first-world countries. In the United States, more than 11,000 new cases are diagnosed each year, with nearly 4,000 deaths annually.

Symptoms: Early cervical cancer does not generally produce any distinguishable signs or symptoms. Abnormalities found in screening tests are the most common and effective method for detecting the presence of precancerous and cancerous cervical cells. As untreated disease progresses, symptoms may include unusual vaginal bleeding (after intercourse, between periods, postmenopausal); watery, bloody, and foul-smelling vaginal discharge; pelvic pain; or pain during intercourse.

Screening and diagnosis: Extensive cervical screening programs designed to detect early, precancerous cervical changes are well established in most developed countries. Exfoliative cytology (Pap test) is the primary component of these programs, although molecular HPV deoxyribonucleic acid (DNA) testing is also commonly incorporated.

Five-Year Survival Rates for Cervical Cancer, by Stage

Stage	*Survival Rate (%)*
IA	95+
IB1	90
IB2	80-85
IIA/B	75-78
IIIA/B	47-50
IV	20-30

Colposcopy is a second-level diagnostic procedure used as a follow-up to abnormal screening results.

Named after the physician who developed the procedure (Papanikolaou), exfoliative cytology, or Pap test, is a screening procedure involving the collection and microscopic evaluation of cervical cells. During a routine pelvic examination, cervical cells are collected by broom, brush, spatula, or other means. These cells are either smeared directly onto a microscope slide (as in the traditional, "dry" Pap smear) or transferred into a liquid medium to concentrate the cells for subsequent transfer onto a slide. This new liquid-based cytology has demonstrated greater test sensitivity because more cells can be analyzed.

The HPV DNA test is a molecular analysis of a cervical sample to determine the presence of HPV and its type. This test is used in conjunction with an abnormal Pap test as an additional diagnostic tool.

A colposcopy is a pelvic examination in which a light source and binocular microscope are used to enable a direct magnified inspection of the patient's cervix, vagina, and vulva. Application of a weak acetic acid solution also serves to highlight any suspicious abnormalities.

Following abnormal screening results, additional tests may be ordered to confirm diagnosis and determine how far the cancer has spread (staging):

- Biopsy: Analysis of a small section of tissue collected from the cervix
- Proctoscopy: Visual inspection of the rectum for the presence of cancer
- Imaging (such as X ray, magnetic resonance imaging, computed tomography, positron emission tomography): Patient/organ appropriate imaging to inspect for cancer spread (metastasis)

Cervical cancer is staged based on tumor size, invasive nature, and degree of metastasis (spread to lymph nodes/organs). Cervical cancer is staged with the International Federation of Gynecology and Obstetrics (FIGO) system:

- Stage 0: Carcinoma in situ; superficial cancer is detected in the cervical lining.
- Stage I: Cancer has invaded the cervix but has not spread.
- Stage IA: Microscopic amounts of cancer cells are present.
- Stage IA1: Cancer invasion is less than 3 millimeters (mm) deep and less than 7 mm wide.
- Stage IA2: Cancer invasion is between 3 and 5 mm deep and less than 7 mm wide.
- Stage IB: Cancer is greater than 5 mm deep and greater than 7 mm wide.
- Stage IB1: Cancer is visible but less than 4 centimeters (cm).
- Stage IB2: Cancer is visible and greater than 4 cm.
- Stage II: Cancer has spread beyond the cervix but is contained within the pelvis.
- Stage IIA: Cancer has spread to the upper part of the vagina.
- Stage IIB: Cancer has spread to the parametrial tissue (next to the cervix).
- Stage III: Cancer has spread to the lower part of the vagina or the pelvic wall.
- Stage IIIA: Cancer has spread to the lower third of the vagina.
- Stage IIIB: Cancer has spread to the pelvic wall or blocks urine flow.
- Stage IV: Cancer has spread to nearby organs.
- Stage IVA: Cancer has spread to the bladder or rectum.
- Stage IVB: Cancer has spread to more distant organs.

Treatment and therapy: Treatment of cervical cancer largely depends on disease stage. The three treatment options are surgery, radiation, and chemotherapy.

Surgical removal is used primarily for nonmetastatic lesions. Cryosurgery uses a metal probe cooled with liquid nitrogen to freeze cancerous cells. Laser surgery uses a laser to burn (vaporize) cancerous cells. In conization, a thin, heated wire (LEEP, or loop electrosurgical excision procedure) or surgical/laser knife (cold knife cone biopsy) removes the affected tissue. Rarely used as a sole treatment, conization aids in diagnosis before additional surgery or alternative treatment. In a hysterectomy, the degree of the removal of uterine tissue (simple vs. radical) depends on the stage and patient circumstances.

Radiation employs high-energy X rays to kill cancer cells, either externally (external beam radiation) or internally via a radioactive capsule (brachytherapy).

Chemotherapy uses anticancer drugs (such as cisplatin, paclitaxel, topotecan, ifosfamide, or fluorouracil) taken orally or intravenously to treat metastasized cancer.

Prognosis, prevention, and outcomes: Early detection through effective screening programs offers a high probability for complete cancer eradication. Continued adherence to annual cervical screening and healthy habits is integral to continued remission.

A new vaccine, Gardasil, approved by the Food and Drug Administration offers protection against the most dangerous, high-risk HPV types 16 and 18. It also protects against types 6 and 11, which cause genital warts. For greatest efficacy, the vaccine should be administered before the patient has become sexually active. The Federal Advisory Committee on Immunization Practices (ACIP) recommends vaccination for girls aged eleven and twelve. The committee also recommends that nonvaccinated women from age thirteen to twenty-six receive catch-up vaccinations. Although the American Cancer Society (ASC) agrees with the initial vaccination protocol, it recommends catch-up vaccinations for young women aged thirteen to eighteen only. ACS recommends that older women discuss the potential benefit of the vaccination with regard to their personal risk factors for previous exposure to HPV.

Pam Conboy, B.S.

For Further Information

Devita, Vincent T., Jr., Samuel Hellman, and Steven A. Rosenberg, eds. *Cancer: Principles and Practice of Oncology*. 7th ed. Philadelphia: Lippincott Williams & Wilkins, 2005.

Saslow, D., et al. "American Cancer Society Guideline for Human Papillomavirus (HPV) Vaccine Use to Prevent Cervical Cancer and Its Precursors." *CA: A Cancer Journal for Clinicians* 57 (2007): 7-28.

Stewart, Bernard W., and Paul Kleihues, eds. *World Cancer Report*. Lyon, France: IARC Press, 2003.

Other Resources

American Cancer Society
http://www.cancer.org

American College of Obstetricians and Gynecologists
http://www.acog.org

American Society for Colposcopy and Cervical Pathology
http://www.asccp.org

Gynecologic Cancer Foundation
http://www.thegcf.org

International Agency for Research on Cancer
http://www.iarc.fr

National Cancer Institute
http://www.cancer.gov

National Cervical Cancer Coalition
http://www.nccc-online.org

World Health Organization
http://www.who.org

See also: Afterloading radiation therapy; Antiviral therapies; Benign tumors; Biological therapy; Birth control pills and cancer; Carcinomas; Carcinomatosis; Colposcopy; Conization; Diethylstilbestrol (DES); Endometrial cancer; Exenteration; Fertility drugs and cancer; Gynecologic cancers; Human Papillomavirus (HPV); Hysterectomy; Hystero-oophorectomy; Infectious cancers; Loop Electrosurgical Excisional Procedure (LEEP); Pap test; Pelvic examination; Pregnancy and cancer; Vaccines, preventive; Vaginal cancer; Virus-related cancers

▶ Childhood cancers

Category: Diseases, Symptoms, and Conditions
Also known as: Childhood neoplasms, Childhood malignancies

Related conditions: Leukemia, lymphoma, brain cancer, neuroblastoma, osteosarcoma, retinoblastoma, rhabdomyosarcoma

Definition: Childhood (or pediatric) cancers are an ensemble of cancers that occur in individuals who are between the ages of 0 to 19 years of age. Most children's cancer centers treat patients up to age 20. The twelve major types of childhood cancers vary by type of histology, site of origin, race, sex, and age. They are leukemias, lymphomas, brain and spinal tumors, sympathetic nervous system tumors, retinoblastoma, kidney tumors, liver tumors, bone tumors, soft-tissue sarcomas, gonadal and germ-cell tumors, epithelial tumors, and other and unspecified malignant tumors. The most common types are leukemias and lymphomas.

Risk factors: Childhood cancers result from noninherited mutations or changes in the genes of developing cells. Some risk factors have been associated with different types of childhood cancers such as acute lymphocytic leukemia (ALL) and acute myelogenous leukemia (AML).

If a child has an identical twin who was diagnosed with ALL or AML before the age of six, the child has a 20 to 25 percent greater risk of developing the illness. Nonidentical twins and other siblings of children with leukemia have two to four times the average risk of developing the illness. Children with Down syndrome, Klinefelter syndrome, or other genetic syndromes and those who have received drugs following organ transplants also are at greater risk of developing leukemia. Children whose mothers had x-rays during pregnancy and children who were exposed after birth to diagnostic medical radiation from computed tomography scans also have an increased risk of some cancers. Children who have received radiation therapy or chemotherapy for other types of cancer have an increased risk of developing leukemia within an eight-year period following treatment. Studies of possible environmental risk factors, including parental exposure to cancer-causing chemicals, prenatal exposure to pesticides, childhood exposure to common infectious agents, and living near a nuclear power plant, have so far produced mixed results. About 5 percent of all cancers in children are the result of inherited mutations associated with certain familial syndromes. Examples of such syndromes that increase the risk of childhood cancer are Li-Fraumeni syndrome, Beckwith-Wiedemann syndrome, Fanconi anemia syndrome, Noonan syndrome, and von Hippel-Lindau syndrome.

Etiology and the disease process: In childhood leukemia, an abnormal amount of white blood cells, or leukocytes, is produced in the bone marrow; these cells invade the bloodstream and deplete the body's ability to fight infection. As the disease progresses, it affects the body's ability to produce red blood cells and platelets, resulting in anemia, bleeding disorders, and continued risk of infection from the overproduction of white blood cells.

Lymphocytes are infection-fighting white blood cells that are made and stored in the lymph nodes (organs in the neck, groin, abdomen, chest, and armpits), spleen, thymus, tonsils, and bone marrow. In lymphoma, the white blood cells of the lymphatic system grow abnormally, producing cancerous cells called Reed-Sternberg cells. Although Hodgkin disease is most often seen in children aged fifteen or older, nodular lymphocyte predominance (LP) is more common in younger children, accounting for about one-fifth of the incidence of most Hodgkin disease in children. Non-Hodgkin lymphoma (NHL) occurs more often in boys than girls and most often between the ages of two and ten. Unlike the non-Hodgkin lymphoma seen in adults, most cases of NHL in children are of the fast-growing, aggressive type (such as Burkitt lymphoma, non-Burkitt lymphoma, and lymphoblastic lymphoma).

Another common type of childhood cancer, neuroblastomas (solid tumors), often begins in one of the adrenal glands above the kidneys; the tumors can also can arise in nerve tissues in the neck, abdomen, pelvis, or chest. While the cause of neuroblastomas is unknown, they are believed to arise from anomalies during the normal development of the adrenal glands.

Existing scientific data continues to suggest that possibly in conjunction with other risk factors infection plays a critical role in the development of childhood ALL. However, no specific bacterial- or viral-associated infections are definitively associated with the disease.

Incidence: In the United States cancer continues to be the leading disease-related cause of death among children and adolescents. At the beginning of 2014, an estimated 10,450 children and adolescents, ages 0 to 19 years, were newly diagnosed with cancer and 1,350 died from such cancers. Also in the United States, the incidence of childhood cancer generally is approximately 125 per million persons, with slightly increased rates in males and white children. Cancer rates remain higher for children under five years of age and those between the ages of fifteen and nineteen.

The National Cancer Institute (NCI), reports leukemias as the most common of cancers occurring in childhood (25 percent). Of these, 60 percent were cases of acute lymphocytic leukemia (ALL), and 38 percent were acute myelogenous leukemia (AML). Most childhood leukemias are diagnosed under the age of 8 years, with reports of peak incidences ranging from 2–3 years to 2–5 years. The next most common type of tumors are those of the CNS (17%) followed by neuroblastoma (7%) which is the most common form of solid tumor occurring outside the brain in children. Non-Hodgkin lymphoma (NHL) (6%) is described as tumors originating from lymphoid tissues primarily of lymph nodes. Wilms tumor (6%) is referred to as a nephroblastoma and is the most common childhood abdominal malignancy. This tumor affects one or both kidneys and seen in children between two and three years of age. Hodgkin disease is next in commonality (5%) and defined as a unique neoplasm in which the malignant cell, called the Reed-Stenberg cell (RSC), represents only a small proportion of cells constituting the bulk of the tumor. Rhabdomyosarcoma (3%) develops in cells that become mature voluntary muscle and is noted as the most common soft-tissue sarcoma seen in children. Retinoblastoma (3%) affecting the eye is next common followed by osteosarcoma (3%), thought to arise from a primitive mesenchymal bone-forming cell.

Improvements in the survival rates of leukemias, Hodgkin disease, and sarcomas can be traced to the use of aggressive therapy and the prudent use of blood products, use of cytokines, and improved supportive care to prevent and treat infections. However the incidence and mortality rates of childhood cancers differ worldwide and depend on how extensive data is reported. Incidences vary from as high as 155 per million persons in Nigeria to 40 per million persons in the Indian population of Fiji. Rates for the United States are thought to be more accurate because 94% of all patients with cancer are reportedly seen at one of the institutions of the Children's Oncology Group (COG).

Symptoms: The symptoms of childhood cancer vary by type, may mimic symptoms of other illnesses, and may include unexplained weight loss; headaches; vomiting; increased swelling or pain in bone, joints, back, or legs; a detectable lump or mass in the abdomen, pelvis, chest, armpit, or neck; unusual bleeding, bruising, or rash; recurring infections; sudden and persistent eye or vision changes; nausea; a whitish color behind the pupil; tiredness; pallor; and recurring and persistent fevers.

A child in the early stages of leukemia may not have these symptoms but may exhibit other changes in behavior, such as lacking the usual energy to engage in activities, and irritability. Additionally, child leukemia patients might display easy bruising, unusual bleeding, frequent nose bleeds, bleeding gums, repeated, frequent infections, fever that lasts for several days, loss of appetite, weight loss swollen lymph nodes, bloated or tender stomach, swollen liver or spleen, and night sweats.

A painless swelling of the lymph nodes, fever, and fatigue are often symptoms of both Hodgkin disease and non-Hodgkin lymphoma. The type of Hodgkin disease most often seen in young adults ages fifteen and older is associated with these symptoms: swollen lymph node in the neck, groin, or armpit; lethargy and weakness; facial swelling; night sweats; unexplained fever and weight loss; abdominal pain or swelling; difficulty breathing; and pain. Non-Hodgkin lymphoma may progress quickly in children, with many initially diagnosed at Stage III or IV, so these children may first complain of abdominal pain, fever, or constipation or decreased appetite originating from an abdominal mass.

Neuroblastoma, or a cancer of the sympathetic nervous system, the most common type of cancer in infants, is usually seen as a lump or mass in the abdomen causing swelling, discomfort, pain, or a feeling of fullness. A neuroblastoma can also occur in the pelvis, neck, or eye. Often the neuroblastoma may spread to bone, causing pain, limping, weakness, numbness, or inability to walk. In about one-quarter of cases, the child may develop fever; less common symptoms include rapid heartbeat, flushed skin, sweating, irritability, high blood pressure, and diarrhea.

Screening and diagnosis: There are no tests that screen for childhood cancers such as leukemia or lymphoma; however, there are standard tests for diagnosing them. Typically, a parent notices a change in a child's behavior and brings the child to the doctor, who will conduct a complete physical and examine the child for enlargement of the lymph nodes, liver, or spleen. If a blood cancer such as leukemia is suspected, the doctor will order a complete blood count (CBC) with differential. A fraction of patients with leukemia may have a normal blood test result when diagnosed. Suspicious cases must have a bone marrow test to confirm the diagnosis of leukemia.

If Hodgkin disease or non-Hodgkin lymphoma is suspected, the physician will do a thorough exam and order a CBC and a chest X ray. If the diagnosis of lymphoma is confirmed, the doctor may refer the child to a specialist, such as a pediatric hematologist or oncologist, for further diagnostic tests such as a biopsy of the tumor to differentially diagnose the type of lymphoma, a bone marrow aspirate, or an imaging test such as a computed tomography (CT) scan.

Neuroblastomas are relatively rare, and screening for them in children with no symptoms is not believed to decrease mortality from the disease, so no screening test is conventionally used. Most neuroblastomas are detected within the first six months of life. A doctor who suspects an infant of having a neuroblastoma will order a urinalysis, which will reveal a higher-than-normal concentration of metabolites from the body's breakdown of catecholamine neurotransmitters. If the physical exam and urine chemistry results indicate a neuroblastoma, the doctor will proceed to order other tests, such as an X ray, CT scan, abdominal ultrasound, CBC, blood test of liver and kidney function, bone scan, metaiodobenzylguanidine (MIBG) scan, and bone marrow aspiration.

Staging is used to describe the disease at the time of diagnosis and to help the doctor determine the type of therapy, its course, and its prognosis. Leukemia, unlike other childhood cancers, is staged based on its presence and proliferation in organs other than its presence in the bone marrow and blood. Other factors in staging include sex, race, organ spread, types of leukemic cells, presence of abnormal chromosomes, and response to treatment within seven to fourteen days of inception. Staging to assess a child's prognosis seems to be more important in children with ALL than in those with AML. Age and white blood cell count (WBCC) are important factors in staging ALL, with children younger than one and older than ten at highest risk (having a high white blood cell count of 50,000 cells per cubic millimeter).

Lymphoma is staged based on the extent of the disease. Stage I lymphoma is limited to one primary area of the lymph node or organ, while Stage IV indicates the lymphoma has spread to one or more tissues or organs outside the lymphatic system.

Neuroblastomas are staged I to IV-S, with Stage I being a tumor that is visible, is localized, and can be removed, and Stage IV being a cancer that has spread to distant lymph nodes or other parts of the body. In Stage IV-S, limited to a child less than one year of age, the cancer has spread to skin, liver, or bone marrow but not to bone. Alternatively, neuroblastomas may be staged on the basis of low, intermediate, and high risk, depending on the features of the cancer cells, the age at which the child is diagnosed, and the stage of the disease.

Treatment and therapy: Childhood cancers are treated with surgery, chemotherapy, radiation therapy, or a combination of two or more therapies. Cancers in children, unlike those in many adults, typically are fast growing and respond well to chemotherapy. Children are often treated in children's cancer centers, which tend to offer new therapies and the latest treatment with clinical trials. The NCI recommends that children with cancer be treated by a multidisciplinary team consisting of a pediatric oncologist and other specialists and that all children be considered for clinical trials to test the effectiveness of existing treatments and evaluate the benefits and side effects of experimental treatments. The American Cancer Society (ACS) recommends that parents ask their pediatric cancer team about the potential side effects of treatment before the regimen begins. Side effects include hair loss, fatigue, risk of infection, easy bruising or bleeding, vomiting, diarrhea, bone marrow changes leading to anemia, lower white blood cell counts leading to reduced ability to fight infections, and a reduction in platelet production.

Treatment for the most common forms of cancer seen in children, acute lymphocytic leukemia (ALL) and acute myelogenous leukemia (AML), consists of three phases: induction, consolidation, and maintenance. Once the cancer is staged by risk group, induction therapy is designed to induce remission such that leukemic cells are no longer present in bone marrow, normal cells return, and blood counts return to normal. The month-long treatment, often performed in the hospital, is intense because of the risk of serious infection, but more than 95 percent children with ALL who receive this treatment experience remission. Although the cancer is in remission, consolidation treatment lasting four to six months and maintenance therapy lasting at least two years are required to destroy all cancerous cells. These intravenous chemotherapies are coupled with intrathecal chemotherapy (drugs injected into the fluid surrounding the brain and spinal cord) to destroy cancer cells that may have spread to the central nervous system. In addition, radiation therapy may be directed at the brain or spinal cord if the leukemia was present in cerebrospinal fluid at the time of diagnosis; however, the side effects and long-term effects of radiation to the brain are such that this type of radiation therapy is avoided whenever possible. Low-risk ALL has the highest cure rate, 85 to 95 percent of all cases.

In all age groups, Hodgkin lymphoma is highly sensitive to chemotherapy and irradiation and was the first cancer to be cured with radiation therapy alone or with a combination of several chemotherapeutic agents.

The three main types of therapy for Hodgkin disease are radiation therapy to decrease tumors and destroy cancerous cells; chemotherapy or systemic drug therapy; and bone marrow and peripheral blood transplants, particularly for those whose disease recurs. The four types of non-Hodgkin lymphoma seen in children (Burkitt, lymphoblastic, anaplastic large-cell lymphoma, and large B-cell lymphoma) may be localized in a swollen lymph node, but often the disease has spread to other organs at the time of diagnosis.

Some neuroblastomas go away without treatment, while others commonly require surgery. Approximately half of the tumors spread to bone and bone marrow, requiring chemotherapy, radiation therapy, stem cell transplantation, or immunotherapy. The location of the tumor, age of the child, and diffusion of the tumor are factors in determining the recommended treatment

Prognosis, prevention, and outcomes: Overall, death rates have declined and five-year survival rates have increased for most types of childhood cancers. The increase in survival rates is attributable to new treatments resulting in cures or long-term remission for many children with cancer. Although the majority of cancers respond well to treatment, some will recur and require the child's doctor to develop a new treatment plan. The most commonly reported longevity statistic is the five-year survival rate, or the percentage of children with cancer who live at least five years after diagnosis.

According to the American Cancer Institute the 5-year survival rates for the most recent time period (2005-2011) for the more common childhood cancers are:

Acute lymphocytic leukemias: 89%, Acute myelogenous leukemias: 65%, Brain and other central nervous system tumors: 72%, Wilms tumors: 92%, Hodgkin lymphomas: 98%, Non-Hodgkin lymphomas: 89%, Rhabdomyosarcomas: 69%, Neuroblastomas: 78%, Retinoblastomas: 97%, Osteosarcomas: 69%, Ewing sarcomas: 78%.

Children with cancer respond to chemotherapies and tolerate treatment better than adults do, making their prognosis bright. However, children who survive cancer may have long-term effects that require lifelong follow-up. These late or delayed effects can include hormonal disturbances in the endocrine system causing short stature, problems in puberty, thyroid or fertility disturbances, secondary learning difficulties, and other health consequences of the disease or treatment. Published data on long-term survivors of childhood cancers indicate that those most at risk of developing secondary sarcomas (cancers of connective or supportive tissue such as in bone, fat, or muscle) are children whose primary cancer was in soft tissue, bone, or renal tissue, or was Hodgkin disease. Because sarcomas can occur anywhere in the body and are more difficult to detect, long-term aggressive follow-up of childhood cancer patients is critical to their staying healthy.

Susan H. Peterman, M.P.H.
Updated by: Jeffrey P. Larson PT, ATC

For Further Information

Eiser, Christine. (2004). Children with cancer: *The quality of life*. Mahwah, N.J.: Lawrence Erlbaum Associates.

Fromer, Margot Joan. (1998). *Surviving childhood cancer: A guide for families*. Oakland, CA: New Harbinger.

Keene, Nancy. (2002). *Chemo, craziness, and comfort: My book about childhood cancer*. Washington, D.C.: Candlelighters.

Langton, Helen. (2000). *The child with cancer: Family-centered care in practice*. New York: Baillière Tindall.

O'Connor, S. M., & Boneva, R. S. (2007). Infectious Etiologies of Childhood Leukemia: Plausibility and Challenges to Proof. *Environmental Health Perspectives,* 115(1): 146–150. http://doi.org/10.1289/ehp.9024

Botha, M. H., & Kruger, T. F. (2012). A review of the incidence and survival of childhood and adolescent cancer and the effects of treatment on future fertility and endocrine development.(Report). *South African Journal of Obstetrics and Gynaecology*. South African Medical Association. Retrieved March 02, 2016 from HighBeam Research: https://www.highbeam.com/doc/1G1-288874072.html

Other Resources

Candlelighters Childhood Cancer Foundation
http://www.candlelighters.org

The Leukemia and Lymphoma Society
http://www.lls.org

Memorial Sloan-Kettering Cancer Center
http://www.mskcc.org

U.S. Cancer Statistics Working Group. United States Cancer Statistics: 1999–2012 Incidence and Mortality Web-based

Report. Atlanta: U.S. Department of Health and Human Services, Centers for Disease Control and Prevention and National Cancer Institute; 2015
www.cdc.gov/uscs.
http://www.cancer.org/

Children's Oncology Group (COG)
www.childrensoncologygroup.org

National Children's Cancer Society, Inc.
www.children-cancer.org

See also: Acute Lymphocytic Leukemia (ALL); Bone cancers; Breast cancer in children and adolescents; Craniopharyngiomas; Craniosynostosis; Cryptorchidism; Denys-Drash syndrome and cancer; Ependymomas; Family history and risk assessment; Genetics of cancer; Hereditary polyposis syndromes; Hodgkin disease; Juvenile polyposis syndrome; Leukemias; Medulloblastomas; Nephroblastomas; Neuroblastomas; Non-Hodgkin lymphoma; Pediatric oncology and hematology; Peutz-Jeghers Syndrome (PJS); Pheochromocytomas; Pineoblastomas; Pleuropulmonary blastomas; RB1 gene; Retinoblastomas; Rhabdomyosarcomas; Rothmund-Thomson syndrome; Spinal axis tumors; Spinal cord compression; Vaginal cancer; Von Hippel-Lindau (VHL) disease; Wilms' tumor; Wilms' tumor Aniridia-Genitourinary anomalies-mental Retardation (WAGR) syndrome and cancer; Yolk sac carcinomas; Young adult cancers

▶ Chordomas

Category: Diseases, Symptoms, and Conditions
Also known as: Chordocarcinomas, chordoepitheliomas

Related conditions: Sarcomas

Definition: Chordomas are cancerous bone tumors that can occur anywhere along the spinal cord, most commonly at the base of the skull, at the base of the spine (sacrum), or in the tailbone (coccyx).

Risk factors: There are no known risk factors. Bone injury, environment, diet, medications, and genetics do not appear to play a role in the development of chordomas.

Etiology and the disease process: Chordomas develop in leftover pieces of cells from the notochord, a flexible, rod-shaped structure that forms during early fetal development and precedes the spine.

Incidence: Chordomas are rare. Most cases have been reported in persons age forty to seventy. Sacrum chordomas are more common in men; chordomas at the skull base are more common in women.

Symptoms: Symptoms develop gradually and depend on the tumor site. Tumors near the skull base can cause headaches, face pain, and vision problems. Tumors in the lower spine and tailbone area may lead to leg weakness, leg or groin numbness, constipation, impotence, and bowel and bladder dysfunction. A tailbone chordoma may manifest with a noticeable mass. Chordomas in the upper part of the spine may cause hoarseness and swallowing problems.

Screening and diagnosis: Most chordomas grow slowly and do not spread, and the gradual development of symptoms often results in a delayed diagnosis. Patients often have symptoms for more than a year before diagnosis. Computed tomography and magnetic resonance imaging can reveal bone destruction and tissue damage. Biopsy of the tumor confirms the diagnosis.

Treatment and therapy: Surgery to remove the tumor and surrounding tissue is the best option but often difficult because of the tumor's precarious positioning near the spinal cord and brain. Surgery often results in some type of nerve loss. For example, removing a chordoma from the tailbone can damage the nerves that control bladder and bowel function. Radiation therapy may be used along with surgery to ensure that all cancer cells are destroyed. Chemotherapy does not appear to be an effective treatment for chordomas.

Prognosis, prevention, and outcomes: If cancer cells remain after treatment, a chordoma can recur and spread to other parts of the body, most commonly the lymph nodes, lungs, and liver. The recurrence rate is high. Survival rates depend on the location of the tumor. Persons with chordomas of the skull base tend to have the best prognosis. Overall, about 90 percent of persons with chordomas survive about five to ten years.

Kelli Miller Stacy, ELS

See also: Bone cancers; Spinal axis tumors

▶ Choriocarcinomas

Category: Diseases, Symptoms, and Conditions
Also known as: Chorioblastomas, trophoblastic tumors, chorioepitheliomas, gestational trophoblast neoplasia, gestational trophoblastic disease

Related conditions: Invasive mole

Definition: One of the most dangerous germ-cell cancers, choriocarcinoma is a quick-growing cancer that occurs in a woman's uterus after a pregnancy, miscarriage, or spontaneous abortion. This cancer arises from trophoblastic cells of the placenta and mimics the development of normal placental tissue. The cancer is usually invasive (metastatic), growing so fast that the original tumor outgrows its blood supply and dies, leaving behind only a small scar. For unknown reasons, it metastasizes early to the lungs, liver, and brain.

Risk factors: Pregnant women are at risk.

Etiology and the disease process: Choriocarcinoma is an uncommon cancer that is associated with pregnancy. Choriocarcinomas result from genetic damage to a germ cell. The cancer forms in the trophoblast (placental) cells that surround the baby. About half of all choriocarcinomas arise from a hydatidiform mole, also known as a molar pregnancy, in which a nonviable embryo implants and rapidly grows within the mother's uterus. Approximately one-quarter of choriocarcinomas occur after pregnancy has resulted in the delivery of a normal child. The remainder of cases occur after any type of abortion, ectopic pregnancy, or genital tumor. Most choriocarcinomas form inside the reproductive organs, such as the testes or ovaries, especially in young adults. A few choriocarcinomas arise in sites outside the reproductive organs (extragonadal tumors); these are usually found in young adults and are more common in men.

Incidence: In North America, choriocarcinoma occurs in approximately 1 in 30,000 to 40,000 pregnancies.

Choriocarcinoma is more common in Asian Americans than African Americans, and least common in whites. Choriocarcinoma has been shown to occur following hydatidiform mole (50 percent), normal term pregnancy (25 percent), and spontaneous abortion (25 percent).

Symptoms: The symptoms of a choriocarcinoma vary, depending on where the tumor originates and where it spreads. If the cancer is in the uterus, the most common symptom is bleeding. Cancers in the ovary often have only subtle signs such as widening of the waistline or pain. In the testes, choriocarcinomas can often be felt as small painless lumps. Choriocarcinomas that spread to other organs may reveal their presence as a result of the bleeding or complications from bleeding that occur in their presence. In the brain, this bleeding can cause a stroke. Additional symptoms may include irregular vaginal bleeding, uneven swelling of the uterus, persistently high human chorionic gonadotropin (HCG) levels, or localized pain.

Screening and diagnosis: Most choriocarcinomas produce human chorionic gonadotropin, a hormone normally found only during pregnancy. The presence of HCG in the blood can help in diagnosing this cancer and monitoring the success of treatment. Choriocarcinomas are usually referred to a doctor who specializes in cancer treatment (an oncologist). To diagnose this tumor, the doctor will do a physical examination and examine the internal organs with X rays or ultrasounds. Choriocarcinomas may not be biopsied before being treated because they tend to bleed heavily. Choriocarcinomas can be detected using ultrasound, X rays, computed tomography (CT), magnetic resonance imaging (MRI) scans, or positron emission tomography (PET) scans.

Treatment and therapy: After making the initial diagnosis, the oncologist will take a careful history and perform an examination to rule out metastasis (spread to other organs). Chemotherapy is the treatment of choice. Choriocarcinoma is one of the tumors that is most sensitive to chemotherapy. The cure rate, even for metastatic choriocarcinoma, is about 90 percent. Almost all patients without metastases can be cured; however, metastatic disease to the kidneys, liver, or brain can be fatal. The chemotherapy regimen is generally EMA-CO: etoposide, methotrexate, actinomycin D, cyclosphosphamide, and vincristine (Oncovin). A hysterectomy (surgical removal of the uterus) is rarely required; however, a hysterectomy may be offered to patients over forty years of age or those desiring sterilization. It may be required for those with severe infection and uncontrolled bleeding.

Prognosis, prevention, and outcomes: No known means of prevention exists; however, early detection of the symptoms and prompt medical treatment can improve the odds of survival. Although careful monitoring after the removal of a hydatidiform mole or the termination of pregnancy may not prevent the development of choriocarcinoma, it is essential in early identification of the condition, which improves outcome. The prognosis for choriocarcinomas in the uterus is very good. Although these tumors have often spread throughout the body, chemotherapy results in a cure or remission in at least 85 to 90 percent of cases. Women who have had choriocarcinomas often go on to have normal pregnancies and deliveries. Choriocarcinomas in sites other than the uterus have a poorer prognosis. These tumors tend to spread quickly and do not always respond well to chemotherapy. Although treatment can be effective, the outcome usually depends on how widely the cancer is dispersed. Generally, the prognosis is worse if the cancer can be found in the liver or brain, if HCG levels are high, or if the original tumor developed outside the gonads. However, about two-thirds of women who initially have a poor outlook go into remission (a disease-free state).

Thomas L. Brown, Ph.D.

For Further Information

Baker, Vicki V. "Gestational Trophoblastic Disease." In *Clinical Oncology*, edited by Martin D. Abeloff et al. 2d ed. Philadelphia: Churchhill Livingstone, 2000.

Berkowitz, Ross S., and Donald P. Goldstein. "Gestational Trophoblast Neoplasia." In *Practical Gynecologic Oncology*, edited by Jonathan S. Berek and Neville F. Hacker. 4th ed. Philadelphia: Lippincott Williams & Wilkins, 2004.

Vinay, Kumar, Abul K. Abbas, and Nelson Fausto. *Robbins and Cotran Pathological Basis of Disease*. 7th ed. Philadelphia: Elsevier/Saunders, 2005.

Other Resources

Eyes on the Prize.org
http://www.eyesontheprize.org/index.shtml

My Molar Pregnancy.com
http://www.geocities.com/thornfield8998/molar.html

See also: Germ-cell tumors; Gestational Trophoblastic Tumors (GTTs); Human Chorionic Gonadotropin (HCG); Hydatidiform mole; Pituitary tumors; Teratocarcinomas

▶ Chronic Lymphocytic Leukemia (CLL)

Category: Diseases, Symptoms, and Conditions
Also known as: Chronic lymphoid leukemia

Related conditions: Acute lymphocytic leukemia, acute myeloid leukemia, chronic myeloid leukemia

Definition: Chronic lymphocytic leukemia (CLL) is a cancer of the white blood cells. A lymphocyte is a type of white blood cell made in the bone marrow that helps fight infection. For unknown reasons, the bone marrow begins to make lymphocytes that develop abnormally, causing this fast-growing type of cancer. In this disease name, "chronic" means that the disease does not progress as rapidly as acute lymphocytic leukemia.

Risk factors: There are few risk factors for CLL. Past research has concluded that the risk of developing CLL is not affected by environmental factors. However, research is ongoing as to whether exposure to herbicides and insecticides increases the risk of CLL. About half the people who develop CLL have chromosomal abnormalities, such as deletions on a chromosome or an extra chromosome. People with close relatives who have CLL have a slightly increased risk of developing this disease. Risk increases with age; patients with CLL are rarely under the age of forty-five and are generally over the age of sixty. Men are more likely to develop CLL than women, and whites and those of Russian Jewish or Eastern European Jewish descent are more likely to develop it than those of other racial and ethnic backgrounds.

Etiology and the disease process: CLL starts in a single white blood cell (lymphocyte). These CLL cells begin to multiply and crowd out the normal white blood cells. The CLL cells accumulate in the bone marrow, but they do not stop normal blood cell production quite as much as some other types of leukemia. Slow-growing CLL may cause only minimal changes in the blood for years. Some patients begin to produce an antibody during the CLL disease process that works against their body's own red blood cells and causes a severe type of anemia. In a small number of CLL patients, the disease changes and begins to act like a more aggressive type of lymphoma or leukemia. In a very small number of CLL patients, throughout the disease process, CLL begins to act like acute lymphocytic leukemia (ALL).

Incidence: About 15,340 people in the United States were diagnosed with CLL in 2007. Most with CLL are more than fifty years old.

Symptoms: Symptoms of CLL usually develop slowly. Patients may find out they have this type of slow-growing cancer after getting blood tests for another condition. Symptoms may include anemia, bleeding easily, bone pain, bruising easily, fever, joint pain, loss of appetite, night sweats, pain or a feeling of fullness below the ribs, shortness of breath, swollen liver, swollen lymph nodes, swollen spleen, tiredness, unexplained or repeated infections, and weight loss.

Screening and diagnosis: There is no screening test for CLL. Blood and bone marrow tests are necessary to diagnose CLL. These tests look for abnormal lymphocyte cells. A bone marrow aspirate test (using a long needle to take marrow out of the bone) and a bone marrow biopsy (surgical removal of some bone marrow) are two possible tests. The bone marrow aspirate test looks for abnormal cells in the bone marrow and can also be used for other types of analysis. A bone marrow biopsy can show how much disease is already in the bone marrow. The results of these tests help determine which type of drug therapy to use and how long treatment should last. Another test that may be performed, immunophenotyping, helps determine whether the increased lymphocytes in the blood are monoclonal (came from a single malignant cell). This can help distinguish CLL from other types of diseases that cause increased lymphocytes in the blood.

Depending on where the cancer started and the results of testing, CLL may be categorized into B-cell CLL (the most common type), T-cell CLL (which generally behaves more like other T-cell cancers than like CLL), or NK-cell CLL. B-cell CLL may be divided into further subtypes based on whether genetic mutations have occurred. As these mutations may affect how rapidly the disease progresses, this further division may help doctors determine treatment and which patients will benefit from earlier treatment. These subdivisions may also give a general idea of the progression and outcome of the disease, such as what effect the disease will have on marrow and blood cell development and what other organs, such as kidneys, bowels, or liver, may be affected. Researchers are investigating whether these subdivisions of CLL are actually different types of cancer.

Staging of CLL involves evaluating the number of CLL cells; whether the liver, lymph nodes, or spleen are enlarged; and whether the red blood cell or platelet counts

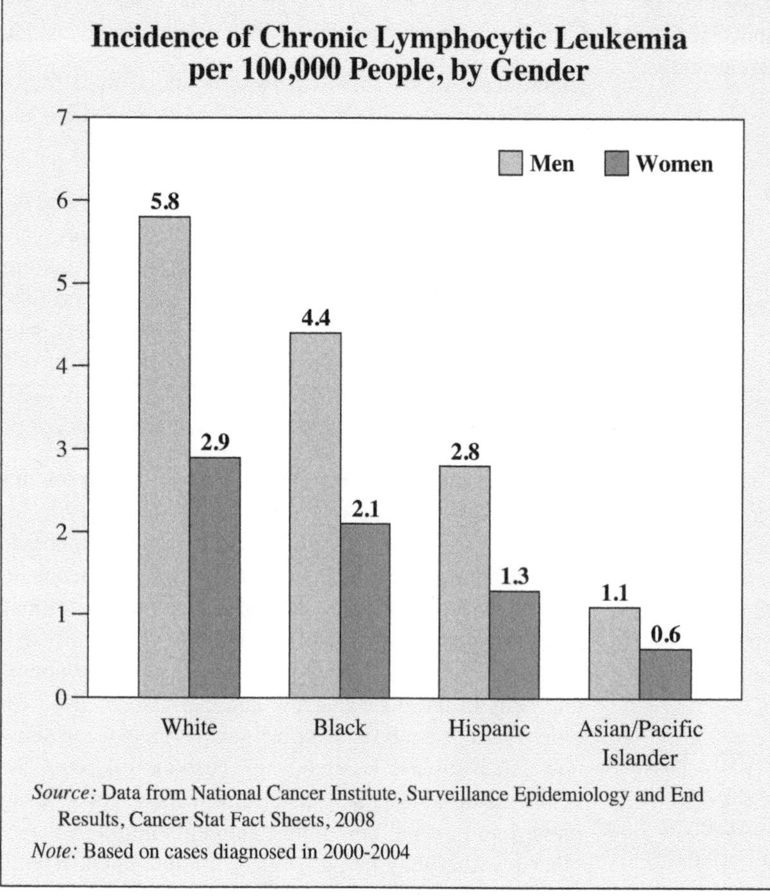

Source: Data from National Cancer Institute, Surveillance Epidemiology and End Results, Cancer Stat Fact Sheets, 2008

Note: Based on cases diagnosed in 2000-2004

are low. In the Rai system, used commonly in the United States, CLL is divided into five stages:

- Stage 0: Large numbers of lymphocytes in the blood but no other symptoms
- Stage I: Large numbers of lymphocytes in the blood and enlarged lymph nodes
- Stage II: Large numbers of lymphocytes in the blood, enlarged liver or spleen, possibly enlarged lymph nodes
- Stage III: Large numbers of lymphocytes in the blood, too few red blood cells (anemia), possibly enlarged lymph nodes, liver, or spleen
- Stage IV: Large numbers of lymphocytes in the blood, too few platelets, possibly too few red blood cells, and possibly enlarged lymph nodes, liver, or spleen

Treatment and therapy: Patients diagnosed with CLL may not need treatment immediately. They may have good health for several years without any treatment at all. However, doctors will want to watch and wait—closely follow patients with CLL to ensure that the CLL is not getting worse. This allows patients to avoid the side effects of treatment until treatment is necessary.

However, some patients will need treatment near the time of diagnosis because these patients have had the disease for some time and it is progressing or because they have a faster-growing type of CLL. Treatment may become necessary when the number of CLL cells rapidly becomes higher, the number of normal cells becomes lower, anemia becomes worse, the lymph nodes or spleen have enlarged, or symptoms have become bothersome to patients.

Treatment involves slowing the growth of CLL cells, keeping patients well enough to carry out daily activities, and protecting patients from infections, because the abnormal white cells are not able to fight infection. CLL is usually treated with chemotherapy or monoclonal antibody therapy. Both these therapies involve the use of certain drugs or drug combinations to kill abnormal lymphocytes.

A bone marrow or cord blood transplant may help some CLL patients. A transplant is a high-risk procedure, however, and probably will not be used unless a patient has a fast-growing type of CLL, is younger than fifty-five years of age, and has a close relative who is a good transplant match. Older patients or patients with slow-growing CLL are not good transplant candidates.

CLL is not usually treated with radiation therapy. However, radiation may be used if a large mass of lymphocytes is blocking an important part of the body, such as the kidneys, stomach, intestines, or throat. In a small number of CLL patients, surgery to remove the spleen (splenectomy) can help relieve pressure if the spleen is filled with too many CLL cells.

If patients with CLL have problems fighting infections, they may be treated with antibiotics. If infections become a chronic problem, patients may be treated with injections of a protein found in the blood that fights infections (immunoglobulin).

Follow-up treatment for CLL involves regular doctor visits and continuing lab tests to make sure the CLL cells are not beginning to increase rapidly. These doctor visits also help find any side effects from treatment. Patients who have had CLL are at increased risk for developing some other cancers, such as lung, colon, or skin cancer, and patients should be screened for these conditions during follow-up visits.

Prognosis, prevention, and outcomes: There is no cure for CLL and no known way of preventing the disease. However, many patients, especially those with slow-growing forms of this disease, may live for many years in good health. Survival rates range from one year to more than twenty or thirty years depending on stage and form of disease. The five-year survival rate of CLL patients is greater than 70 percent.

Marianne M. Madsen, M.S.

For Further Information

Caligaris-Cappio, F., and R. Dalla-Favera, eds. *Chronic Lymphocytic Leukemia*. New York: Springer, 2005.

Faguet, G. B. *Chronic Lymphocytic Leukemia: Molecular Genetics, Biology, Diagnosis, and Management*. Totowa, N.J.: Humana Press, 2003.

Parker, James N., and Philip M. Parker, eds. *The Official Patient's Sourcebook on Chronic Lymphocytic Leukemia: A Revised and Updated Directory for the Internet Age*. San Diego, Calif.: Icon Health, 2002.

Other Resources

Chronic Lymphocytic Leukemia Foundation
http://www.cllfoundation.org

Leukemia and Lymphoma Society
http://www.leukemia-lymphoma.org

National Cancer Institute
Chronic Lymphocytic Leukemia Treatment
http://www.cancer.gov/cancertopics/pdq/treatment/CLL

See also: Acute Lymphocytic Leukemia (ALL); Acute Myelocytic Leukemia (AML); Agent Orange; Blood cancers; Chronic Myeloid Leukemia (CML); Hairy cell leukemia; Hemolytic anemia; Immunoelectrophoresis (IEP); Leukemias; Lymphocytosis; Monoclonal antibodies; Richter syndrome; Side effects; Staging of cancer

▶ Chronic Myeloid Leukemia (CML)

Category: Diseases, Symptoms, and Conditions
Also known as: Chronic granulocytic leukemia, chronic myelocytic leukemia, chronic myelogenous leukemia

Related conditions: Acute lymphocytic leukemia, acute myeloid leukemia, chronic lymphocytic leukemia, chronic myelomonocytic leukemia, chronic neutrophilic leukemia, juvenile myelomonocytic leukemia, other myeloproliferative disorders such as essential thrombocythemia, myelofibrosis, and polycythemia vera

Definition: Chronic myeloid leukemia (CML) is one of the four types of leukemia, cancers of the white blood cells. Patients with CML have a growth of malignant bone marrow cells, and these bone marrow cells begin to accumulate in the blood. Usually, these patients have a chromosome abnormality called the *BCR-ABL* cancer gene. "Chronic" means this cancer is more slow growing than an acute type of cancer. "Myeloid" is the type of white blood cell that is affected.

Risk factors: About 95 percent of people with CML have a chromosome abnormality called the Philadelphia chromosome (named after the city where it was first documented). The Philadelphia chromosome occurs when a piece of chromosome 22 breaks off at a gene called *BCR*. If a piece of chromosome 9 breaks at a gene called *ABL* and switches with the break in chromosome 22, the *BCR-ABL* cancer gene forms. This gene somehow instructs cells to make a protein that leads to CML. This gene appears only in the cells that form blood and is not passed on to other family members. This switch in chromosomes may be affected by very high levels of radiation (such as in atomic bomb survivors) or high-dose radiation therapy for other kinds of cancers. However, most people with CML do not have these risk factors, and others who have these risk factors do not develop CML.

Etiology and the disease process: Like all leukemias, CML begins with a change in a single cell. At diagnosis, patients may be feeling well. Usually, the body makes more white blood cells only when fighting an infection, and when the infection has passed, the number of white blood cells returns to normal. However, if this disease is not treated, the white blood cells begin to increase rapidly and start to circulate in the blood, causing swelling of the liver and spleen. The number of *BCR-ABL* cancer genes in the body increases. The disease may progress to a phase in which the patient has a low red blood cell count (anemia) and the platelets are not able to function properly. Eventually the ability of the white blood cells to fight infection is affected.

Incidence: About 4,500 people in the United States were diagnosed with CML in 2007. Though children may have CML, it is very uncommon; only about 2 percent of CML patients are children. Most CML occurs in adults. It is slightly more common in men than women. The risk of getting this cancer increases with age; most patients are adults older than age sixty.

Symptoms: Symptoms of CML usually develop slowly. Patients may find they have this type of cancer after getting blood tests for another condition. Symptoms may include anemia (low red blood cell count), bleeding easily, bone pain, bruising easily, fever, loss of appetite, night sweats, pain or a feeling of fullness below the ribs (especially in the upper left abdomen), paleness, shortness of breath, stomach pain, swollen liver, swollen spleen, tiredness, unexplained or repeated infections, weakness, and weight loss.

Screening and diagnosis: There is no screening test for CML. Generally, CML can be diagnosed from an examination of the blood cells. However, bone marrow tests may be done to look for changes not seen in the blood. Cytogenetic tests (tests that analyze a cell's chromosomes) may also be used to confirm the diagnosis by looking for the *BCR-ABL* cancer gene. The results of these tests help determine which type of drug therapy to use and how long treatment should last.

CML has three phases that are determined by how many immature leukemia cells (blasts) are in the bone marrow and blood:

- Chronic phase: Most patients, about 85 percent, are in this stage when their CML is diagnosed. During this time, the blood and bone marrow have less than 5 percent blasts. Red blood cells and platelets are affected; however, white blood cells are still fighting infection. This stage may last for years.
- Accelerated phase: During this phase, there are more than 5 percent but less than 30 percent blasts in the blood and bone marrow. Patients may begin to feel ill. They may have anemia, the number of platelets in the blood may drop, and the white cells may either increase or decrease. The number of blast cells begins to increase, and the spleen may swell. At this phase, the disease is progressing, and patients are likely to move into the next phase.
- Blast crisis phase: In this phase, there are more than 30 percent blasts in the blood and bone marrow. Patients in this phase often have infections. They may also be short of breath or tired and have stomach pain, bone pain, or bleeding. The number of blast cells in the blood and bone marrow increases, and the number of red cells and platelets drops. At this phase, CML may begin to act more like an acute leukemia.

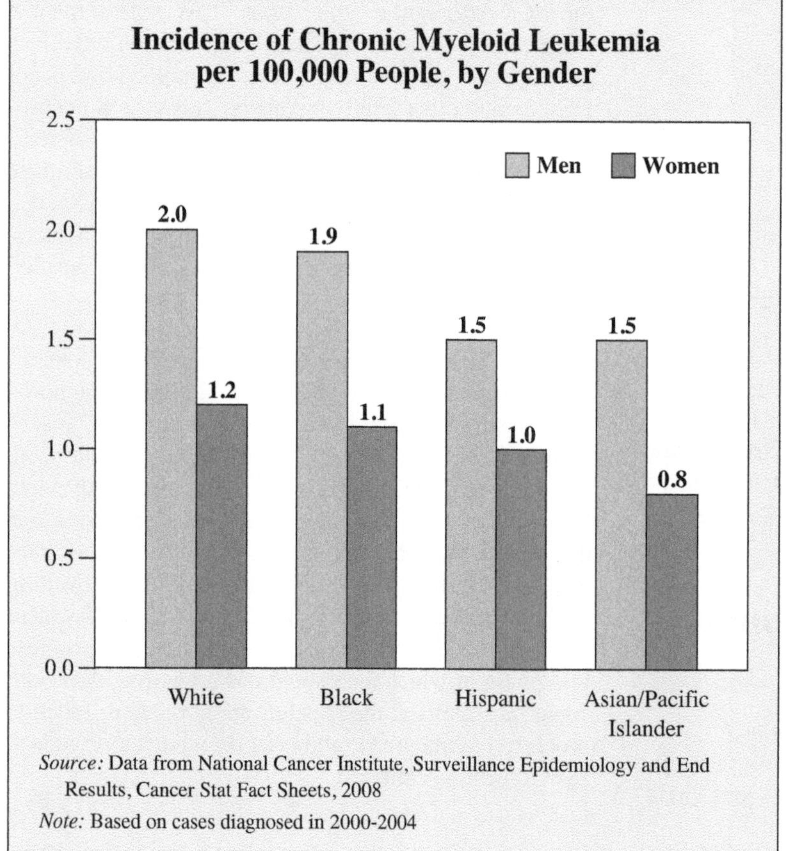

Source: Data from National Cancer Institute, Surveillance Epidemiology and End Results, Cancer Stat Fact Sheets, 2008

Note: Based on cases diagnosed in 2000-2004

Treatment and therapy: Drugs or chemotherapy are usually used to achieve treatment goals for patients with CML. These goals include bringing the red blood cell and platelet counts back to normal and eliminating all the cells with the *BCR-ABL* gene. This treatment also helps shrink the spleen back to normal size. Treatment does not cure CML. However, patients usually achieve remission, during which they feel well and are able to return to normal activities. If treatment is stopped, the symptoms are likely to flare up again. This may also happen if a patient becomes resistant to the drug treatment.

Another possible treatment for CML is to have white blood cells removed from the blood (leukapheresis). This may help if a patient has a very high white blood cell count, so high that the white blood cells are interfering with blood flow to parts of the body, such as the brain.

Monitoring whether treatment is working is important with this disease. Patients will continue to have blood tests to see if red blood cell, white blood cell, and platelet counts are returning to normal. A blood test or bone marrow biopsy (surgically removing some bone marrow) can show whether the *BCR-ABL* gene count is decreasing. Cytogenetic tests such as fluorescent in situ hybridization (FISH) or polymerase chain reaction (PCR) may be used to monitor the level of *BCR-ABL* genes. Other tests, such as computed tomography (CT) scans or ultrasounds, may be used to see how this cancer is affecting other parts of the body, such as the spleen.

A bone marrow or cord blood transplant may help some CML patients. A transplant is a high-risk procedure but is the only cure for CML. Whether a patient is a good candidate for a bone marrow transplant depends on the patient's age and overall health, how the patient is responding to treatment with drugs, and how well donor cells and patient cells match. Transplants are generally more successful in younger patients and in those patients who are still in the chronic phase.

Prognosis, prevention, and outcomes: There is no known way to prevent CML, though promising drugs are being tested. A bone marrow transplant is currently the only cure for CML; however, many patients can control CML with drug therapy.

Outcomes for this disease depend on many factors, including age, size of spleen, and blood cell counts. The median survival rate for CML is four to six years. However, when the disease has moved into the accelerated phase, survival is usually less than one year. When this disease has moved into the blast crisis phase, survival rates drop to only a few months.

Marianne M. Madsen, M.S.

For Further Information

Cortes, Jorge, and Michael Deininger, eds. *Chronic Myeloid Leukemia*. New York: Informa Healthcare, 2007.

Lackriz, Barb. *Adult Leukemia: A Comprehensive Guide for Patients and Families*. Cambridge, Mass.: O'Reilly, 2001.

Talpaz, Moshe, and Hagop M. Kantarjian, eds. *Medical Management of Chronic Myelogenous Leukemia*. New York: Dekker, 1998.

Other Resources

CMLHelp.org
http://www.cmlhelp.org

Leukemia and Lymphoma Society
http://www.leukemia-lymphoma.org

National Cancer Institute
Chronic Myelogenous Leukemia Treatment
http://www.cancer.gov/cancertopics/pdq/treatment/CML

See also: Acute Lymphocytic Leukemia (ALL); Acute Myelocytic Leukemia (AML); Biological therapy; Bone Marrow Transplantation (BMT); 1,4-Butanediol dimethanesulfonate; Chronic Lymphocytic Leukemia (CLL); Computed Tomography (CT) scan; Genetics of cancer; Leukapharesis; Leukemias; Myeloproliferative disorders; Tyrosine kinase inhibitors

▶ Cold nodule

Category: Diseases, Symptoms, and Conditions
Also known as: Hypofunctioning thyroid nodule

Related conditions: Thyroid cancer, Hashimoto or de Quervain's thyroiditis

Definition: A cold or hypofunctioning nodule is a focal area of decreased uptake of radiotracer on a nuclear medicine thyroid scan that may correlate with a thyroid nodule felt on routine physical examination of the thyroid gland performed by a doctor.

Risk factors: The risk factors for a cold nodule are the same as those for thyroid cancer, including previous radiation to the neck area as therapy for acne or for enlarged tonsillar tissue, a family history of thyroid cancer, and exposure to radioiodine in childhood.

Etiology and the disease process: About 80 to 90 percent of solitary thyroid nodules are hypofunctioning. Although malignant thyroid tumors do not concentrate radioisotopes well and can therefore manifest as cold thyroid nodules, only about 10 to 20 percent of cold thyroid nodules occurring in young patients and about 5 percent of cold nodules occurring in adult patients are malignant. The remainder consist of cysts, inflammatory nodules of either Hashimoto or de Quervain's thyroiditis, hemorrhagic benign nodules, or degenerative nodules.

Incidence: The annual incidence of cold thyroid nodules in the general population is 5.2 per 100,000 young people and 55.9 per 100,000 adults.

Symptoms: Symptoms include enlargement of the thyroid gland or a palpable lump or nodule within the gland. Physical findings suggestive of a malignant nodule in the thyroid include lymphadenopathy in the neck, size of the nodule, fixation to adjacent structures, or tracheal deviation.

Screening and diagnosis: A cold nodule on a nuclear medicine scan may be composed of solid or cystic material or a combination of both as shown by thyroid ultrasound. Ultrasound is not especially useful for differentiating benign from malignant nodules of the thyroid unless multiple tiny echogenic foci are seen throughout the nodule, suggestive of microcalcifications. However, it is useful in guiding fine needle aspiration of the nodule. Neither computed tomography (CT) nor magnetic resonance imaging (MRI) helps distinguish benign from malignant thyroid nodules unless there is cervical adenopathy or local invasion.

Treatment and therapy: Biopsy of the nodule is usually recommended using fine needle aspiration under ultrasound guidance to obtain tissue for pathologic evaluation. If the pathology from the biopsy shows malignant cells, then surgical removal of the nodule is warranted.

Prognosis, prevention, and outcomes: If the nodule is benign, the prognosis is excellent. If the nodule is found to contain cancerous cells, then the prognosis depends on the stage and type of thyroid cancer found at surgery.

Debra B. Kessler, M.D., Ph.D.

See also: Thyroid nuclear medicine scan

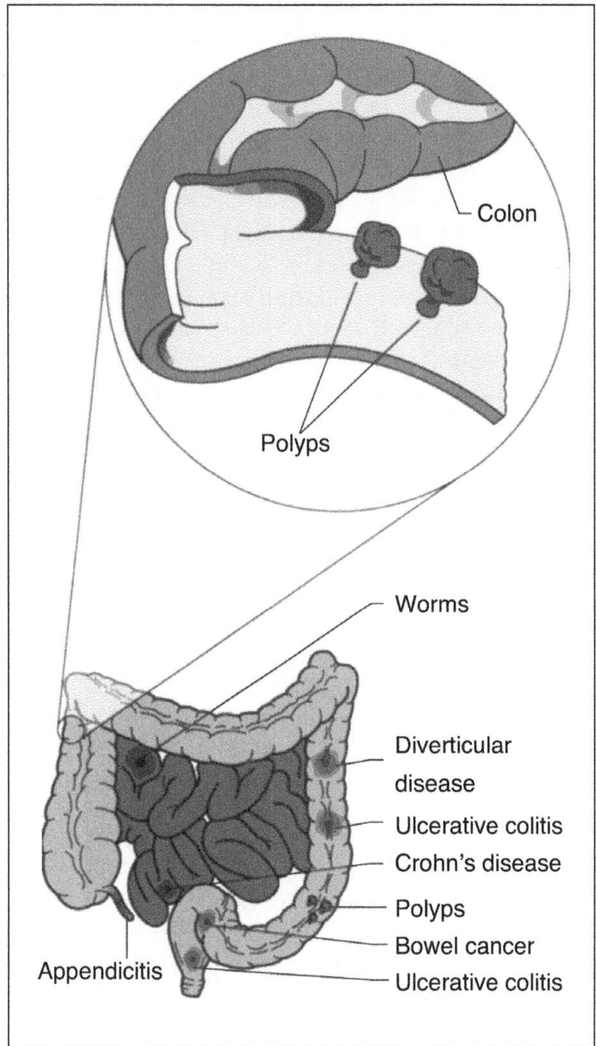

Polyps and other intestinal disorders.

▶ Colon polyps

Category: Diseases, Symptoms, and Conditions
Also known as: Colorectal polyps

Related conditions: Familial adenomatous polyposis (FAP), Gardner syndrome, colon cancer

Definition: Colon polyps are extra clumps of tissue that grow inside the large intestine. Most polyps are benign, but some can turn into cancer.

Risk factors: People older than age fifty and those with a family or personal history of colon polyps or colon cancer are more likely to develop these growths. Ulcerative colitis and Crohn disease increase a person's risk of polyps. Genetic mutations play a role in a small number of colon polyp cases.

A high-fat diet, alcohol consumption, smoking, excess weight, and a lack of exercise have also been linked to an increased risk for colon polyps.

Etiology and the disease process: Polyps are caused by abnormal cell growth. They may be smaller than a pebble or larger than a golf ball. Some are flat; others have a domelike shape. The larger the polyp, the more likely it will turn cancerous.

There are three types of colon polyps: adenomatous, hyperplastic, and inflammatory. Adenomatous polyps may turn into cancer if they grow larger than a quarter inch wide. Hyperplastic polyps are rarely cancerous. Inflammatory polyps may develop after a flare-up of inflammatory bowel disease.

Incidence: Persons over age sixty with normal risk factors have a 1 in 4 chance of developing a polyp. Colon polyps afflict more men than women.

Symptoms: There may be no symptoms. However, some polyps, particularly larger ones, can cause constipation or diarrhea, blood in the stool, rectal bleeding, or crampy abdominal pain.

Screening and diagnosis: A doctor may feel a rectal polyp during a rectal exam, but a physical exam is usually normal. Other tests used to screen for polyps include barium enema, sigmoidoscopy, or colonoscopy. Cancer experts recommend that persons age fifty and older at normal risk be screened every ten years with a colonoscopy. Alternatively, screening with sigmoidoscopy or barium enema may be done every five years. People at increased risk for polyps may need screenings more often.

Treatment and therapy: Polyps can be removed during a colonoscopy or sigmoidoscopy or surgically through the abdomen. A biopsy of the polyp determines if it is cancerous.

Prognosis, prevention, and outcomes: A low-fat diet rich in fruits and vegetables and foods high in calcium and folate may reduce the risk of colon polyps. Other forms of prevention include regular exercise, losing excess weight, avoiding alcohol, and not smoking.

Kelli Miller Stacy, ELS

See also: Adenomatous polyps; Cholecystectomy; Colonoscopy and virtual colonoscopy; Colorectal cancer; Colorectal cancer screening; Desmoid tumors; Duodenal carcinomas; Gastric polyps; Gastrointestinal cancers; Gastrointestinal oncology; Hereditary mixed polyposis syndrome; Hereditary polyposis syndromes; Juvenile polyposis syndrome; Polypectomy; Polyps; Rectal cancer; Sigmoidoscopy

▶ Colorectal cancer

Category: Diseases, Symptoms, and Conditions
Also known as: Colon cancer, rectal cancer, intestinal cancer

Related conditions: Familial polyposis

Definition: Colorectal cancer (CRC) is cancer of the colon, which is also called the large intestine, and the rectum. The cells of the colon and rectum become abnormal and lose the defining characteristics of normal intestinal cells and their ability to divide in a controlled way.

These cells grow rapidly and form tumors. The large intestine includes the ascending colon, transverse colon, and sigmoid colon. The rectum and anus follow the sigmoid colon, where solid waste (feces or stool) exits the body.

Carcinoma, a type of cancer originating from epithelial cells of the colorectal mucosa, is the most common cell type found in CRC. Epithelial cells normally line the digestive system, glands, and make up the top layers of skin. Intestinal epithelial cells vary somewhat from those in other parts of the body. More than 90% of colorectal carcinomas are adenocarcinomas. Other rare types of colorectal carcinomas include neuroendocrine, squamous cell, adenosquamous, spindle cell and undifferentiated carcinomas.

Risk factors: Increasing age is associated with the likeliness of colorectal cancer diagnosis and increases progressively after the age of 40, followed by a sharp rise after the age of 50. A family history of colorectal cancer is another risk factor as up to 20% of people who develop colorectal cancer have other family members who have been affected by this disease. Familial polyposis, ulcerative colitis, and Crohn disease also increase risk of CRC. The reasons for the increased risk are not clear, but it likely due to inherited genes, shared environmental factors, or some combination of these. Diet strongly influences the risk of colorectal cancer, and changes in food habits might reduce up to 70% of this cancer problem. Diets high in fat, especially animal fat, are a major risk factor for colorectal cancer. The implication of fat as a possible etiologic factor is linked to the concept of the typical Western diet, which favors the development of a bacterial flora capable of degrading bile salts to potentially carcinogenic compounds. Physical inactivity and excess body weight are reported to account for about a fourth to a third of colorectal cancers.

Etiology and the disease process: Some changes take place in the colon before cancer develops. First, a small area of precancerous cells forms on the surface of the intestine. These cells can mutate into cancerous cells and will continue to grow in both directions outward from the surface and inward though deeper layers of tissue that form the multiple layers of the intestinal wall. As the abnormal growth invades these layers, it can encroach on blood vessels and lymph nodes, from which cancer cells

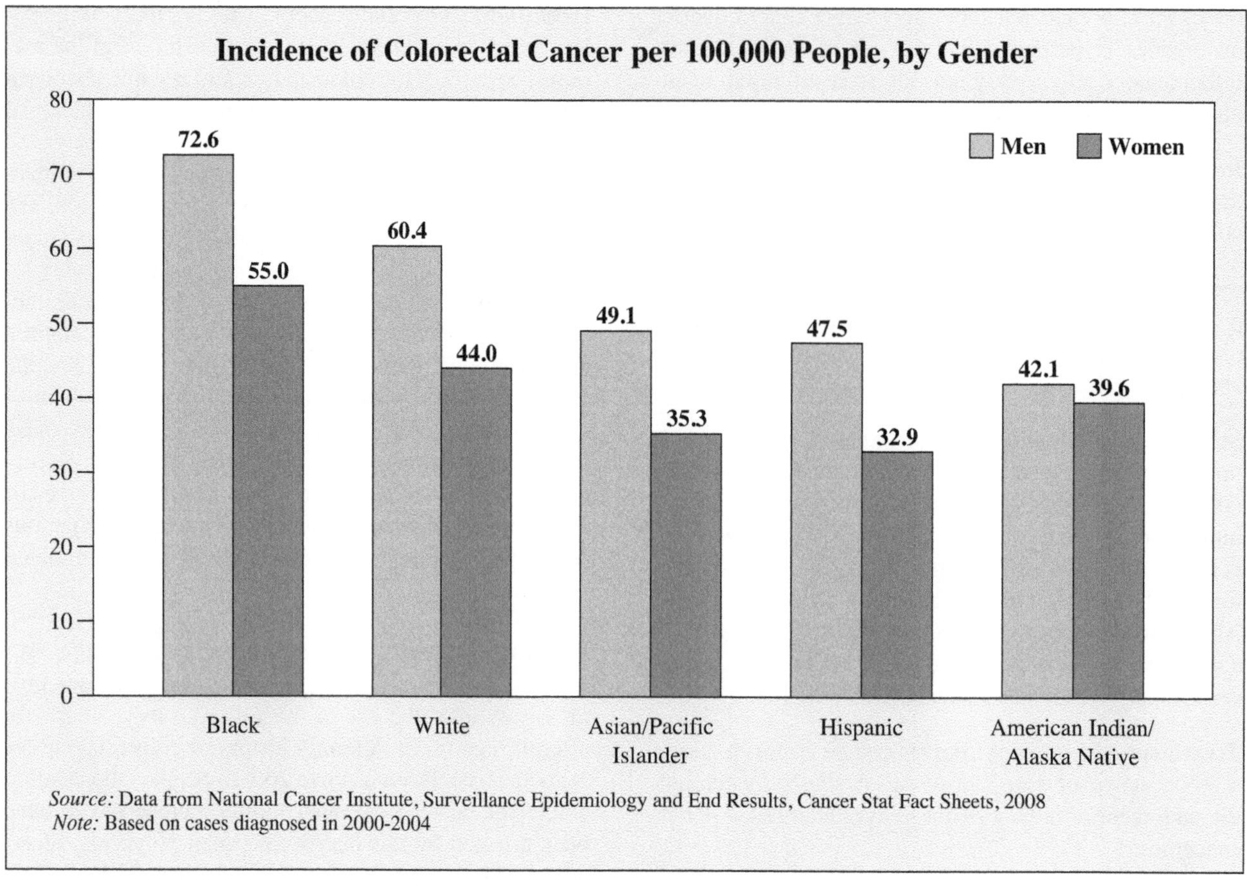

Source: Data from National Cancer Institute, Surveillance Epidemiology and End Results, Cancer Stat Fact Sheets, 2008
Note: Based on cases diagnosed in 2000-2004

can travel to the liver or other organs. Liver metastases are common with advanced disease.

The most common large intestine abnormality is noncancerous growths called polyps. Polyps grow into the intestine from its walls. Some polyps have a stalk. Polyps usually grow in the sigmoid colon and the rectum. Adenomatous polyps (derived from glandular tissue) are more likely to become malignant (cancerous). Approximately 25 percent of people with colon cancer have polyps somewhere else in the large intestine. Polyps are removed unless there are so many of them that it is better to remove a section of the large intestine containing the polyps. Frequent examination of the large intestine is necessary to watch for new growth. The most extreme measure to prevent the growth of more polyps is the surgical removal of the rectum and anus. In such cases, a surgical opening is made in the abdominal wall (ileostomy), where solid waste can be collected in a pouch (colostomy bag).

Familial polyposis is a hereditary condition. People with familial polyposis are genetically predisposed to grow one hundred or more precancerous adenomatous polyps in the large intestine. Cases of colorectal cancer due to this condition appear before the age of forty, unlike colorectal cancers due to other causes, which have a higher rate of incidence with advancing age. The lifetime risk of developing a colorectal adenoma is nearly 19% in the U.S. population. Nearly 95% of sporadic colorectal cancers develop from these adenomas.

Incidence: Colorectal cancer is the third most common cancer for men and women in the United States and other Western countries. It is also the third leading cause of death. In 2014, an estimated 71,830 men and 65,000 women were diagnosed with colorectal cancer and 26,270 men and 24,040 women were predicted to succumb to the disease. Greater than one-third of all deaths (29% in men and 43% in women) will occur in individuals aged 80 years and older.

Just prior to 2014, there were projected to be 136,830 individuals newly diagnosed with colorectal cancer and 50,310 colorectal cancer deaths in the United States. Approximately 60% of cases and 70% of deaths occur in those aged 65 years and older. Among women, almost 30% of cases and more than 40% of deaths will occur in those aged 80 years and older, compared with approximately 20% of cases and 30% of deaths among men.

Men, in general, have higher incidence rates per 100,000 people than women: Black men have the highest rate at 72.6 per 100,000; whites, 60.4; Asian/Pacific Islanders, 49.1; Hispanics, 47.5; and American Indian/Alaska natives, 42.1. Among women, black women have the highest incidence rates at 55 per 100,000, followed by white women, 44.0; American Indian/Alaska natives, 39.6; Asian/Pacific Islanders, 35.3; and Hispanics, 32.9. Trends in colorectal cancer incidence for men and women from 1975 to 2004 show a decline for all races and ethnicities.

Symptoms: There are no symptoms of early colorectal cancer. Screening is the most important component in prevention and early detection. Symptoms such as weight loss, constipation, blood in the stool, and liver disease indicate a more advanced stage of disease.

Screening and diagnosis: There are several tests for screening and diagnosis. The type and frequency of testing depend on the patient's age and medical history. A yearly fecal occult blood test/fecal immunochemical test (FOBT/FIT) is recommended in people age fifty or older. A physician decides which additional test double-contrast barium X ray, flexible sigmoidoscopy, or colonoscopy should be given to each person, starting at age fifty and every five to ten years after for those without new symptoms.

- Fecal occult blood test (FOBT): Three fecal samples taken at different times are placed on special cards that are sent to the laboratory for testing. The presence of blood in the sample indicates that further testing is required. A positive FOBT does not necessarily mean cancer. Blood can come from hemorrhoids, a noncancerous polyp, or inflammatory bowel diseases such as Crohn disease or ulcerative colitis.
- Fecal immunochemical test (FIT): A relatively new test, also known as an immunochemical fecal occult blood test (iFOBT), to detect blood in the feces. The advantage to this test is that the patient is not required to restrict certain foods and medications before collecting the sample. Also, early evidence indicates that the FIT might be more specific in detecting blood than the FOBT.
- Double-contrast barium X ray: An X ray of the colon and rectum using barium for contrast. Growths, narrowing of the colon, and evidence of inflammation can be seen, as the barium outlines the large intestine. Biopsies and polyp removal are not possible with this procedure.
- Flexible sigmoidoscopy: The sigmoidoscope is a flexible tube with a light and a tiny camera at the tip. The instrument is introduced into the rectum. Polyps, other growths, and evidence of inflammation can be seen in the lower one-third of the intestine and rectum. Biopsies (tiny samples of abnormal tissue) can be taken of tissue that appears abnormal. Studies have shown that people who have regular screening with sigmoidoscopy after age 50 years have a 60 to 70 percent lower risk of death due to cancer of the rectum and lower colon than people who do not have screening.
- Colonoscopy: The colonoscope is a flexible tube with a light and tiny camera at the tip. The patient is given "conscious sedation" and frequently sleeps though the procedure. The tube is introduced through the rectum and is passed into all three sections of the large intestine. Biopsies of abnormalities can be taken. The colonoscopy is the only test that visualizes the entire colon and allows for biopsy of abnormalities. Studies suggest that colonoscopy reduces deaths from colorectal cancer by about 60 to 70 percent.
- Cologuard: This test detects tiny amounts of blood in stool (with an immunochemical test similar to FIT) as well as nine DNA biomarkers in three genes that have been found in colorectal cancer and precancerous advanced adenomas.

If a biopsy is positive for cancer, further testing is required to see if the cancer has spread. The process is called staging.

- Stage 0: Very early cancer is present on the innermost layer of the intestine.
- Stage I: Cancer is in the inner layers of the colon.
- Stage II: Cancer has spread through the muscle wall of the colon.
- Stage III: Cancer has spread to the lymph nodes.
- Stage IV: Cancer has spread to other organs.

Treatment and therapy: Treatment options vary according to disease stage and the age and general health of the patient. The main treatment categories are surgery, chemotherapy, radiation therapy, and targeted therapy (specifically targeting cancer cells by stimulating the immune system). More than one of these treatments may be used. Many patients choose to get a second opinion, which allows them to have increased confidence in the treatment option that they have chosen with their physician or to explore other options. It is very important that colorectal cancer patients ask questions necessary to feel confident that they understand the disease and treatment. Patients are advised to take a trusted friend or family member to appointments and write down questions at home to ask their physician.

Surgery is the primary treatment. The type of surgery depends on the stage of disease. Laparoscopic surgery, which involves a small incision in the abdomen, can remove some Stage 0 and Stage 1 tumors and cancerous polyps (polypectomy). Surgery in the early stages can be curative. Surgical procedures range from polypectomy, often performed during a colonoscopy, to resection (removal) of major sections of the large intestine or rectum. When resection is performed, up to one-third of the intestine is removed. The ends of each section are then attached (anastomosis) where there is healthy tissue on each side. Cancer of the rectum and anus may require colectomy, a process in which the surgeon removes part or all of the colon, brings a normal section of the large intestine through an opening in the abdomen, and attaches a bag to collect solid waste.

Radiation therapy focuses high-energy beams directly into the tumor from outside the body, killing the cancer cells. Radiation usually follows surgery to remove a large mass or tumor. Radiation therapy is very precise and can be focused on small areas of tumor cells not seen during surgery. There are times when radiation is used before surgery to shrink a tumor and ease removal.

Radiation for colon cancer is performed with a linear accelerator. Precision calculations determine the most direct path to the tumor cells while damaging the fewest normal cells. Treatment lasts only a few minutes per day and might continue for several weeks.

Endocavitary radiation treatment for cancer of the rectum and anus is performed internally. A small, handheld device is introduced into the rectum, where the dose of radiation can more directly reach the cancer cells.

Side effects from radiation include skin irritation, nausea, bladder irritation, bowel incontinence, diarrhea, rectal irritation, and fatigue. Sexual dysfunction can occur in men and women.

Chemotherapy involves several strategies. It can be used after surgery when all evidence of cancer is gone, or it can work to prevent a return of the cancer, which is called adjuvant chemotherapy. Drugs used to treat colorectal cancer include fluorouracil (5-FU), capecitabine (Xeloda), oxaliplatin (Eloxatin), and irinotecan (Camptosar).

Systemic chemotherapy is the introduction into the body of toxic, cancer-fighting chemicals, which find cancer cells and kill them. Cancer cells divide more rapidly than normal cells. Chemotherapy drugs get inside the cancer cells more rapidly and kill them. A targeted variation is injecting chemotherapy drugs directly into an artery supplying blood to an organ (liver) that contains tumor cells.

Side effects of chemotherapy are due to the toxicity of the drugs, which kill cancerous and noncancerous cells. Common side effects are severe diarrhea, low blood counts, nausea, and vomiting. Newer medications are available to control the nausea and vomiting.

Targeted therapy exploits unique abnormalities of cancer cells other than just rapid cell division. Proteins called monoclonal antibodies selectively find the cancer cells and kill them. There are fewer side effects, possibly from less damage to normal cells. Targeted therapy is not without side effects or danger. Lung scarring, rashes, fatigue, infection, and allergic reactions are all realities with this therapy. Monoclonal antibody and target therapy drugs include bevacizumab (Avastin), cetuximab (Erbitux), and panitumumab (Vectibix).

Oral Pharmaceutical Drugs for CRC include Lonsurf, a tablet that combines the drugs trifluridine and tipiracil hydrochloride. Lonsurf treats patients with metastatic colorectal cancer whose disease progressed after standard treatments. The drug combination was previously known as TAS-102.

Biologic therapy. These treatments utilize substances made from living organisms to treat disease. These substances may occur naturally in the body or may be made in the laboratory. Some biological therapies stimulate or suppress the immune system to help the body fight cancer, infection, and other diseases. Other biological therapies attack specific cancer cells, which may help keep them from growing or kill them. They may also lessen certain side effects caused by some cancer treatments. Types of biological therapy include immunotherapy such as vaccines, cytokines, and some antibodies.

Prognosis, prevention, and outcomes: People who are aware of their family history for colorectal cancer or polyps are in a good position to lessen their chances for contracting colorectal cancer. High-fat, low-fiber diets are implicated in higher rates of CRC, but the mechanism is not known. People who eat lean meat, smaller portions of meat, and more vegetables and grains have lower rates of CRC. Physical activity also seems to be important.

It is imperative that beginning at age fifty, yearly FOBT/FIT testing is performed and that colonoscopy, flexible sigmoidoscopy, or double-contrast barium X ray is also performed every five to ten years. The main reason people do not have these screening tests are concerns about the colon-cleansing procedure before testing, unease about taking fecal samples for the FOBT, and embarrassment.

Excellent prognosis or cure is associated with early detection. Stages 0, I, II, and III are potentially curable. Colorectal cancer that has not spread (metastasized) or invaded the intestinal wall has a greater chance for cure. More than 90 percent of patients receiving treatment during the early stages will survive at least five years. Some 39 percent of colorectal cancer is found in the early stages.

Stage IV cancer has spread to organs such as the liver, ovaries, lungs, or peritoneum. Surgery is performed not to cure the cancer but to prevent the colon from becoming blocked by the tumor. Liver metastases have been successfully removed through surgery. There have been some cures from this procedure, but this stage of disease is difficult to cure. Multiple therapies are used with Stage IV disease and include targeted therapies, chemotherapy, freezing tumors, and radiation.

Janet R. Green
Updated by: Jeffrey P. Larson PT, ATC

For Further Information

Brown, Gina. (2007). *Colorectal cancer.* New York: Cambridge University Press.

Cassidy, Jim, Johnston, Patrick, & van Cutsem, Eric. (Eds.). (2007). *Colorectal cancer.* New York: Informa Healthcare.

Fleming, M., Ravula, S., Tatishchev, S. F., & Wang, H. L. (2012). Colorectal carcinoma: Pathologic aspects. *Journal of Gastrointestinal Oncology,* 3(3), 153–173. http://doi.org/10.3978/j.issn.2078-6891.2012.030

Haggar, F. A., & Boushey, R. P. (2009). Colorectal cancer epidemiology: Incidence, mortality, survival, and risk factors. *Clinics in Colon and Rectal Surgery,* 22(4), 191–197. http://doi.org/10.1055/s-0029-1242458

Holen, Kyle, & Chung, Ki Young. (2008). *Dx/Rx: Colorectal cancer.* Sudbury, MA: Jones and Bartlett.

O'Reilly, Derek A., & Poston, Graeme J. (2007). Classification of colorectal liver metastases. *Advances in Gastrointestinal Cancer.* Retrieved February 26, 2016 from HighBeam Research: https://www.highbeam.com/doc/1G1-171137590.html

Other Resources

American Cancer Society
http://www.cancer.org

Centers for Disease Control and Prevention
http://www.cdc.gov

Colon Cancer Alliance
http://www.ccalliance.org

MayoClinic.com
http://www.mayoclinic.com

National Cancer Institute
http://www.cancer.gov

Susan Cohan Kasdas Colon Cancer Foundation
http://www.coloncancerfoundation.org

U.S. Food and Drug Administration
10903 New Hampshire Avenue
Silver Spring, MD 20993
1-888-INFO-FDA (1-888-463-6332)

See also: Adenomatous polyps; Anal cancer; APC gene testing; Bethesda criteria; Colon polyps; Crohn disease; Cyclooxygenase 2 (COX-2) inhibitors; Desmoid tumors; Diverticulosis and diverticulitis; DPC4 gene testing; Duodenal carcinomas; Enteritis; Enterostomal therapy; Epidermoid cancers of mucous membranes; Gardner syndrome; Gastric polyps; Gastrointestinal cancers; Hemorrhoids; Hereditary mixed polyposis syndrome; Hereditary polyposis syndromes; Inflammatory bowel disease; Juvenile polyposis syndrome; MLH1 gene; MSH genes; Peutz-Jeghers Syndrome (PJS); PMS genes; Polyps; Rectal cancer

▶ Comedo carcinomas

Category: Diseases, Symptoms, and Conditions
Also known as: Ductal carcinoma in situ (DCIS), high nuclear grade or poorly differentiated DCIS

Related conditions: Spontaneous nipple discharge, Paget disease

Definition: Comedo carcinoma is a type of ductal carcinoma in situ (very-early-stage breast cancer), which accounts for approximately 22 to 45 percent of all breast cancers diagnosed with mammography. Most cases appear after the age of fifty-five and may persist for years without a palpable abnormality. Ductal carcinoma in situ (DCIS) refers to a family of cancers that occur in the breast ducts. There are two categories of DCIS, noncomedo and comedo. The high grade or comedo type represents 40 percent of all DCIS and on pathologic evaluation appears as pluglike necrotic material that can be expressed from the ducts of the cut pathology specimen. On mammography, often a linear branching or casting pattern of microcalcifications is visible.

Risk factors: Risk factors include increasing age, having few children and the first child after the age of thirty, obesity, a history of atypical hyperplasia or of breast carcinoma, and having a mother or sibling with breast cancer.

Etiology and the disease process: In comedo carcinoma, cancer forms in the breast ducts. The comedo form of DCIS has dead cells (necrosis) that plug the center of the breast duct. It tends to grow fast and has a higher risk of invasive cancer than noncomedo DCIS.

Incidence: Ductal carcinoma in situ is becoming increasingly common, accounting for 22 to 45 percent of newly diagnosed cases of breast cancer. The comedo type represents about 40 percent of the cases and carries a poorer prognosis.

Symptoms: Most patients are asymptomatic. Less commonly, DCIS appears as a mass with ill-defined or lobulated borders on a mammogram, which may or may not be associated with malignant microcalcifications.

Screening and diagnosis: On a mammogram, comedo carcinoma manifests as clusters of pleomorphic (many-formed), ductally oriented microcalcifications. In the staging system used to classify cancer, DCIS is known as Stage 0 and is sometimes called precancer. It may also be referred to as tumor in situ (Tis), which means that the cancer is noninvasive.

Treatment and therapy: The standard treatment is needle localization and lumpectomy with radiation or simple or modified mastectomy.

Prognosis, prevention, and outcomes: Some 20 to 50 percent of women with comedo carcinoma develop invasive cancer five to ten years after initial diagnosis if the cancer is not removed surgically.

Debra B. Kessler, M.D., Ph.D.

See also: Duct ectasia; Ductal Carcinoma In Situ (DCIS); Invasive ductal carcinomas

▶ Cowden syndrome

Category: Diseases, Symptoms, and Conditions
Also known as: Multiple hamartoma syndrome

Related conditions: *PTEN* hamartoma tumor syndrome (PHTS), Lhermitte-Duclos disease

Definition: Cowden syndrome is an inherited disorder characterized by the presence of multiple tumorlike growths, termed hamartomas. Although these hamartomas are generally benign, or noncancerous, individuals with hamartomas have a predisposition to the development of certain cancers.

Risk factors: Cowden syndrome is inherited in an autosomal dominant pattern and therefore may be inherited from just one parent.

Etiology and the disease process: Cowden syndrome is linked to mutations in the *PTEN* gene. *PTEN* is a tumor-suppressor gene, which normally functions to control cell growth and division. The mutations in *PTEN* may either be inherited or occur spontaneously. Approximately 80 percent of patients with Cowden syndrome have identified mutations in the *PTEN* gene. However, the cause of the condition in the other 20 percent of patients is unknown.

Incidence: The exact incidence of Cowden syndrome is not known but is estimated at 1 in 200,000 individuals.

Symptoms: The major defining symptom of Cowden syndrome is the presence of multiple hamartomas. These growths are generally small and most often occur on the skin and on mucous membranes such as the inside of the nose and mouth. However, hamartomas may also occur on the inner lining of the intestines and within other parts of the body. Also, patients with Cowden syndrome often develop noncancerous breast and thyroid diseases. Another common symptom of Cowden syndrome is macrocephaly, or an enlargement of the patient's head.

Screening and diagnosis: Cowden syndrome is typically diagnosed through recognition of the extensive hamartomas. To help confirm a diagnosis, the *PTEN* gene can be sequenced to identify any mutations.

Treatment and therapy: The hamartomas and other symptoms related to Cowden syndrome are typically not treated; however, the main recommendation is for these patients to continue to be screened to watch for the early development of cancerous lesions.

Prognosis, prevention, and outcomes: Because Cowden syndrome is often an inherited disorder, little can be done to prevent the disease. Patients with Cowden syndrome have a heightened risk of developing certain cancers. These include breast cancer, thyroid cancer, and uterine cancer. However, with routine screening, these tumors may be diagnosed in early stages and therefore often respond well to therapy.

Lisa M. Cockrell, B.S.

See also: Family history and risk assessment; Thyroid cancer; Trichilemmal carcinomas

▶ Craniopharyngiomas

Category: Diseases, Symptoms, and Conditions
Also known as: Rathke pouch tumors, adamantinomas

Related conditions: Endocrinological and neurological dysfunctions

Definition: A craniopharyngioma is a slow-growing, histologically benign tumor that has been found above and below the sella turcica (depression in the upper surface of the sphenoid bone) and in ectopic locations in the brain. Most craniopharyngiomas are found in the sella turcica and the area above it, home to the pituitary gland and hypothalamus. Although generally benign, craniopharyngiomas, like malignant tumors, can metastasize to areas outside the brain. When discovered, they typically range from 1 to 4 inches in size. They grow by expansion and can cause compression of structures such as the optic chiasm and nerves and the pituitary stalk and gland. The three subtypes are adamantinomatous or pediatric type, which is the classic and most common form of this tumor, having primarily a cystic composition, usually with a solid component; papillary or adult type, which has a more encapsulated, solid component that typically has no calcifications; and mixed type, which is composed of transitional features between the adamantinomatous and papillary variants.

Risk factors: The cause of craniopharyngioma is not known, and there are no known environmental or infectious risk factors. More than 50 percent of people with craniopharyngiomas are younger than eighteen (adamantinomatous type), and most cases occur in children between the ages of five and ten. The second most common age range in which craniopharyngioma occurs is between forty and sixty years (papillary). Craniopharyngiomas do not appear to be more prevalent in a particular gender or ethnicity, nor do they appear to be inherited.

Etiology and the disease process: Although the etiology of craniopharyngiomas has not been determined with certainty, several theories exist as to their origin. One theory is that craniopharyngiomas are another form of a congenital tumor known as an epidermoid cyst. (Epidermoid cysts can arise anywhere in the body and are proven to be congenital.) Another theory suggests that they arise from embryonic dental or jaw tissue (dental anlage). A third theory, and the one that seems to be the most popular, purports that craniopharyngiomas are remnants of Rathke's pouch (a depression in the roof of the developing mouth that gives rise to the anterior pituitary) and arise from squamous cell nests found at the junction of the pituitary stalk and the distal portion of the anterior pituitary.

Craniopharyngioma appears as a single, large cyst or multiple cysts filled with a cloudy, proteinaceous, brownish-yellow material that glitters because it contains floating cholesterol crystals. This kind of tumor most frequently arises in the pituitary stalk and projects into the hypothalamus. Craniopharyngioma causes symptoms in three different ways: first, as it grows it increases the pressure on the brain; second, as it enlarges it interferes with the normal function of the pituitary gland; and third, as it grows upward, it damages the optic nerve.

Incidence: Craniopharyngioma is a rarely occurring, nonheritable cancer. According to the National Cancer Data Base, the overall incidence of craniopharyngioma in the United States is 0.13 per 100,000 persons per year. Craniopharyngiomas account for 1 to 3 percent of all intracranial tumors and 4.2 percent of all childhood intracranial tumors. The incidence does not vary by sex or race. Approximately 340 cases of craniopharyngiomas occur annually in the United States, with 96 occurring in children between birth and fourteen years of age. Recurrences usually occur at the primary site. Ectopic and metastatic recurrences are extremely rare and have been reported after surgical removal. Recurrence rates can be as high as 20 percent.

Symptoms: Symptoms frequently develop slowly and become obvious only after the tumor enlarges to about 1.5 inches in diameter. Craniopharyngiomas produce symptoms by compression of adjacent neural structures, leading to endocrine and visual problems; they obstruct cerebrospinal fluid pathways, causing hydrocephalus and increased intracranial pressure, which lead to headaches and nausea.

The most common symptoms are headache (55 to 86 percent of patients), endocrine dysfunction (66 to 90 percent of patients), and visual disturbances (37 to 68 percent of patients). Headaches are slowly progressive, dull, continuous, and positional, becoming severe when endocrine symptoms become obvious. Endocrine dysfunction includes hypothyroidism, adrenal failure, and diabetes insipidus; young patients typically display growth failure and delayed puberty. Nearly three-quarters of patients suffer some sort of damage to the optic pathway.

Other manifestations relate to the various connections of the hypothalamic-pituitary complex and surrounding structures. Tumors located in the thalamus and frontal lobes are often accompanied by corresponding endocrine, autonomic, and behavioral problems, such as hyperphagia and obesity, short-term memory deficits, psychomotor retardation, emotional immaturity, and lethargy.

Screening and diagnosis: Computed tomography (CT) scanning and magnetic resonance imaging (MRI) are the screening methods of choice for craniopharyngioma. MRI, with or without administration of contrast enhancement, is generally preferred over CT scanning but may not be as readily available. Although CT can clearly demonstrate the characteristic calcifications and size of the tumor, MRI can demonstrate the size and extent of the tumor as well as any ventricular involvement. MRI results can confirm cystic features of the tumor. Various MRI sequences, such as fluid-attenuated inversion recovery (FLAIR), gradient echo, and diffusion-weighted imaging, can aid in making the correct diagnosis.

The diagnostic workup for craniopharyngioma also includes complete endocrinological and neuroophthalmological evaluation with visual-field examination and neuropsychological assessment. The endocrinological tests will include serum electrolytes, serum and urine osmolality, thyroid studies, morning and evening cortisol levels, growth hormone levels, and luteinizing and follicle-stimulating hormone levels.

Postoperatively, CT scanning is performed to establish a baseline from which follow-up scans will be judged. MRI is often performed to determine whether there is any residual tumor.

Treatment and therapy: There is no medical therapy per se for craniopharyngioma. There is little debate that the standard treatment of this tumor is surgical excision followed by adjuvant radiotherapy; however, controversy does exist about the optimal degree of excision. Some physicians believe that complete resection is the best treatment and that every effort should be made to remove as much of the tumor as possible. Others advocate a planned partial tumor excision, leaving radiotherapy or radiosurgery to complete the removal. The controversy stems from the fact that nearly all craniopharyngiomas are located in eloquent areas of the brain; removal necessitates maneuvering around very delicate anatomical structures, which, if damaged during the course of tumor removal, could fail to perform normally, leaving the patient with severe deficits. Craniopharyngiomas tend to adhere to the structures and tissues that surround them, making them difficult to excise without disturbing or damaging these other entities. It is especially challenging to resect a craniopharyngioma that is adhering to the pituitary gland, the hypothalamus, or the optic chiasm and nerves. For example, damage to the pituitary gland, which controls the activity of many other endocrine glands, such as the thyroid, the ovaries, and the adrenal glands, can result in a cascade of endocrine-related disorders including hypothyroidism, obesity, diabetes, and, in children, failure to thrive. Damage to the hypothalamus, which controls the activity of the pituitary by releasing various hormones to regulate it, can result in a host of problems from interrupted circadian rhythm to impaired immune system function. Damage to the optic chiasm and optic nerves can cause visual disturbances ranging from mild hemianopsia (in which each eye is able to send images from only half its field of vision to the brain) to complete blindness. Because of these issues, treatment of craniopharyngioma is complex.

The surgical approach used is dictated by the tumor's location. If the predominant portion of the tumor is intrasellar, the approach is usually transsphenoidal (through the sphenoid bone). The transsphenoidal approach is less invasive than craniotomy (in which part of the skull is removed to provide access to the brain) and therefore preferable. Craniotomy is necessary when the predominant component is suprasellar. Certain suprasellar masses may be approached through an extended transsphenoidal craniotomy.

The pterional craniotomy is the standard approach to suprasellar lesions because it allows the surgeon to see the optic nerves and chiasm. A subfrontal approach is used for lesions that are anterior to the optic chiasm, but this may be difficult to determine preoperatively. Cyst aspiration combined with instillation of radioactive isotope phosphorus-32 is the alternative to traditional resection; however, a tumor with significant solid components is not likely to respond to this type of treatment.

Prognosis, prevention, and outcomes: The survival rate for patients who undergo surgery for craniopharyngioma is estimated to be 86 percent at two years and 80 percent at five years postdiagnosis. Survival varies by age group, with excellent survival rates for patients younger than twenty years old and poorer survival rates for those older than sixty-five. Molecular and genetic studies focusing on the treatment and prevention of craniopharyngioma are ongoing.

Keller Kaufman-Fox, B.A.

For Further Information

Chakrabarti, I., A. P. Amar, W. Couldwell, and M. H. Weiss. "Long-Term Neurological, Visual, and Endocrine Outcomes Following Transnasal Resection of Craniopharyngioma." *Journal of Neurosurgery* 102 (2005): 650-657.

Chiou, S. M., et al. "Stereotactic Radiosurgery of Residual or Recurrent Craniopharyngioma, After Surgery, with or Without Radiation Therapy." *Neuro-oncology* 3 (2001): 159-166.

Garrè, M. L., and A. Cama. "Craniopharyngioma: Modern Concepts in Pathogenesis and Treatment." *Current Opinions in Pediatrics* 19 (2007): 471-479.

Merchant, T. E., et al. "Craniopharyngioma: The St. Jude Children's Research Hospital Experience, 1984-2001." *International Journal of Radiation Oncology, Biology and Physics* 53 (2002): 533-542.

Rekate, Harold L. "Craniopharyngioma." *Journal of Neurosurgery (Pediatrics 4)* 103 (2005): 297-298.

Other Resources

MedlinePlus
Craniopharyngioma
http://www.nlm.nih.gov/medlineplus/ency/article/000345.htm

National Cancer Institute
Childhood Craniopharyngioma
http://www.cancer.gov/cancertopics/pdq/treatment/childbrain/Patient/page10

See also: Brain and central nervous system cancers

▶ Craniosynostosis

Category: Diseases, Symptoms, and Conditions

Related conditions: Craniofacial syndromes

Definition: Craniosynostosis is a process resulting in premature closure or fusion of the cranial sutures. The most common site is the sagittal suture, followed by the coronal, lambdoidal, and metopic. This condition results in an abnormally shaped skull and occurs with a male-to-female ratio of 3:1. Approximately 10 percent are familial, resulting from an autosomal dominate inheritance. Other cases are the result of chromosome deletions, duplications, translocations, breaks, missense, or splice-site abnormalities. Prenatal head constraint is hypothesized as a causative factor in some cases. In utero human development proceeds in a normal fashion, with abnormalities becoming apparent at birth or shortly thereafter. The phenotypic presentation is variable. More than one hundred syndromes have been associated with craniosynostosis.

Risk factors: Primary cases of craniosynostosis, in the majority of cases, is the result of spontaneous genetic mutations, although it can also be transmitted genetically from a parent. Children with microcephaly (poor brain growth) are at risk of developing craniosynostosis. Normal brain growth pushes the cranial bones apart at the sutures, but with impaired brain growth, sutures may prematurely fuse.

Etiology and the disease process: Mutations in fibroblast growth factor receptor (*FGFR1*, *FGFR2*, *FGFR3*), *TWIST*, and *MSX2* genes are associated with craniosynostosis development. Fibroblast growth factor receptors affect animal growth, development, and homeostasis. They regulate cell growth, differentiation, migration, and survival. They exert direct influence on the formation of various tissues, organs, and blood vessels and are responsible for wound healing. *FGFR* mutations are directly associated with specific growth and development abnormalities, including the inability to control cell growth leading to tumor formation.

Currently, four *FGFR* mutations have been identified. These mutations produce a variety of results. Germline mutations cause skeletal dysplasia (hypochondroplasia, achondroplasia) and craniosynostosis syndromes (Apert, Beare-Stevenson, Crouzon, Pfeiffer, Jackson-Weiss), while somatic mutations cause a variety of cancers.

Oncogenes and tumor-suppressor genes are located near recombination sites on chromosomes. Thus, when breaks, translocations, deletions, and amplifications occur in these regions, tumor-suppressor genes can be excluded or oncogenes can be amplified. These processes lead to the development of various cancers. *FGFR* mutations have been identified in endometrial, breast, gastric, colorectal, bladder (urothelial), cervical, endometrial, and glial tumors and multiple myeloma. In addition, *FGFR* mutations are implicated in the formation of benign skin lesions such as epidermal nevi and seborrheic keratoses.

Saethre-Chotzen syndrome, an autosomal dominantly inherited form of craniosynostosis, is caused by the mutation of the transcription factor gene *TWIST1*. The protein encoded by this gene is a transcription factor that regulates metastasis and is overexpressed in Saethre-Chotzen syndrome. This abnormality is highly associated with early breast cancer development.

An autosomal dominant *MSX2* defect has been identified as the causative agent in Boston-type craniosynostosis.

Incidence: Craniosynostosis occurs in 1 in 3,000 live births. The association with different syndromes varies from 1 in 25,000 to 1 in 150,000.

Symptoms: Normally, bone growth in the skull occurs at its edges, where the initial skull bones are approximated by fibrous connective tissue. When premature fusion of approximated skull bones occurs, the skull assumes an abnormal shape. Palpation of the sutures, fontanels, and skull bones; measurement of the skull circumference; and observation of the skull shape are performed by the care provider during a physical examination of the individual. Premature suture closure may result in additional symptoms, such as increased intracranial pressure and developmental delay. The individual may exhibit bulging eyes, wide-spaced eyes, a beaked nose, low-set ears, and a small jaw. Certain syndromes may also be associated with hand and limb abnormalities.

Screening and diagnosis: Detection is through physical examination and radiographic techniques including X rays and three-dimensional computed tomography (CT) scans. A CT scan not only can detect suture fusion but also can evaluate the brain for underlying structural abnormalities, thereby assisting the surgeon in planning corrective surgery.

Individuals with craniosynostosis are at risk for having an associated syndrome and for developing various cancers. Because of the high incidence of chromosomal defects, duplications, deletions, and substitutions associated with craniosynostosis, affected individuals are candidates for genetic counseling and chromosomal analysis. Early and consistent screening for cancer leads to diagnosis and treatment in earlier stages of the disease, making a cure more possible.

Treatment and therapy: Surgery is performed to reopen closed sutures and provide a more normal-appearing skull. An open surgical technique is used with multiple suture fusions or if the surgery is performed after the first year of life. This method involves an ear-to-ear incision, removing, reshaping, replacing, and securing the affected bones. For a single fused suture or if surgery is done in the first few months of life, surgical instruments called endoscopes are inserted through small scalp incisions, and small pieces of bone are removed, releasing the suture fusion. These patients then wear a custom-molded helmet for several months. The helmet provides a template for normal skull growth and shape. For other cosmetic issues, the individual may require orthodontic and orthognathic (jaw) surgery to restore normal facial features.

Prognosis, prevention, and outcomes: The prognosis for craniosynostosis is good and improves with early detection and treatment. The morbidity and mortality depend on associated defects as part of a syndrome. Currently, there is no method to prevent autosomal dominant transmission to offspring or to prevent new mutations.

FGFR mutations produce a variety of results. Research is necessary to determine how mutations result in different consequences. If it can be determined how mutations affect outcomes, definitive targeted therapies can be developed. One such proposal is anti-*FGFR* therapy, designed to target the upregulated *FGFR* genes. Because of the associated risk for a variety of cancers, the individual will require ongoing evaluation and screening for carcinogenesis.

Wanda Todd Bradshaw, R.N.C., M.S.N.

For Further Information

Cohen, M. Michael. "Malformations of the Craniofacial Region: Evolutionary, Embryonic, Genetic, and Clinical Perspectives. *American Journal of Medical Genetics* 115 (2002):245-268.

Coumoul, Xavier, and Chu-Xia Deng. "Roles of FGF Receptors in Mammalian Development and Congenital Diseases." *Birth Defects Research* 69 (2003): 286-304.

Hansen, Ruth, et al. "Fibroblast Growth Factor Receptor 2, Gain-of-Function Mutations, and Tumourigenesis: Investigating a Potential Link." *Journal of Pathology* 207 (2005): 27-31.

Ridgway, E. B. "Skull Deformities." *Pediatric Clinics of North America* 5, no. 2 (2004): 359-387.

Other Resources

Children's Craniofacial Association
http://www.ccakids.com

March of Dimes Birth Defects Foundation
http://www.marchofdimes.com

National Institute of Neurological Disorders and Stroke
http://www.ninds.nih.gov/index.htm

See also: Craniotomy; Dry mouth; Mucosa-Associated Lymphoid Tissue (MALT) lymphomas; Nasal cavity and paranasal sinus cancers

▶ Crohn's disease

Category: Diseases, Symptoms, and Conditions
Also known as: Crohn disease, ileitis, ileocolitis, regional enteritis, enteritis

Related conditions: Aphthous ulcers, episcleritis, sclero-conjunctivitis, recurrent iritis, uveitis, erythema nodosum, pyoderma gangrenosum, spondyloarthropathy or spondyloarthritis-ankylosing spondylitis and sacroiliitis, peripheral arthritis, hypercoagulability, secondary amyloidosis, primary sclerosing cholangitis, gallstones, perianal disease, malnutrition, malabsorption, osteoporosis, anemia, lymphoma, cholangiocarcinoma, adenocarcinoma of the gastrointestinal tract, colorectal cancer

Definition: Crohn's disease is a chronic inflammatory condition of the gastrointestinal tract, anywhere from the mouth to the anus, but most commonly at the end of the small intestine called the ileum and in the adjoining large bowel (colon).

Risk factors: Those with a family history of Crohn's disease, a genetic predisposition, or a history of smoking are at greatest risk for this disease.

Etiology and the disease process: Crohn's disease (CD) belongs to the group of diseases known as inflammatory bowel disease (IBD), a generic term for diseases characterized by inflammation in the small and large bowels. Other IBDs are ulcerative colitis (UC) and indeterminate colitis (lymphocytic colitis and collagenous colitis).

Crohn's disease affecting the colon is associated with a higher risk of developing colorectal cancer.

There are many theories about the etiology of Crohn's disease, but the exact cause is unknown. It is known to run in families and be more common in certain ethnicities, suggesting a genetic predisposition. However, no specific reason or factor consistently explains the origin of the disease. The current belief relates Crohn's disease to an inflammatory process. The human immune system protects people from harmful foreign substances (referred to as antigens) in the environment such as bacteria, viruses, and parasites. This protection is provided by cells and various proteins (such as antibodies) through an inflammatory reaction that is a response toward antigens or cell injuries. In Crohn's disease, the immune system reacts abnormally against the affected part of the gastrointestinal tract and causes damage. This inappropriate inflammation leads to the clinical manifestations of Crohn's disease.

Studies have shown that the inflammation related to Crohn's disease is multifactorial and may depend on genetic factors, immune reactions, and environmental cues. A region of human chromosome 16 was found to possibly contain genes that are involved in the abnormal inflammatory response in Crohn's disease. One such gene, known as NOD2/CARD15, was found to be more common in Crohn's disease patients than in the general population. An abnormality in this gene causes a mutation in the gene product (protein) that ultimately weakens the immune system's ability to respond against bacteria in the gastrointestinal tract. This defect somehow causes the immune system to turn against its own gastrointestinal tissues and attack them instead. The runaway immune reaction that characterizes Crohn's disease may be a response to bacterial antigens, or to modified parts of the gastrointestinal tract associated with the inflammation.

Anti-tumor necrosis factor-alpha (TNF-alpha) is a protein produced by the immune system cell called macrophages. TNF is involved in various biological processes and it enhances the ability of white blood cells to defend against infections and other foreign substances. TNF is implicated in many diseases including autoimmune diseases such as Crohn's disease. TNF may be a cause of the inflammation associated with Crohn's disease; it is abnormally elevated in patients with Crohn's disease, causing excessive inflammation with its related adverse effects.

IBDs (Crohn's disease and ulcerative colitis) have similar symptoms, but they also have significant differences. Crohn's disease can affect any part of the gastrointestinal tract, cause inflammation deeply penetrating through the tract linings (full thickness), and show radiographic results suggestive of Crohn's disease. Ulcerative colitis affects the colon and rectum; it can also cause a "backwash" ileitis in the junction of the small and large intestines. Ulcerative colitis inflammation is mainly in the superficial linings of the affected colon and is confined to a part of or all of the colon. The last part of the colon (the rectum) is usually most affected. Tissue sampling can identify the difference between Crohn's disease and ulcerative colitis.

Incidence: Crohn's disease affects approximately one in 300 adults in Europe and North America. In North America, the incidence for Crohn's Disease is 3.1 to 20.2 cases per 100,000 person-years. Based on health insurance claims for 9 million Americans in 2007, the prevalence of Crohn's disease in children younger than 20 years was 43 per 100,000 and in adults was 201 per 100,000. About 20 percent of Crohn's disease cases run in families. Men and women are affected equally, but with slight female predominance in late adolescence and early adulthood. Crohn's disease is more common in people of European and Jewish heritage than those of other ethnicities. The onset of Crohn's disease has two peaks: between the ages of fifteen and thirty and the ages of sixty and eighty. However, most patients are diagnosed before the age of thirty.

Symptoms: There are many manifestations of Crohn's disease, including symptoms within the gastrointestinal tract and outside of it (extraintestinal). Constitutional symptoms of Crohn's disease are fatigue, fever, loss of appetite, and weight loss. Most common gastrointestinal tract symptoms are prolonged diarrhea, with or without rectal bleeding, and abdominal pain (tenderness), usually in the lower right area, which can be mistaken for appendicitis. Malabsorption in the gastrointestinal tract can lead to malnutrition and weight loss, which is related to delayed development and poor growth in children. Mouth ulcers may manifest along with pain in the mouth and gums. Problems of the throat such as pain or difficulty with swallowing can occur if the esophagus is involved.

Patients with Crohn's disease may develop perianal diseases such as fissure in ano (fissures or tears in the lining of the anus) and fistula-in-ano (abnormal connection between the anal intestinal lining and another part of the body, such as the skin, bladder, vagina, or another part of the gastrointestinal tract). Fistulas are most common in the anal region; abscesses (pockets of pus) may be present as a complication. Blockage (obstruction) and perforation of the gastrointestinal tract may occur. Extraintestinal symptoms include eye disorders, skin problems, arthritis, and liver and gallbladder diseases.

Screening and diagnosis: Screening is done through a comprehensive patient history and physical examination. Blood tests will include complete blood count for anemia and assessing markers of inflammation such as erythrocyte sedimentation rate (ESR) and C-reactive protein (CRP) for inflammation. A stool test will be performed to assess gastrointestinal tract bleeding, infection or inflammation (Calprotectin fecal test). Special tests for antibodies, such as antineutrophil cytoplasmic antibodies and anti-Saccharomyces cerevisiae antibodies, may be used if the diagnosis of Crohn's disease is uncertain. Radiographic studies can include upper and lower gastrointestinal series (barium enema). Upper or lower gastrointestinal (GI) endoscopy can identify the affected site, allow tissue sampling (biopsy), and confirm the diagnosis of Crohn's disease. Examples of GI endoscopies that use flexible tubes with light and camera at the ends for visualization include upper GI endoscopy (for the mouth, esophagus, stomach and upper part of the small bowel), enteroscopy (for the small bowel), colonoscopy (for the large bowel) and capsule endoscopy (which uses a pill-like camera for the whole intestine but mainly for the small bowel visualization). The severity of Crohn's disease is diverse, and its activity is described as mild-moderate, moderate-severe, severe-fulminant, and in remission.

Treatment and therapy: Crohn's disease has no cure; however, symptoms can be alleviated. Management of Crohn's disease and its complications may include medications for treatment of symptoms such as antidiarrheal agents (loperamide and diphenoxylate), nutritional support, surgery, or a combination of these modalities. Medications for Crohn's disease include antibiotics such as ciprofloxacin and metronidazole; anti-inflammatory drugs such as corticosteroids, sulfasalazine, and 5-ASA or 5-aminosalicylate (which has uncertain benefits); immunomodulators that inhibit the immune response such as azathioprine, 6-mercaptopurine, and methotrexate; and biologic therapies such as infliximab (Remicade®), adalimumab (Humira®) and certolizumab (Cimzia®), which are antibodies that block tumor necrosis factor (TNF)-alpha activity. A class of biologic therapies called anti-integrin antibodies, such as natalizumab (Tyzabri®) and vedolizumab (Entyvio®), are also effective; these block white blood cells accumulating at the site of inflammation. Another biologic therapy that was recently found to be effective for Crohn's disease management is ustekinumab (Sterlara®). It is a monoclonal antibody that specifically targets proteins involved in inflammation and immune responses. A recent study using an early treatment of combined immunosuppression (immunomodulator + antibody to TNF) showed improved clinical outcomes (decreased need for surgery or hospital admissions and decreased Crohn's disease-related complications). All of these medications may have side effects ranging from nausea, vomiting, and headaches to infection susceptibility and other more serious potential outcomes. The risks and benefits of medications are assessed and modifications implemented on an individual basis.

Regular nutritional assessments are necessary to prevent malnutrition, which can result from malabsorption in the inflamed small and large bowels. Surgical intervention is needed in some cases, such as failure of medical treatment and complications such as obstruction, perforation, nonstop bleeding, abscess, and fistula.

Prognosis, prevention, and outcomes: Crohn's disease is a chronic medical condition. It can manifest in recurrent episodes of the active disease (flares) or remain in remission for variable time periods. Patients with Crohn's disease are monitored closely for related conditions such as associated cancers. Regular cancer screening using colonoscopy is recommended for patients with colonic Crohn's disease ten years after its diagnosis because of its association with colorectal cancer.

Miriam E. Schwartz, M.D., M.A., Ph.D., and Colm A. Ó'Moráin, M.A., M.D., M.Sc., D.Sc.

For Further Information

Kappelman, Michael D., Rifas-Shiman, Sheryl L., Kleinman, Ken, Ollendorf, Dan, Bousvaros, Athos, Grand, Richard J., & Finkelstein, Jonathan A. (2007). The prevalence and geographic distribution of Crohn's disease and ulcerative colitis in the United States. *Clinical Gastroenterology and Hepatology,* 5(12), 1424-1429. An article that reported the estimation of the prevalence of Inflammatory Bowel Diseases (Crohn's Disease and Ulcerative Colitis) in the United States; the study intended to quantify the overall burden of disease and assist the planning for appropriate clinical services.

Khanna, Reena, Bressler, Brian, Levesque, Barrett G., Zou, Guangyong, Stitt, Larry W., Greenberg, Gordon R., ... REACT Study Investigators. (2015). Early combined immunosuppression for the management of Crohn's disease (REACT): a cluster randomised controlled trial. *The Lancet, 386*(10006), 1825-1834. The REACT Study which evaluated using an early treatment of Crohn's Disease with combined immunosuppression (immunomodulator + antibody to TNF); the results showed improved clinical outcomes (decreased need for surgery or hospital admissions and decreased Crohn's disease-related complications).

Lichstenstein, Gary R., Hanauer, Stephen B., Sandborn, William J. & the Practice Parameters Committee of the American College of Gastroenterology. (2009). Management of Crohn's disease in adults. *American Journal of Gastroenterology,* 104(2), 465–483. This is the practice guideline developed by the American College of Gastroenterology for managing Crohn's Disease in adults. This article is available to the public and can be accessed at http://www.nature.com/ajg/journal/v104/n2/full/ajg2008168a.html.

Sandborn, William J. (2014). Crohn's Disease evaluation and treatment: Clinical decision tool. *Gastroenterology,* 147(3), 702-705. This article conveys that the treatment of Crohn's Disease is in evolution and this clinical decision tool is designed to assist clinical providers in their identification, assessment and treatment of patients with Crohn's Disease. This article is available to the public and can be accessed free at http://www.gastrojournal.org/article/S0016-5085%2814%2900918-4/fulltext

Singh, Siddharth & Loftus, Edward V. Jr. (2015). Crohn's disease: REACT to save the gut. The *Lancet,* 386(10006), 1800-1802. This article is a commentary on the most recent findings of the REACT Study that showed high quality evidence supporting the early treatment of Crohn's Disease in community gastroenterology practices using combined immunosuppression with an immunomodulator and antibody to TNF.

U.S. Department of Health and Human Services, National Institutes of Health (NIH).National Institute of Diabetes and Digestive and Kidney Diseases (NIDDK).The National Digestive Diseases Information Clearinghouse (NDDIC). (September, 2014). *Crohn's Disease.* NIH Publication No. 14–3410. Retrieved from http://www.niddk.nih.gov/health-information/health-topics/digestive-diseases/crohns-disease/Pages/facts.aspx. This is a government publication that provides basic information for patients regarding the identification, assessment, diagnosis and treatment of Crohn's Disease.

Other Resources

American Academy of Family Physicians - FamilyDoctor.org
http://familydoctor.org/familydoctor/en/diseases-conditions/inflammatory-bowel-disease.html

American College of Gastroenterology
http://patients.gi.org

American Gastroenterological Association
http://www.gastro.org/patient-care/patient-center

Centers for Disease Control (CDC) and Prevention
http://www.cdc.gov/ibd

Crohn's & Colitis Foundation of America
http://www.ccfa.org

Crohn's and Me Make the Connection
http://www.crohnsandme.com

European Crohn's and Colitis Organisation
http://www.ecco-ibd.eu

European Federation of Crohn's and Ulcerative Colitis Associations
http://www.efcca.org

Irish Society for Colitis and Crohn's Disease
http://www.iscc.ie

National Association for Colitis and Crohn's Disease (UK)
http://www.nacc.org.uk

U.S. National Library of Medicine MedlinePlus
http://www.nlm.nih.gov/medlineplus/crohnsdisease.html

See also: Bacteria as causes of cancer; Cholecystectomy; Colon polyps; Colonoscopy and virtual colonoscopy; Colorectal cancer; Colorectal cancer screening; Duodenal carcinomas; Enteritis; Gastrointestinal cancers; Ileostomy; Inflammatory bowel disease; Leiomyosarcomas; Pancolitis; Small intestine cancer

▶ Cushing syndrome and cancer

Category: Diseases, Symptoms, and Conditions
Also known as: Cushing's syndrome, hypercortisolism, hyperadrenocorticism

Related conditions: Polycystic ovary syndrome, pseudo-Cushing's syndrome

Definition: Cushing syndrome is an endocrine disorder that results from prolonged exposure of the body to high levels of the hormone cortisol.

Risk factors: People who take exogenous steroids, like arthritics or organ transplant patients, and families that show an inherited tendency to develop endocrine gland tumors are at risk of developing Cushing syndrome.

Etiology and the disease process: The adrenal glands lie on top of the kidneys, and the hormone cortisol is made by the outer layer (cortex) of the adrenal glands. Cortisol maintains blood sugar levels and blood pressure, reduces the inflammatory response, balances the activity of insulin, and regulates the metabolism of proteins, sugars, and fats. It also helps the body respond to stress and is found in high levels in women in their last three months of pregnancy, highly trained athletes, and people suffering from depression.

Cortisol secretion by the adrenal glands is tightly regulated. A peptide hormone called corticotropin-releasing hormone (CRH) is released into the bloodstream by a portion of the brain called the hypothalamus. CRH signals to the anterior lobe of the pituitary gland, which lies just below the hypothalamus, to release a protein hormone called adrenocorticotropin (ACTH). Circulating ACTH signals to the adrenal cortex cells to release cortisol. Normal blood cortisol levels shut off CRH and ACTH release by the hypothalamus and anterior lobe of the pituitary gland, respectively. Perturbation of this negative feedback control loop can abnormally increase blood cortisol levels.

Particular tumors of the anterior lobe of the pituitary (pituitary adenomas) that secrete increased amounts of ACTH cause most cases of Cushing syndrome (Cushing disease). Tumors outside the pituitary also can secrete increased amounts of ACTH (ectopic ACTH syndrome). Lung tumors cause more than half these cases. Sometimes adrenal gland tumors can cause Cushing syndrome. Adrenocortical carcinomas cause high blood cortisol levels and rapid onset of symptoms.

Incidence: The majority of Cushing syndrome cases are due to exogenous glucocorticoids. The annual incidence of endogenous Cushing syndrome is estimated at 10 to 15 cases per 1 million individuals.

Symptoms: Symptoms of Cushing syndrome include rapid weight gain concentrated around the face (moon face) and trunk; excessive sweating; thinning of the skin that causes easy bruising, poor healing, and stretch marks; muscle weakness, particularly in the shoulders and hips; excessive hair growth in women; and fat pad deposition on the back of the neck and collar bone (buffalo hump). Excess cortisol also causes insomnia, infertility, and psychological disturbances that range from euphoria to psychosis and also commonly include depression, anxiety, and panic attacks. Complications include bone loss and osteoporosis, high blood pressure, kidney stones, type II diabetes, and unusual infections as a result of suppression of the immune system.

Screening and diagnosis: The urinary free cortisol (UFC) test determines free cortisol concentrations in the urine over a twenty-four-hour period. Urinary cortisol concentrations higher than three to four times the normal level (50 to 100 micrograms a day) are highly suggestive for Cushing syndrome. However, measuring cortisol in saliva at nighttime has become more popular. High salivary cortisol levels are also indicative of Cushing syndrome.

The dexamethasone suppression test determines the location of the abnormality. Dexamethasone mimics the physiological effects of cortisol, inhibiting ACTH release by the anterior lobe of the pituitary gland and decreasing cortisol production. If an ectopic source of cortisol production exists, then dexamethasone administration should not decrease blood or urine cortisol levels. Low-dose and high-dose dexamethasone tests are combined, and if there is no change in cortisol levels before and after dexamethasone administration for either test, an adrenal or ectopic ACTH-producing tumor is indicated. No change for the low-dose test and normal suppression in the high-dose test indicate a pituitary tumor. The CRH stimulation test further distinguishes between pituitary and ectopic ACTH-producing tumors. After an injection of CRH, patients with pituitary adenomas usually experience a rise in blood levels of ACTH and cortisol, but those with ectopic ACTH syndrome and cortisol-secreting adrenal tumors show no such response.

If the endocrine tests are positive for Cushing syndrome, computed tomography scans of the chest and abdomen or magnetic resonance imaging of the pituitary gland can detect tumors of the adrenal glands or pituitary gland that might be producing excessive cortisol or ACTH.

Treatment and therapy: Reducing the use of corticosteroid drugs can ameliorate the symptoms of exogenous Cushing syndrome. In the case of endogenous Cushing syndrome, surgery is recommended for tumors producing ACTH or cortisol. Radiation therapy is sometimes required to completely extirpate the tumor. Drugs that reduce cortisol production such as ketoconazole (Nizoral), mitotane (Lysodren), or metyrapone (Metopirone) can normalize cortisol blood levels and are given before surgery for those who are quite ill or to those for whom surgery and radiation were not completely successful.

Prognosis, prevention, and outcomes: If left untreated, Cushing syndrome is lethal, but with treatment, most patients experience some relief of symptoms and cortisol normalization.

Michael A. Buratovich, Ph.D.

For Further Information

Blevins, Lewis, S., ed. *Cushing's Syndrome.* New York: Springer, 2002.

Gaillard, Rolf C., ed. *The ACTH Axis: Pathogenesis, Diagnosis, and Treatment.* New York: Springer, 2003.

Parker, James N., and Philip M. Parker, eds. *The Official Patient's Sourcebook on Cushing's Syndrome: A Revised and Updated Directory for the Internet Age.* San Diego, Calif.: Icon Health, 2002.

Walsh, Mary. *Cushing's Syndrome, A Patient Guide: One Woman's Journey.* Rye, N.Y.: New Mill Press, 2001.

Zuckerman, Eugenia, and Julie R. Ingelfinger. *Coping with Prednisone (and Other Cortisone-Related Medicines): It May Work Miracles, but How Do You Handle the Side Effects?* 2d ed. New York: St. Martin's Griffin, 2007.

Other Resources

MedlinePlus
Cushing Syndrome
http://www.nlm.nih.gov/medlineplus/ency/article/000410.htm

National Endocrine and Metabolic Diseases Information Services
Cushing's Syndrome
http://www.endocrine.niddk.nih.gov/pubs/cushings/cushings.htm

See also: Adrenal gland cancers; Adrenocortical cancer; Carney complex; Endocrine cancers; Hepatomegaly; Hormonal therapies; Neuroendocrine tumors; Paraneoplastic syndromes; Pituitary tumors; Urinanalysis

▶ Cutaneous breast cancer

Category: Diseases, Symptoms, and Conditions

Related conditions: Inflammatory breast cancer (IBC), melanoma of the breast, Paget disease of the breast

Definition: Cutaneous breast cancer is the metastatic spread of a primary breast cancer to the skin. The most common site of skin metastases is to the affected breast, but it may also metastasize to the axilla, back, scalp, face, neck, extremities, around the ear, and above the clavicle.

Risk factors: Although cutaneous cancer can occur with many types of cancer, it is most common with breast cancer and is associated with a history of breast cancer. It is not known why some breast cancers metastasize to the skin.

Etiology and the disease process: Cutaneous breast cancer develops when the cancer cells invade the bloodstream or lymphatic system. For cutaneous cancer to develop, the cancer cells must evade the body's immune defenses and then settle on the skin, where they invade the tissue.

Incidence: Cutaneous breast cancer is relatively rare. It is estimated that from 0.7 to 10.4 percent of breast cancer patients will develop skin metastases.

Symptoms: The symptoms of cutaneous breast cancer are changes in the skin, most commonly over the site of the primary breast cancer or on the mastectomy incision. There are several types of cutaneous lesions that can develop. The most common are reddened nodules (lumps) and papules (pimple-like lesions). There may also be purple papules, nodules, and plaques (flat, raised patches). Sometimes only a reddened, raised patch develops. The patch appears inflamed and has a defined margin. The last type is a large, purple plaque that has infiltrated the tissue.

Screening and diagnosis: There is no screening in particular for cutaneous breast cancer. A diagnosis of cutaneous breast cancer is verified by skin biopsy. Cutaneous breast cancer is not staged as a separate entity because it is a sign of metastases of breast cancer and indicates Stage III or IV breast cancer.

Treatment and therapy: Cutaneous breast cancer may be surgically excised, treated with photodynamic therapy, or cryotherapy (freezing). Systemic chemotherapy may be administered, or a topical cream called imiquimod 5 percent (Aldara) may be applied. Treatment is performed to improve the patient's quality of life.

Prognosis, prevention, and outcomes: Because it is a sign of advanced breast cancer, the presence of cutaneous breast cancer is indicative of a poor prognosis. There is no way to prevent it.

Christine M. Carroll, R.N., B.S.N., M.B.A.

See also: Breast cancer in men; Clinical Breast Exam (CBE); Comedo carcinomas; Ductal Carcinoma In Situ (DCIS); Invasive ductal carcinomas; Nipple discharge

▶ Cutaneous T-Cell Lymphoma (CTCL)

Category: Diseases, Symptoms, and Conditions
Also known as: Anaplastic large-cell lymphoma, cutaneous anaplastic large-cell lymphoma, granulomatous slack skin, lymphomatoid papulosis, lymphoproliferative disorder, pagetoid reticulosis, reticulum cell sarcoma of the skin, Woringer-Kolopp disease

Related conditions: Adult T-cell leukemia and lymphoma, follicular mucinosis, mycosis fungoides, non-Hodgkin lymphoma, peripheral T-cell lymphoma, Sézary syndrome

Definition: Cutaneous T-cell lymphoma (CTCL) is a type of non-Hodgkin lymphoma that mainly affects the skin. It is an uncontrolled growth of T cells, a type of white blood cell. "Cutaneous" means that this disease affects the skin. Sézary syndrome is a type of CTCL in which the skin, lymph nodes, and blood are all affected. Mycosis fungoides is another kind of CTCL in which only the skin and lymph nodes are affected.

Risk factors: What causes CTCL is not known. Usually people with lymphomas have some type of gene mutation; however, if there is an exact mutation associated with this type of cancer, it is still unknown. In some patients, this disease may be associated with a preexisting allergic condition or a viral infection. Currently, researchers are investigating whether there is a connection between this disease and viruses and whether environmental factors have any association with this disease.

Etiology and the disease process: Most types of non-Hodgkin lymphoma do not affect the skin. However, CTCL is different in that it mostly affects skin cells. This disease often starts with a rash that itches, sometimes to the point of interrupting sleep, or very dry skin. It may progress to red, scaly patches on the skin, called plaques, that spread to larger areas of skin. The skin may also have tumors that may become infected or turn into bloody sores. This disease may progress to the lymph nodes and, in advanced cases, can spread to the spleen, liver, and intestines. In some cases, this type of lymphoma may begin to act like a more aggressive Hodgkin lymphoma.

Incidence: CTCL is quite rare. In the United States, only about 1,500 new cases of CTCL are diagnosed each year. People between the ages of forty and sixty are most likely to get this type of cancer, and children rarely have it. Men are twice as likely as women to develop CTCL, and it is slightly more common in African Americans than in those of other racial backgrounds.

Symptoms: Symptoms of CTCL include a rash; red, scaly, itchy skin; and skin tumors.

Screening and diagnosis: A physical examination is helpful in diagnosing CTCL. However, since CTCL's effect on the skin is similar to that of many other conditions, a diagnosis of CTCL involves a biopsy of the affected skin. This skin is then examined under a microscope to determine if T cells are growing abnormally. Diagnosis may also involve blood tests to determine if the cancer has spread to the blood system. Computed tomography (CT) or magnetic resonance imaging (MRI) scans may be used to look at lymph nodes to determine if the disease has spread to them.

One type of staging of CTCL involves three stages; however, the disease does not always progress through these stages.

- Pretumor stage: Small raised patches appear on the skin, usually on the breast or buttocks, though they may appear anywhere. These patches may resemble eczema. Most patients never progress beyond this stage.
- Plaque stage: Red patches appear on the skin, and sometimes there is no hair growth in these patches. These irregularly shaped patches, called plaques, may appear anywhere on the body but are usually on the face or buttocks or in the skin folds.
- Tumor stage: Tumors, or raised lumps, begin to appear on the skin. These tumors and the plaques may become ulcers (bleeding sores). Sometimes the lymph nodes are affected at this stage, and occasionally, the cancer affects internal organs such as the spleen, liver, or lungs at this stage.

This disease may also be called Sézary syndrome, especially if it progresses to the point of having many abnormal lymphocytes in the blood. Sometimes in Sézary syndrome, the entire skin is red, thick, swollen, and itchy.

Non-Hodgkin lymphomas are often graded into low grade (slow growing) or high grade (fast growing). CTCL is a low-grade non-Hodgkin lymphoma.

Another type of staging of the disease, associated particularly with Sézary syndrome, is as follows:

- Stage I: Only parts of the skin are affected with a red, scaly rash. There are no tumors, and lymph nodes are normal.
- Stage II: The lymph nodes are normal or enlarged but have no cancerous cells, and the skin has red, scaly rash but no tumors, or the lymph nodes are normal or enlarged but do not contain cancerous cells, and the skin has tumors.
- Stage III: Most of the skin is affected by the red, scaly rash, but the lymph nodes, either normal or enlarged, do not contain cancerous cells.
- Stage IV: In addition to the skin rash, either cancer cells are in the lymph nodes or cancer cells have spread to other organs.

Treatment and therapy: Treatments for CTCL involve treating the skin either topically (on the surface), systemically (through the blood), or a combination of both. Treatment may control the disease, but if a patient does not continue treatment, the disease may recur.

If only small areas of the skin are affected, the disease can be treated by radiotherapy or electronic beam radiation. High-energy rays are directed at the affected skin, killing the abnormal lymphocytes while minimizing the damage to the healthy cells. This treatment is most effective during the early stages of the disease. It may also be used on the entire body if the cancer has not spread below the outer layer of the skin.

Another type of topical therapy is UVB (ultraviolet light B) therapy. The patient's skin is exposed to UVB, which can help slow down the growth of skin cells.

CTCL can also be treated by a type of chemotherapy in which drugs are applied directly to the skin using a cream, gel, or ointment. If the cancer becomes much worse or is not responding to other types of therapy, conventional chemotherapy, where drugs are injected into the blood-stream, may also be used.

Photochemotherapy, a combination therapy, may be used if the cancer affects a large area of skin. A patient takes certain drugs that make the skin very sensitive to a type of ultraviolet light called ultraviolet light A. After the drugs have had time to affect the tumors, the skin is exposed to ultraviolet light A, which kills the tumors in the skin.

Researchers are investigating oral drugs and immunotherapy (therapy that uses the body's own immune system to fight the disease) that may be useful for CTCL patients.

Prognosis, prevention, and outcomes: CTCL may stay only in the skin for several years, and many patients can lead normal lives for quite some time while controlling the disease with treatment.

Outcomes for CTCL depend on the type of disease the patient has, how quickly the disease is progressing, and how well the patient is responding to therapy.

Prognosis for patients with mycosis fungoides is usually good, as this type of CTCL usually affects only the skin, and patients are generally diagnosed early in the disease process. These patients have a median survival rate of more than twelve years. Those with Sézary syndrome generally have a more limited prognosis with a median survival of five years as this disease extends into the blood system. Patients whose internal organs are affected have a median survival of two to four years.

Marianne M. Madsen, M.S.

For Further Information

Greer, John P., et al., eds. *Wintrobe's Clinical Hematology*. 11th ed. Philadelphia: Lippincott Williams & Wilkins, 2004.

Souhami, Robert, et al., eds. *Oxford Textbook of Oncology*. 2d ed. New York: Oxford University Press, 2002.

Zackheim, Herschel, ed. *Cutaneous T-cell Lymphoma: Mycosis Fungoides and Sézary Syndrome*. Boca Raton, Fla.: CRC Press, 2005.

Other Resources

Cutaneous Lymphoma Foundation
http://www.clfoundation.org

Leukemia and Lymphoma Society
http://www.leukemia-lymphoma.org

Lymphoma Information Network
http://www.lymphomainfo.net

See also: Mycosis fungoides; Sézary syndrome

▶ Denys-Drash syndrome and cancer

Category: Diseases, Symptoms, and Conditions
Also known as: DDS

Related conditions: Wilms' tumor (WT), Frasier syndrome, WAGR syndrome

Definition: Denys-Drash syndrome is a rare disorder that usually causes kidney failure by the age of three, malformed sex organs, and often Wilms' tumor. It is caused by a *WT1* gene mutation and was named for two pediatricians, Pierre Denys and Allan Drash, who initially described this condition.

Risk factors: The primary risk factor is having a relative with a *WT1*-related disorder.

Etiology and the disease process: Denys-Drash syndrome originates with the mutation of the *WT1* gene's chromosome 11, band p13. Children with Denys-Drash syndrome are usually born with kidney disease, which becomes apparent several weeks after birth through eighteen months. Malignant Wilms' tumor growth in one or two kidneys occurs in approximately 90 percent of Denys-Drash patients. Cancer occasionally extends from the kidneys into the livers, lungs, and lymph nodes.

Incidence: The precise number of Denys-Drash syndrome cases is uncertain, with an estimated 160 cases from the late 1960's through the early twenty-first century. U.S. physicians diagnose approximately 500 children annually with Wilms' tumors, which represent 95 percent of kidney cancers affecting children and 6 percent of pediatric cancers.

Symptoms: Denys-Drash syndrome patients often exhibit symptoms commonly associated with kidney disorders and Wilms' tumors, including swollen abdomens, elevated blood pressure, and bloody urine. Both male and female Denys-Drash syndrome patients have abnormal external or internal genitalia.

Screening and diagnosis: Physicians test young children born with genitalia irregularities for Denys-Drash syndrome. Chromosome analysis verifies *WT1* gene mutations. During infancy, biopsies and blood tests detect problems with kidneys. Computed tomography (CT) scanning, magnetic resonance imaging (MRI), or ultrasounds of abdomens locate tumors. Pediatricians apply the National Wilms' Tumor Study Group (NWTS) staging system's five stages to determine effective treatments.

Treatment and therapy: Medical strategies to combat Denys-Drash syndrome primarily consist of surgery, radiation, or chemotherapy, either separately or combined to impede growth and eliminate malignancies. Some Denys-Drash syndrome patients undergo kidney transplantation and dialysis. Additional pharmaceutical and dietary therapies reduce blood pressure and aid kidney functioning.

Prognosis, prevention, and outcomes: Denys-Drash syndrome patients often develop infections, circulatory problems, and additional cancers that exacerbate their condition. Preventive options include replacing kidneys with healthy transplants and routine screening for malignancies. Kidney failure causes the death of approximately two-thirds of Denys-Drash syndrome patients by age three. In contrast, approximately 90 percent of patients treated solely for Wilms' tumor survive.

Elizabeth D. Schafer, Ph.D.

See also: Nephroblastomas; Wilms' tumor; Wilms' tumor Aniridia-Genitourinary anomalies-mental Retardation (WAGR) syndrome and cancer

▶ Depression

Category: Diseases, Symptoms, and Conditions; Social and Personal Issues
Also known as: Major depression, major depressive disorder, reactive depression, adjustment disorder with depressed features, depression with psychotic features

Related conditions: Anxiety disorder, mood disorder, first episode depression, chronic depression, depression in remission

Definition: Depression is a common cognitive state conceptualized as a range from transient, nonclinical low mood and sadness which remits quickly, to a chronic, life-threatening clinical disorder requiring aggressive intervention by a mental health professional. Depression can lead to significant impairment of an individual's ability to function and is a leading cause of disability worldwide. Clinical depression might co-occur with cancer, but it is not considered typical or expected, which contradicts the belief that depression and cancer "understandably" go hand in hand. However, depression is one of the most common mental health complications in cancer patients.

Risk factors: Depression is most common among cancer patients with advanced disease symptoms that are not treated or inadequately treated. It commonly coexists with anxiety. Most cancer patients manifest transient symptoms of depression that are responsive to support; reassurance; and information about what to expect regarding the course, treatment, and prognosis of their disease. Other cancer patients experiencing unremitting or recurrent depression require aggressive monitoring and intervention. The following list depicts risk factors that favor the development of clinical depression within the context of a cancer diagnosis:

- Family history of depression
- Past history of depression, depression treatment, psychiatric hospitalization, or psychiatric/personality disorder
- History of unusual, eccentric behavior
- Confusion (may be indicative of an organically based depression)
- Maladaptive coping style
- Dysfunctional family coping or complex family issues
- Limited social support
- Financial problems including lack of insurance or large copayment/deductible expense
- Multiple roles, obligations, and stressors
- Advanced cancer
- Treatment resulting in disfigurement or loss of function
- Presence of significant caretaking role (dependent children, parents, others)
- Inadequate symptom management
- Treatment that has a depressionogenic effect (certain chemotherapies, steroids, narcotics)

Etiology and the disease process: Clinical depression, cancer related or not, consists of a complex interaction of factors. These include genetic predisposition to aberrant neurochemical states that precede or result from an inadequate stress response combined with a distorted, negatively-biased cognitive style or worldview that is learned and reinforced early in life. This multidimensional framework indicates a need for combined psychopharmacologic and psychotherapeutic treatment approaches that are well supported in the medical literature. Clinical depression can present as a single episode, be chronic and unremitting, or occur over time with periods of remissions and exacerbations.

Cancer patients' quality of life is intricately affected by an illness that may present comorbid to the physical manifestation of cancer. Depression is one example of such a comorbid presentation. Regardless of current classification (mood dysregulation disorder, major depressive disorder, or persistent depressive disorder) life management of cancer conditions typically do not exist without psychological influences (either cause or effect). In fact, ten to twenty percent of cancer patients will present with depressive symptoms, regardless of cancer stage or venue of diagnosis. After consideration of cancer treatments, and in consultation with the oncology provider team, both psychological and pharmacological treatments are effective.

Incidence: Incidence and Prevalence rates vary and depend on the population studied, site and stage of cancer, and method used to diagnosis depression. Depression prevalence rates among cancer patients range from 5 percent (lower than the general population rates) to 90 percent (higher than the general population rates). Studies that use established diagnostic criteria (DSM) report rates of depression of about 25 percent. Rates of depression are highest among patients with advanced cancer and in studies in which stringent diagnostic guidelines are not used.

Symptoms: Symptoms of depression in cancer populations include the following:

Affective Symptoms	*Neurovegetative symptoms*
• Persistent sad mood • Loss of interest or pleasure in typically pleasurable activities • Feelings of guilt, worthlessness, helplessness • Crying, not easily comforted • Frequent thoughts of death or suicide	• Trouble concentrating, indecisiveness • Appetite change • Diminished energy that may be mixed with restlessness and anxiety • Fatigue, loss of energy • Insomnia or hypersomnia

Diagnosis of cancer-related depression relies heavily on the presence of affective symptoms. Neurovegetative symptoms (physical and environmental changes) that characterize depression in physically healthy individuals are not good predictors of depression in cancer patients because cancer and its treatment produce similar symptoms. Additional behaviors suggestive of depression include refusal, indecisiveness, or noncompliance with treatment; persistent anxiety and sadness; unresponsiveness to usual support; unremitting fear associated with procedures; excessive crying; hopelessness that does not diminish over time; an abrupt change in mood or behavior; eccentric behavior or confusion; and excessive guilt or self-blame for illness.

Screening and diagnosis: A formal diagnosis of depression is based on fulfillment of criteria outlined in the American Psychiatric Association's *Diagnostic and Statistical Manual of Mental Disorders: DSM-5* (2013). The diagnostic subtypes of depression include major depressive disorder (severe depression that includes symptoms observed during the same 2-week period and is particularly amenable to pharmacologic treatment), disruptive mood dysregulation disorder, adjustment disorder (severe recurrent temper outburst manifested verbally), dysthymia (chronic, low-level depression that pervades an individual's personality and daily life), and substance/medication-induced depressive disorder. Major depression and adjustment disorder are common diagnoses among individuals with cancer. In genetically predisposed individuals, dysthymia usually precedes a cancer diagnosis or occurs for the first time following cancer diagnosis.

Depressive symptoms not severe enough or of sufficient duration to achieve diagnostic status are the most common type of depressive phenomena in individuals with cancer. Because a formal diagnosis is not present, these symptoms are often ignored despite a common, negative life management impact. More research on the simultaneous occurrence of cancer and depression is needed, including symptom profiles, clinical treatment trials, and related outcomes.

A number of tests screen for depression, but they have not been consistently incorporated into clinical cancer care. Nonpsychiatric providers fail to diagnose and treat depression in as many as 50 percent of cancer patients with depressive disorders. Obstacles to recognizing depression include inadequate provider knowledge of diagnostic criteria, competing treatment priorities in oncology settings, time limitations in busy offices, concern about the stigma associated with a psychiatric diagnosis, limited reimbursement, and uncertainty about the value of screening mechanisms for co-occurring diagnosis and treatment. In general, regardless of whether screening measures are used, if symptoms do not remit in a reasonable time frame, evaluation of depressive symptoms by a mental health professional should be sought.

Treatment and therapy: Psychosocial interventions can have an important effect on the overall adjustment of patients and their families to cancer and its treatment. Factors contributing to the diagnosis of depression should influence the treatment approach. Treatments include psychopharmacologic treatment, individual psychotherapy, group therapy, family therapy, marital therapy, or some therapeutically appropriate combination of these.

Antidepressant medication should be chosen on the basis of diagnostic subtype, treatment response, and side effect profile. Major depression is commonly treated with one of several classes of antidepressant medication, commonly a selective serotonin reuptake inhibitor (SSRI) or a selective serotonin and norepinephrine reuptake inhibitor (SSNRI). Dosages are typically lower than required in non-co-occurring individuals and can positively affect other symptoms that the patient might be experiencing, such as pain and anxiety. In the oncology setting, a multimodal treatment approach is most effective in treating depression and can have a positive impact on a range of psychosocial and medical outcomes.

Prognosis, prevention, and outcomes: Left untreated, depression can produce a range of negative outcomes including diminished quality of life, noncompliance with treatment, and diminished survival. Depression can be prevented in some individuals by providing preemptive counseling, education, support, and information about resources. Early recognition and treatment offer the best hope for rapid remission. Modern therapies are effective in treating depression even among cancer patients who are in progressive and terminal stages of illness. Treatment can vastly improve quality of life and diminish suffering; thus routine screening and treatment should be a universal aspect of comprehensive cancer care.

Jeannie V. Pasacreta
Updated by: Daniel L. Yazak, D.E.D.

For Further Information

Akechi, T., & Furukawa, T.A. (2016). Depressed with cancer can respond to antidepressants, but further research is needed to confirm and expand on these findings. *Evidence Based Mental Health.* Retrieved from http://ebmh.bmj.com on February 11, 2016.

Burger-Szabo, A., Gabos-Greu, M., Theodor, M., Hajnal, F., Ferencz, M, Gabos-Grecu, C., & Gabos-Grecu, I. (2015). Pain and distress in cancer patients. *Acta Medica Marisensis,* 61(3): 213-216. doi: 10.1515/amma-2015-0057.

Dong, S.T., Butow, P.N., Tong, A., Agar, M., Boyle, F., Forster … Lovell, M.R. (2016). *Support Care Cancer,* 24: 1374-1386. doi: 10.1107/s00520-015-2913-4.

Hendrix, C.C., Bailey,Jr., D.E., Steinhauser, K.E., Olsen, M.K., Stechuchak, K.M., Lowman, S.G. … Tulsky, J.A. (2016). Effects of enhanced caregiver training program on cancer caregiver's self-efficacy, preparedness, and psychological well-being. *Support Care Cancer,* 24: 327-336. doi: 10.1007/s00520-015-2797-3.

Hinz, A., Mehnert, A., Kocalevent, R.-D., Brahler, E., Forkman, T., Singer, S., & Schulte. (2016). Assessment of depression severity with the PHQ-9 in cancer patients and in the general population. *Psychiatry,* 16(22): doi: 10.1186/s12888-016-0728-6.

Hulbert-Williams, N., Neal, R., Morrison, V., Hood, K., & Wilkinson, C. (2012). Anxiety, depression, and quality of life after cancer diagnosis: What psychosocial variables best predict how patients adjust? *Psycho-Oncology,* 21: 857-867. doi: 10.1002/pon.1980.

Krug, K., Miksch, A., Peters-Klimm, F. Engeser, P., & Szecsenyi, J. (2016). Correlation between patient quality of life in palliative care and burden of their family caregivers: A prospective observational cohort study. *BMC Palliative Care,* 15(4). doi: 10.1186/s12904-016-0082-y.

Moseholm, E., Rydaho-Hansen, S., Lindhardt, B.O. (2016). Under diagnostic evaluation for possible cancer affects the health-related quality of life in patients presenting with non-specific symptoms. *PLOS ONE,* 11(2). doi: 10.1371/journal.pone.0148463.

Russell, B., Collins, A., Dowling, A., Dally, M., Gold, M., Murphy, M. … Philip, J. (2016). Predicting distress among people who care for patients living longer with high-grade malignant glioma. *Support Care Cancer,* 24: 43-51. doi: 10.1007/s00520-015-2739-0.

Watanabe, N., Horikoshi, M., Yamada, M., Shimodera, S., Akechi, T., Miki, K. … Furukawa, T.A., (2015). Adding smartphone-based cognitive behavior therapy to pharmacotherapy for major depression (FLATT project): Study protocol for a randomized controlled trial. *BioMed Central,* 16(293). doi: 10.1186.s13063-015-0805-z.

Other Resources

Abramson Cancer Center of the University of Pennsylvania
http://www.oncolink.org/resources

American Psychosocial Oncology Society
http://www.apos-society.org

Cancer Care
http://www.cancercare.org

National Institute of Mental Health Depression.
http://www.nimh.nih.gov/health/topics/depression/index.shtml

Substance Abuse and Mental Health Services Administration
http://www.samhsa.gov

See also: Anxiety; Appetite loss; Benzodiazepines; Elderly and cancer; End-of-life care; Exercise and cancer; Fatigue; Grief and bereavement; Hormonal therapies; Integrative oncology; Living with cancer; Medical marijuana; Opioids; Pain management medications; Palliative treatment; Personality and cancer; Psycho-oncology; Psychosocial aspects of cancer; Self-image and body image; Survivorship issues

▶ Dermatofibrosarcoma Protuberans (DFSP)

Category: Diseases, Symptoms, and Conditions
Also known as: Bednar tumor, familial dermatofibrosarcoma protuberans, fibrosarcomatous tumors with attenuated dermal surfaces, fibrosarcomatous progression, fibrosarcoma of the skin, metastatic dermatofibrosarcoma protuberans, progressive and recurring dermatofibroma

Related conditions: Dermatofibroma, epidermal inclusion cyst, fibrosarcoma, giant cell fibroblastoma, fibrous histiosytoma, keloid and hypertrophic scar, lymphoma, malignant melanoma, metastatic carcinoma of the skin, morphea

Definition: Dermatofibrosarcoma protuberans (DFSP) is a rare type of skin cancer that affects the inner layer of the skin (dermis). "Derma" means that it affects the skin. "Protuberans" means that it sticks out (protrudes) above the skin.

Risk factors: There is no known cause of DFSP. In a minority of patients, about 10 percent, some type of trauma, such as a burn, scar, or injection site, has occurred at the site where the disease develops. Laboratory studies seem to show that a type of chromosome mutation tends to help the previous skin damage evolve into this type of cancer. In this chromosome mutation, material from chromosomes 17 and 22 somehow combine to form another chromosome or switch material from one chromosome to another. However, many people with this chromosome mutation do not develop DFSP, and many who have DFSP do not have this chromosome mutation.

Etiology and the disease process: DFSP is a very slow-growing cancer. It usually starts as a small, hardly noticeable lump on the skin, which may remain that way for several years. It may then get larger and develop into a sore, or plaque, that is irregularly shaped, can vary in color (it may be red-brown, red-blue, or simply a bit darker than the surrounding skin), and bulges out. This lump may be tender or bleed, or it may be painless. This type of cancer most often occurs on the body, arms, or legs. It very rarely occurs on the neck or head.

Rarely, DFSP may appear as a thickened area of skin or a soft depressed area of skin. This type of DFSP may go unnoticed for quite some time, until it has grown big enough for a patient to notice, and so may have spread far underneath the skin. This type of DFSP is difficult to diagnose as it looks very similar to other skin diseases.

DFSP does not generally spread beyond the original tumor site. However, the tumors are very aggressive in that they move out underneath healthy skin. The tumor may be much larger under the surface than it appears to be from the top of the skin. This makes DFSP a difficult cancer to completely eliminate because the distance the tumor has spread underneath the top layer of skin may make it difficult to remove the entire tumor, and cells that are left behind tend to grow into another tumor. In rare cases, this cancer may spread to lymph nodes or into the bloodstream, where it may spread to the lungs, heart, brain, or bones.

Incidence: This type of cancer is relatively rare, having a rate of about 4 new cases per 1 million people each year. DFSP occurs slightly more often in men than in women. Though it may occur in persons of any race, blacks develop this cancer at almost twice the rate whites do. An uncommon variant called Bednar tumor occurs mostly in black patients. This cancer occurs most often in people between the ages of twenty and fifty. It is very rarely found in newborns, children, or the elderly (those over eighty years old).

Symptoms: DFSP appears as a small, red-brown or red-blue tumor on the skin that may develop into a larger, irregularly shaped lump. This lump may feel rubbery or firm. It is attached under the skin so it does not move around when touched. Usually, the lump is not painful. It may develop into a patch of several lumps or nodules.

Screening and diagnosis: There is no screening test or staging system for DFSP. Because the appearance of the skin in a patient with DFSP can be similar to that of a patient with many other conditions, a diagnosis involves a biopsy of the affected skin. This skin is examined under a microscope to determine if cells are growing abnormally. There is no blood test available for determining whether a patient has DFSP. Usually, imaging tests such as computed tomography (CT) or magnetic resonance imaging (MRI) are not used in diagnosis unless the tumors are suspected to have spread into the lymph system or into other body areas.

Treatment and therapy: Surgery is generally the first line of treatment for this type of cancer. Usually, the tumor itself and a large amount of skin around it must be removed to ensure that the entire tumor, growing under the skin where it cannot be seen, is removed. This type of surgery is called wide excision.

Mohs micrographic surgery (MMS) is often used because this type of surgery allows a surgeon to view the edges of the skin through a microscope during surgery. While removing the tissue around the edges of the tumor, the surgeon can keep checking to make sure the skin around the tumor site has no more cancerous cells. Once no more cancerous cells are present in the tissue at the edges of the surgery site, the surgeon can stop removing skin. This can help ensure removal of the entire tumor.

When surgery is used to remove DFSP tumors, the surgical site is often large. Depending on the amount of skin removed, a patient may need skin grafts to close the surgery site. The tumors often have ragged edges and unusual shapes, making removal of the entire tumor difficult. As a result, DFSP has a high rate of recurrence. Any cancerous cells left behind tend to grow into another tumor.

If the cancer is large or its removal would cause serious cosmetic damage, such as a scar on the face or in another exposed area, radiation therapy may be used. In radiation therapy, the skin is exposed to high-energy rays that destroy the cancerous cells while doing as little damage as possible to the surrounding healthy tissues. Radiation therapy may also be used as a follow-up to surgery.

Chemotherapy is rarely used with DFSP, as it has proven to be relatively ineffective. Researchers are developing oral medications and molecular-level therapies to treat this type of cancer. Oral medications may be able to target the specific cancerous cells and kill them while causing few, if any, side effects to the rest of the body. Molecular-level therapies use the body's own natural defenses to target and kill cancerous cells.

Prognosis, prevention, and outcomes: This type of cancer usually does not spread, but it has a high rate of recurrence: In about 20 percent of DFSP patients, the cancer returns in the same place. Usually, this is because the first occurrence of the cancer was not completely removed. Because of this high rate of recurrence, it is important that patients continue to receive follow-up care. Recurrence usually happens within three years, and patients should be seen regularly during that period to assess any tumor sites to ensure that cancerous cells left behind during surgery have not begun to grow.

If the cancer has spread into the lymph nodes or bloodstream, as it does in only about 3 percent of cases, the prognosis is much worse than if the cancer has been contained to tumors in the skin, with death usually occurring within two years. Prognosis is even worse with the variation of this cancer called fibrosarcomatous progression, because this variation is a much more aggressive type of cancer. Older patients (over fifty years old) are more likely to have a poorer outcome than those who are younger.

Marianne M. Madsen, M.S.

For Further Information

Agnew, Karen L., Barbara A. Gilchrist, and Christopher B. Bunker. *Skin Cancer*. Oxford, England: Health Press, 2005.

Du Vivier, Anthony, and Phillip H. McKee. *Atlas of Clinical Dermatology*. 3d ed. Edinburgh: Churchill Livingston, 2002.

Hunter, John, John Savin, and Mark Dahl. *Clinical Dermatology*. 3d ed. Malden, Mass.: Blackwell, 2002.

Other Resources

DermNet NZ
http://www.dermnetnz.org/lesions/dfsp.html

Skin Cancer Foundation
http://www.skincancer.org

See also: Fibrosarcomas, soft-tissue; Sarcomas, soft-tissue

▶ Desmoid tumors

Category: Diseases, Symptoms, and Conditions
Also known as: Aggressive fibromatosis

Related conditions: Familial adenomatous polyposis (FAP), Gardner syndrome

Definition: Desmoid tumors are tumors of the tissue surrounding muscle that may develop anywhere in the body, but often in the abdomen.

Risk factors: Familial adenomatous polyposis (FAP), an inherited syndrome in which thousands of polyps are found in the colon, is a risk factor as well as surgical trauma, pregnancy and childbirth, and exposure to high levels of hormones.

Etiology and the disease process: In many cases the cause of desmoid tumors is not known; however, they may be related to trauma (especially surgical trauma) or to hormones. There is a known genetic association between desmoid tumors and familial adenomatous polyposis.

Incidence: Desmoid tumors are uncommon, with an approximate annual incidence of 2 to 4 cases per 1 million people. Desmoid tumors are more frequent in women than in men. The tumors are usually found in individuals between the ages of ten and forty. Individuals with familial adenomatous polyposis have a 4 to 20 percent chance of developing a desmoid tumor.

Symptoms: A desmoid tumor is usually a painless mass; it may be felt as a lump. Pain may develop if nerves, muscles, or organs are affected by the growing tumor. Tumors in the abdomen can cause abdominal pain, a change in bowel habits, or rectal bleeding.

Screening and diagnosis: Ultrasound imaging is used initially to examine soft-tissue tumors. A computed tomography (CT) scan or magnetic resonance imaging (MRI) may be used subsequently. The diagnosis of desmoid tumor is made by biopsy.

Treatment and therapy: Surgery to remove the tumor is the best treatment, but radiation or drug therapy may also be used either alone (if the tumor is inoperable) or in combination with surgery. Drug therapy may range from aspirin or COX-2 inhibitors (including celecoxib) to hormonal therapy (such as tamoxifen, toremifene, raloxifene, or progesterone). Low-dose chemotherapy for one year or high-dose chemotherapy for a shorter period may be used when other therapies have failed or when the tumor is fast growing or causes symptoms. If there are no symptoms, watchful waiting (observation without treatment) could be appropriate.

Prognosis, prevention, and outcomes: Desmoid tumors are benign and very rarely spread from the site of the original tumor. However, they are locally aggressive and local recurrence rates can be as high as 70 percent. Recurrence is monitored by repeat MRI. Individuals with desmoid tumors should be tested for mutations of the *APC* gene.

Vicki Miskovsky, B.S., R.D.

See also: Fibrosarcomas, soft-tissue; Gardner syndrome; Hereditary polyposis syndromes

▶ Desmoplastic Small Round Cell Tumor (DSRCT)

Category: Diseases, Symptoms, and Conditions
Also known as: Desmoplastic sarcoma, desmoplastic cancer

Related conditions: Solid tumor, testicular cancer, ovarian cancer

Definition: A desmoplastic small round cell tumor (DSRCT) is a rare but highly aggressive tumor usually appearing in the abdomen and surrounding lymph nodes.

Risk factors: There are no known risk factors that have been identified as specific for the DSRCT.

Etiology and the disease process: The tumors in DSCRT appear to arise from early developmental cells in childhood. The cell of origin for this tumor is unknown. The tumor shows characteristics of epithelial, mesenchymal, and neural differentiation. The tumor can metastasize through lymph nodes or the bloodstream primarily into areas of the abdomen including the spleen, diaphragm, liver, and intestines. Other sites include the lungs, central nervous system, bones, uterus, bladder, genitals, abdominal cavity, and the brain.

Incidence: DSCRT is extremely rare, usually occurring in men in their twenties.

Symptoms: The most common symptoms include abdominal pain, abdominal mass, and gastrointestinal obstruction.

Screening and diagnosis: Patients are often misdiagnosed at onset of symptoms, and the rapid growth of the tumor cells can lead to an advanced stage (in which the cancer has spread to lymph nodes and other organs) before being diagnosed. Confirmation of DSCRT is usually done by biopsy. Identification of a genetic abnormality in chromosomes 11 and 22 has been useful in confirming the diagnosis of the tumor.

Treatment and therapy: Because the tumors involve a large portion of the abdomen, surgery is rarely an option. Patients have some success with high doses of chemotherapy and radiation therapy.

Prognosis, prevention, and outcomes: The prognosis of patients diagnosed with desmoplastic round cell tumors is very poor, with fewer than 20 percent surviving more than two to three years. Research has shown that a genetic abnormality called translocation is apparent in chromosomes 11 and 22, and scientists continue to study the pathogenesis of this tumor and various chemical agents to find which are most effective against the tumor.

Robert J. Amato, D.O.

For Further Information

Johanson, Paula. *Frequently Asked Questions About Testicular Cancer*. New York: Rosen, 2008.
Kurth, Karl H., Gerald H. Mickisch, and Fritz H. Schröder. *Renal, Bladder, Prostate, and Testicular Cancer: An Update*. New York: Parthenon, 2001.
Parker, James N., and Philip M. Parker, eds. *The Official Patient's Sourcebook on Testicular Cancer: A Revised and Updated Directory for the Internet Age*. San Diego, Calif.: Icon Health Publications, 2002.

See also: Fibrosarcomas, soft-tissue

▶ Diarrhea

Category: Diseases, Symptoms, and Conditions
Also known as: Dysentery, intestinal flu

Related conditions: Colorectal cancer, gastrointestinal disease

Definition: Diarrhea is the passage of frequent loose or liquid stools. Diarrhea is usually characterized by the passage of loose stools more than three to four times in one day.

Risk factors: Diarrhea may occur as a result of cancer treatment, such as chemotherapy or other cancer medications; radiation therapy to the pelvis, rectum, or abdomen; or surgery. Diarrhea may be the result of an underlying condition, including central nervous system disorders, bowel obstruction, diverticulitis (outpouchings of the colon), and hernia. Diarrhea may be a sign of gastric cancer, colon cancer, rectal cancer, bowel cancer, and other cancers, and it also may occur on the growth or spread of these types of cancer.

Lactose intolerance and certain medications, such as antibiotics, can increase the risk of diarrhea. Anxiety about cancer or cancer treatment also can contribute to the development of diarrhea.

Etiology and the disease process: Chemotherapy and radiation therapy can cause changes in the function of the intestines, including increased or decreased peristalsis (the wavelike contraction of the muscles to propel the contents of the intestines through the digestive tract). An increase in peristalsis can cause stool to move faster through the intestines, leading to diarrhea or cramping. Chemotherapy also can change the normal bacteria in the intestines, causing diarrhea.

Dehydration is a concern for patients who have diarrhea. Dehydration occurs when more fluid is lost than is taken in, and the body does not have enough water and other fluids to carry out its normal functions. Signs of mild dehydration include dry mouth, weakness, dizziness, and fatigue. Signs of severe dehydration require immediate medical attention and include extreme thirst; irritability and confusion; very dry mouth, skin, and mucous membranes; decreased urination; low blood pressure; rapid heartbeat; and fever.

Incidence: Diarrhea is very common among patients undergoing cancer treatments, particularly those receiving certain chemotherapy drugs as well as radiation to the stomach or abdomen. The National Cancer Institute reports that 25 percent of patients experience severe diarrhea.

Symptoms: Symptoms of diarrhea include the passage of frequent loose or liquid stools more than three times in one day. Other symptoms that accompany diarrhea include urgency to have a bowel movement, bloating, and nausea.

Symptoms range from moderate to severe, and vary among patients. Symptoms can impede cancer treatment, resulting in a delay, dose reduction, or discontinuation of therapy.

Changes in stool frequency, consistency, volume, or the presence of blood, mucus, or pus in the stool may indicate an underlying disease. If diarrhea occurs more than six times a day, or does not resolve within twenty-four hours after taking prescribed antidiarrheal medications, the patient should call the prescribing physician.

Screening and diagnosis: A thorough review of the patient's medical history and a physical exam are performed, and stool tests can be performed to identify blood and bacterial, fungal, parasitic, or viral pathogens. Diagnostic tests may include upper endoscopy, upper gastrointestinal series (barium swallow), abdominal X rays, sigmoidoscopy, and colonoscopy.

Treatment and therapy: Symptom management is critical to avoid an interruption in the delivery of cancer treatment. A registered dietitian can provide nutritional therapy to help the patient develop an eating plan that meets dietary requirements while reducing side effects, helping to make treatment more tolerable. In some cases, antidiarrheal medications are prescribed. First-line treatment includes loperamide and diphenoxylate/atropine. Second-line treatment for persistent, chronic diarrhea includes octreotide subcutaneous injections. It is important for patients to ask their physician first before self-treating diarrhea and related symptoms, as some over-the-counter remedies could interfere with cancer treatment.

Conservative techniques to manage diarrhea include the following:

- Increasing fluid intake to prevent dehydration
- Eating bland foods in small amounts
- Following a clear liquid diet of juices and broth until symptoms subside
- Avoiding spicy, high-fat, and sugary foods
- Eating small, frequent meals
- Eating slowly and chewing food completely before swallowing
- Taking medication with food, unless advised otherwise
- Avoiding high-fiber foods and dairy products
- Avoiding caffeine and alcoholic beverages
- Including high-potassium foods, as advised by the doctor

In addition to these recommendations, relaxation techniques such as deep breathing and guided imagery may help. Patients should follow their physician's specific guidelines for managing treatment side effects and should call the doctor when symptoms are severe or persist for more than twenty-four hours. When necessary, nutritional supplements also may be recommended to ensure sufficient caloric and nutrient intake.

Prognosis, prevention, and outcomes: Diarrhea can be effectively managed with conservative treatments and medications and is generally relieved when cancer treatments are completed. There usually are no long-term effects of gastrointestinal symptoms that are properly managed, according to the American Cancer Society.

Hospitalization is recommended for patients with severe dehydration or diarrhea that results in the inability to maintain adequate hydration or nutrition and for patients with chronic diarrhea that does not resolve within twenty-four hours after taking prescribed antidiarrheal medications.

Left untreated, chronic diarrhea can cause significant morbidity and mortality because of nutritional deficiencies, and fluid and electrolyte imbalances may lead to potentially life-threatening dehydration or impaired kidney function.

Although cancer treatments can result in diarrhea that may be temporarily unpleasant to the patient, the potential side effects, if adequately managed under a physician's care, should be measured against the cancer-fighting benefits of a particular treatment.

Angela M. Costello, B.S.

For Further Information

Field, Michael, ed. *Diarrheal Diseases*. New York: Elsevier, 1991.

Kogut, Valerie, and Sandra Luthringer. *Nutritional Issues in Cancer Care*. Philadelphia: Oncology Nursing Society, 2005.

Scott-Brown, Martin, Roy A. J. Spence, and Patrick G. Johnston, eds. *Emergencies in Oncology*. New York: Oxford University Press, 2007.

Other Resources

American Cancer Society
http://www.cancer.org

American College of Gastroenterology
http://acg.gi.org

National Cancer Institute
http://www.cancer.gov

National Institute of Diabetes and Digestive and Kidney Diseases
National Digestive Diseases Clearinghouse
http://digestive.niddk.nih.gov/index.htm

See also: Adrenal gland cancers; Angiogenesis inhibitors; Anthraquinones; Antidiarrheal agents; Antinausea medications; Chemotherapy; Crohn disease; Diverticulosis and diverticulitis; Gastrointestinal cancers; Gastrointestinal complications of cancer treatment; Inflammatory bowel disease; Laxatives; Rectal cancer; Side effects; Symptoms and cancer; Weight loss

▶ Disseminated Intravascular Coagulation (DIC)

Category: Diseases, Symptoms, and Conditions
Also known as: Consumptive coagulopathy

Related conditions: Bleeding, thrombosis

Definition: Disseminated intravascular coagulation (DIC) is a condition that prevents the body from regulating blood clotting. Small blood clots develop throughout the body, and substances needed for clotting become depleted. This systemic coagulation and resulting inability to form clots can lead to organ failure and hemorrhage (excessive bleeding). DIC can be chronic and develop over time, or arise acutely and require emergency intervention.

Risk factors: The clotting cascade associated with DIC can be brought on by a number of health problems: infection, severe trauma, cancer, complications during pregnancy and childbirth, and some types of snakebite. Patients with solid tumor cancers and acute leukemias have an increased risk. Chronic DIC may be induced or aggravated by various stimuli, including radiation therapy and chemotherapy. Acute DIC is usually associated with infections.

Etiology and the disease process: DIC occurs when an overabundance of clotting factors are released into the bloodstream in response to tissue damage. Widespread clotting occurs within the microvasculature throughout the body. The excessive clotting can damage organs and, paradoxically, "uses up" clotting factors and platelets (clotting cells) such that the blood can no longer clot normally.

Incidence: Some 10 to 15 percent of patients with metastatic cancer show evidence of DIC, and it is present in approximately 15 percent of patients with acute leukemia.

Symptoms: Acute DIC symptoms include bleeding, sudden bruising, shortness of breath, and low urine output from kidney damage. Chronic DIC may produce no symptoms at all or only minimal bleeding or clotting.

Screening and diagnosis: No single test is used to diagnose DIC. Blood tests include a D-dimer test (test for a certain breakdown product of blood clots), prothrombin time (measure of blood-clotting tendency), fibrinogen level (level of a protein needed for blood to clot), and complete blood count. The physician will look at the patient's clinical symptoms (bleeding, bruising, and so on) along with available blood tests to make a diagnosis.

Treatment and therapy: Treatment for DIC involves treatment for the underlying cause. Supportive care with platelets and clotting factors will be used to stop excessive bleeding. Transfusions of blood cells may be necessary to replace blood that has been lost. In some cases, heparin (a blood thinner) may be used to stop the cascade of clotting events.

Prognosis, prevention, and outcomes: Prognosis will be primarily determined by the underlying condition that led to DIC and the severity of the DIC itself. For patients with sepsis and severe trauma, the presence of DIC may increase the risk of death by 1.5 to 2 times.

Melanie Hawkins, B.S.N., R.N., O.C.N.

See also: Acute Lymphocytic Leukemia (ALL); Acute Myelocytic Leukemia (AML); Leukemias; Mesothelioma; Paraneoplastic syndromes

▶ Diverticulosis and diverticulitis

Category: Diseases, Symptoms, and Conditions
Also known as: Diverticular disease

Related conditions: Perforated bowel, bowel obstruction, chronic constipation, peritonitis, gastrointestinal bleeding, colon cancer

Definition: Diverticulosis is a condition in which an outpouching occurs in an area of the colon. This area of outpouching is known as a diverticulum. Occasionally a diverticulum becomes infected or inflamed, leading to a condition known as diverticulitis.

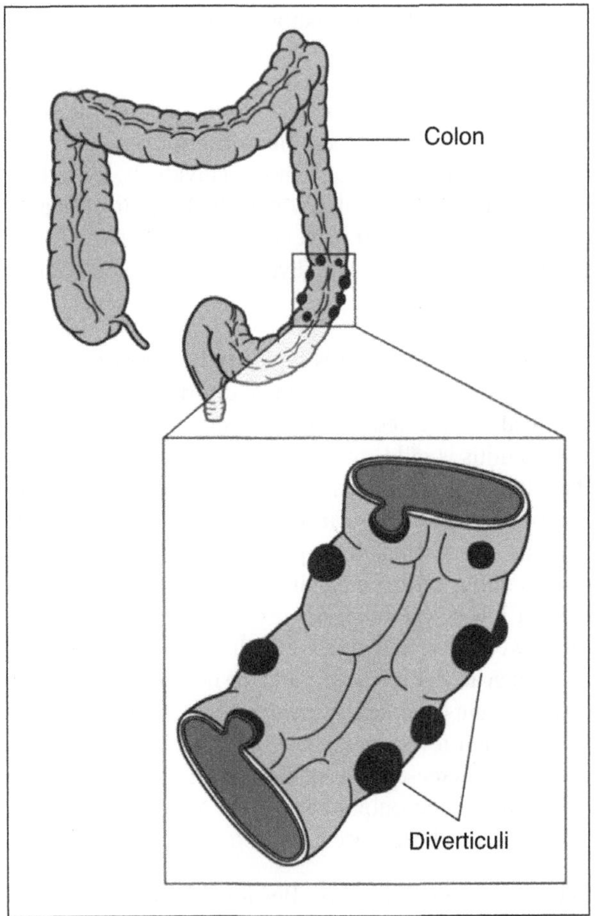

Diverticulitis, a condition in which outpouchings on the colon wall become inflamed, is a risk factor for cancer.

Risk factors: Risk factors include a low intake of dietary fiber and chronic constipation.

Etiology and the disease process: Inadequate intake of dietary fiber is thought to contribute to the development of diverticulitis. When fiber is lacking in the diet, there is less residue in the fecal matter. Reduced residue narrows the bowel lumen, increasing intraluminal pressure during defecation.

A diverticulum results when high intraluminal pressure is exerted on an area of weakness in the gastrointestinal wall, where blood vessels enter. High pressure causes layers of the wall in the area of weakness to herniate through the muscular wall, forming a diverticulum.

Fecal material, undigested food, and bacteria collect in the diverticulum, forming a hard mass that diminishes blood flow to the diverticulum. The diverticulum becomes inflamed and infected, causing fever and lower abdominal pain. If this condition is left untreated, an abscess may develop and the intestinal wall may perforate.

Incidence: According to the National Institutes of Health, diverticular disease affects about 2.5 million people in the United States. Of those individuals, more than 600,000 require hospitalization annually for treatment of the disease. About 20 percent of those diagnosed with diverticulosis will develop diverticulitis at some point in their lives.

Symptoms: Diverticulosis typically produces no symptoms. Symptoms occur when a diverticulum becomes inflamed or infected and diverticulitis develops. When diverticulitis is mild, symptoms include moderate pain in the left lower abdomen and low-grade fever. The inflammation may also cause irritability and spasticity of the adjoining abdominal wall, producing diarrhea. In acute diverticulitis, severe cramping pain suddenly occurs in the left lower abdomen. Anorexia, nausea, constipation, fever, weakness, and abdominal distension may also occur. When an abscess occurs and the bowel perforates, abdominal pain becomes severe and abdominal rigidity develops. High fever, chills, low blood pressure, increased heart rate, decreased level of consciousness, diarrhea, and diminished urine output also occur. Without immediate treatment, death may occur.

Screening and diagnosis: Because diverticulosis does not produce symptoms, it is commonly discovered during testing for another disorder. It is also commonly found during colonoscopy for routine colon cancer screening.

When symptoms prompt a visit to a health care provider, diverticulitis is diagnosed through physical examination and diagnostic testing. The health care provider will begin by taking a medical history, asking questions about the onset and severity of symptoms, bowel habits, dietary intake, and medications. The health care provider may also perform a digital rectal examination to check for a mass or blockage. A small stool sample may be obtained to check for occult blood (blood that is not visible to the eye).

The health care provider may also order a blood test, known as a complete blood count, to check for signs of infection and bleeding. Blood cultures may be ordered to determine whether the infection has spread to the blood. An abdominal computed tomography scan, commonly referred to as an abdominal CT scan, may be performed to detect diverticulitis and can reveal an abscess. A barium enema may also be performed. An abdominal X ray may show free air under the diaphragm, indicating that perforation has occurred. When acute diverticulitis subsides, the health care provider may order a colonoscopy to determine the extent of disease and to rule out other disorders.

Diverticulitis may be a risk factor for contracting certain types of cancer, and it can make cancers of the colon more difficult to properly diagnose.

Treatment and therapy: Treatment for diverticular disease depends on the severity of disease. Diverticulosis is commonly treated with a high-fiber diet. Increasing fiber in the diet softens stools and decreases the pressure within the colon so that fecal material moves through freely. Twenty to thirty-five grams of fiber should be consumed each day. A psyllium dietary fiber supplement may also be recommended. Fluid intake should also be increased to two liters per day, if other medical conditions allow. Exercise also helps increase the rate of stool passage.

Mild diverticulitis may be treated with a liquid diet to rest the bowel until symptoms subside, followed by a high-fiber diet. Antibiotics such as metronidazole, ciprofloxacin, levofloxacin, or co-trimoxazole may be prescribed for seven to ten days. A mild analgesic such as acetaminophen may also be recommended. If discomfort is caused by spasm, an antispasmodic such as oxyphencyclimine may be prescribed.

Severe diverticulitis may require hospitalization for administration of intravenous antibiotics and fluids. If the infection does not subside with antibiotic therapy, surgical intervention may be necessary. Emergency surgery may also be necessary if a fistula or perforation occurs. Surgery involves removing a portion of the colon and clearing the abdominal cavity. Because infection is present, the colon cannot be reconnected until the infection is cleared. Therefore the surgeon must create a temporary colostomy. A second surgery is required to reconnect the colon after the infection is gone.

Prognosis, prevention, and outcomes: With early recognition and treatment, prognosis is good. According to the National Institutes of Health, approximately 3,300 deaths occurred as a result of diverticular disease in 2002.

Collette Bishop Hendler, R.N., M.S.

For Further Information

Black, P. and C. Hyde. *Diverticular Disease*. Hoboken, N.J.: John Wiley & Sons, 2005.

Kruis, W., et al. *Diverticular Disease: Emerging Evidence in a Common Condition*. Norwell, Mass.: Springer and Falk Foundation, 2006.

Munden, Julie, et al. *Pathophysiology Made Incredibly Easy!* 4th ed. Philadelphia: Lippincott Williams & Wilkins, 2008.

Other Resources

MedlinePlus
Diverticulosis
http://www.nlm.nih.gov/medlineplus/tutorials/diverticulosis/htm/index.htm

National Digestive Diseases Information Clearinghouse
Diverticulosis and Diverticulitis
http://digestive.niddk.nih.gov/ddiseases/pubs/diverticulosis/

See also: Antidiarrheal agents; Colonoscopy and virtual colonoscopy; Colorectal cancer; Colorectal cancer screening; Crohn disease; Cruciferous vegetables; Diarrhea; Enterostomal therapy; Fecal Occult Blood Test (FOBT); Fiber; Gastrointestinal cancers; Gastrointestinal complications of cancer treatment; Hemorrhoids; Immunochemical Fecal Occult Blood Test (iFOBT); Inflammatory bowel disease; Laxatives; Nuclear medicine scan; Nutrition and cancer prevention; Obesity-associated cancers; Pancolitis; Sigmoidoscopy; Small intestine cancer; Upper Gastrointestinal (GI) series

▶ Down syndrome and leukemia

Category: Diseases, Symptoms, and Conditions
Also known as: Trisomy 21 and cancer of white blood cells

Related conditions: Transient leukemia (TL), transient myeloproliferative disorder, transient abnormal myelopoiesis

Definition: Down syndrome and Blood cancers Individuals with Down syndrome have three copies of chromosome 21 instead of two. Those with Down syndrome have a significant risk of developing certain forms of leukemia. Leukemia is a blood cancer in which cancerous changes take place in marrow cells that form lymphocytes (white blood cells).

Risk factors: Children with Down syndrome have a 10 to 20 times greater risk of developing leukemia than other children. They develop acute lympholastic leukemia and two types of megakaryoblastic leukemia: transient leukemia(TL) and acute megakaryoblastic leukemia (AMKL). Down syndrome children have a 500 times greater risk of developing AMKL than other children and about 10 percent of newborns with Down syndrome develop TL.

Etiology and the disease process: In TL and AMKL, blasts (immature blood cells) accumulate in blood and bone marrow, and white blood cell differentiation is abnormal. TL in the newborn goes into remission within a few months. Of those who had TL, 20 to 30 percent will develop AMKL later in life. The relationship between Down syndrome and increased risk for leukemia is not completely understood. However, it has been observed that—in addition to having trisomy for chromosome 21—children who develop TL have mutations in the transcription factor GATA1, which plays an important role in the normal development of red blood cells, megakaryocytic, and basophilic cell lines. The GATA1 gene' (also known as a hematopoietic growth factor) is on the X chromosome. It is thought that additional mutations must occur for AMKL to develop.

Incidence: The incidence of Down syndrome is 1 in 800, and 1 in 95 Down syndrome children will develop leukemia, compared with 1 in 2,000 children in general.

Symptoms: As with other leukemias, the symptoms associated with Down syndrome leukemias include fatigue, skin pallor, bruising, bleeding, difficulty in wound healing, enlarged lymph nodes, and joint pain.

Screening and diagnosis: Analysis of the blood is done in children with Down syndrome to test for signs of leukemia. In TL in Down syndrome, analysis of blood and bone marrow shows variable numbers of blasts. The acute leukemia cell produces nonfunctional leukemia cells that crowd out normal cells.

Treatment and therapy: Children with Down syndrome and leukemia are typically treated with chemotherapy. Blasts of Down syndrome TL are sensitive to low doses of cytosine arabinoside. Children with Down syndrome and leukemia are more sensitive than other children to some drugs used in chemotherapy, such as methotrexate, so Down syndrome children must be carefully monitored for drug toxicity. Down syndrome children are also at an increased risk of developing acute myeloid leukemia. Such children have an increased risk of cardiotoxicity if treated with the usual dose of anthracycline. However, they can be treated successfully with a lower dose of anthracycline.

Additionally, a study comparing Down syndrome children with and without leukemia showed a reduced verbal intelligence in those who were treated for leukemia.

Prognosis, prevention, and outcomes: Down syndrome TL neonates have a 15 percent risk of developing a potentially fatal liver disease and an increased risk of developing cardiopulmonary failure and spleen necrosis. Though Down syndrome children are at an increased risk of developing leukemias, they have a reduced risk of developing solid tumors.

Susan J. Karcher, PhD

For Further Information

American Journal of Medical Genetics. (2014). Connection found between lack of PRC2 gene and B-cell acute lymphoblastic leukemia. *American Journal of Medical Genetics Part A,* 164(8): x-xi.

Dana-Farber Cancer Institute. (2014, April). Link between Down syndrome, leukemia uncovered. *ScienceDaily.* www.sciencedaily.com/releases/2014/04/140420131810.htm

Heft, E., & Blanco, J. G. (2016). Anthracycline-related cardiotoxicity in patients with acute myeloid leukemia and Down syndrome: A literature review. *Cardiovascular Toxicology,* 16(1): 5-13.

Oncology Times. (2014). Reasons identified for link between Down syndrome and leukemia. *Oncology Times,* 36(10): 66-67.

Roncadin, C., Hitzler, J., Downie, A., Montour-Proulx, I., Alyman, C., Cairney, E., & Spiegler, B. J. (2015). Neuropsychological late effects of treatment for acute leukemia in children with Down syndrome. *Pediatric Blood Cancer,* 62: 854–858.

Xavier, A. C., Edwards, H., Dombkowski, A. A., Balci, T. B., Berman, J. N., Dellaire, G., ... Taub, J. W. (2011). A unique role of GATA1s in Down syndrome acute megakaryocytic leukemia biology and therapy. *PLoS ONE,* 6(11): e27486. doi:10.1371/journal.pone.0027486.

See also: Acute Lymphocytic Leukemia (ALL); Acute Myelocytic Leukemia (AML); Blood cancers; Childhood cancers; Cytogenetics; Genetic testing; Myelodysplastic syndromes; Ultrasound tests

▶ Dry mouth

Category: Diseases, Symptoms, and Conditions

Also known as: Xerostomia, Sjögren syndrome, cotton mouth (slang), oral dryness, aptyalism, asialia, stomatitis sicca, Zagari disease

Related conditions: Tooth decay, canker sores and mouth sores, geographic tongue, gum sensitivity, gingivitis, halitosis (bad breath), dysphagia (difficulty swallowing), dry eyes, nasal dryness, nosebleeds

Definition: Dry mouth is an insufficient amount of saliva and moisture that would otherwise naturally lubricate and rinse the oral cavity.

Risk factors: Many medications (prescription and over the counter) can cause dry mouth: antihistamines, antidepressants, antianxiety drugs, antihypertensive drugs, decongestants, sinus medications, pain medications, asthma and allergy medications, diuretics, and Parkinson's medications. Chemotherapy or radiation treatments (particularly radiation therapy to the head and neck regions) also can cause this condition. Diseases and disorders that increase the risk of dry mouth include Parkinson's disease, thyroid disorders, cancer, diabetes, human immunodeficiency virus (HIV) and acquired immunodeficiency syndrome (AIDS), Sjögren syndrome, stroke, systemic lupus erythematosus (SLE), increased progesterone levels, and decreased estrogen levels. Other factors that amplify dry mouth include smoking tobacco or marijuana, hormone imbalances, mouth breathing, dry air environment, drinking strong citrus juices, vitamin or mineral deficiencies, anxiety and stress, alcohol consumption, high fevers, stones or tumors in the salivary ducts, hyperventilation, nasal obstruction, vomiting or diarrhea, and excessive sweating.

Etiology and the disease process: Saliva contains enzymes that help break down and rinse away food particles and liquids. It also neutralizes acids and sugars in the mouth. Inadequate lubrication causes a dry mouth environment. When a person loses the ability to produce the normal amount of saliva, plaque and bacteria build up and adhere to the teeth, causing rapid, extensive decay and serious oral infections. Oral infections have the potential to interfere with planned cancer treatment therapies.

Incidence: In general, dry mouth issues are more frequent in men; however, they also are more common in women during menopause and postmenopause. Dry mouth syndrome increases with the number of medications taken by an individual. Dry mouth can also be caused by an autoimmune disease called Sjögren syndrome. Approximately 4 million people are diagnosed each year with Sjögren syndrome. Approximately one-third to one-half of all cancer patients develop dry mouth complications because of radiation therapy, chemotherapy, and medication treatments.

Symptoms: Symptoms include a dry or fissured tongue, a dry oral cavity, chapped or cracked lips, difficulty swallowing, increased risk of tooth decay, increased chance of mouth sores, bad breath (halitosis), increased gum sensitivity, gingivitis, bleeding gums, a burning sensation in the mouth, a dry throat, dry eyes, and increased oral infections.

Screening and diagnosis: The patient is the first to notice symptoms. Friends and relatives often hear the lack of saliva within the patient's speech and notice an unpleasant mouth odor. Dentists often note the dryness during dental exams and discover an increase in the number of cavities.

Treatment and therapy: Patients should drink plenty of liquids during meals and sip on water between meals to help rinse away food particles, make it easier to swallow, and neutralize any oral debris. Sipping on soda all day or sucking on sugary hard candies in an effort to alleviate dry mouth should be avoided. Instead, patients may eat sugar-free candy or chew sugarless gum to help stimulate their natural salivary secretions. They should also eat healthy foods including those with natural oils such as peanuts, peanut butter, and fish. Patients should avoid coffee and tea that have sugar or creamers added. They should stop smoking, avoid all tobacco products, and stop drinking alcohol. Patients should brush twice daily, floss after snacks and meals, and use alcohol-free fluoride mouth rinses. Some patients may need hormone replacement therapy (HRT) or vitamin supplements. They may also use artificial saliva substitutes or fluoride gels such as PreviDent, Biotene, or PerioGard.

Prognosis, prevention, and outcomes: Dry mouth can be a temporary or permanent situation depending on its cause. Radiation therapy can permanently damage salivary glands, and chemotherapy can cause saliva to become thick. Patients may reduce dry mouth symptoms by changing their medications; however, they should check with their doctor before changing or discontinuing any medications. Using water rinses, saliva substitutes, and fluoride rinses without alcohol will help alleviate dry mouth symptoms, strengthen teeth, and fight future tooth decay. Serious oral infections and extensive decay may result in loss of teeth and difficulty wearing dentures. Maintaining excellent oral hygiene is a challenge with dry mouth issues. More frequent dental exams and cleanings are necessary to check for decay. By avoiding the triggers that provoke dry mouth and using the recommended treatments, dry mouth may be manageable.

Suzette Buhr, R.T.R., C.D.A.

For Further Information

American Dental Association. *ADA Guide to Dental Therapeutics*. 4th ed. Chicago: Author, 2006.

Litin, Scott C., Jr., ed. *Mayo Clinic Family Health Book*. 3d ed. New York: HarperResource, 2003.

National Institutes of Health. *Dry Mouth*. NIH Publication 99-3179. Bethesda, Md.: Author, 1999.

Shafer, William G., Maynard K. Hine, and Barnet M. Levy. *A Textbook of Oral Pathology*. 4th ed. Philadelphia: W. B. Saunders, 1983.

Waal, Isaac van der. *Diseases of the Salivary Glands Including Dry Mouth and Sjögren's Syndrome: Diagnosis and Treatment*. New York: Springer-Verlag, 1997.

Other Resources

American Cancer Society
http://www.cancer.org

American Dental Association
http://www.ada.org

National Institutes of Health
National Institute of Dental and Craniofacial Research
http://www.nidcr.nih.gov/HealthInformation/DiseasesAndConditions/DryMouthXerostomia/DryMouth.htm

What Causes Dry Mouth?
http://www.drymouth.info/consumer/whatcausesDM.asp

See also: Aids and devices for cancer patients; Antidiarrheal agents; Antinausea medications; Appetite loss; Diarrhea; End-of-life care; Endoscopic Retrograde Cholangiopancreatography (ERCP); Graft-Versus-Host Disease (GVHD); Hysterectomy; Lambert-Eaton Myasthenic Syndrome (LEMS); Mucositis; Opioids; Radiation therapies; Sjögren syndrome; Smoking cessation; Taste alteration; Weight loss

▶ Duct ectasia

Category: Diseases, Symptoms, and Conditions
Also known as: Plasma cell mastitis, mastitis obliterans, comedomastitis, secretory disease of the breast

Related conditions: Periductal mastitis

Definition: Duct ectasia is a benign condition in which the mammary milk ducts (small tubes that carry breast milk to the nipple) fill with fluid and become plugged and inflamed.

Risk factors: Duct ectasia is more common in women with a history of periductal mastitis (infection of the breast ducts), cigarette smoking, an inverted nipple, and more than one pregnancy. The hormonal changes that occur with aging increase a woman's risk of developing duct ectasia, as does a lack of vitamin A.

Etiology and the disease process: Duct ectasia appears to start with an inflammatory process (the body's response to irritation or injury), similar to an infection. A duct fills with fluid from the blood plasma, the lymph system, and the circulatory system. Lipids (fatty substances) and dead cells block the fluid from draining and lead to a buildup of the fluid in the duct. This causes the duct to dilate and become hardened.

Incidence: Duct ectasia typically develops in women who are in their forties or fifties and are in perimenopause or menopause.

Symptoms: Duct ectasia may appear as a lump in the breast or as an infection, marked by redness, swelling, pain, hardness, and fever. There may be a nipple discharge that is tan, white, greenish, or black. Sometimes, the nipple is inverted.

Screening and diagnosis: Duct ectasia is diagnosed by physician examination of the nipple discharge, breast self-examination, mammography, or breast ultrasound. Although the symptoms usually provide the necessary information for diagnosing duct ectasia, in some instances it may be necessary to biopsy the affected area of the breast.

Treatment and therapy: The treatment for duct ectasia usually involves medication. The patient is given an antibiotic based on the culture and sensitivity of the nipple discharge. Warm, moist compresses are applied to the affected breast area three to four times a day for ten to fifteen minutes. The patient should wear a supportive bra and sleep on the unaffected side. In rare instances, it is necessary to incise (surgically open) and drain the infected duct.

Prognosis, prevention, and outcomes: There is no method for preventing duct ectasia. Because duct ectasia is a benign problem, recovery is generally complete. Some women do have multiple incidences of duct ectasia. This condition does not increase a woman's risk of developing breast cancer.

Christine M. Carroll, R.N., B.S.N., M.B.A.

See also: Breast cancer in pregnant women; Comedo carcinomas; Ductal Carcinoma In Situ (DCIS); Lumps; Nipple discharge; Ultrasound tests

▶ Ductal Carcinoma In Situ (DCIS)

Category: Diseases, Symptoms, and Conditions
Also known as: Stage 0 breast cancer

Related conditions: Breast cancer, Paget disease of the nipple

Definition: Ductal carcinoma in situ (DCIS) is a noninvasive form of breast cancer occurring in the ducts that are responsible for secreting milk. It is the most common type of noninvasive breast cancer, and because it is nonmetastatic, most patients survive their disease.

Risk factors: Reproductive risk factors include women who never had a full-term pregnancy, had their first pregnancy after age thirty, started menstruation early, or had a late menopause. The use of oral contraceptives and postmenopausal estrogen-progestin replacement therapy (more than five years) has been shown to increase the risk of breast cancer. Having a family history of early-onset or bilateral disease and carrying the breast cancer susceptibility gene *BRCA1* or *BRCA2* increase the risks as well. Breast cancer risk increases with age, with most cases occurring in women over the age of sixty. The following are factors that reduce the risk of breast cancer: physical activity (exercise), multiple pregnancies, breast-feeding, and early removal of both ovaries.

Etiology and the disease process: Not all DCIS lesions become invasive breast cancer, but most invasive lesions are preceded by DCIS. Most of the genetic changes present in invasive breast cancer are already present in DCIS, suggesting that if left untreated, these tumors would indeed become invasive.

Incidence: The National Cancer Institute estimates that 12.7 percent of women born today will be diagnosed with breast cancer at some time in their lives. DCIS is the most common type of breast cancer, representing 21 percent of all newly diagnosed cases and as many as 30 to 50 percent of new breast cancers diagnosed by mammography. In 2005, there were estimated to be more than 60,000 new cases of DCIS in the United States. The use of mammography has greatly increased the detection and diagnosis of DCIS, leading to an increased rate of survival for those women whose lesions are detected early.

Symptoms: Most breast cancers do not cause any pain, making them hard to detect. However, any change in the size or shape of the breast, change in the look or feel of the breast or nipple, or any lump or thickening in or near the breast or underarm area may be a symptom of breast cancer. Other more obvious changes include nipple discharge, tenderness, an inverted nipple, and ridges in or pitting of the breast (when the skin looks like that of an orange).

Screening and diagnosis: Because this disease can remain symptomless, monthly self-examination of the breasts after the age of twenty, yearly checkups, and regular mammographies after the age of forty are crucial to early detection. Most of the new cases of DCIS detected by mammography are not detectable by examination alone.

Once DCIS is detected, tissue is sampled using fine needle aspiration (FNA) biopsy or core needle biopsy. According to the standard staging system, DCIS is a Stage 0 breast cancer. Pathologic analysis will determine the classification of the tumor, its size and margins, and if the tumor is hormone dependent. These criteria are then further classified as follows:

- Grade I (low grade): Non-high grade without necrosis (the tumor cells look similar to normal cells, and the tumor may be solid, cribiform, or papillary)
- Grade II (medium grade): Non-high grade with necrosis
- Grade III (high grade): Very quickly growing tumor with the cells in the center of the duct becoming starved from the blood supply; described as "comedo"

Treatment and therapy: Treatment will vary from case to case depending on the size and grade of the tumor and whether there is a family history of breast cancer. Typically, once diagnosis is confirmed, a lumpectomy is performed to remove the entire area of the DCIS and a marginal area of normal breast tissue around it. This is followed by radiation to the whole breast to kill cancer cells outside the surgical margin and to reduce the risk of the cancer coming back. In some cases a mastectomy, in which the entire breast is removed, may be recommended if the DCIS covers a very large area or multiple areas of the breast, or if the patient has a family history of breast cancer or a known gene abnormality (*BRCA1* or *BRCA2*). Because this type of cancer has not invaded into the normal tissue, chemotherapy is not needed for DCIS. If the tumor tests positive for hormone receptors, hormonal therapy (tamoxifen and aromatase inhibitors) can be used to lower the risk of recurrence.

Prognosis, prevention, and outcomes: Because DCIS is a precancerous or preinvasive lesion, the prognosis is very good. Less than 1 percent will die from this disease. It is possible that an invasive focus not found at the time of diagnosis will later develop into metastatic disease, but the likelihood is small. About 40 to 50 percent of local recurrences are invasive and 10 to 20 percent of patients will develop metastases and die from their disease. The more aggressive the therapy, the lower the rate of mortality. Additional treatment, including surgery, radiation therapy, antiestrogen therapy, or a combination of these, will reduce the chances of recurrence of the disease.

Terry J. Shackleford, Ph.D.

For Further Information

Hunt, Kelly K., Geoffrey L. Robb, Eric A. Strom, and Naoto T. Ueno. *Breast Cancer*. M. D. Anderson Cancer Care Series. New York: Springer, 2001.

Link, John. *Breast Cancer Survival Manual: A Step-by-Step Guide for the Woman with Newly Diagnosed Breast Cancer*. 4th ed. New York: Holt, 2007.

"The Picture Problem: Mammography, Air Power, and the Limits of Looking." *The New Yorker*, December 13, 2004. http://www.gladwell.com/2004/2004_12_13_a_picture.html.

Roses, Daniel F. *Breast Cancer*. Philadelphia: Elsevier, 2005.

Shockney, Lille D. *Navigating Breast Cancer: A Guide for the Newly Diagnosed*. Sudbury, Mass.: Jones & Bartlett, 2006.

Other Resources

American Cancer Society
http://www.cancer.org

Breastcancer.org
http://www.breastcancer.org

National Cancer Institute
Breast Cancer
http://www.cancer.gov/cancertopics/types/breast

Susan G. Komen for the Cure
http://www.komen.org

University of Texas, M. D. Anderson Cancer Center
Breast Cancer
http://www.mdanderson.org/diseases/breastcancer/

See also: Breast cancer in children and adolescents; Breast cancer in men; Breast cancers; Comedo carcinomas; Ductal lavage; Ductogram; Invasive ductal carcinomas; Lobular Carcinoma In Situ (LCIS); Medullary carcinoma of the breast; Mucinous carcinomas; Progesterone receptor assay; Tubular carcinomas

▶ Duodenal carcinomas

Category: Diseases, Symptoms, and Conditions
Also known as: Small intestine cancer

Related conditions: Crohn disease, celiac disease, colon polyps

Definition: Duodenal carcinoma is a cancer of the duodenum, the first (upper) part of the small intestine.

Risk factors: Risk factors include Crohn disease, celiac disease, familial adenomatous polyposis (FAP), exposure to radiation, smoking, alcohol consumption, and a diet high in fats or high in salted, pickled, or smoked foods.

Etiology and the disease process: Genetic disposition, environmental exposures, and lifestyle are all potential root causes of duodenal carcinoma. The duodenum is the first part of the small bowel that is exposed to ingested chemicals that may be carcinogenic and to pancreatic biliary juices that may also be carcinogens. There are five types of small intestine cancers (adenocarcinoma, sarcoma, carcinoid tumors, gastrointestinal stromal tumors, and lymphoma). The most common type of duoendal carcinoma is adenocarcinoma.

Incidence: Duodenal carcinoma is a relatively rare cancer that makes up less than 1 percent of gastrointestinal cancers.

Symptoms: The symptoms of duodenal carcinoma may include abdominal pain, weight loss, bloating, cramping, blood in stools, and less commonly anemia and jaundice.

Screening and diagnosis: There may be a considerable amount of time between the identification of nonspecific symptoms (such as abdominal pain and bloating) and the diagnosis of duodenal carcinoma. A physical exam, medical history, X rays of the abdomen, abdominal ultrasound, a barium contrast study, and an upper gastrointestinal series may be used in the diagnosis. Small intestine adenocarcinomas are staged beginning with adenocarcinoma in situ, Stage I (the cancer has invaded the connective tissue or muscular layer of the bowel), Stage II, Stage III (the cancer has spread to regional lymph nodes), and Stage IV (the cancer has spread to distant organs).

Treatment and therapy: Surgery is the usual treatment, but surgical removal of a duodenal tumor can be difficult because of the area in which it is located. Surgery to bypass the area of the tumor (connecting the stomach to an area of the intestine beyond the mass) is sometimes necessary. Chemotherapy and radiation therapy are sometimes used to try to shrink the cancer or if the cancer has spread.

Prognosis, prevention, and outcomes: Individuals with duodenal carcinoma should be monitored after treatment for signs and symptoms of recurrence and should have abdominal computed tomography (CT) scans every six months.

Vicki Miskovsky, B.S., R.D.

See also: Cholecystectomy; Gallbladder cancer; Gastric polyps; Gastrinomas; Gastrointestinal cancers; Gastrointestinal oncology; Multiple endocrine neoplasia type 1 (MEN 1); Pancreatitis; Percutaneous Transhepatic Cholangiography (PTHC); Small intestine cancer; Upper Gastrointestinal (GI) endoscopy; Upper Gastrointestinal (GI) series; Zollinger-Ellison syndrome

▶ Dysplastic nevus syndrome

Category: Diseases, Symptoms, and Conditions
Also known as: Atypical mole syndrome, dysplastic mole, Clark's nevus

Related conditions: Malignant melanoma, familial atypical mole and melanoma (FAMM) syndrome

Definition: Dysplastic nevus syndrome is a skin condition characterized by the presence of numerous atypical nevi, or moles.

Risk factors: White men and women with light-colored hair and freckled skin are believed to be at high risk for dysplastic nevi, especially with excessive sun exposure. Dysplastic nevi are strongly linked to melanoma: The presence of the former may signify an increased risk for developing the latter. Individuals with a family history of dysplastic nevi, with numerous dysplastic nevi on their bodies, and with at least two family members diagnosed with melanoma, are almost certain to develop melanoma. This is called familial atypical mole and melanoma (FAMM) syndrome.

Etiology and the disease process: Dysplastic nevi are abnormally growing moles. Whether ultraviolet exposure plays a significant role in their development is still a subject for debate. Dysplastic nevi are, however, associated with frequent and severe sunburns, a family history of dysplastic nevi, and weakened immunity (for example, due to cancer chemotherapy).

Incidence: In the United States, dysplastic nevi are present in 2 to 5 percent of the white population. In other countries, such as Australia, New Zealand, Germany, and Sweden, dysplastic nevi are clinically diagnosed in as much as 18 percent of the adult white population. This condition rarely occurs in individuals of Middle Eastern, black, or Asian descent. No gender predilection exists; the condition may start manifesting as early as childhood.

Symptoms: Unlike common moles, atypical nevi are asymmetrical; have uneven shades of tan, brown, red, or pink; have irregular borders; and are greater than 5 millimeters in diameter. Atypical moles are frequently found on the back, chest, abdomen, scalp, arms, or legs, but they can sometimes arise on unexposed areas such as the breasts or buttocks.

Screening and diagnosis: A thorough examination of the patient's skin surface and a detailed family history are important in screening for dysplastic nevi. An excisional biopsy and histological analysis of the tissue sample will differentiate between dysplastic nevi and malignant melanoma.

Treatment and therapy: There is no definitive treatment for dysplastic nevi. Surgical removal of dysplastic moles does not guarantee against the development of melanoma.

Prognosis, prevention, and outcomes: Individuals with dysplastic nevi syndrome should avoid prolonged sun exposure without sunscreen protection. Regular skin examinations will help monitor for any suspicious changes in dysplastic nevi.

Ophelia Panganiban, B.S.

See also: Carney complex; Choriocarcinomas; Craniosynostosis; Gestational Trophoblastic Tumors (GTTs); Hereditary cancer syndromes; Human Chorionic Gonadotropin (HCG); Hydatidiform mole; Melanomas; Moles; Sjögren syndrome; Skin cancers

▶ Edema

Category: Diseases, Symptoms, and Conditions
Also known as: Lymphedema, fluid retention

Related conditions: Cancers of the breast, colon, ovary, uterus, and testicles

Definition: Edema, known as fluid retention, results from the accumulation of fluid in certain tissues, leading to swelling. In lymphedema, lymph (a fluid containing a high amount of lymphocytes, or white blood cells) accumulates in tissues because the excess fluid and proteins cannot be returned into the circulation. Edema can result in decreased mobility of the affected limb, as well as pain, risk of infection, and poorer quality of life.

Risk factors: The main risk factor for edema is surgery for breast and other cancers in which removal of the primary tumor may lead to removal of nearby lymph nodes.

Etiology and the disease process: Cancer-related edema either is caused directly by the cancer or is a result of treatment. In some cases, cancer cells may build up in the neighboring lymph nodes, blocking the flow of the lymphatic fluid. Cancer patients may also have poor nutritional intake, in part because of loss of appetite and metabolic disorders, and their bodies may not have sufficient amounts of protein to function normally. If the kidneys are impaired, they will not be able to properly rid the body of salt through the urine. This leads to an increased amount of salt in the body, causing water to be retained and leading to edema.

Edema can also be the result of the drugs that cancer patients receive. Chemotherapy drugs associated with an increased risk of edema include cyclosporine, docetaxel, gemcitabine, imatinib, and thalidomide. Additional anticancer agents known to cause edema include corticosteroids, anabolic steroids, progestins, and nonsteroidal anti-inflammatory agents. In addition, some treatments may directly affect the lymphatic system. For example, in breast cancer patients, the neighboring axillary lymph nodes may be affected either by targeted radiation therapy or surgical removal (known as node dissection). Disrupting the lymphatic system is a cause of lymphedema.

Incidence: Edema in the arm is a common side effect in breast cancer patients, especially if they have received radiation therapy or had a lymph node removed. The reported incidence depends on the type of breast cancer therapy administered and the time since treatment. Based on an analysis of multiple studies in which women received a variety of surgical procedures and adjuvant therapies, it is estimated that approximately 1 in 4 women may develop arm edema after treatment for breast cancer. Moreover, the frequency of lymphedema rises over time since treatment.

Symptoms: The symptom of edema is swelling of the limbs.

Screening and diagnosis: Edema may be diagnosed by measuring limbs; a difference of more than 2 centimeters between the circumference of the normal and affected limbs would indicate edema. Bioelectrical impedance (to quantify the fluid accumulation) and lymphoscintigraphy (to visualize the lymphatic system) may also be used.

Treatment and therapy: Treatment for edema can be broken down into three categories: diet, supportive therapy, and pharmacological therapy.

Reducing the amount of dietary salt consumed may help to manage edema. Patients should avoid foods that are high in salt or sodium, including canned soups, canned or processed meats, prepared mixes and foods (including frozen dinners and fast foods), snack foods (pretzels, potato chips, olives, cheeses, pickles), and high-salt seasonings (bouillon cubes, seasoned salts, soy sauce, Worcestershire sauce, and premixed spice packets).

Supportive therapies are also important in treating edema. Elevating affected limbs above the heart may help reduce swelling. Other strategies include wearing elastic compression stockings or sleeves, which help to return the excess fluid into the circulation. Massage, compression pumps, and specialized physical therapy and exercise regimens may also be effective. Less frequently used methods include electrically stimulated lymphatic drainage (such as uniform or sequential compression with either pneumatic or hydrostatic pressure devices) and surgery (such as surgical excision of the affected area, insertion of a lymphatic-venous shunt, or liposuction).

Diuretics are a commonly prescribed medication to reduce edema, since they inhibit the ability of the kidneys to reabsorb and retain salt, leading to the elimination of more salt and water in the urine. Loop diuretics, named because they target the loop of Henle within the kidney tubules, include furosemide (Lasix), torsemide (Demedex), and butethamide (Bumex). Thiazide diuretics may also be used, but they may cause potassium to be excreted in the urine. Potassium-sparing diuretics include spironolactone (Aldactone), triamterene (Dyrenium), and amiloride (Midamor).

Elizabeth A. Manning, Ph.D.

For Further Information

Bourgeois, P., O. Leduc, and A. Leduc. "Imaging Techniques in the Management and Prevention of Posttherapeutic Upper Limb Edemas." *Cancer* 83 (December 15, 1998): 2805-2813.

Cohen, S. R., D. K. Payne, and R. S. Tunkel. "Lymphedema: Strategies for Management." *Cancer* 92 (August 15, 2001): 980-987.

Erickson, V. S., et al. "Arm Edema in Breast Cancer Patients." *Journal of the National Cancer Institute* 93, no. 2 (January 17, 2001): 96-111.

Mortimer, P. S. "The Pathophysiology of Lymphedema." *Cancer* 83 (1998): 2798-2802.

Petrek, J. A., P. I. Pressman, and R. A. Smith. "Lymphedema: Current Issues in Research and Management." *CA: A Cancer Journal for Clinicians* 50, no. 5 (September/October, 2000): 292-307.

Other Resources

Huntsman Cancer Institute
Edema
http://www.hci.utah.edu/patientdocs/hci/drug_side_effects/edema.html

MedicineNet.com
Edema
http://www.medicinenet.com/edema/article.htm

National Cancer Institute
Lymphedema
http://www.cancer.gov/cancertopics/pdq/supportivecare/lymphedema/healthprofessional

See also: Beckwith-Wiedemann Syndrome (BWS); Lymphangiosarcomas; Lymphedema; Magnetic Resonance Imaging (MRI); Mastectomy; Nephroblastomas; Rhabdomyosarcomas

▶ Embryonal cell cancer

Category: Diseases, Symptoms, and Conditions
Also known as: Embryonal cancer

Related conditions: Testicular cancer, germ-cell tumor

Definition: Embryonal cell cancer is a malignant germ-cell tumor that occurs most often in the testes and accounts for about 40 percent of testicular tumors. Under the microscope, these tumors may resemble tissues of early embryos. This type of tumor can grow rapidly and spread outside the testicle.

Risk factors: Birth defects such as male infants with undescended testis (chryptorchidism) can lead to embryonal cancer.

Etiology and the disease process: Embryonic cells grow in the embryo, and some develop into germ cells that make up the reproductive system in men and women. These embryonic germ cells follow a midline path through the body after development and descend into the pelvis as ovarian cells or into the scrotal sac as testicular cells.

Embryonal cell cancer results when the reproductive germ cell develops abnormally into cancerous cells. Differing from the other types of testicular cancers, embryonal carcinoma can have several of the properties of an abnormally developed fetus.

Incidence: Embryonal cell cancer is very rare, accounting for approximately 40 percent of all testicular tumors, which occur in less than 1 percent of the male population. Embryonal carcinomas are usually seen in men age twenty-five to thirty-five but have also affected youths in their late teens. The chances of an embryonal carcinoma spreading from one testicle to the other are less than 1 percent. Embryonal carcinoma in the ovaries of females is extremely rare and usually occurs before the age of thirty.

Symptoms: Patients with embryonal cell cancer usually have a tumor, swelling, or mass that can be felt or seen, or an abnormal shape, or irregularity in, testicular size.

Screening and diagnosis: Diagnostic procedures for embryonal cell cancer may include biopsy of the tumor; blood tests, including testing for tumor markers and a complete blood count (CBC) to determine the size, number, and maturity of different blood cells within the blood; and multiple imaging studies such as computed tomography (CT), magnetic resonance imaging (MRI), ultrasound, and X ray.

Treatment and therapy: Specific treatment for germ-cell tumors is determined by the patient's age, overall health, medical history, and the extent of the disease. Surgery is generally performed to remove the malignant cells, and patients may undergo chemotherapy or radiation to reduce the risk of recurrence of cancerous cells.

Prognosis, prevention, and outcomes: With all testicular cancers, strategies employing surgery, chemotherapy, or radiation therapy (either alone or in combination) have created cure rates approaching 100 percent for low-stage or early disease and more than 85 percent for more advanced tumors. Early detection by performing monthly testicular self-exams can greatly improve the chances of curing the cancer.

Robert J. Amato, D.O.

See also: Beckwith-Wiedemann Syndrome (BWS); Cryptorchidism; Germ-cell tumors; Kidney cancer; Rhabdomyosarcomas; Teratocarcinomas; Testicular cancer; Testicular self-examination; Yolk sac carcinomas

▶ Endocrine cancers

Category: Diseases, Symptoms, and Conditions

Related conditions: Prolactinoma, acromegaly, gigantism, pituitary adenoma, thyroid cancer (papillary, medullary, follicular, C-cell, anaplastic), parathyroid adenoma, parathyroid carcinoma, pheochromocytoma, insulinoma, glucagonoma, somatostatinoma, multiple endocrine neoplasia (MEN) type 1 (Wermer syndrome), MEN type 2A (Sipple syndrome), MEN type 2B, carcinoid tumor, islet cell tumor, Cushing disease

Definition: Endocrine cancers are a group of benign and malignant growths that originate from the tissues of the endocrine glands. The endocrine glands are responsible for regulating a number of bodily functions, including cellular metabolism, growth, development of male and female primary and secondary sex characteristics, the menstrual cycle, water and sodium balance, calcium distribution, and blood pressure. A number of functions also relate to reactions to stressors, which include the fight-or-flight response and immune system modulation.

The endocrine system is related functionally to the nervous system in that it maintains the long-term equilibrium of vital organ systems. Complex feedback loops at the pituitary (secondary) or hypothalamic (tertiary) level as well as physiologic demands normally regulate hormone secretion. The hypothalamus-anterior pituitary axis regulates several glands, including the adrenal cortex, thyroid gland, and reproductive system. The hypothalamus-posterior pituitary axis directly regulates physiologic functions such as breast milk ejection and uterine contraction, and stimulates water retention in the kidneys. The autonomic axis regulates body functions in response to stress and injury and includes the adrenal medulla, the juxtoglomerular apparatus in the kidney, and the alpha and beta islet cells in the pancreas. The parathyroid gland does not belong to any axis. Endocrine cancers can alter this equilibrium, leading to potentially life-threatening conditions in extremis.

Risk factors: The risk factors for developing an endocrine cancer depend on the cellular origin of the cancer and the stimulus that promotes cancer cell proliferation, and they can generally be classified as environmental or hereditary. Environmental risk factors may include exposure to radiation as in the case of thyroid cancers. Although spontaneous cases do arise, such as in cases of parathyroid adenomas and insulinomas, other endocrine cancers arise as part of a distinct clinical syndrome with multiple endocrine gland involvement.

The most prominent risk factor for the development of hereditary endocrine tumors is a genetic predisposition. The MEN syndromes are autosomal dominant, with a 50 percent probability of offspring inheriting the disease.

Etiology and the disease process: The transformation of a normal endocrine cell into a cancerous cell is often caused by a single or a number of additive unrepaired gene alterations that prevent uncontrolled cellular division and programmed cell death. These cancer cell transformations do not differ much from the transformation of cells in other organs and have common etiologic agents such as the tumor-suppressor gene *TP53*. However, specific tumor-suppressor gene mutations are responsible for the genesis of certain endocrine cancers. MEN 1 originates from either a mutation within the embryonic crest cell or inactivation of the tumor-suppressor gene *MEN1*, located on the long arm of chromosome 11 (11q13). MEN 2A, 2B, and familial medullary thyroid carcinoma originate from a mutation in the *RET* proto-oncogene, located on the long arm of chromosome 10 (10q11.2). *MEN1* tumor-suppressor gene mutations, along with changes in the *RET* proto-oncogene, have also been implicated in sporadic medullary thyroid carcinoma cases. Papillary thyroid cancer genesis has been attributed to mutations in the *PTC* and *TRK-A* genes, in conjunction with the *RET* proto-oncogene and *RAS* oncogene, respectively.

Endocrine cancers may be functional or nonfunctional. Functional endocrine cancers are so named because the hormone secretions from the cancer cells have the same effect on the same target organs as do hormones from normal endocrine cells. These cancer cell hormones may be structurally identical or slightly altered. Functional endocrine cancers do not respond in a normal fashion to the inhibitory feedback mechanisms in normal endocrine cells. Although some cancers lack receptors that decrease or halt hormone secretion, other cancers may be stimulated by their own secretions in a way that resembles the inhibitory mechanisms of some endocrine glands. Nonfunctional endocrine cancers do not secrete hormones or hormone-like molecules. They may be derived from hormone-secreting cells but are more often derived from stromal tissue (tissue surrounding supporting tissue). They may nonetheless interfere with normal gland function by compressing or infiltrating surrounding tissue.

Incidence: According to the American Cancer Society, about 25,520 new cases of endocrine cancer were reported in 2004, or less than 1 in 10,000 people. By affected organ, thyroid cancers are the most common of all endocrine cancers, followed by pituitary gland cancers. Specific data regarding the rarer cancers are sparse. Some endocrine cancers such as thyroid cancer tend to appear in individuals older than fifty years.

Symptoms: Symptoms of endocrine cancer are generally related to both the indirect effects of malignancy—such as fever, malaise, anorexia, weight loss, or paraneoplastic syndrome—and the direct and gland-specific effects of the tumor. The specific symptoms of endocrine cancers are classically related to the endocrine gland axis from which they originate, wherein serum measurements of the hormones causing symptoms directly or indirectly follows. For example, a tumor in the thyroid gland causing symptoms of increased cellular metabolism (sweating, irritability, palpitations, irregular heartbeats, heat intolerance) may be confirmed by measurements of both thyroid-stimulating hormone (TSH) and thyroid hormone. Alternately, a TSH tumor would be suspected in a patient who exhibits hyperthyroid symptoms but has a normal thyroid gland, being mindful of the loss of the inhibitory feedback mechanism in these tumors. Other endocrine cancers may require a combination of laboratory tests relating to their functional status in addition to

Stage at Diagnosis and Five-Year Relative Survival Rates for Thyroid Cancer, 1996-2004

Stage	*Cases Diagnosed (%)*	*Survival Rate (%)*
Localized[a]	59	99.7
Regional[b]	34	96.9
Distant[c]	5	56.0
Unstaged	3	89.3

Source: Data from National Cancer Institute, Surveillance Epidemiology and End Results, Cancer Stat Fact Sheets, 2008

[a]Cancer still confined to primary site

[b]Cancer has spread to regional lymph nodes or directly beyond the primary site

[c]Cancer has metastasized

hormone levels. For example, a simple parathyroid gland tumor secreting parathyroid hormone-like substances may manifest in a patient with recurrent kidney stones and heart rhythm disturbances from a high serum calcium with a correspondingly low phosphorus level because of bone demineralization.

Symptom overlap is more often present because of the different possible locations of a tumor along the hypothalamic-pituitary-target organ axis, requiring an exhaustive diagnostic workup. For instance, an anterior pituitary tumor such as a prolactinoma may have the symptoms of milk production and cessation of menses in a nonpregnant woman. Similarly, a gonadotropic hormone-secreting tumor or gonadotropin-releasing hormone (GnRH) tumor in the hypothalamus may also halt the menstrual cycle.

Endocrine cancers can also manifest by compressing or infiltrating adjacent tissue and structures, altering their function. An example is anterior pituitary tumors, which may initially manifest as a partial blindness termed bilateral hemianopsia (involving the right and left visual fields of the right and left eyes, respectively) in which right and left optic nerve fibers are compressed as they cross below the anterior pituitary. The specific pituitary cells may be nonfunctional or secrete excess hormones that can affect the axis accordingly. Posterior pituitary tumors may also manifest in this fashion. Other cancers may remain undetected or grow to large sizes (as with ovarian cancers).

The hereditary multiple endocrine neoplasia (MEN) syndromes consist of two main variants, MEN 1 and MEN 2. MEN 1 has pituitary, parathyroid, and pancreas involvement. MEN 2A manifests as medullary thyroid cancer (MTC), pheochromocytoma, an adrenal medulla tumor, and parathyroid hyperplasia (overproliferation). MEN 2B is essentially type 2A without parathyroid involvement and with the addition of mucosal neuromas and gut ganglioneuromas (nerve cell tumors) with a Marfanoid body habitus (long limbs and fingers, flexible joints, lens dislodgement, and mitral valve prolapse). Isolated MTC may also be familial and is less aggressive compared with MEN-associated MTC.

Screening and diagnosis: As clinical symptoms and signs of endocrine cancers can vary widely from textbook-style presentations, diagnosis is generally oriented toward confirming clinical suspicions through routine laboratory tests and tests measuring hormone levels. Although interpretation of some tests—such as thyroid function tests and a twenty-four-hour urine collection for catecholamine metabolites of epinephrine and norepinephrine (metanephrine, vanillylmandelic acid, or VMA) for a suspected pheochromocytoma—may be straightforward, other tests approach diagnosis by process of elimination. Tests that require such multiple steps include the dexamethasone suppression test and the progesterone challenge test. The dexamethasone suppression test involves a screening of a twenty-four-hour urine collection for cortisol as well as evaluation of the anterior pituitary (Cushing syndrome) and adrenal cortex hormone levels in response to low and high doses of dexamethasone. The progesterone challenge is similar in that it assesses the onset of bleeding with administration of suppressing doses of estrogen and progesterone to assess the presence of an androgen-secreting tumor, among other, nontumor-related diseases. These tests may also be used to assess baseline glandular functioning. Tumor markers such as cancer antigen 125 (CA 125) for ovarian cancer are rarely used alone to confirm diagnoses, although they can be used to monitor for disease recurrence.

Visualization of a suspected cancer is carried out as much as possible. Imaging studies provide information for determining whether surgery is possible. If surgery is a plausible option, imaging studies provide surgeons with a means by which to plan their approach. Conventional imaging studies include computed tomography (CT) and magnetic resonance imaging (MRI). Organ-specific studies such as thyroid scans or

OctreoScans for islet cell tumors rely on tumor uptake of radiolabeled substances to disclose their location. Thyroid scans also help determine the presence of hormone activity, which is absent in most thyroid cancers. Occasionally, local or distal spread of tumors may occur, in which case more comprehensive imaging studies of probable areas of spread, such as the chest, abdomen, pelvis, or head, are conducted.

A biopsy of tumors with high-yield procedures such as fine needle aspiration of thyroid nodules or masses can greatly aid in planning future treatment. Occasionally, this may be done during an operation through frozen section, in which a tumor specimen is frozen and thinly sliced for microscopic evaluation by a pathologist.

Formal, regular screening is not usually done because of the rareness of these cancers but may be conducted when patients have a family history of multiple endocrine gland involvement. Although tumors that are hereditary have a clear genetic etiology, routine genetic testing such as that for *RET* is reserved for patients with medullary thyroid cancer.

Treatment and therapy: Treatment of endocrine cancers generally consists of surgical removal of the lesions alongside chemotherapy or radiotherapy. Medical therapies are often limited but nonetheless essential in reducing complications. These include ensuring the control of other diseases and correcting blood pressure and fluid and electrolyte derangements, particularly in patients in whom the thyroid, parathyroid, pancreatic islet cells, and adrenal glands are involved. The surgical approach for endocrine cancers usually conforms to the relevant local anatomy while achieving optimal visualization even if the surgical field may be quite limited. For instance, a transsphenoidal approach to the pituitary gland involves making a surgical "window" through the posterior aspect of the mouth, as opposed to thyroid surgery at the base of the neck. Spread to neighboring structures may entail lymph node sampling conforming to the lymph drainage within the area of the tumors in addition to removal of secondary sites of spread wherever possible. Chemotherapy and radiotherapy are instituted for most endocrine cancers to eliminate remaining tumor cells not removed by surgery and thus decrease the chance for recurrence.

Prognosis, prevention, and outcomes: The 2004 ratio of deaths to incidence in the United States from endocrine cancers irrespective of cause was estimated at 9.6 percent. Total deaths from endocrine cancers from the same year were estimated at 2,440. Most endocrine cancers have high five-year survival rates approaching 95 percent or more. Thyroid cancers in particular have high five-year survival rates, around 96 percent if detected early. As with all other cancers, this may drop to 5 percent in advanced disease involving more malignant variants (medullary, follicular, anaplastic). Cancers that are detected late, such as ovarian or adrenal cancers, have correspondingly lower survival rates of 50 percent and 40 percent, respectively.

Complications from surgery include bleeding, marked reduction or total loss of endocrine gland function, or interruption of hypothalamic-pituitary axis equilibrium. Hormone replacement therapy may eventually be lifelong, particularly in thyroid and pituitary gland cancers. Preventive measures include proper radiation shielding of neck and genital areas.

Aldo C. Dumlao, M.D.

For Further Information

Braverman, Lewis E. *Diseases of the Thyroid.* 2d ed. Totowa, N.J.: Humana Press, 2003.

Clark, Orlo H. *Endocrine Tumors.* Hamilton, Ont.: BC Decker, 2003.

Kelloff, Gary, Ernest T. Hawk, and Caroline C. Sigman. *Cancer Chemoprevention.* Totowa, N.J.: Humana Press, 2005.

Other Resources

American Cancer Society
http://www.cancer.org

Cancer Index
Endocrine Malignancies
http://www.cancerindex.org/clinks2e.htm

Stanford Cancer Center
Endocrine Cancers
http://cancer.stanford.edu/endocrine/

See also: Adrenal gland cancers; Adrenocortical cancer; Endocrinology oncology; Endometrial cancer; Fertility drugs and cancer; Gynecologic cancers; Gynecologic oncology; Hormonal therapies; Human growth factors and tumor growth; Multiple endocrine neoplasia type 1 (MEN 1); Multiple endocrine neoplasia type 2 (MEN 2); Neuroendocrine tumors; Pancreatic cancers; Parathyroid cancer; Pituitary tumors; Thyroid cancer

▶ Endometrial cancer

Category: Diseases, Symptoms, and Conditions
Also known as: Uterine corpus cancer, uterine cancer

Related conditions: Obesity, hypertension, polycystic ovary syndrome, endometrial hyperplasia

Definition: Endometrial cancer is cancer of the endometrial cells that line the uterus, which is the female organ in which the fetus develops. Estrogen, a female hormone, is a primary growth signal for the endometrium (lining of the uterus). When endometrial cells are exposed to increased levels of estrogen for long periods of time and when they acquire certain genetic mutations, they can become cancerous.

Risk factors: Certain demographic characteristics—being over the age of fifty, being white, and never having been pregnant—can contribute to the risk of endometrial cancer. Long-term exposure to estrogen may also affect the incidence of endometrial cancer. Estrogen exposure can be in the form of hormone replacement therapy (commonly used to control menopause-related symptoms) or tamoxifen (an estrogen-like drug used to prevent or treat breast cancer). Increased exposure to estrogen can also occur in women who began menstruation early (before the age of twelve) or reached menopause late (after the age of fifty). Because estrogen can be produced in fatty tissue, being overweight can increase the risk of endometrial cancer. Furthermore, obesity-related conditions, such as type 2 diabetes and high blood pressure, may increase the risk. Finally, many diseases may also be associated with an elevated risk of endometrial cancer, including endometrial hyperplasia (a noncancerous condition characterized by overgrowth of the endometrium), a history of breast or ovarian cancer, and hereditary nonpolyposis colorectal cancer (a disease caused by mutations in deoxyribonucleic acid, or DNA, repair genes).

Etiology and the disease process: Within the female reproductive system, the ovaries are responsible for producing the hormones estrogen and progesterone. The levels of these hormones fluctuate each month, allowing the endometrium to thicken (because of endometrial cell growth) at the beginning of the monthly menstruation cycle in preparation for an egg to be fertilized and implanted within the uterus. At the end of the monthly cycle, the endometrium is shed if pregnancy does not occur. Because estrogen is responsible for stimulating the growth of endometrial cells, too much estrogen may lead to too much cell growth.

Age at Death for Uterine Cancer, 2001-2005

Age Group	*Percentage Diagnosed*
Under 20	0.0
20-34	0.4
35-44	2.2
45-54	8.1
55-64	18.4
65-74	26.4
75-84	28.7
85 and older	15.9

Source: Data from National Cancer Institute, Surveillance Epidemiology and End Results, Cancer Stat Fact Sheets, 2008

Note: The median age of death from 2001 to 2005 was seventy-three, with an age-adjusted death rate of 4.1 per 100,000 women per year.

Genetic changes may also contribute to the transformation of normal cells into cancerous cells. Endometrial cancer can be divided into type 1 and type 2 carcinomas based on their relationship with estrogen and how the cells look under a microscope. Type 1 carcinoma, which accounts for 70 to 80 percent of all endometrial cancer cases, is estrogen dependent and associated with the inactivation of *PTEN* (a tumor-suppressor gene) and mutations in DNA repair genes, *KRAS* (a gene that encodes a proto-oncogene), and beta-catenin (a protein). In the less prevalent (but more aggressive) type 2 carcinoma, which follows an estrogen-independent pathway, major genetic changes within endometrial cells include mutations in *TP53* (another tumor-suppressor gene) and overexpression of human epidermal growth factor receptor 2/neu (HER2/neu). When cells have tumor-suppressor genes and DNA repair genes that are not functional, they lose the ability to regulate growth and cell division, as well as the ability to fix additional mutations that may arise. Expressing excess growth factor receptors also means that cells may grow and divide more quickly and may not respond when cellular signals try to stop proliferation.

Incidence: In women, endometrial cancer is the fourth most common cancer (after breast, lung, and colon cancers). Some 95 percent of uterine cancers are endometrial; the other 5 percent are due to cancerous muscle or myometrial cells within the uterus. The American Cancer Society estimated that in 2007 more than 39,000 new cases would arise and about 7,400 people would die from endometrial cancer in the United States.

Symptoms: The most common symptoms in endometrial cancer are pelvic pain and vaginal bleeding between menstrual periods or after menopause.

Screening and diagnosis: Screening tests such as a pelvic exam, a Pap smear (to check for cervical cancer), and a transvaginal ultrasound (to determine if the endometrium is too thick) may be performed. Blood tests can look for lower red blood cell counts (possibly indicating loss of blood from the uterus) and for raised levels of cancer antigen 125 (CA 125, a protein that is associated with tumors of the endometrium and ovaries).

To make a diagnosis, a tissue sample from the uterine lining should be removed and analyzed under the microscope. Tissue samples can be obtained either by a biopsy or by dilation and curettage (D&C). A D&C is a more invasive procedure for obtaining endometrial tissue and may be done if the biopsy did not obtain a large enough sample or if the biopsy was positive for cancer and a confirmation is needed.

Endometrial cancer is staged using the International Federation of Gynecology and Obstetrics (FIGO) cancer staging system, as follows:

- Stage I: The tumor is only in the uterus.
- Stage II: The cancer has spread from the body of the uterus to the cervix.
- Stage III: The cancer has spread outside the uterus but not outside the pelvis (and not to the bladder or rectum). Lymph nodes in the pelvis may contain cancer cells.
- Stage IV: The cancer has spread into the bladder or rectum, or it has spread beyond the pelvis to other parts of the body.

Treatment and therapy: Women with endometrial cancer may undergo surgical removal of the uterus, in a procedure known as a hysterectomy. Often, the uterus is removed along with the Fallopian tubes and ovaries as well as neighboring lymph nodes to ensure that all of the cancerous cells have been removed. Although this is the standard treatment for women already in menopause and no longer fertile, women of childbearing age need to consider the outcome of this surgery as they will lose the ability to have a child. For Stage I endometrial cancer, surgery to remove the uterus has been shown to be 90 percent effective.

Radiation therapy, where high-dose X rays are used to kill cancer cells, may be used after surgery to prevent the formation of or treat existing cancer cells outside the uterus. Radiation may also be used in place of surgery if women refuse a hysterectomy or if a tumor is growing rapidly, associated closely with muscle cells in the uterus, or is highly vascularized (with lots of blood vessels infiltrating the tumor). Radiation therapy can be delivered either conventionally (the standard external X ray) or as brachytherapy (internal radiation to target only the inner lining of the uterus). Although brachytherapy has fewer side effects than conventional radiation therapy, its effects are only local, so it cannot be used if the cancer has spread outside the uterus.

Hormone therapy is often used when cancer has spread outside the uterus. Synthetic progestin, which is a form of progesterone, is used to inhibit the growth of cancerous endometrial cells. Although this therapy may be associated with higher risks of recurrence than surgical removal of the uterus, this option is attractive to women who still want to have children or who were diagnosed in a very early stage. Chemotherapy may also be used to kill cancer cells that have spread beyond the uterus.

Prognosis, prevention, and outcomes: To prevent endometrial cancer (both initial and recurrent cases), taking hormones with progesterone may help slow or inhibit the growth of endometrial cells. Women may undergo hormone therapy with progestin or take birth control pills. Women who take birth control pills have a reduced risk of endometrial cancer for up to ten years after discontinuing oral contraceptives. As with other cancers, living a healthy lifestyle is important in reducing the risk of cancer. This includes maintaining a healthy weight (as obesity is a risk factor for developing endometrial cancer) and exercising regularly.

For endometrial cancer, the five-year survival rates for women receiving the proper treatment are approximately 75 to 95 percent for women diagnosed at Stage I, 50 percent for Stage II, 30 percent for Stage III, and less than 5 percent for Stage IV.

In a study analyzing recurrence rates across sixteen studies, the overall risk of recurrence was 13 percent, and this was even less in low-risk patients who were diagnosed with Stage I or II cancers or who did not have associated diseases known to increase the risk of endometrial cancer. This study also showed that about 70 percent of recurrences were accompanied by symptoms, and 68 to 100 percent of these recurrences occurred within about a three-year span after the follow-up visit.

Elizabeth A. Manning, Ph.D.

For Further Information

Canavan, T. P., and N. R. Doshi. "Endometrial Cancer." *American Family Physician* 59, no. 11 (June, 1999): 3069-3077.

Fung-Kee-Fung, M., et al. "Follow-Up After Primary Therapy for Endometrial Cancer: A Systematic Review." *Gynecologic Oncology* 101, no. 3 (June, 2006): 520-529.

Liu, F. S. "Molecular Carcinogenesis of Endometrial Cancer." *Taiwanese Journal of Obstetrics and Gynecology* 46, no. 1 (March, 2007): 26-32.

Robertson G. "Screening for Endometrial Cancer." *Medical Journal of Australia* 178, no. 12 (June 16, 2003): 657-659.

Sherman, M. E. "Theories of Endometrial Carcinogenesis: A Multidisciplinary Approach." *Modern Pathology* 13, no. 3 (March, 2000): 295-308.

Other Resources

MayoClinic.com
Endometrial Cancer
http://www.mayoclinic.com/health/endometrial-cancer/DS00306/DSECTION=1

National Cancer Institute
Endometrial Cancer
http://www.cancer.gov/cancertopics/types/endometrial

See also: Antiestrogens; 1,4-Butanediol dimethanesulfonate; CA 125 test; Chemoprevention; Colposcopy; Computed Tomography (CT) scan; Conization; Dilation and Curettage (D&C); Endometrial hyperplasia; Endoscopy; Family history and risk assessment; Geography and cancer; Ginseng, panax; Gynecologic cancers; Herbs as antioxidants; Hormonal therapies; Hormone Replacement therapy (HRT); Hysterectomy; Hysterography; Hystero-oophorectomy; Hysteroscopy; Isoflavones; Leiomyomas; Leiomyosarcomas; Mitochondrial DNA mutations; *MLH1* gene; *MSH* genes; Nutrition and cancer prevention; Obesity-associated cancers; Pap test; Transvaginal ultrasound; Uterine cancer

▶ Endometrial hyperplasia

Category: Diseases, Symptoms, and Conditions
Also known as: EH, endometrial neoplasia, endometrial intraepithelial neoplasia

Related conditions: Endometrial cancer

Definition: Endometrial hyperplasia is the abnormal proliferation of the cells that comprise the inner cell lining of the uterus (endometrium). The endometrium is the tissue layer in which a fertilized ovum implants itself and divides. It consists of glands and surrounding supportive tissue (stroma) and is rich in blood, from which the developing embryo derives oxygen and nutrients through the placenta.

Risk factors: Risk factors for endometrial hyperplasia are related to lifetime exposure to excess estrogen and include estrogen therapy without progesterone, tamoxifen therapy, late menopause, no history of childbirth, infertility or failure to ovulate, obesity, and obesity-related diseases (diabetes, hypertension). A known hereditary nonpolyposis colon cancer (HNPCC) genetic mutation carrier or a woman with a strong family history of colon cancer is at high risk not only for hyperplasia but for cancer as well.

Etiology and the disease process: Endometrial hyperplasia is primarily caused by estrogen stimulation of the endometrial glands. These glands then proceed to multiply and enlarge. Abnormal endometrial hyperplasia may eventually arise from normal cyclic estrogen stimulation. However, there may be sources of excess estrogen independent of the menstrual cycle involved in abnormal endometrial proliferation, such as granulosa cell tumors, polycystic ovary syndrome (PCOS), tamoxifen therapy, or use of estrogen-containing birth control pills. Estrogen stimulation alone results in an unstable endometrial bed, which is prone to breakdown and bleeding. Over time, excessive endometrial stimulation and rapid cell division increase the chance of cell mutations that ultimately predispose the woman to cancer.

Incidence: In women with documented abnormal uterine bleeding, 20 percent was caused by endometrial hyperplasia. The incidence may be as high as 25 percent in postmenopausal women on estrogen hormone replacement therapy (HRT); 36 to 49 percent in nonmenstruating, nonovulating women whose condition is the result of PCOS or other undetermined cause; and close to 50 percent in hypertensives and diabetics, although concomitant obesity as a source of excess estrogen formation may account for this according to other studies.

Symptoms: Abnormal uterine bleeding is the main symptom associated with endometrial hyperplasia. The bleeding, compared with the woman's normal menstrual cycle, may be characterized as excessive in amount, duration, frequency, or a combination of these. Painless spotting or bleeding from the vagina in a postmenopausal woman is the most common symptom reported in endometrial cancer. In premenopausal women, heavy menstrual bleeding can be confused with physiologic hyperplasia that occurs during the menstrual cycle. Bleeding between periods may also raise the suspicion of endometrial hyperplasia, although extrauterine masses producing excess estrogen or intrauterine masses such as polyps or fibroids bleeding into the uterine cavity must also be considered. Symptoms accompanying long-standing significant blood loss include fatigue due to anemia. On examination of the pelvis, an enlarged uterus in a nonpregnant or postmenopausal woman may also suggest hyperplasia. This may or may not be accompanied by abnormal findings in the ovaries, Fallopian tubes, and supporting ligaments.

Screening and diagnosis: The American Cancer Society currently has no screening recommendations for endometrial hyperplasia. Further testing is carried out in patients who exhibit a high clinical suspicion for endometrial cancer, particularly postmenopausal women over forty years of age. These tests include an endometrial biopsy and an optional pelvic ultrasound when a mass is detected on physical examination. An adequate endometrial biopsy is the standard by which the endometrium is evaluated for cellular characteristics suggestive of precancer.

Diagnosis of endometrial hyperplasia and type are dependent on microscopic examination of the biopsy sample. The biopsy sample, containing glands and tissue surrounding these glands (stroma), is examined and classified according to the proportion of glands to stroma, morphology of the glands, and cellular characteristics suggestive of precancer (cellular atypia).

Simple, enlarged glands seen within a larger proportion of stroma pose about a 1 percent risk of progression to endometrial cancer. More complex glands possessing more cellular outpouchings than the previous type and a paucity of stroma pose a 3 to 5 percent risk. Simple and complex type glands with atypical cell characteristics (dark-staining cells with large nuclei and little cytoplasm) pose an 8 to 10 percent and 25 to 30 percent risk, respectively.

Treatment and therapy: The type of treatment depends on the classification of the hyperplasia irrespective of atypia and, in premenopausal women, the desire to bear children after treatment. Cyclic progestin therapy is used for premenopausal women with no atypical cell findings on biopsy or for those with atypical findings who still wish to bear children. Treatment takes place over three to six months using progesterone contraceptives that can be taken by mouth, such as megestrol acetate and medroxyprogesterone acetate. Intramuscular medroxyprogesterone acetate and levonorgestrel via an intrauterine device (IUD) may also be used for three months and five years, respectively. Follow-up with endometrial biopsies is done every six months to check for recurrence. Discontinuation of progestin depends on the absence of symptoms and a normal biopsy.

A total hysterectomy is the recommended course of action in premenopausal women who no longer desire to bear children or are no longer of childbearing age, and in postmenopausal women with findings of atypia on endometrial biopsy.

Prognosis, prevention, and outcomes: A substantial number of patients diagnosed with endometrial hyperplasia with and without atypical cells found on biopsy spontaneously regress (50 percent and 80 percent, respectively). However, treatment as described above should be strongly considered.

Aldo C. Dumlao, M.D.

For Further Information

Boston Women's Health Book Collective. *Our Bodies, Ourselves: Menopause.* New York: Simon & Schuster, 2006.

Goodwin, Scott C., Michael S. Broder, and David Drum. *What Your Doctor May Not Tell You About Fibroids: New Techniques and Therapies—Including Breakthrough Alternatives to Hysterectomy.* New York: Warner Books, 2003.

Rosenthal, Sara M. *The Gynecological Sourcebook.* 4th ed. New York: McGraw-Hill, 2003.

Other Resources

American College of Obstetricians and Gynecolgists
Endometrial Hyperplasia
http://www.medem.com/MedLB/article_detaillb.cfm?article_ID=ZZZ7Z2GWQMC&sub_cat=9

National Cancer Institute
What You Need to Know About Cancer of the Uterus
http://www.nci.nih.gov/cancertopics/wyntk/uterus/page3

See also: Dilation and Curettage (D&C); Endometrial cancer; Granulosa cell tumors

▶ Endotheliomas

Category: Diseases, Symptoms, and Conditions
Also known as: Hemangioendotheliomas, hemangiosarcomas, angiosarcomas, hemangiomas, meningiomas

Related conditions: Soft-tissue sarcoma, benign tumors

Definition: Endothelioma is a general term used to describe malignant or benign neoplasms of endothelial tissue (the cells that line blood vessels or lymphatic channels). These tumors can arise in any part of the body and often are referred to by terms specific to their location. For example, meningioma or dural endothelioma is a type of benign brain tumor, hepatic angiosarcoma or hemangioendothelioma is a type of liver cancer, and hemangioma is a tumor that often develops on or just under the skin. All fall under the somewhat broader heading of soft-tissue sarcomas.

Risk factors: There are no readily identifiable risk factors particular to malignant endothelioma (angiosarcoma), although several risk factors associated with soft-tissue sarcomas in general have been identified. These include exposure to chlorophenols in wood preservatives and phenoxyacetic acid in herbicides, exposure to ionizing radiation, and very rare genetic predispositions in some families. Infantile hemangiomas do not appear to have a hereditary origin, and no known food, medication, or activity during pregnancy has been identified as a risk factor.

Etiology and the disease process: The etiology of malignant endothelioma is obscure, although tumors have been known to develop as complications from a preexisting condition. Lymphedema resulting from radical mastectomy may trigger the development of angiosarcoma, and radiation-induced angiosarcomas have developed many years following successful radiotherapy for visceral carcinomas and Hodgkin disease. Environmental carcinogens such as vinyl chloride and thorium dioxide have been shown to induce hepatic hemangioendothelioma. Once initiated in the lining of the blood vessels, the tumor spreads rapidly and builds its own blood vessel network.

The causes of infant and neonatal benign hemangioma are also unknown, although some studies have implicated the process of estrogen signaling in hemangioma proliferation. Other studies suggest that an interaction between fetal skin and the maternal placenta may trigger the tumor formation.

Incidence: Less than 1 percent of newly diagnosed cancers are soft-tissue sarcomas. Of these, only about 2 percent are classified as hemangiosarcomas or angiosarcomas. The annual incidence of soft-tissue sarcomas in the United States is approximately 2 to 3 cases per 1 million people. Hemangiomas, on the other hand, are the most common benign childhood tumors, occurring in approximately 4 to 10 percent of children with northern European backgrounds, although they are much less prevalent in children with other ethnic backgrounds. They are common in twin pregnancies, and the incidence may be as high as 25 percent in premature infants weighing less than 1,000 grams. Female children are three to five times more likely to be affected than male children.

Symptoms: Symptoms vary greatly depending on tumor location. Soft-tissue sarcomas of the extremities usually present as painless swellings that grow at a moderately rapid pace. Abdominal and thoracic endotheliomas may grow to large masses before detection. Neurologic symptoms may result from the compression of lumbar or pelvic nerves, and in the case of liver, heart, or bowel tumors, organ function may be compromised as the tumors grow. Up to one-third of patients may present with anemia or other evidence of recent hemorrhage, including gastrointestinal bleeding, hemothorax, or persistent hematoma.

Infantile hemangiomas present a more predictable growth pattern. Although occasionally present at birth, most arise during the first few weeks after birth and grow rapidly over the next several months. This is followed by a gradual shrinking, which may occur over a period of one to seven years. Regression appears to be complete in 50 percent of children by the age of five and in essentially all children by the age of twelve.

Screening and diagnosis: Diagnosis of malignant endothelioma in most cases is based on surgical biopsy and direct histological examination of tumor tissue. The characteristic network of blood vessels usually provides an unambiguous identification. Screening tests for industrial workers exposed to vinyl chloride are available, but screening programs for people exposed to other environmental carcinogens are not generally available because of the rarity of this type of cancer. Staging of these tumors generally follows the guidelines established by the American Joint Committee on Cancer. These stages are based on the size of the tumor (T), the degree of spread to regional lymph nodes (N), and spread to distant lymph nodes and organs (metastasis, M) as well as its grade.

Treatment and therapy: Treatment of malignant endothelioma varies considerably depending on tumor location, although surgical removal with wide margins (2 centimeters, or cm) is recommended whenever possible. However, surgery may be inadvisable for a massive tumor or one extending into vital structures. In these cases and sometimes following successful surgery, chemotherapy, radiation therapy, or both are often recommended. Two recent studies report the successful treatment of patients with advanced epithelioid hemangioendothelioma using the new antiangiogenic agents, sunitinib malate and pazopanib. Both of these drugs are oral multi-target tyrosine kinase inhibitors that target the vascular endothelial growth factor receptors produced by the tumor cells. This is a promising alternative approach when conventional chemotherapy does not lead to significant improvement.

Most infantile hemangiomas disappear without treatment, often leaving no visible marks or scars. Occasionally in the case of large affected areas, cosmetic surgery may be indicated. Oral corticosteroids may be prescribed, and small raised lesions may be treated by the direct injection of corticosteroids. In cases of incomplete resolution or for flat, superficial lesions in cosmetically significant areas, pulsed dye laser therapy can be useful.

Prognosis, prevention, and outcomes: Malignant endotheliomas, like most soft-tissue sarcomas, are clinically aggressive, often difficult to treat, and have a high rate of local recurrence and metastasis. The prognosis is relatively unfavorable, with reported five-year survival rates generally less than 50 percent.

Jeffrey A. Knight, Ph.D.

For Further Information

DeVita, Vincent T., Lawrence, Theodore S., & Rosenberg, Steven A. (Eds.). (2015). *DeVita, Hellman, and Rosenberg's cancer: Principles & practice of oncology* (10th ed.). Philadelphia: Wolters Kluwer.

Goldblum, John R., Folpe, Andrew L., & Weiss, Sharon W. (2014). *Enzinger and Weiss's soft-tissue tumors* (6th ed.). Philadelphia: Elsevier Saunders.

Weinberg, Robert A. (2013). *The biology of cancer* (2nd ed.). New York: Garland Science.

Other Resources

Angiosarcoma Support Organization
http://www.angiosarcoma.org/

Liddy Shriver Sarcoma Initiative
http://liddyshriversarcomainitiative.org
MayoClinic.com.

Angiosarcoma
http://www.mayoclinic.com/health/angiosarcoma/AN00841

National Cancer Institute
Soft Tissue Sarcoma.
http://www.cancer.gov/cancertopics/types/soft-tissue-sarcoma/

See also: Angiosarcomas; Ewing sarcoma; Fibrosarcomas, soft-tissue Hemangiosarcomas; Meningiomas; Sarcomas, soft-tissue

▶ Enteritis

Category: Diseases, Symptoms, and Conditions
Also known as: Radiation enteritis

Related conditions: Crohn disease, irritable bowel syndrome

Definition: Enteritis is an inflammation of the small or large intestine or both. Enteritis can be acute (short term) or chronic (long lasting).

Risk factors: In cancer patients, enteritis is caused by radiation therapy to the abdomen, pelvic area, or rectum. Radiation therapy is given either to treat an inoperable tumor or as an adjunct to surgery or chemotherapy. The likelihood of developing radiation enteritis depends on multiple factors, including:

- where the radiation was targeted
- strength and frequency of radiation treatment
- tumor size
- amount of bowel (large or small intestine) exposed to radiation
- whether radiation therapy is given at the same time as chemotherapy
- presence of radioactive implants to target tumors
- patient health and nutritional status

Generally, the higher the dose and frequency of radiation and the larger the amount of intestine exposed, the more likely the individual is to develop radiation enteritis. Patients who have diabetes, high blood pressure, poor nutritional status, or conditions that interfere with blood flow to the intestines are more likely to develop radiation enteritis.

Etiology and the disease process: Enteritis is an inflammation of the bowel. In noncancer patients, acute enteritis most often occurs because the individual has consumed food or water contaminated with bacteria or viruses that irritate the intestine. Chronic enteritis occurs from gastrointestinal disorders such as Crohn disease. Radiation enteritis is a specific type of enteritis that occurs as the result of radiation therapy during cancer treatment.

Radiation is used to kill rapidly dividing cancer cells. However, it also kills normal cells, especially those that divide frequently. The cells lining both the large and small intestine tend to divide often and can be substantially damaged by exposure to radiation necessary to treat cancer occurring in the abdomen and pelvis.

As the cells lining the wall of the intestine are damaged, the digestive function is disrupted, and water and nutrients are no longer efficiently absorbed. In acute radiation enteritis, the changes to the cells are reversible and the condition usually clears up a month or two after radiation therapy stops. In chronic radiation enteritis, the cellular damage continues. Symptoms usually improve for a time, but recur between six and eighteen months after radiation therapy has been completed. Damage to the intestinal lining in chronic radiation enteritis is permanent, and symptoms are difficult to control.

Incidence: There is controversy over how many people develop radiation enteritis. Some studies have found that almost all patients exposed to abdominal radiation develop some acute symptoms, while other studies have recorded rates of about 35 percent. This variation is probably due to different techniques and doses used at different cancer centers. Of those people who develop acute symptoms, between 5 and 15 percent develop chronic problems.

Symptoms: Many symptoms of acute and chronic radiation enteritis are similar. They include crampy abdominal pain, nausea, vomiting, watery or bloody diarrhea, mucous discharge, and bleeding from the rectum. Individuals with chronic enteritis also lose weight, have vitamin deficiencies, and pass loose, fatty or greasy stools. Occasionally with chronic enteritis, the intestine may become obstructed or a perforation (hole) may develop.

Screening and diagnosis: For acute radiation enteritis, diagnosis is made on the basis of symptoms appearing shortly after radiation therapy has begun. For chronic radiation enteritis, observation of symptoms and a patient history are used for diagnosis. In chronic enteritis, tests are done to rule out a return of the tumor or other conditions that could cause similar symptoms.

Treatment and therapy: Radiation enteritis is treated by managing the symptoms. Dietary changes include avoiding spicy, fatty, and high-fiber foods, alcohol, and milk products, because the intestine often loses the ability to make the enzyme lactase, which is needed to digest milk. Diarrhea is treated with antidiarrheal medicines such as bismuth subsalicylate (Kaopectate), diphenoxylate and atropine (Lomotil), anhydrous morphine (Paregoric), or loperamide (Imodium). Fluid intake is increased to compensate for fluids lost with diarrhea. Antispasmodics may also be given to slow contractions in the bowel. Nutritional counseling is important, especially in chronic enteritis, because the bowel loses the ability to absorb nutrients. Nutritional supplements and digestive aids are often given. Surgery to remove the damaged portion of the bowel in chronic enteritis is controversial.

Prognosis, prevention, and outcomes: Symptoms of acute radiation enteritis usually continue two to three weeks after radiation therapy has finished. Within a few months, symptoms usually disappear completely, and the cells lining the intestine return to normal. In chronic radiation enteritis, the cells lining the intestinal wall are permanently damaged, and symptoms continue indefinitely, although treatment may help to control them. Nutritional counseling and modified diet can help reduce some symptoms of the disorder.

Martiscia Davidson, A.M.

For Further Information

Dodd, Marilyn J. *Managing the Side Effects of Chemotherapy and Radiation*. 2d ed. San Francisco: Regents University of California School of Nursing, 2001.

Keane, Maureen, and Daniella Chace. *What to Eat if You Have Cancer*. 2d ed. New York: McGraw-Hill, 2007.

Smith, Tom. *Coping with Bowel Cancer*. London: Sheldon Press, 2006.

Staritz, M., et al., eds. *Side Effects of Cancer Chemotherapy on the Gastrointestinal Tract*. Boston: Kluwer Academic, 2003.

Other Resources

MedlinePlus

Radiation Enteritis
http://www.nlm.nih.gov/medlineplus/ency/article/000300.htm

National Cancer Institute
Gastrointestinal Complications
http://www.cancer.gov/cancertopics/pdq/supportivecare/gastrointestinalcomplications/patient

See also: Colorectal cancer; Crohn disease; Gastrointestinal cancers; Gastrointestinal complications of cancer treatment; Inflammatory bowel disease; Small intestine cancer

▶ Eosinophilic leukemia

Category: Diseases, Symptoms, and Conditions
Also known as: Primary eosinophilia, hypereosinophilic syndrome (HES)

Related conditions: Myelogenous leukemias

Definition: Eosinophilic leukemia is a malignancy of blood-forming cells in which eosinophils (a type of white blood cell) are the prominent neoplastic leukocytes.

Risk factors: Some forms have a genetic basis originating with chromosomal abnormalities (*FIP1L1-PDGFRA* fusion gene). However, most cases are idiopathic (of unknown origin).

Etiology and the disease process: Leukemias are neoplastic lymphoproliferative diseases that involve bone marrow cells. The specific type of leukemia depends on which particular cell, usually in the leukocyte/white blood cell lineage. The abnormality generally begins in the early blast (immature) cell stage and results in an uncontrolled proliferation of the cells. Eosinophilic leukemias involve the specific white cell known as an eosinophil, a bilobed white cell that stains with the dye eosin.

Incidence: Eosinophilic leukemia is considered a subcategory of chronic myelogenous leukemias, a group of diseases with an annual incidence of 1 to 2 cases per 100,000 people. The specific number categorized as hypereosinophilic syndrome is not determined, due to its rarity.

Symptoms: Symptoms are often general, categorized as "flulike" symptoms. These include an unexplained fever, swollen lymph nodes, and unexplained fatigue.

Screening and diagnosis: Screening is generally not carried out for leukemias. The extent of chromosomal abnormalities is occasionally used to determine prognosis. Diagnosis is based on the microscopic observation of immature or abnormal leukocytes, in particular, early-stage eosinophils, using either blood samples or bone marrow biopsies.

Treatment and therapy: Treatment is based on the extent or stage of the disease and may involve a variety of procedures. The treatment of choice begins with chemotherapy involving the use of antiproliferative drugs such as vincristine or cyclophosphamide either orally or intravenously. Most chemotherapeutic drugs produce side effects such as nausea or a lowering of the blood count. Steroids are sometimes included with treatment as a means to reduce such effects.

Other methods of treatment include surgery—removal of the spleen, a site of neoplastic cell production or accumulation—and radiation therapy. Radiation therapy has proven most useful as a palliative treatment rather than one that effects a "cure." Biological therapy, the use of interferon-alpha, as a means to stimulate an immune response against the neoplasm may also be included in treatment.

Prognosis, prevention, and outcomes: Since the genetic basis for eosinophilic leukemia is unknown, there is no known means of prevention. Prognosis depends on the effectiveness of treatment, the maturation stage of precursor cells, and the extent of neoplastic cell infiltration into other organs. Survival may be measured in months, or in some cases remission may last for decades.

Richard Adler, Ph.D.

See also: Leukemias; Myeloproliferative disorders

▶ Ependymomas

Category: Diseases, Symptoms, and Conditions

Related conditions: Glial tumors and gliomas

Definition: An ependymoma is a central nervous system cancer that arises from the ependymal cells that line the fluid-containing ventricles and central canal of the brain and spinal cord, respectively. Ependymomas are a type of glial cell tumor and are collectively derived from the cells that provide support and nourishment to neural cells. Ependymomas account for 3 percent of all glial cell tumors and 6 to 9 percent of all primary central nervous system tumors.

Risk factors: The most salient risk factor relates to a genetically mediated transformation of normal ependymal cells into tumor cells. A history of neurofibromatosis type 2 is associated with the development of spinal ependymomas. Neurofibromatosis type 2, an autosomal dominant syndrome, is caused by a mutation in the *NF2* gene manifesting with skin lesions (café-au-lait spots) and bilateral hearing loss from acoustic nerve tumor growth. Familial occurrences of isolated ependymomas have also been documented.

Etiology and the disease process: Ependymomas originate from the transformation of an ependymal cell. Although no single aberration has been implicated, involvement of chromosome 22 has been most commonly implicated, the same chromosome that bears the *NF2* tumor-suppressor gene (22q12). Changes seen in genetic studies include translocation (removal and subsequent reattachment of a chromosomal segment to another chromosome), deletion of the long arm (22q), or monosomy (absence of one half of a chromosome pair). One family study has narrowed down this region (22pter-22q11.2), suggesting that a tumor-suppressor gene may be responsible. Other aberrations in several other chromosomes were noted in other studies.

Incidence: Ependymomas have two incidence peaks: in early childhood and in adulthood. The mean age of ependymoma occurrence in childhood is at five years, peaking again during adulthood at a mean age of thirty-four. However, a substantial number of ependymomas in children, 30 percent of all childhood cases, manifest before age three. By location, ependymomas in the brain are seen more commonly in children (90 percent of cases), while spinal (intramedullary) tumors are more commonly seen in adults (60 percent of cases).

Symptoms: Obstruction of the flow of cerebrospinal fluid (CSF) within the fourth ventricle, with resulting pressure buildup and tissue compression, usually occurs. Brain stem involvement may be seen as irritability or lethargy. Cerebellar symptoms denoting involvement may be seen as frequent loss of balance and dizziness. Occasional cerebrum involvement may manifest as personality and behavioral changes or one-sided body weakness or paralysis. Symptoms of increased pressure include nausea, vomiting, morning headache, and vision changes. Physical examination findings may include papilledema (swelling of both optic nerves), limb incoordination with voluntary movements, cranial nerve VI to X compression signs such as eye movement (nystagmus, lateral gaze weakness or paralysis), facial movement, speech and swallowing abnormalities, and increase in head circumference in babies less than two years of age. Spinal cord manifestations roughly correspond with the affected nerve root level, ranging from pain to sensory deficits, weakness, paralysis, loss of reflexes, and muscle wasting.

Screening and diagnosis: There are no routine screening tests available for ependymomas. Clinical history, physical examination, and neuroimaging tests such as magnetic resonance imaging (MRI) or computed tomography (CT) can suggest an ependymoma. These tumors are seen as intraventricular or intramedullary masses that closely match or are darker in contrast to surrounding tissue. Clues that may aid in distinguishing a tumor from normal tissue include cystic formations, calcifications, hemorrhage, or necrosis. The final diagnosis of the type of ependymoma is mainly pathological, when a tissue sample is examined microscopically and classified according to the World Health Organization classification for ependymal tumors. Grade I includes subependymomas and myxopapillary ependymomas; grade II includes cellular, papillary, and clear-cell ependymomas, and grade III ependymomas are of the anaplastic (malignant) variety.

Treatment and therapy: Treatment of ependymomas includes surgical removal, radiation therapy, and chemotherapy. The most important factor in a good prognosis is surgical removal, in which a gross total resection is done irrespective of tumor location, removing the entire primary tumor. Postoperative radiotherapy and chemotherapy—a regimen of cisplatin, etoposide, carboplatin, vincristine, and mechlorethamine or of ifosfamide, carboplatin, and etoposide (ICE)—are carried out to prevent recurrence. Radiotherapy is preferred over chemotherapy except in malignant cases. Restoration of normal cerebrospinal fluid circulation through the ventricles and central canal is a secondary objective if assessment of cerebrospinal fluid shows poor outflow postoperatively. This may be achieved with the addition of a device diverting excess cerebrospinal fluid to the abdominal cavity (ventriculoperitoneal shunt).

Prognosis, prevention, and outcomes: The overall five-year survival rate for all ependymoma patients is 50 percent. Children have a much lower five-year survival rate (14 percent) when compared with adults (76 percent) because of where children's tumors are typically located. Prognosis depends on several predictors, the most significant being the extent of tumor resection. Five-year survival rates approach 70 percent in gross total resection as opposed to 30 to 40 percent in partial resection irrespective of tumor grade. Other factors include amount of remaining tumor, tumor grade, age, infratentorial location, local spread to the brain stem, metastases, and rate of recovery.

Complications associated with surgery in posterior fossa (cerebellar) resections include cerebellar mutism (speech deficits or absence with cerebellar deficits) and long-term neurologic deficits.

Aldo C. Dumlao, M.D.

For Further Information

Dempsey, Sharon. *My Brain Tumour Adventures: The Story of a Little Boy Coping with a Brain Tumour.* London: Jessica Kingsley, 2003.

Parker, James N., and Philip M. Parker, eds. *The Official Patient's Sourcebook on Adult Brain Tumors: A Revised and Updated Directory for the Internet Age.* San Diego, Calif.: Icon Health, 2002.

_______. *The Official Patient's Sourcebook on Childhood Ependymoma: A Revised and Updated Directory for the Internet Age.* San Diego, Calif.: Icon Health, 2002.

Other Resources

Cancer Backup

Ependymoma

http://www.cancerbackup.org.uk/Cancertype/Brain/Typesofbraintumour/Ependymoma

National Cancer Institute

Childhood Ependymoma Treatment

http://www.cancer.gov/cancertopics/pdq/treatment/childependymoma/patient/

See also: Brain and central nervous system cancers; Carcinomatous meningitis; Craniotomy; Gliomas; Simian virus 40; Spinal axis tumors

▶ Epidermoid cancers of mucous membranes

Category: Diseases, Symptoms, and Conditions

Related conditions: Squamous cell carcinoma, skin cancers, head and neck cancers, nasopharyngeal cancer, laryngeal cancer, nasal cavity and paranasal sinus cancers, oral and oropharyngeal cancers, gastrointestinal cancers, urinary system cancers

Definition: Epidermoid cancers of mucous membranes are squamous cell malignancies in tissues in which glands produce mucosal fluids to protect epithelial cells and assist various physiological functions. These membranes line the interiors of body cavities, organs, and structures that connect either directly or indirectly to external skin openings. Some references to epidermoid cancers of mucous membranes limit them to head and neck cancers. Since the mid-nineteenth century, medical literature has mentioned epidermoid cancers in other mucous membranes, which are extensive throughout the torso, including respiratory, gastrointestinal, and genitourinary tracts.

Risk factors: Nicotine exposure increases people's risk for developing epidermoid malignancies in mucous membranes in the mouth, larynx, and pharynx. Alcohol consumption exacerbates epidermoid cancer risks. Oncology experts have associated epidermoid cancers of mucous membranes with such carcinogens as asbestos and industrial by-products, including sawdust.

Medical professionals have connected these cancers to diets containing large amounts of salt and preservatives, which can damage mucous membranes. They have also tied these cancers to periodontitis and the Epstein-Barr virus. Some researchers hypothesize that the human papillomavirus (HPV) might cause epidermoid cancer in mucous membranes. Investigators have studied how pemphigoid, an autoimmune condition causing blistering of mucous membranes, possibly affects patients' vulnerability to cancer.

Etiology and the disease process: Epidermoid carcinomas form in squamous cells both in external skin tissues and internal membrane tissues in organs and cavities. Squamous cell carcinomas develop in the outer epithelial layer of membranes when routine cell division and replacement and sometimes epithelial cell production of keratin proteins deviate and extra abnormal cells and keratin accumulate. Malignant squamous cells typically first appear as lesions known as erythroplasia if they are red or brown and leukoplakia if they are white. Tumors grow and spread into other epithelial layers. For example, epidermoid tumors in lungs begin in respiratory passage membranes, then extend to adjacent organs or lymph nodes.

Incidence: Squamous cell carcinomas associated with external skin cancers, with an estimated 400,000 diagnoses in the United States yearly, occur more frequently than they develop in mucous membranes. Statistics for each type of mucous membrane affected by epidermoid cancers vary. More than 90 percent of various head and neck cancers consist of squamous cell carcinomas. Some 30 percent of non-small-cell lung cancer cases diagnosed involve squamous cell carcinomas. Men are more susceptible than women to developing epidermoid cancers in mucous membranes. These malignancies tend to occur after the age of fifty.

Symptoms: Many patients locate lumps in their neck or detect lesions on their lips or inside their mouth. These oral sores as well as others in mucous membrane tissues do not undergo the normal healing processes. Epidermoid cancers in mucous membranes may cause sore throats and affect how people chew, swallow, and speak. Swollen or numb sinus, jaw, or neck areas; impaired hearing; respiration difficulties; and altered sensory abilities are other symptoms. Some patients experience problems with how dentures fit.

Screening and diagnosis: Health professionals, including dentists, screen patients for potential membrane cancers and collect tissue or fluid samples for laboratory testing. Diagnostic procedures include computerized imaging and scanning, endosonography, and other tests. Physicians differentiate epidermoid carcinomas in mucous membranes from keratin cysts and mucosal melanomas.

Oncologists stage most epidermoid cancers of mucous membranes with the TNM (tumor/lymph node/metastasis) system, devising designations that expand the four basic stages to describe lymph node impact more precisely in terms of tumor size, extent of metastasis, and location relative to nodes. Various types of mucous membrane epidermoid cancers have specific staging criteria, such as which vocal cord is affected.

Treatment and therapy: Many physicians use radiation, chemotherapy, and surgical treatment to remove tumors, lymph nodes, or affected organs. Radiation and chemotherapy without surgery enables patient to continue normal activities and capabilities by retaining such body parts as their larynx, which is essential for speech. Some oncologists deliver chemoradiation intravenously to tumors. Researchers have tested the potential for using herpes simplex virus type 1 to treat tumors in mucous membranes.

Speech and physical therapists, nutritionists, prosthodontists, plastic surgeons, and other specialists enhance treatment of epidermoid cancers in mucous membranes. Psychologists offer emotional support because an estimated 40 percent of mucous membrane cancer patients suffer intense depression.

Prognosis, prevention, and outcomes: Patients with epidermoid cancers in mucous membranes are most likely to survive if their malignancies are detected at an early stage, with an estimated 90 percent survival rate. Medical professionals estimate that more than 50 percent of cases, however, remain undiagnosed until tumor growth has expanded to later stages, increasing fatalities within five years of diagnosis, compared with other cancers.

Elizabeth D. Schafer, Ph.D.

For Further Information

Egan, Conleth A., et al. "Anti-Epiligrin Cicatricial Pemphigoid and Relative Risk for Cancer." *The Lancet* 357, no. 9271 (June 9, 2001): 1850.

Gallegos-Hernández, José-Francisco, et al. "The Number of Sentinel Nodes Identified as Prognostic Factor in Oral Epidermoid Cancer." *Oral Oncology* 41, no. 9 (October, 2005): 947-952.

Sonis, Stephen T., Douglas E. Peterson, Deborah B. McGuire, and David A. Williams, eds. "Mucosal Injury in Cancer Patients: New Strategies for Research and Treatment." *Journal of the National Cancer Institute Monographs* 29 (2001): 1-54.

Other Resources

American Cancer Society

Detailed Guide: Oral and Oropharyngeal Cancer
http://www.cancer.org/docroot/CRI/CRI_2_3x.asp?dt=60

National Cancer Institute

Head and Neck Cancer: Treatment
http://www.cancer.gov/cancertopics/treatment/head-and-neck

See also: Gastrointestinal cancers; Head and neck cancers; Laryngeal cancer; Lung cancers; Mucinous carcinomas; Nasal cavity and paranasal sinus cancers; Oral and oropharyngeal cancers; Salivary gland cancer; Skin cancers; Squamous cell carcinomas; Throat cancer; Urinary system cancers

▶ Erythroplakia

Category: Diseases, Symptoms, and Conditions
Also known as: Oral cancer

Related conditions: Leukoplakia

Definition: Erythroplakia is a precancerous soft, reddened patch found on the floor of the mouth, the tongue, or the soft palate.

Risk factors: Smoking and alcohol consumption, especially in combination, are known risk factors for erythroplakia; use of smokeless tobacco and smoking marijuana also are considered potential risk factors.

Etiology and the disease process: A history of smoking and use of alcohol may be an underlying cause of erythroplakia, but sometimes there is not an identifiable cause. This type of oral lesion has a high rate of developing cancer.

Incidence: Oral cancers usually appear in older adults (over sixty years) and represent approximately 3 percent of all malignancies in men and approximately 2 percent of all malignancies in women.

Symptoms: There may be no early symptoms other than the reddened patch; some lesions may be mixed with white patches (this is called erythroleukoplakia). Later symptoms may include bleeding, loose teeth, and a change in the fit of dentures.

Screening and diagnosis: Early detection is important, and screening exams should be performed by primary care physicians and dentists. When a suspicious reddened patch is found in the mouth, a biopsy is taken; this can be done by the primary care physician or by a head and neck specialist. Oral tumors are staged using the TNM system that describes the size of the primary tumor (T), the involvement of the regional lymph nodes (N), and whether the cancer has spread (metastasis, M). A numerical rating is assigned to each letter, and a stage grouping of 0-IV is assigned based on the ratings for the three categories.

Treatment and therapy: Excision of the oral cancer is usually the necessary treatment; radiation therapy may be used alone or in combination with surgical treatment. The treatment team is multidisciplinary and may include a head and neck surgeon, an oral and maxillofacial pathologist, a general pathologist, a radiation oncologist, a neuroradiologist, a reconstructive surgeon, a medical oncologist, a general dentist, an oral and maxillofacial surgeon, a maxillofacial prosthodontist, a dental hygienist, a nurse specialist, a speech pathologist, a nutritionist, and a tobacco cessation counselor.

Prognosis, prevention, and outcomes: The prognosis of oral cancers depends on the pathology findings and the extent of the lesion. A complete head and neck evaluation should be done to look for other cancers. As tobacco and alcohol use are known risk factors, avoiding or ceasing use will help prevent erythroplakia.

Vicki Miskovsky, B.S., R.D.

See also: Alcohol, alcoholism, and cancer; Chewing tobacco; Leukoplakia; Oral and oropharyngeal cancers

▶ Esophageal cancer

Category: Diseases, Symptoms, and Conditions
Also known as: Cancer of the esophagus

Related conditions: Barrett esophagus

Definition: Esophageal cancer is a disease caused by a malignant tumor that forms in the tissues of the esophagus. The two main types are adenocarcinoma and squamous cell carcinoma.

Risk factors: Gastroesophageal reflux disease (heartburn) causes about one-third of all esophageal cancers, particularly adenocarcinoma. Tobacco use of any form and heavy alcohol consumption are major risk factors for squamous cell carcinoma. Individuals who both smoke and drink excessively have a synergistic (greater than additive) risk of developing esophageal cancer. People with a diet low in fruits and vegetables have a higher incidence of esophageal cancer, and there is evidence that a high intake of refined cereals and red and processed meats can be detrimental as well. Obese people have a greater risk for adenocarcinoma, primarily through an increased incidence of acid reflux disease.

Etiology and the disease process: The esophageal wall has several layers. The inner lining is called the mucosa and has two parts: the epithelium and lamina propria. The epithelium consists of thin, flat squamous cells. The submucosa lies under the mucosa, followed by two layers of muscle. The esophageal wall is connected to various lymph nodes.

Esophageal tumors begin in the epithelial layer. Risk factors such as tobacco use and heavy alcohol consumption may case squamous cell carcinoma. This cancer tends to spread linearly across the submucosal layer.

Adenocarcinoma occurs largely because of chronic acid reflux and develops mainly in the lower esophagus. Acid reflux occurs when the lower esophageal sphincter between the stomach and esophagus malfunctions and allows gastric contents to reflux back into the esophagus. Acid reflux can cause inflammation and erosion of the epithelium. When the healing process takes place, the squamous cells can be replaced by glandular cells that look like the cells that line the stomach. This abnormal epithelium is termed Barrett esophagus. Although this abnormal epithelium is more resistant to acid reflux, a person with the condition is at higher risk to develop adenocarcinoma. When adenocarcinoma develops, it spreads by penetration through the full thickness of the esophageal wall. Both types of esophageal cancer can spread via the lymph nodes and eventually throughout the body.

Incidence: Each year about 13,200 people in the United States are diagnosed with esophageal cancer, and 12,500 die of the disease. The risk of developing esophageal cancer increases with age, with the highest incidence between ages fifty-five and seventy. Men are two to four times more likely to contract the disease than women are. Blacks are six times more likely than whites to acquire squamous cell carcinoma, while adenocarcinoma is four times more frequent in whites than in blacks. Adenocarcinoma has increased more than fourfold in the United States over the last thirty years. People with Barrett esophagus have a highly increased risk for developing adenocarcinoma, estimated between thirty and one hundred times normal. Certain regions of the world have a very high incidence of squamous cell carcinoma, such as northern Iran and northern China.

Symptoms: The most common symptom of esophageal cancer is dysphagia (difficulty in swallowing). Dysphagia primarily involves solid foods and can progress rapidly in severity (over a period of weeks to months). This symptom does not usually appear until at least half of the esophagus is blocked by a tumor. Weight loss can occur because of reduced food intake or muscle wasting from cancer-caused changes in metabolism. Other symptoms such as hoarseness, pain in the chest or throat, or vomiting of blood can be caused by tumor spread.

Screening and diagnosis: When a patient complains of symptoms to the physician, many diagnostic tests are available. A barium swallow begins with a patient drinking a barium solution that coats the normally smooth surface of the esophageal lining. Subsequent X rays can reveal early cancers that appear as small, round bumps or flat, raised areas. Advanced cancers reveal larger irregular areas and a narrowing of the esophagus.

Upper endoscopy or esophagoscopy is a procedure involving the use of a flexible viewing tube called an endoscope. The doctor can view suspicious growths and abnormalities in the esophagus and take biopsies for laboratory examination.

Endoscopic ultrasound involves attaching a small ultrasound probe to the endoscope. The probe sends very sensitive sound waves that penetrate deep into tissues. This technique can determine how far the tumor has spread into the tissues.

Stage at Diagnosis and Five-Year Relative Survival Rates for Esophageal Cancer, 1996-2004

Stage	*Cases Diagnosed (%)*	*Survival Rate (%)*
Localized[a]	24	33.7
Regional[b]	30	16.9
Distant[c]	30	2.9
Unstaged	16	10.8

Source: Data from National Cancer Institute, Surveillance Epidemiology and End Results, Cancer Stat Fact Sheets, 2008

[a]Cancer still confined to primary site

[b]Cancer has spread to regional lymph nodes or directly beyond the primary site

[c]Cancer has metastasized

Computed tomography (CT) is used to determine the extent (stage) of the cancer, rather than an initial diagnosis. The CT scan takes many X-ray images as it rotates around the body. A computer then translates this information into thin sections of the body. The scans can show tumors in the esophagus, lymph nodes, and other organs where the cancer may have spread.

A positron emission tomography (PET) scan involves injecting a small amount of radioactive glucose tracer into the patient's vein. The tumors show up brighter on the resultant scan. The PET scan indicates the presence or absence of malignancy based on the increased metabolic activity of tumors. PET scans can detect cancer before the anatomic and structural changes shown by tumors have time to develop. This test is valuable in detecting cancer spread to distant lymph nodes or throughout the body.

The progression of esophageal cancer is described by staging classification systems. The National Cancer Institute uses the following staging system:

- Stage 0: The cancer is confined to the epithelial layer. It is also called carcinoma in situ, meaning "in place."
- Stage I: Cancer has spread to the submucosal layer.
- Stage IIA: Cancer has spread to the muscle layer or to the outer wall of the esophagus.
- Stage IIB: Cancer may have spread to any of the first three layers of the esophagus and to nearby lymph nodes.
- Stage III: Cancer has spread to the outer walls of the esophagus and may have spread to tissues or lymph nodes near the esophagus.

• Stage IVA: Cancer has spread to nearby or distant lymph nodes.
• Stage IVB: Cancer has spread to distant lymph nodes or organs in other parts of the body.

Treatment and therapy: Surgery is the most common treatment for esophageal cancer; however, there are many risks involved. The surgeon removes the cancerous part of the esophagus and may remove lymph nodes and part of the stomach if the cancer is advanced. Surgery is mainly useful for Stages 0 to I, when it is most likely to be curative. If surgery is contemplated for Stages III and IV, it is usually done in combination with other therapies such as chemotherapy and radiation. Surgery is not feasible for cancers that have spread beyond the esophagus. Radiation is most effective when used with other therapies. Radiation is used to relieve symptoms of dysphagia, or in combination with chemotherapy to shrink tumors before surgery. Radiation used alone is rarely curative.

Chemotherapy helps to sensitize cancer cells to radiation, so chemotherapeutic agents are often used in combination, with or without surgery. The most effective agent is cisplatin. Fluorouracil has synergistic activity with cisplatin so is often used in combination. Other chemotherapeutic agents showing promise include paclitaxel, irinotecan, and oxaliplatin. Chemotherapy alone is rarely curative.

Photodynamic therapy can be used to treat very early cancers that are on or just under the epithelial lining. It is also used for palliative therapy to alleviate dysphagia. A nontoxic chemical is injected into the blood and allowed to accumulate in the tumor. A special laser light is focused on the tumor through an endoscope. The light converts the chemical to a toxic form that kills tumor cells.

Prognosis, prevention, and outcomes: Esophageal cancer is a very deadly cancer with an overall curative success of less than 10 percent. By the time symptoms appear, the disease is incurable in half the cases. The benefit of a screening program to detect esophageal cancer at an earlier stage has not been demonstrated. Even monitoring patients with gastrointestinal reflux disease for the presence of Barrett esophagus has not been shown to improve survival rate.

The best preventive measures are to minimize the risk factors.

David A. Olle, M.S.

For Further Information

Koshy, Mary, et al. "Multiple Management Modalities in Esophageal Cancer." *The Oncologist* 9 (2004): 137-159.

Rankin, Sheila C., ed. *Carcinoma of the Esophagus*. New York: Cambridge University Press, 2008.

Sharma, Prateek, and Richard Sampliner, eds. *Barrett's Esophagus and Esophageal Adenocarcinoma*. 2d ed. Malden, Mass.: Blackwell, 2006.

Other Resources

American Cancer Society
http://www.cancer.org

MayoClinic.com
Esophageal Cancer
http://www.mayoclinic.com/health/esophageal-cancer/DS00500

National Cancer Institute
Esophageal Cancer
http://www.cancer.gov/cancertopics/types/esophageal/

See also: Alcohol, alcoholism, and cancer; Bacteria as causes of cancer; Barium swallow; Barrett esophagus; Cardiomyopathy in cancer patients; Cigarettes and cigars; Endoscopy; Esophagectomy; Esophagitis; Fanconi anemia; Gastrointestinal cancers; Gastrointestinal oncology; Oral and oropharyngeal cancers; Stent therapy; Thoracotomy; Upper Gastrointestinal (GI) endoscopy

▶ Esophagitis

Category: Diseases, Symptoms, and Conditions
Also known as: Inflammation of the esophagus

Related conditions: Gastroesophageal reflux disease (GERD), Barrett esophagus, heartburn (pyrosis), difficulty swallowing (dysphagia), painful swallowing (odynophagia)

Definition: Esophagitis is a general condition in which the esophagus, the muscular tube connecting the mouth to the stomach, is inflamed. Different medical conditions are associated with esophagitis, including GERD, a condition in which the stomach contents flow backward into the esophagus, and nonreflux esophagitis. Serious gastrointestinal complications of esophagitis include a narrowing of the esophagus (strictures), ulcers, and in rare cases a risk of esophageal cancer.

Risk factors: Factors that may increase the risk of developing esophagitis include pregnancy, obesity, scleroderma, smoking, alcohol, caffeine, chocolate, fatty or spicy foods, spinal cord injury, and certain medications (such as nonsteroidal anti-inflammatory drugs, or NSAIDs, including aspirin and ibuprofen).

Etiology and the disease process: The etiology of esophagitis differs depending on the cause of the inflammation. In GERD-associated esophagitis, a backflow (reflux) of acidic fluid from the stomach (containing gastric acid, pepsin, and sometimes bile) to the esophagus causes irritation of the epithelium (the cells lining the esophagus). In some instances, a premalignant condition called Barrett esophagus can develop, which can increase the risk of developing esophageal cancer. However, the risk of esophageal cancer in patients with Barrett esophagus is relatively small: less than 1 percent of Barrett esophagus patients a year.

Nonreflux esophagitis may be caused by infection (viral, bacterial, fungal, or parasitic organisms), chemicals (ingestion of a caustic chemical or medication), radiation therapy (physically damaging the lining of the esophagus leading to inflammation and ulceration), or in rare instances immune-mediated disorders (eosinophilic esophagitis).

Incidence: Esophageal reflux symptoms are estimated to occur in 33 to 44 percent of the general population on a monthly basis with up to 7 to 10 percent of people having daily symptoms. Radiation esophagitis occurs in up to 80 percent of patients receiving radiation therapy to the esophagus.

Symptoms: The most common symptom is heartburn (pyrosis). Other common symptoms of esophagitis include upper abdominal discomfort, nausea, bloating, and fullness. Less common symptoms of esophagitis include dysphagia, odynophagia, cough, hoarseness, wheezing, and vomiting of blood (hematemesis).

Screening and diagnosis: A physician can establish a diagnosis of GERD based on patient history alone. However, if symptoms are severe or do not respond to treatment, the physician may order diagnostic tests designed to determine mucosal injury, amount of reflux, and pathophysiology, including barium X-ray series, endoscopy, an ambulatory acid (pH) probe test, and an esophageal impedance test.

During a barium X-ray series, the patient drinks a barium solution that, through a series of X rays, provides a picture of the shape and condition of the esophagus, stomach, and upper intestine (duodenum). X rays can also reveal a hiatal hernia, an esophageal narrowing, or a growth.

During an endoscopy, or an esophagogastroduodenoscopy (EGD), a flexible tube with a light and camera (endoscope) is inserted down the throat and can reveal inflammation of the esophagus or stomach. A biopsy may also be taken during an EGD to test for Barrett esophagus, esophageal cancer, or the presence of a bacterium that may cause peptic ulcers.

An ambulatory acid (pH) probe test can identify when and for how long stomach acid flows back into the esophagus. A flexible tube (catheter) is inserted through the nose into the esophagus to position a probe in the esophagus just above the stomach. The other end of the catheter is attached to a small computer that records acid measurements. The probe remains in place for one or two days while measurements are recorded.

The esophageal impedance test is similar to the ambulatory acid probe test except that it measures whether gas or liquids reflux back into the esophagus.

Treatment and therapy: The goals of treatment are to provide symptom relief, heal ulcerations, and prevent complications. Reflux esophagitis is managed with over-the-counter agents, such as H2-receptor antagonists (cimetidine, ranitidine, famotidine, nizatidine) and with lifestyle changes such as altering eating habits (for example, avoiding alcohol, caffeine, carbonated beverages, chocolate, fatty foods, or overly large meals), ceasing to smoke cigarettes, and sleeping with the head of the bed elevated by about 4 to 6 inches. Proton pump inhibitors (omeprazole, lansoprazole, pantoprazole, esomeprazole, or rabeprazole) are frequently prescribed and appear effective at relieving symptoms and healing erosive esophagitis in up to 90 percent of patients.

Infectious esophagitis is treated with antibiotics, whereas glucocorticoids are effective in patients with immune-mediated esophagitis. Radiation esophagitis treatment involves symptom management (similar to reflux esophagitis) and prevention (radioprotectors, varying treatment doses and schedules). For severe cases, a temporary feeding tube can be inserted into the stomach or surgery may be required to treat the injuries. To treat pain associated with esophagitis, a prescription analgesic can be gargled with and swallowed.

Prognosis, prevention, and outcomes: Though the response to therapy may be different depending on the specific cause of the esophagitis, the disorders that cause esophagitis usually respond to treatment.

Anita P. Kuan, Ph.D.

For Further Information

Icon Health. *Esophagitis: A Medical Dictionary, Bibliography, and Annotated Research Guide to Internet References*. San Diego, Calif.: Author, 2004.

Parkman, Henry, and Robert S. Fisher, eds. *The Clinician's Guide to Acid/Peptic Disorders and Motility Disorders of the Gastrointestinal Tract*. Thorofare, N.J.: SLACK, 2006.

Yamada, T., ed. *Textbook of Gastroenterology*. 4th ed. Philadelphia: Lippincott Williams & Wilkins, 2003.

Zoler, Mitchel L., and Robert Finn. "Drug Update: Gastroesophageal Reflux Disease." *Family Practice News* 32, no. 9 (2002): 25.

Other Resources

Cleveland Clinic Health Information Center
Esophagitis
http://www.clevelandclinic.org/health/health-info/docs/2800/2896.asp?index=10138

International Foundation for Functional Gastrointestinal Disorders
http://aboutgimotility.org/

MayoClinic.com
GERD
http://www.mayoclinic.com/health/gerd/DS00967

MedlinePlus
Esophagitis
http://www.nlm.nih.gov/medlineplus/ency/article/001153.htm

See also: Alcohol, alcoholism, and cancer; Bacteria as causes of cancer; Barium swallow; Barrett esophagus; Candidiasis; Cardiomyopathy in cancer patients; Cigarettes and cigars; Endoscopy; Esophageal cancer; Esophagectomy; Fanconi anemia; Gastrointestinal cancers; Gastrointestinal oncology; Hematemesis; Oral and oropharyngeal cancers; Stent therapy; Stomatitis; Thoracotomy; Upper Gastrointestinal (GI) endoscopy

▶ Estrogen-receptor-sensitive breast cancer

Category: Diseases, Symptoms, and Conditions
Also known as: Estrogen-receptor-positive breast cancer, hormone-dependent breast cancer

Related conditions: Breast cancer, fibroadenomas, breast cysts, fibrocystic breasts

Definition: Estrogen-receptor-sensitive breast cancer is the diagnosis given for a breast cancer that is driven by estrogen stimulation. It is by far the most common type of breast cancer. Breast cancer cells are primarily epithelial. About 75 percent of breast cancers originate in the ducts of the breast, in which cells are larger than normal epithelial cells and exhibit a variety of patterns, and 15 percent originate in the lobules, in which cells are smaller, uniform, and appear in rows. Rare, invasive cancers compose the remaining 10 percent.

Risk factors: Age and gender are the strongest risk factors, with about 75 percent of cases occurring in women over age fifty, although younger women tend to have more aggressive tumors. Early menstruation (before age twelve), late menopause (after age fifty-five), and reproductive history (late pregnancy) are associated with higher risk, possibly because of the longer lifetime exposure to growth-stimulating estrogen. Inherited mutations in the tumor-suppressor genes *BRCA1* and *BRCA2* and a family history of the disease can increase risk as well.

Etiology and the disease process: Although the cause of estrogen-receptor-sensitive breast cancer is unknown, estrogen appears to be involved with the proliferation and progression of the disease. Estrogen is produced by the ovaries, adrenal glands, and some fat tissue. In normal breast cells, especially the milk glands, estrogen stimulates cell division both directly and through its influence on other hormones (such as progesterone) and growth factors. Researchers believe that higher than normal amounts of estrogen can increase the rate of cell division (and the risk for chance mutations) and trigger the proliferation of cells already harboring genetic mutations. Even after cancer has developed, estrogen-receptor-sensitive cells depend on estrogen stimulation for continued growth and possibly for survival.

Incidence: Estrogen-receptor-sensitive breast cancer is the most common cancer in women in the United States (excluding nonmelanoma skin cancers). After steadily increasing during the previous two decades, breast cancer incidence began to decrease between 2001 and 2003 from approximately 100 to 75 per 100,000 in the United States, with a couple hundred thousand cases diagnosed each year and a little over 1 million cases worldwide.

Symptoms: The classic symptom for this type of cancer is a palpable lump in the breast. Other symptoms include a noticeable difference in breast size or shape, breast swelling, nipple discharge or inversion, dimpling of the skin, orange peel consistency of skin, and enlarged lymph nodes in the area of the armpit or collarbone.

Breast Cancer Stages

Stage	*Tumor Size*	*Node Involvement*	*Metastasis*
I	Less than 2 centimeters	No	No
IIA, IIB	2-5 centimeters	Possible	No
IIIA, IIIB, IIIC	More than 5 centimeters; cancer may extend to chest wall	Possible for IIIA; most likely for IIIB and IIIC	No
IV	N/A	N/A	Yes

Screening and diagnosis: The breast self-exam in combination with the clinical exam and mammogram, during which X rays are taken of the breasts to detect masses too small to feel, are the best screening tools available. Newer options include ultrasound, which can differentiate between cysts and solid tumors and is useful in diagnosing younger women who typically have higher breast density; magnetic resonance imaging (MRI), used to visualize tumor size and locate additional tumors; and computer-aided detection (CAD), which scans a mammogram for undetected tumors. In the future, nuclear medicine studies may be utilized as additional screening and diagnostic tools.

Biopsy is necessary to confirm cancer, and the type of biopsy selected depends on size, location, and number of masses, as well as the patient's medical history. A fine-needle aspiration biopsy uses a very thin needle to draw out fluid from abnormal tissue, a core biopsy uses a larger needle to remove a tissue sample, a Mammotome (or vacuum-assisted) biopsy inserts a probe that suctions and slices several tissue samples, and surgical biopsy removes all or part of the abnormal tissue. Surgical biopsy may be ultimately necessary for confirmation of cancer.

Tumors are described using the TNM (tumor/lymph node/metastasis) classification system, which corresponds with four main breast cancer stages.

Treatment and therapy: Treatment options include a breast-conserving lumpectomy (removal of the tumor and part of the surrounding tissue) or a modified radical mastectomy (removal of the breast, lymph nodes, and fatty tissue associated with the breast and lining of the chest). Both surgeries are a drastic improvement over the disfiguring Halstead radical mastectomy that was used until the 1970's. Postoperative radiation is recommended, followed with chemotherapy, which consists of a combination of cyclophosphamide (Cytoxan), methotrexate or doxorubicin (Adriamycin), and 5-fluorouracil (5-FU). Because this type of breast cancer responds to hormone stimulation, hormone therapy that antagonizes the estrogen receptor (either tamoxifen or one of the newer aromatase inhibitors) is used in addition to chemotherapy.

Prognosis, prevention, and outcomes: Due to increased screening and the advantages of hormone therapy, survival rates are greater than 80 percent for women with estrogen-receptor-sensitive breast cancer. Mortality has decreased since the 1980's from 33 deaths per 100,000 to 25 deaths, although it remains the second leading cause of cancer deaths in women. (Lung cancer is the first.)

Because the cause is unknown, preventive measures are difficult to outline. Researchers are investigating possible links between estrogen-receptor-sensitive breast cancer and oral contraceptives, environmental factors, silicone implants, obesity, hormone replacement therapy, smoking, alcohol, and lack of exercise.

Amber L. Fields, M.S.

For Further Information

DeGregorio, Michael W., and Valerie J. Wiebe. *Tamoxifen and Breast Cancer*. New Haven, Conn.: Yale University Press. 1996.

Hartmann, Lynn C., and Charles L. Loprinzi. *Mayo Clinic Guide to Women's Cancers*. New York: Kensington, 2005.

Ricks, Delthia. *Breast Cancer Basics and Beyond*. Alameda, Calif.: Hunter House Books, 2005.

Other Resources

American Cancer Society
http://www.cancer.org

BreastCancer.org
http://www.breastcancer.org

National Cancer Institute
http://www.cancer.gov

See also: Antiestrogens; Breast cancers; Estrogen Receptor Downregulator (ERD); Hormonal therapies; Hormone receptor tests; Hormone replacement therapy (HRT); Phytoestrogens; Progesterone receptor assay; Receptor analysis

▶ Ewing sarcoma

Category: Diseases, Symptoms, and Conditions
Also known as: Ewing's sarcoma, Ewing sarcoma of the bone, extraosseus Ewing sarcoma, extraskeletal Ewing sarcoma, Ewing tumor, Ewing angioendothelioma, Ewing endothelial sarcoma, Ewing syndrome, malignant primary bone tumor, red bone marrow tumor, neural tumor

Related conditions: Primitive neuroectodermal tumor, peripheral primitive neuroectodermal tumor, Askin's tumor, osteosarcoma

Definition: Ewing sarcoma is a rare disease involving cancer cells found in bones and soft tissue. It usually occurs in the pelvis, ribs, arm bone (humerus), shoulder blade, or leg bone (femur). It gets its name from James Ewing, who in the 1920's first described the disease as being separate from other known types of cancers such as lymphoma or neuroblastoma. Ewing noticed that this type of cancer responded well to radiation. It belongs to a group of tumors sometimes called the Ewing family of tumors because of the close molecular relationship between these kinds of tumors.

Risk factors: More than 90 percent of people who develop this disease have an unusual rearrangement between chromosomes: A piece of chromosome 11 and a piece of chromosome 22 have switched places (called a gene translocation). However, this translocation is not inherited or passed on genetically, so family members of those affected with Ewing sarcoma have no more risk of developing the cancer than the general population does.

Male teenagers are most often diagnosed with this disease. The cancer is thought to be linked somehow to the rapid growth that occurs during puberty. Whites are more likely to develop this disease than are Asians and African Americans.

Very rarely, Ewing sarcoma can develop as a secondary tumor in patients who have had radiation therapy for another type of cancer.

Etiology and the disease process: Because this cancer occurs most often during the teenage years, there may be a link between the onset of puberty and early stages of this disease.

Ewing sarcoma usually starts in a bone, though it can start in soft tissue. The most common starting place for these tumors is in the pelvis or in the leg bones. The tumors may then spread to the chest cavity, other bones, bone marrow, lungs, kidneys, or heart when tumor cells enter the bloodstream and travel elsewhere in the body. This disease may also spread to the central nervous system or lymph nodes, but this is much less common.

Incidence: This disease occurs most often in male children and teenagers, mostly between ten and twenty years old. However, female children and teenagers also develop this disease. In the United States, this cancer affects children less than three years of age at a rate of 0.3 per million and teenagers between the ages of fifteen and nineteen at a rate of 4.6 per million. People over the age of twenty-five rarely develop this type of cancer. Experts estimate that in the United States each year about 200 new cases of this cancer are diagnosed in children and about 20 in adults. These tumors make up about 30 percent of the bone cancers in children.

Symptoms: Symptoms of Ewing sarcoma involve pain (which may be worse at night), swelling (especially when the tumor is located in the long bones of the arm or leg), redness, tenderness, stiffness, a mass that grows quickly and may feel warm, or a bone that breaks unexpectedly. Some patients have fever, fatigue, anemia, or weight loss. Numbness, tingling, or paralysis can also be symptoms if the tumor is located near nerves.

Screening and diagnosis: Because this disease is so rare, no screening is recommended. When Ewing sarcoma is suspected, doctors generally use X rays to determine if there is a suspicious growth. A magnetic resonance imaging (MRI) scan or blood tests also may be helpful in making a diagnosis. If Ewing sarcoma is suspected, two additional tests are used to see if the disease has spread: a computed tomography (CT) scan, which usually includes the lungs to see if the disease has spread there, and a bone scan.

Ewing sarcoma may initially be mistaken for a bone infection (osteomyelitis) or another type of bone cancer (osteosarcoma). A sample of the tumor (biopsy) is necessary to confirm the diagnosis of Ewing sarcoma. A biopsy may be performed with a fine needle, taking only a small sample of the tumor, or by surgery, where all or a large part of the tumor is removed. Sometimes, bone marrow also is biopsied to determine if the disease has spread there.

There is no formal staging for Ewing sarcoma. Gauging the extent of this disease is done by simply determining whether the cancer has spread into other tissues.

Treatment and therapy: Ewing sarcoma is usually a very aggressive disease. By the time of diagnosis, nearly all patients with Ewing sarcoma have some spreading of the disease throughout the body. Most patients are treated with chemotherapy, sometimes before and after surgery, to ensure treatment of any tumors throughout the body.

Surgery or radiation may also be used at the local site of the main tumor if the tumor can be removed without damaging vital organs. Sometimes surgery involves removing bones, which can be replaced or rebuilt with artificial bones or bone grafts. With Ewing sarcoma, radiation therapy usually involves radiation that comes from a machine outside the body rather than from implanted radiation seeds. Radiation therapy can shrink large tumors to alleviate symptoms if the tumor cannot be removed with surgery.

Other types of treatment may include rehabilitation, including occupational or physical therapy. Patients may also need supportive care to help with side effects of chemotherapy, radiation, or surgery. Some patients may benefit from a transplant of blood stem cells or bone marrow.

Diagnosis of Ewing sarcoma usually occurs during the teenage years, sometimes an already turbulent period. Surgery may cause disfigurement during a period of life when looks are very important. Support groups in which teens meet other people with this condition may be especially helpful in dealing with the psychological trauma that this disease can cause.

Generally, patients with Ewing sarcoma benefit from treatment at a children's hospital or medical center with doctors who have experience treating pediatric cancers.

Prognosis, prevention, and outcomes: The prognosis for patients with this disease depends on how far the disease has spread, the size and location of the main tumor, and how responsive the tumors are to chemotherapy. For patients who at diagnosis show no signs of the spread of the disease and choose an aggressive course of treatment involving chemotherapy, surgery, and radiation, survival rates at five years are 70 to 75 percent. However, at diagnosis, at least 15 percent of these patients already have cancer throughout their bodies, generally because symptoms are so vague and nonspecific. These patients have a five-year survival rate of 30 percent. Children under the age of eleven, female children and teenagers, those with smaller tumors, and those who have tumors below the elbow or below the calf have the highest survival rates.

People who have had Ewing sarcoma need continual follow-up care. Even if the cancer is treated and its spread stopped, it often develops again in the place where it first arose and tends to spread throughout the body. Health issues may spring up later that are caused by the type of treatment given. These issues may involve heart and lung problems, slowed or decreased growth and development, and problems with sexual development. It is important for a patient who has had this disease to be regularly monitored for these types of concerns.

There is no known way to prevent Ewing sarcoma. However, not everyone with the gene translocation develops this disease. Scientists are investigating why the gene translocation causes the disease only in some people to see if there are ways to block this cancer from forming. Research is also under way to determine new and improved techniques for diagnosing this cancer earlier in the disease process.

Marianne M. Madsen, M.S.

For Further Information

Icon Health. *Ewing's Sarcoma: A Medical Dictionary, Bibliography, and Annotated Research Guide to Internet References*. San Diego, Calif.: Author, 2004.

Pappo, Alberto S., ed. *Pediatric Bone and Soft Tissue Sarcomas*. New York: Springer, 2005.

Theroux, Nicole. *Ewing's Sarcoma Family of Tumors: A Handbook for Families*. Glenview, Ill.: Association of Pediatric Oncology Nurses, 1999.

Other Resources

Cancer Index

Ewing's Sarcoma: Frequently Asked Questions
http://www.cancerindex.org/ccw/faq/ewings.htm

The Cure Our Children Foundation

Ewing's Sarcoma and Pediatric Cancer Support Group Resources Page
http://www.cureourchildren.org

Ewing's Research Foundation

http://www.letsbeatthis.org

National Cancer Institute

Ewing Family of Tumors Treatment

http://www.cancer.gov/cancertopics/pdq/treatment/ewings/healthprofessional

See also: Amputation; Bone cancers; Limb salvage; Neuroectodermal tumors; Pediatric oncology and hematology; Spinal axis tumors; Tumor markers; Young adult cancers

▶ Eye cancers

Category: Diseases, Symptoms, and Conditions
Also known as: Intraocular cancers, uveal cancers

Related conditions: Retinal detachment, angle-closure glaucoma

Definition: Eye cancers are malignant tumors of the eye, which is made up of the globe, the orbit, and the adnexal structures. The globe (or eyeball) is filled with a fluid called vitreous humor and contains the retina and the uvea. The uvea consists of the iris (pigmented area surrounding the pupil), choroid (pigmented lining of the eyeball that brings blood to the retina and the front of the eye), and ciliary body (made up of the cells producing the aqueous humor and the muscles that control the shape of the lens). Cancers that develop in the globe (retina and uvea) are called intraocular cancers. The orbit is made up of the tissues surrounding the eyeball, including the muscles that control the directional movement of the globe and the nerves of the eye. Tumors in these tissues are called orbital cancers. The adnexal structures consist of the eyelids and the tear glands. Cancers that occur in these structures are called adnexal cancers.

Risk factors: For intraocular melanoma, the risk factors include advanced age (the peak age is seventy), being white, and having light (blue or green) eye color, fair skin, and the ability to tan. For retinoblastoma in children, 10 percent of patients have retinoblastoma in their family history. If the disease is passed from parent to child, the child often has retinoblastoma in both eyes.

Etiology and the disease process: The most common intraocular or uveal eye cancers are melanomas, although these are rare, with approximately 4.3 new cases per 1 million people. Most intraocular melanomas initially do not cause any symptoms, but as the tumor grows, symptoms may include distortion of the pupil, blurred vision, and decreased visual acuity caused by secondary retinal detachment. Extensive retinal detachment can be accompanied by secondary angle-closure glaucoma. Other tumors that can resemble intraocular melanomas in clinical presentation are metastatic carcinoma, posterior scleritis, and benign tumors such as nevi and hemangiomas. This should be considered when making a diagnosis of intraocular melanoma.

Approximately 90 percent of intraocular melanomas occur in the choroid and are called choroidal melanomas. Choroidal melanomas are primary intraocular cancers, that is, cancers that originate in the eye. They initiate from pigmented cells in the choroid and have the potential to become malignant (metastasize to other organs). The remaining intraocular melanomas are melanomas of the iris. These tumors often grow from pigmented spots in the iris that may be present for many years before developing into tumors. They are relatively slow growing and rarely metastasize, and therefore are associated with a better prognosis than choroidal melanomas.

Another kind of intraocular cancer is intraocular lymphoma, which can be either Hodgkin disease or non-Hodgkin lymphoma. These lymphomas typically originate in the lymph nodes but can also originate in the stomach, lungs, and eye. Primary intraocular lymphomas are rare and are always of the non-Hodgkin type. These cancers usually occur in elderly or immunosuppressed people.

Adnexal tumors affecting the eyelid include basal cell carcinomas, which constitute 85 to 95 percent of all malignant eyelid tumors; squamous cell carcinoma; sebaceous cell carcinoma; and malignant melanoma. Basal cell carcinomas and squamous cell carcinomas are most common in elderly people with fair skin. Basal cell carcinomas commonly occur in the inner part of the lower eyelid and are often nodular, appearing as raised pearly bumps with tiny blood vessels. Sebaceous cell carcinomas originate in the eyelid tear glands in elderly people and can be highly malignant, returning after removal and invading the eye socket and lymph nodes. Malignant melanomas are associated with unusual or changing pigmentation. Tumors of the conjunctiva can be squamous cell carcinoma, malignant melanoma, or lymphoma.

Secondary intraocular cancers originate in other organs in the body and spread (metastasize) to the eye. Breast and lung cancers are most likely to metastasize to the eye, especially the uvea. Tumors can also metastasize from the prostate, kidneys, thyroid, and the gastrointestinal tract, though this occurs less frequently than metastasis from the breast and lung.

Retinoblastoma is the most common form of eye cancer in children. It is most common in children younger than the age of five, and affects boys and girls in equal proportion. Approximately 75 percent of retinoblastoma cases are unilateral (affecting one eye). Some 90 percent of patients do not have a family history of retinoblastoma.

Incidence: In 2008, about 2,390 adults were estimated to be diagnosed with cancer of the eye and orbit and 240 were estimated to die of the cancer. The incidence of intraocular melanomas, the most common form of intraocular cancer, is approximately 4.3 new cases per 1 million people. Retinoblastoma affects 1 in every 15,000 to 30,000 live babies per year, with 350 new cases annually. It affects all races with similar frequency.

Symptoms: Symptoms of intraocular tumors may include distortion of the pupil, blurred vision, bulging eyes, watery eyes, pain in or around the eye (rare), and decreased visual acuity caused by secondary retinal detachment. Extensive retinal detachment may be accompanied by secondary angle-closure glaucoma. Other symptoms may include floaters, where spots, flashes, or wavy lines appear in the visual field; loss of peripheral vision, where objects to the side cannot be seen; and a pigmented spot on the iris that enlarges with time (this could be a sign of iris melanoma). Symptoms of retinoblastoma include a white pupil reflex (leukocoria or cat's-eye reflex) instead of the normal black pupil or red reflex.

Screening and diagnosis: Diagnosis of eye tumors can be performed by means of an eye examination with an ophthalmoscope or slit lamp. This is the single most important diagnostic test for eye tumors. For example, most choroidal melanomas can be diagnosed by visual examination of the pupil for the presence of tumors. Choroidal melanomas range in shape and pigmentation, from dark brown to unpigmented. However, most choroidal melanomas are brown to gray-green in color and have a dome or nodular shape.

Other tumors may need additional tests, which include echography or ultrasound, in which sound waves are directed at the eye from a small probe placed on the eye. The reflection patterns are then analyzed to determine if tumors are present. Another diagnostic technique is called fluorescein angiography and involves the introduction of eye drops that cause pupil dilation followed by the injection of a fluorescent dye into a vein in the arm. The dye passes through the blood vessels in the back of the eye and a camera takes a series of photographs, from which the physician can determine if a tumor is present. Echography and fluorescein angiography can also be used to distinguish between eye tumors and hemorrhages or macroaneurysms that may occur in the choroid or below the retinal epithelium.

Stage at Diagnosis and Five-Year Survival Rates for Eye and Orbit Cancer, 1996-2004

Stage	*Cases Diagnosed (%)*	*Survival Rate (%)*
Localized[a]	75	86.7
Regional[b]	9	68.7
Distant[c]	4	70.4
Unstaged	12	77.6

Source: Data from National Cancer Institute, Surveillance Epidemiology and End Results, Cancer Stat Fact Sheets, 2008
[a]Cancer still confined to primary site
[b]Cancer has spread to regional lymph nodes or directly beyond the primary site
[c]Cancer has metastasized

The most invasive diagnostic test that can be performed is the eye biopsy. This involves inserting a long narrow-bored needle into the eye and extracting tissue for examination with a microscope. The risk of ocular mortality associated with an eye biopsy, however, is a serious drawback to this diagnostic test and influences many physicians to use alternative means of diagnosis.

Staging of intraocular tumors involves determining the tumor thickness (apical height) and width (basal diameter). Tumor sizes are classified as small (apical height of 1 millimeter, or mm, to 3 mm, basal diameter equal to or greater than 5 mm), medium (apical height of 2 mm to 10 mm, basal diameter less than 16 mm), large (apical height greater than 10 mm, basal diameter equal to or greater than 16 mm), and diffuse (horizontal, flat growth pattern and tumor thickness 20 percent or less than the greatest basal dimension). Diffuse tumors are rare and have a poorer prognosis. Physicians also determine if the tumor has metastasized and, if so, to what extent. Metastasis of the tumor to preauricular, submandibular, or cervical lymph node regions indicates that subconjunctival extension has occurred. Systemic metastasis usually occurs first in the liver and may also occur in the lung, bone, and subcutaneous sites. Metastasis or spreading of the cancer to the optic nerve, eye socket, or meninges is very rare and is called extraocular extension. The American Joint Committee on Cancer has developed a method for intraocular cancer staging. Metastasis of retinoblastoma tumors is rare but when it occurs, tumors can spread to the brain, central nervous system, and bones.

Treatment and therapy: One of the most commonly used methods of treating eye cancers is radiation therapy, which can shrink tumors but usually does not eliminate them entirely. It can take two forms: plaque radiation therapy and external-beam, charged-particle radiation therapy. Plaque radiation therapy uses plaques with radioactive pellets on one side and gold coating on the other side. An incision is made in the conjunctiva, and plaques are sewn to the outside of the eye directly over the tumor with the side coated with radioactive pellets facing the tumor. Plaque radiation therapy has a five-year control rate of more than 90 percent but has the disadvantage of a high risk of secondary cataracts. External-beam, charged-particle radiation therapy involves irradiating tumors with precisely focused radiation from a cyclotron, a piece of equipment that is available only at specialized centers. This type of therapy specifically kills tumor tissue without damaging surrounding healthy eye tissue and appears to have a control rate similar to that of plaque radiation therapy. The drawbacks are the need for specialized equipment with limited availability, the need for patient cooperation during the procedure (the eye needs to be held still so that the radiation beam can be directed at the tumor), and the possibility of anterior-segment complications.

Other treatments include local tumor resection, which is used for ciliary body or anterior choroidal tumors that have smaller basal dimensions and greater thickness. The eye tumor can also be treated with chemotherapy, which is administered intravenously and delivered to the eye through the bloodstream. In cases in which treatment of the tumor is unsuccessful, surgery may be required to remove the eye (enucleation). The empty eye socket can then be filled with an eyeball implant made of synthetic material.

Newer treatments include photocoagulation with white light and laser radiation, transpupillary thermotherapy, and cryotherapy. Photocoagulation involves the destruction of small tumors by directing light through the pupil into the tumor. Newer photocoagulation techniques use a diopexy probe that directs the light through the wall of the eye instead of through the pupil. This method can be used alone or together with plaque radiation therapy and cryotherapy. Cryotherapy involves applying a penlike probe to the sclera just next to the tumor and freezing the tumor while the patient is under local or general anesthesia. This usually has to be repeated multiple times before the tumor is destroyed and can cause swelling of the eye and eyelids.

Prognosis, prevention, and outcomes: The prognosis of intraocular cancers depends on several factors, including cell type, tumor size, location of the anterior margin, the extent of ciliary body involvement, extraocular extension, and tumor recurrence. Cell type is the most commonly used factor for predicting cancer prognosis. Intraocular melanomas usually consist of spindle cells and epithelioid cells. Spindle cells have less potential for metastasis than epithelioid cells, and a tumor that is mostly made up of spindle cells is considered to have a better prognosis than one that consists mostly of epithelioid cells.

Recurrent melanoma always has a poor prognosis, regardless of cell type or stage. The treatment selected depends on the tumor size, age and health of the patient, site of recurrence, and previous treatment.

The prognosis for retinoblastoma is usually very good, with most children (more than 95 percent) surviving to live normal lives.

Ing-Wei Khor, Ph.D.

For Further Information

"Malignant Melanoma of the Uvea." In *AJCC Cancer Staging Manual*, edited by Frederick L. Greene et al. 6th ed. New York: Springer-Verlag, 2002.

Singh, A. D., L. Bergman, and S. Seregard. "Uveal Melanoma: Epidemiologic Aspects." *Ophthalmology Clinics of North America* 18 (2005): 75-84.

Other Resources

American Cancer Society
What Is Eye Cancer?
http://www.cancer.org/docroot/CRI/content/CRI_2_4_1x_What_is_eye_cancer_74.asp?sitearea=

Bascom Palmer Eye Institute
Ocular Oncology
http://www.eyecancermd.org/eye_cancers.html

Cancer Help UK
Symptoms of Eye Cancer
http://www.cancerhelp.org.uk/help/default.asp?page=18546

Collaborative Ocular Melanoma Study
About Choroidal Melanoma
http://www.jhu.edu/wctb/coms/general/about-mm/coms1.htm

Eyecancernetwork
http://www.eyecancer.com

Memorial Sloan-Kettering Cancer Center
Retinoblastoma
http://www.mskcc.org/mskcc/html/2867.cfm

National Cancer Institute
Intraocular (Eye) Melanoma Treatment
http://www.cancer.gov/cancertopics/pdq/treatment/intraocularmelanoma/healthprofessional

See also: Eyelid cancer; Gonioscopy; Lacrimal gland tumors; Neurofibromatosis type 1 (NF1); Ophthalmic oncology; Orbit tumors; Retinoblastomas; Rhabdomyosarcomas; Rothmund-Thomson syndrome; Sjögren syndrome

▶ Eyelid cancer

Category: Diseases, Symptoms, and Conditions

Related conditions: Eye cancers

Definition: Eyelid cancer can occur as one of a variety of types of cancer that begin on or around the eyelid. The most common types of eyelid cancer are slow to spread and can often be successfully be treated with surgery to remove the tumor followed by eyelid reconstruction.

Risk factors: The main risk factors for eyelid cancer are light skin tone, skin that easily burns or freckles, and frequent exposure to the sun. Eyelid cancer is most common in people over the age of fifty. Men are affected slightly more often than women. Individuals who have skin around the eye that has been sunburned, burned, or that has been injured because of a disease or infection are believed to be at higher risk for eyelid cancer. A history of other skin cancers is also thought to increase the risk.

Etiology and the disease process: There are four main types of eyelid cancers. Basal cell carcinoma and squamous cell carcinoma are usually slow growing and do not tend to spread to other areas of the body. Sebaceous gland carcinoma and malignant melanoma are more aggressive, faster growing, and much more likely to spread. Basal cell carcinoma is a cancer that develops in the lower epidermis. Squamous cell carcinoma begins in the top layer of the epidermis. Sebaceous gland carcinoma arises in the glands of the eyelid. Melanoma begins in the very bottom layer of the epidermis in the cells called melanocytes. From these beginnings, eyelid cancer can spread to the lymph nodes, areas around the eyelid, and to other areas of the body.

Incidence: Eyelid cancer is not a very common form of cancer. According to the American Society of Clinical Oncology, in the United States the annual rates of eyelid cancer are 19.6 cases for every 100,000 men, and 13.3 cases for every 100,000 women. The most common form of eyelid cancer is basal cell carcinoma, which makes up between 85 and 95 percent of reported cases of eyelid cancer. Sebaceous cell carcinoma makes up about 5 percent of reported cases, sebaceous gland carcinoma between 1 and 5 percent of cases, and malignant melanoma a little less than 1 percent of cases.

Symptoms: The main symptom of eyelid cancer is usually an abnormality in the skin of the eyelid or the surrounding area. Often, the eyelid cancer presents as a small bump, sometimes with small red veins in it. The area may differ in color from the surrounding skin and may seem to change colors or grow in size. The eyelashes in the affected area may be missing. There may be a sore that is crusted over or will not heal, or a tear that does not seem to heal properly. Other possible symptoms include swelling or thickening of the eyelid, and an eyelid infection that will not go away or keeps returning. There is often no pain associated with the discolored or bumpy area.

Screening and diagnosis: The ophthalmologist will determine if the suspicious bump or discoloration is cancerous. If cancer seems likely, a biopsy will be performed. During the biopsy some or all of the suspected lesion is removed. It is then sent to a lab, where a pathologist performs tests and examines it under a microscope to determine if cancer is present and, if so, the type and possible extent. Eyelid cancer is staged based on the size of the tumor, if the cancer has spread to the nearby lymph nodes, and whether it has spread to any other parts of the body.

Treatment and therapy: For many cases of eyelid cancer, especially basal cell carcinomas, the biopsy procedure may actually be all the treatment required. If it is determined that the biopsy removed all the cancerous tissue, no other procedures may be necessary. Most eyelid cancers are treated primarily with surgery. Other procedures, such as cryosurgery, in which the cancerous cells are frozen off, may be necessary. If the cancer has spread to any other parts of the body, appropriate treatment will be required. Radiation and chemotherapy are not usually required for eyelid cancers that have not spread. Because surgical removal of the cancerous tissue is usually the primary treatment option, reconstructive surgery is frequently required after the cancer has been removed.

Prognosis, prevention, and outcomes: The prognosis for cases of eyelid cancer that are caught early is generally very good. According to the American Society of Clinical Oncology, estimates indicate a cure rate of up to 95 percent for basal cell carcinoma. The prognosis for each person depends on the stage at which the cancer was diagnosed and other factors. Sebaceous cell carcinoma is not always treatable with as much success as basal cell carcinoma, because it is more likely to have spread and has a higher incidence of recurrence. Malignant melanoma is most likely to not be treatable successfully because of its tendency to spread to other areas of the body quickly. The best way to prevent eyelid cancer is to take the precautions that are generally recommended to prevent any form of skin cancer, such as avoiding prolonged exposure to intense sun, wearing UV-protective sunglasses, and always wearing sunscreen.

Helen Davidson, B.A.

For Further Information

Albert, Daniel M., and Arthur Polans, eds. *Ocular Oncology*. New York: Marcel Dekker, 2003.

Bospene, Edwin B., ed. *Eye Cancer Research Progress*. New York: Nova Science, 2007.

Fekrat, Sharon, and Jennifer S. Weizer, eds. *All About Your Eyes*. Durham, N.C.: Duke University Press, 2006.

Other Resources

Eyecancernetwork

Squamous Carcinoma of the Eyelid

http://www.eyecancer.com/patient/Condition.aspx?nID=54&Category=Eyelid+Tumors&Condition=Squamous+Carcinoma+of+the+Eyelid

Vision Channel

Skin Cancer of the Eyelids

http://www.visionchannel.net/skincancer/index.shtml

See also: Eye cancers; Gonioscopy; Lacrimal gland tumors; Neurofibromatosis type 1 (NF1); Ophthalmic oncology; Orbit tumors; Retinoblastomas; Rothmund-Thomson syndrome; Sjögren syndrome

▶ Fallopian tube cancer

Category: Diseases, Symptoms, and Conditions

Also known as: Fallopian tube adenocarcinoma, Fallopian tube sarcoma, Fallopian tube mixed mesodermal tumor, broad ligament tumor

Related conditions: Cancer of the uterus, cancer of the ovary, peritoneal carcinomatosis

Definition: Fallopian tube cancer is a rare cancer in one of the Fallopian tubes, which lie on both sides of the top of the uterus (womb). These tubes serve as the site of fertilization for oocytes (eggs) released from the ovary and sperm ascending from the vagina, and then as passageways by which the zygote (fertilized egg) returns to the uterus to implant and where the fetus grows and develops. Cancer of the Fallopian tube is primary (originating in the Fallopian tube) in 10 to 20 percent of cases; the majority of Fallopian tube cancers, however, are metastatic from the ovary, uterus, or gastrointestinal tract (stomach and intestines).

Risk factors: The major risk factors for Fallopian tube cancers are thought to be chronic inflammation in the form of endometriosis or pelvic infections, although this has not been proven. Other possible risk factors include a history of infertility and low parity (fewer than two children). Fallopian tube cancer is a disease of older women, diagnosed at an average age of fifty-nine years, with those diagnosed ranging between ages twenty-six and eighty-five. Oral contraceptive use and pregnancy may reduce a woman's risk of Fallopian tube cancer.

Etiology and the disease process: Based on molecular studies, cancer of the Fallopian tube and ovary share abnormalities of the genes *TP53* and *ERBB-2*, suggesting similar genetic risks and environmental factors.

Incidence: Fallopian tube cancer is the rarest cancer involving the female genital tract, accounting for approximately 1 percent of all gynecologic malignancies. The incidence of Fallopian tube cancer in the United States is 3.6 cases per million women per year, with approximately 300 cases diagnosed in the United States each year. Any woman's individual lifetime risk of Fallopian tube cancer is therefore small.

Symptoms: For the most part, cancer of the Fallopian tube is a disease without specific symptoms. Symptoms that are associated with cancer of the Fallopian tube include an abnormal, watery vaginal discharge or excessive bleeding; such symptoms occur in approximately 50 percent of those with Fallopian tube cancer. Pain and a palpable pelvic mass are infrequently associated with Fallopian tube cancer. Occasionally, the pain associated with Fallopian tube cancer mimics appendicitis.

Screening and diagnosis: No routine screening exists or is recommended for Fallopian tube cancer. Most often, the diagnosis of Fallopian tube cancer is made at the time of exploratory surgery to evaluate the patient's symptoms, such as pelvic pain or a mass. Aside from nonspecific symptoms and the triad of symptoms in postmenopausal women (pelvic pain, a pelvic mass, and vaginal bleeding or discharge), the diagnosis should be suspected when cancer cells show up on microscopic evaluation of vaginal discharge with a negative Pap smear and biopsy of the uterus. An abdominal mass can be further evaluated with a pelvic ultrasound, computed tomography (CT) scan, magnetic resonance imaging (MRI), or a laparoscopic examination of the pelvis (outpatient surgery performed through the belly button with a small, lighted instrument). Definitive diagnosis of primary Fallopian tube cancer, as opposed to metastatic cancer, requires that the tumor be contained within the cavity of the Fallopian tube (lumen), the lining of the Fallopian tube (mucosa) be involved with the tumor, and a transition be demonstrated between the portion of the tube involved and that not involved with cancer. Cancer of the Fallopian tube is based on International Federation of Gynecology and Obstetrics (FIGO) staging. Stage 0 is cancer limited to the lining of the Fallopian tube (mucosa). Stage I is cancer limited to one tube with extension into the muscular layer of the tube but not to the external surface of the tube. Stage II cancer involves one or both tubes with extension beyond the Fallopian tube. Stage III cancer involves one or both tubes with spread beyond the pelvic cavity. Stage IV cancer involves one or both Fallopian tubes with distant metastases (for example, the lungs). Unlike ovarian cancer, which is usually advanced at the time of diagnosis, approximately 50 percent of Fallopian tube cancers are Stage I or II at the time of diagnosis, and 50 percent are Stage III or IV.

Treatment and therapy: Because Fallopian tube cancer is generally diagnosed during surgery, staging is performed at that time to determine the extent of disease so that optimal treatment can be offered. Treatment includes a hysterectomy (removal of the uterus), a bilateral salpingo-oophorectomy (removal of both Fallopian tubes and ovaries), inspection of the surfaces of the lining of the abdominal cavity (the peritoneum) for cancer cells, sampling of lymph nodes, and removal of the omentum (a fatty layer covering the intestines).

For Stage I disease, surgery alone is recommended unless the peritoneum is positive. In that case, postoperative radiation or chemotherapy is offered. For Stages II through IV, postoperative chemotherapy is the standard treatment. A second laparoscopy is often performed on completion of chemotherapy or radiation therapy to confirm control of the disease. A blood test, the cancer antigen 125 (CA 125), can be ordered to monitor disease recurrence.

Prognosis, prevention, and outcomes: The five-year survival for all stages of Fallopian tube cancer is approximately 40 to 50 percent.

Patients diagnosed with Stage I Fallopian tube cancer have five-year survival rates of 65 percent; those with Stage II, 50 to 60 percent; and those with Stages III and IV, 10 to 20 percent.

D. Scott Cunningham, M.D., Ph.D.

For Further Information

Ajithkumar, T. V., A. L. Minimole, M. M. John, and O. S. Ashokkumar. "Primary Fallopian Tube Carcinoma." *Obstetrics and Gynecological Survey* 60 (2005): 247-252.

Pectasides, D., and T. Economopoulos. "Fallopian Tube Carcinoma: A Review." *Oncologist* 11 (2006): 902-912.

Other Resources

Abramson Cancer Center of the University of Pennsylvania

Fallopian Tube Cancer: The Basics
Http://www.oncolink.com/types/article.cfm?c=6&s=49&ss=801&id=9502

Eyes on the Prize

Gynecologic Cancer: Fallopian Tube Cancer
http://www.eyesontheprize.org/FAQ/gynca/fall_tube.html

See also: Adenomatoid tumors; *BRCA1* and *BRCA2* genes; Culdoscopy; Endometrial cancer; Endometrial hyperplasia; Exenteration; Family history and risk assessment; Fertility issues; Gynecologic cancers; Gynecologic oncology; Hormonal therapies; Hysterectomy; Hystero-oophorectomy; Leiomyomas; Oophorectomy; Ovarian cancers; Ovarian cysts; Pelvic examination; Salpingectomy and salpingo-oophorectomy; Uterine cancer

▶ Fanconi anemia

Category: Diseases, Symptoms, and Conditions
Also known as: Fanconi's anemia, FA, aplastic anemia with congenital abnormalities

Related conditions: Leukemia, liver tumors, brain tumors, and cancers of the head, neck, esophagus, and female reproductive system

Definition: Fanconi anemia is a rare inherited disease that affects bone marrow, resulting in reduced blood cell production. It is not the same as Fanconi syndrome, which is a rare kidney disorder.

Bone marrow is the central part of the bones in which blood cells are produced. Red blood cells transport oxygen to the cells, white blood cells protect the body against infection, and platelets cause wounds to clot. Damage to the bone marrow decreases the production of all these types of blood cells.

Having this condition predisposes people to developing several kinds of cancers, including acute myelocytic leukemia (AML) and squamous cell carcinoma. These cancers will arise in a person with Fanconi anemia at a much earlier age than the cancers would normally occur.

Risk factors: Fanconi anemia is a recessive inherited disease, which means that both parents must have the disease genes for their children to develop it. Each child who has two parents with the disease genes will have a 25 percent chance of developing the condition.

Etiology and the disease process: Fanconi anemia is an inherited disease that stems from changes, called mutations, in genes. Genes hold the instructions for cells to make different proteins, which carry out various functions throughout the body. In people with Fanconi anemia, defective genes prevent the production of proteins that are needed for cells to work normally.

Incidence: Although the exact number of people with Fanconi anemia is unknown, it is estimated that between 1 in 100 and 1 in 600 people carry the genetic defect responsible for the condition. Approximately 1 in 360,000 people are born with the disease. The symptoms of Fanconi anemia most often emerge when a child is between the ages of three and twelve, although symptoms can stay dormant until later in life. The disease occurs equally in both genders and among all races; however, there is a higher risk among people of Ashkenazi Jewish descent. Between 18 and 20 percent of people with Fanconi anemia develop leukemia.

Symptoms: Because the disease results in fewer white blood cells, it leaves a person more susceptible to infections. A lower red blood cell count leads to fatigue, and the reduction in platelets can interfere with normal blood clotting. The first signs of the disease are often nosebleeds or bruising. People who have Fanconi anemia may have stunted growth; misshapen, missing, or extra thumbs; abnormal arm, hip, spine, or rib bones; a small head or eyes; kidney problems; an abnormal stomach, esophagus, or intestinal tract; mental retardation; and learning disabilities. Patches of unevenly colored skin (café-au-lait spots) are also common. Men may have smaller than normal genitals. People with Fanconi anemia are more likely to develop leukemia, as well as cancers of the head, neck, and esophagus. Women with the disease are at greater risk for cancers of the reproductive tract.

Screening and diagnosis: The primary test for Fanconi anemia is a chromosome breakage test, which mixes the patient's white blood cells with special chemicals to see whether the chromosomes break more easily than they should.

Doctors can also diagnose the disease by removing a sample of bone marrow with a needle through a procedure known as bone marrow aspiration and examining that sample under a microscope to look for signs of low blood cell production. Another method is a bone marrow biopsy, in which a small needle inserted into the bone removes a piece of bone marrow for testing. Often patients will also have a complete blood count to look for low numbers of white blood cells, red blood cells, and platelets. Other screening methods include developmental tests and a kidney ultrasound. If there is a family history of Fanconi anemia, the condition can be diagnosed before a child is born using amniocentesis and chorionic villus sampling (CVS).

Treatment and therapy: A bone marrow transplant can treat blood cell problems, although it cannot reduce the risk of developing cancer or other problems (such as bone malformations) associated with Fanconi anemia. The bone marrow transplant is most likely to be successful if taken from a matched sibling.

Patients may take artificial versions of male hormones called androgens, which improve red blood cell counts and may also help improve white blood cell counts in certain patients. Taking hemopoietic growth factors, such as erythropoietin, also can increase blood counts, as can having a blood transfusion. Researchers are looking into whether gene therapy to correct the genetic mutation might one day benefit patients with Fanconi anemia.

Prognosis, prevention, and outcomes: Because this is an inherited disorder, there is no way to prevent it, although it is possible to screen a fetus for the disease while still in the womb.

The average life expectancy for someone with Fanconi anemia is age twenty-two, although survival can vary from one person to another. New research and improved bone marrow transplantation outcomes are prolonging the life spans of many individuals with this disease.

Stephanie Watson, B.S.

For Further Information

Frohnmayer, Lynn. *Fanconi Anemia: A Handbook for Families and Their Physicians*. Eugene, Oreg.: Fanconi Anemia Research Fund, 2000.

Schindler, D., and H. Hoehn. *Fanconi Anemia: A Paradigmatic Disease for the Understanding of Cancer and Aging*. Basel, Switzerland: S. Karger, 2007.

Shamin, Ahmad, and Sandra H. Kirk, eds. *Molecular Mechanisms of Fanconi Anemia*. New York: Springer, 2006.

Other Resources

Fanconi Anemia Research Fund
http://www.fanconi.org

MedlinePlus
Fanconi's Anemia
http://www.nlm.nih.gov/medlineplus/ency/article/000334.htm

See also: Acute Lymphocytic Leukemia (ALL); Acute Myelocytic Leukemia (AML); Anemia; Aplastic anemia; Blood cancers; Genetics of cancer; Myelodysplastic syndromes; Nijmegen breakage syndrome; Urinalysis

▶ Fatigue

Category: Diseases, Symptoms, and Conditions
Also known as: Asthenia, tiredness, exhaustion, lack of energy

Related conditions: Anemia

Definition: Fatigue describes a condition of tiredness that has many interrelated physical and emotional factors and impairs a patient's feeling of well-being. Fatigue related to cancer or cancer treatment is a persistent sense of tiredness that can cause distress and depression and affect a patient's ability to continue normal daily aspects of living. While patients with cancer may have fatigue as a chronic condition, this fatigue is not the same as "chronic fatigue syndrome." Cancer-related fatigue differs from the fatigue of overwork or excessive exercise as it is not relieved by sleep or rest.

It should be noted, however, that each patient is unique and that some cancer patients do not report cancer-related fatigue; other patients report having only mild to moderate cancer-related fatigue for a short period of time.

Risk factors: In the setting of cancer, fatigue may be caused by the type of cancer and its stage, chemotherapy or radiation therapy, stress, anemia, depression, chronic pain, lack of sleep, lack of proper nutrition, nausea and vomiting, infections, dehydration and electrolyte imbalance, and weight loss.

Etiology and the disease process: The causes of fatigue in patients with cancer are not clearly understood and appear to be multiple. Fatigue can be one of the first symptoms of the presence of cancer and can also be an indication of disease progression. The disease of cancer itself can cause fatigue, primarily through the release of cytokines, which are thought to induce fatigue, the increased need of cancer cells to maintain their high rate of metabolism, and the alteration of hormone levels. The stress of having cancer also can be the cause of fatigue. Treatments can lead to fatigue as the body tries to deal with the insult of cytotoxins or radiation and tries to rebuild cells after treatment. Many biological therapies (those that attempt to strengthen the patient's immune system to fight cancer) have flulike symptoms, including fatigue, as side effects. Medication used as supportive care (for example, to treat depression or vomiting) can cause fatigue. Another cause of fatigue is lack of sleep, which may be caused by pain, emotional issues, depression, and anxiety. Poor nutrition, caused by lack of interest in food or an inability to eat because of mucositis, diarrhea, nausea, or vomiting, has been implicated in fatigue. Surgery for cancer may be the cause of fatigue, which often lessens as the patient recuperates and heals. One way that cancer can cause fatigue is by spreading to bone marrow, where it destroys red blood cell production and leads to anemia, the most commonly reported cause of fatigue. Both chemotherapy and radiation therapy can destroy bone marrow and cause anemia.

Incidence: Depending on the type of cancer and its treatment, approximately 15 to 95 percent of patients with cancer report feeling mentally and physically fatigued.

Symptoms: Fatigue is manifested by extreme tiredness and inability to perform normal daily functions. Fatigue can then lead to other symptoms, such as depression or poor nutrition (if the patient is unable to shop for groceries or cook). Because of the nature of cancer-related fatigue and its interactions with risk factors and other conditions, it is difficult to pinpoint a single symptom. Common symptoms, however, can include dizziness, confusion, inability to think clearly, loss of balance, being bedridden for more than one day, and worsening conditions (for example, increased vomiting, pain, or depression).

Screening and diagnosis: Because of the complex nature of cancer-related fatigue and its many presumptive causes, it is necessary to carefully rule out causes before effective treatment can occur. It is imperative to understand the pattern of fatigue, including when it started, how long it lasted, and how it changed the patient's daily activity pattern. If fatigue was reported only after radiation therapy, for example, depression and other medications could be ruled out as the cause. The kind of cancer and its stage is important to know, as are known treatment-related symptoms. The side effects of chemotherapeutic agents or other medications may be instructive in determining the cause of fatigue. The health care provider should understand the patient's sleep patterns before starting treatment for cancer as well as during treatment for cancer. It is important to know if the patient's eating habits have changed. Patients should be screened for depression, as this is a common cause of fatigue. Patients may be depressed because of their cancer or because they fear losing their jobs, are having financial difficulties, or are upset about their inability to perform their normal daily activities.

Anemia, which is a common cause of fatigue, can be determined through blood tests. Depression scores can be determined through the use of various screens. No staging is available, however, for grading cancer-related fatigue.

Treatment and therapy: To be treated properly, the source of fatigue—whether is it physical, emotional, or psychological—must be determined. Because anemia is the most common cause of fatigue, blood tests generally are done to check for low red blood cell counts, low hemoglobin concentration, or both. Anemia can be corrected by blood transfusions or by administration of an erythropoiesis-stimulating protein, such as epoetin alfa.

Fatigue due to lack of sleep, depression, or poor nutrition generally can be helped by administration of supportive care, such as drugs, or correction of an underlying cause, such as the inability to shop for and prepare food.

Patients may be able to help themselves by being aware of what causes their fatigue. It may be important to schedule regular naps or limit the number of visitors. It is important to save energy for important tasks and to ask for help with other tasks. Energy levels may be maintained by scheduling regular eating times, including healthy snacks, limiting caffeine and alcohol, and drinking increased amounts of fluids. Some patients report that mild to moderate exercise also helps fight cancer-related fatigue, allows for a better frame of mind, and increases the ability to sleep at night. Exercise can include aerobic or resistance training. Relief of cancer-related fatigue may also come from practicing yoga or meditation. Research suggests that psychosocial interventions, such as group or individual therapy, education, stress management, or support groups, also have a positive effect on cancer-related fatigue.

Prognosis, prevention, and outcomes: Because cancer-related fatigue is often caused by many overlapping factors, it is difficult to predict which patients will be most affected. Fatigue may subside once treatments are completed and the patient's bone marrow has recovered. Fatigue may increase as the cancer stage progresses and the cancer spreads in the body.

MaryAnn Foote, M.S., Ph.D.

For Further Information

Hofman, Maarten, et al. "Cancer-Related Fatigue: The Scale of the Problem." *The Oncologist* 12 (May, 2007): 4-10.

Morrow, G. R. "Cancer-Related Fatigue: Causes, Consequences, and Management." *The Oncologist* 12 (May, 2007): 1-3.

Ryan, J. L., et al. "Mechanisms of Cancer-Related Fatigue." *The Oncologist* 12 (May, 2007): 22-34.

Other Resources

American Cancer Society
Exercise to Keep Active
Http://www.cancer.org/docroot/MIT/MIT_2_ 1x_ExerciseToStayActive.asp

Anemia.com
http://www.anemia.com

MedlinePlus
Anemia
http://www.nlm.nih.gov/medlineplus/anemia.html

National Cancer Institute
Fatigue

http://www.cancer.gov./cancerinfo/pdq/supportivecare/fatigue/Patient/page2

See also: Aids and devices for cancer patients; Anxiety; Chemotherapy; Home health services; Hospice care; Living with cancer; Palliative treatment; Psychosocial aspects of cancer; Radiation therapies; Relationships; Side effects; Stress management; Support groups; Symptoms and cancer

▶ Fever

Category: Diseases, Symptoms, and Conditions
Also known as: Hyperpyrexia

Related conditions: Infection and sepsis in cancer treatment, myelosuppression, neutropenia

Definition: Fever is a pyrogen-mediated elevation of the core body temperature. This is in distinction to hyperthermia, which is an unregulated rise in core temperature as occurs in heat stroke. Pyrogens may originate outside the body (exogenous) or be produced within the body (endogenous). The exogenous pyrogens are typically microorganisms or their toxins and products but also include drugs, antigen-antibody complexes, and other substances. Endogenous pyrogens are various chemicals produced by host cells and are called cytokines.

Risk factors: Fever may be caused by cancer. Although many types of malignant neoplasms may cause fever, some of the most common are lymphomas, leukemias and preleukemias, and renal cell carcinoma. However, fever in cancer patients is more often a consequence of treatment than of the cancer. The protective barrier provided by the skin and mucous membranes may be breached by surgery or vascular catheter placement, providing entrance points for invading microbes, which produce infection and fever. A similar phenomenon may result from chemotherapeutic cancer drugs that destroy not only the cancer cells but also oral and mucous membrane lining cells, inducing mucositis. Drugs may also kill bone marrow cells (myelosuppression and neutropenia), which impairs bodily defense mechanisms against infectious agents. The vascular catheters used to administer drugs, intravenous fluids, and blood components are risks for infection, and the risk increases the longer the catheter is left in place. Administration of blood components can produce fever through a variety of mechanisms.

The antibiotics used to treat infection, like many other drugs, may produce fever, complicating therapy. Some antibiotics, such as sulfonamides and chloramphenicol, can cause neutropenia and fever. Finally, antibiotics may alter the normal flora of the patient, allowing overgrowth of problem organisms. Fungi, such as those of the *Candida* species, may overgrow on the skin and in the gastrointestinal tract, causing infection. An anaerobic-toxin-producing bacterium called *Clostridium difficile* can overgrow in the colon, causing fever and diarrhea.

Venous thrombosis can also cause fever. Some cancers, especially adenocarcinomas, are associated with a hypercoagulable state. Venous stasis may be a consequence of an obstructing tumor mass or lymphadenopathy, immobility (bedrest or surgery), and dehydration. Some antineoplastic drugs can result in endothelial injury. All these factors can contribute to the formation of fever-associated thrombi.

Etiology and the disease process: Fever is a complex process and is not completely understood. The process is initiated by the production of endogenous pyrogens or cytokines. Cytokines are polypeptide proteins that are produced by host cells, probably mononuclear macrophages. Cytokines, including interleukin-1, tumor-necrosis factor, and interleukin-6, produce the rapid onset of fever by acting directly on the brain (hypothalamus). The release of cytokines is induced by the exogenous pyrogens or some endogenous molecules. Exogenous pyrogens are usually microbes and their products (including toxins). An example of an endogenous molecule would be a complement-binding antigen-antibody complex. Finally, the hypothalamus produces prostaglandin E2, which orchestrates physiologic changes that increase core temperature.

Fever is an adaptive response that, for the most part, is beneficial. Increased temperature is associated with increased production of antibacterial substances (superoxides and interferon), increased neutrophil migration, and increased T-cell proliferation, all of which are beneficial in the fight against invading microbes. Nonetheless, fever is metabolically demanding, and prolonged fever can be deleterious to the patient. High fever can damage organs and contribute to circulatory collapse or failure.

Incidence: The relationship between fever and cancer may be examined by looking first at fever in patients who are not diagnosed with cancer or any other causative disease process and second at fever in patients with a specific cancer that has already been diagnosed.

In patients with an undiagnosed fever or fever of undetermined origin, an underlying malignancy has been found to be causative in 9 to 30 percent of patients. Lymphoreticular neoplasms, such as Hodgkin disease and non-Hodgkin lymphoma, are the most common. The age of patients with fever of undetermined origin influences the percentage of neoplasms: Children tend to have fewer cancers and more infections, while elderly adults tend to have higher percentages of cancers.

The incidence of fever in patients in whom cancer is already diagnosed varies widely, as it depends on many variables, including the type and severity of the cancer, treatments employed, and comorbid illnesses. Fever is a common problem in cancer patients.

Symptoms: At the onset of a fever, body heat is conserved by vasoconstriction, and the patient initially feels cool, especially in the hands and feet. Shivering occurs when muscles act to produce heat. Finally, the patient feels warm as the higher setpoint for core temperature is reached. Sweating and vasodilatation (flushing) occur only with heat loss and the subsequent falling temperature.

Screening and diagnosis: For patients with fever of undetermined origin, a detailed history and careful physical examination are important and can provide critical information. Sometimes fever patterns themselves can be revealing. A sudden onset of fever, particularly if preceded by rigors or chills, is indicative of bacteremia or fungemia. Pel-Epstein fever is associated with Hodgkin disease and is characterized by three to ten days of fever followed by three to ten days without a fever. An initial battery of laboratory and radiologic tests is followed by an ordering sequence of more tests depending on the results of previous tests. Ultimately, a biopsy of an abnormal mass, lymph node, or bone marrow is usually required for diagnosis of a specific cancer as a cause of a fever with an undetermined origin.

Patients with previously diagnosed cancer present equally challenging problems in the determination of fever etiology. The most serious immediate issue is to determine if the patient has a life-threatening infection, and empiric antibiotic therapy is commonly administered as a safeguard. After a thorough history is taken and a physical examination is conducted, the patient will undergo screening blood and urine tests, radiologic studies, cultures of blood, and other tests to determine the possible sources of infection. If there are no indications of infection and empiric antibiotic therapy has no beneficial effect, then noninfectious causes must be sought. Drugs, venous thrombosis, and neoplastic fever are all possible. When other causes of fever have failed to be detected by any means and neoplastic fever appears likely, treating the patient with the nonsteroidal anti-inflammatory agent naproxen can aid in the diagnosis. Naproxen appears to have a unique ability to suppress tumor fever but not significantly effect fevers of nonneoplastic origin.

Treatment and therapy: Antipyretic therapy is generally provided only when the patient is uncomfortable or the fever is causing problems such as cardiovascular failure due to fever-induced tachycardia. The fever is not routinely treated because it is a continuing clue to the underlying diagnosis; treatment of the cause of the fever leads to final resolution.

Complicating infections are treated with antibiotics, and associated catheters and other foreign bodies are removed whenever possible. If infection is associated with neutropenia, granulocyte colony-stimulating factor is administered to restore the neutrophil numbers. Drugs are discontinued when necessary, and blood clots are removed or treated. Neoplastic fever can be treated with naproxen while the cancer is being removed or treated with other measures.

Prognosis, prevention, and outcomes: The prognosis depends on many factors but is often related to the ability to successfully control infection in the cancer patient with fever. Correspondingly, unresolved immunosuppression or uncontrolled neoplastic growth can render infections difficult or impossible to resolve. For most patients, successful treatment can be accomplished once a specific etiology for the fever has been established.

Prevention is mainly directed at infections complicating cancers and antineoplastic therapies. Careful management of vascular catheters, minimization of immunosuppressive periods, and prophylactic antibiotics during critical times can all help prevent infections and fever.

H. Bradford Hawley, M.D.

For Further Information

Chang, Jae C., and H. Bradford Hawley. "Neutropenic Fever of Undetermined Origin (N-FUO): Why Not Use the Naproxen Test?" *Cancer Investigation* 13 (1995): 448-450.

Cunha, Burke A., ed. "Fever." *Infectious Disease Clinics of North America* 10 (1996): 1-222.

Dinerello, Charles A., and Jeffrey A. Gelfand. "Fever and Hyperthermia." In *Harrison's Principles of Internal Medicine*, edited by Dennis L. Kasper et al. 16th ed. New York: McGraw-Hill, 2005.

Mackowiak, Philip A., ed. *Fever: Basic Mechanisms and Management*. 2d ed. Philadelphia: Lippincott Williams & Wilkins, 1997.

Murray, Henry W., ed. *FUO: Fever of Undetermined Origin*. New York: Futura, 1988.

Other Resources

American Cancer Society
Fever
http://www.cancer.org/docroot/MBC/content/MBC_2_3X_Fever.asp?sitearea=MBC

National Cancer Institute
Fever, Sweats, and Hot Flashes
http://www.cancer.gov/cancertopics/pdq/supportivecare/fever/Patient/page2

See also: Candidiasis; Coughing; Cytokines; Fatigue; Infection and sepsis; Mucositis; Myelosuppression; Nausea and vomiting; Neutropenia; Night sweats; Nonsteroidal Anti-Inflammatory Drugs (NSAIDs); Pneumonia; Side effects; Symptoms and cancer; Tumor lysis syndrome

▶ Fibroadenomas

Category: Diseases, Symptoms, and Conditions
Also known as: Complex fibroadenomas, juvenile fibroadenomas, giant fibroadenomas

Related conditions: Fibrocystic breast disease, cytosarcoma phyllodes, breast cysts

Definition: Fibroadenomas are benign breast tumors that are characteristically smooth-surfaced, round or oval in shape, and freely movable on palpation (feeling with the fingers). They can range in size from 1 to 15 centimeters (cm). A fibroadenoma consists of homogeneous (closely related) fibrous tissue. In rare instances, a fibroadenoma can contain a breast cancer. This is more likely in a complex fibroadenoma.

A complex fibroadenoma contains several specific tissue changes. They are sclerosing adenosis (hardening of glandular breast tissue) and apocrine metaplasia (conversion of milk-producing cells into an abnormal form). Although a fibroadenoma is not considered a precursor to breast cancer, it is thought that having a complex fibroadenoma slightly increases a woman's risk of developing breast cancer in the future.

Juvenile and giant fibroadenomas occur only in teenagers or young adults and can grow as large as 15 cm. Cytosarcoma phyllodes is a rare type of breast cancer that can occur within a fibroadenoma. Typically, this type of cancer does not spread beyond the breast tissue.

Risk factors: Fibroadenomas require the presence of estrogen to develop and grow, so they occur between menarche and menopause. Generally, after menopause, an existing fibroadenoma will stop growing and may even disappear. If a woman takes estrogen after menopause, she can develop a fibroadenoma.

Etiology and the disease process: A fibroadenoma arises from a single milk duct in the breast and is made up of both glandular (milk-producing cells) and epithelial cells (skin cells that line the duct). There is no fluid inside a fibroadenoma. It develops from an overgrowth of the affected breast tissue. The cause of the overgrowth of tissue is unknown, although estrogen is required for fibroadenoma development.

Fibroadenomas generally stop growing at 2 to 3 cm, although they occasionally grow larger. They may also enlarge during pregnancy and at times of higher estrogen levels during the menstrual cycle.

Immunosuppressive medications appear to have an effect on the growth and development of fibroadenomas. Studies have demonstrated that 50 percent of women who receive the immunosuppressive drug, cyclosporine, after a kidney transplant will develop one or more fibroadenomas.

Incidence: The fibroadenoma is the most common type of benign breast tumor. In women over the age of forty, 8 to 10 percent will develop a fibroadenoma at some time during their lives. Roughly one-third of fibroadenomas are complex fibroadenomas.

Symptoms: In women younger than age forty, fibroadenomas usually appear as palpable (can be felt) breast masses. After age forty, they may be discovered as a palpable breast mass, or they may appear on mammography as a breast mass that is not palpable. Fibroadenomas are not painful.

Screening and diagnosis: Screening is not carried out specifically for fibroadenomas, but some are picked up while screening for breast cancer in women over the age of forty. Breast fibroadenomas may be diagnosed by breast self-examination if they are palpable, or by mammography. On a mammogram, a fibroadenoma appears as a dense area in the breast, and in women over age forty, it may have areas of calcification (mineral deposits). Since it is not possible to determine whether a breast density is a fibroadenoma or breast cancer on mammography, subsequently, a breast ultrasound is performed. On an ultrasound, a fibroadenoma looks like a clear area with defined edges, much as a breast cyst does. The only way to determine whether a density is, indeed, a fibroadenoma is to biopsy it. A biopsy may be performed using a fine needle, a core needle, or surgical incision. A pathologist examines the tissue under a microscope and decides whether it is cancer or a fibroadenoma.

A cancer is present inside 3 percent of fibroadenomas. Typically, these fibroadenomas are larger than usual and have irregular margins that are less clearly defined. In 1 percent of cases, what appears to be a fibroadenoma is actually cytosarcoma phyllodes.

Because a fibroadenoma is not cancer, there is no staging for it. If breast cancer is found within a fibroadenoma, it is staged as a breast cancer.

Treatment and therapy: A fibroadenoma may be totally removed at the time of biopsy by surgical excision or core needle biopsy. If it is not removed, it will be monitored annually for growth and changes by mammography, magnetic resonance imaging (MRI), or ultrasound.

Prognosis, prevention, and outcomes: Since fibroadenomas are benign tumors, the prognosis is excellent for women who develop them. There is a slight increase in the risk of subsequently developing breast cancer. Before menopause, there is no way to prevent a fibroadenoma from developing. After menopause, a woman can prevent a fibroadenoma by avoiding any type of systemic estrogen therapy.

Christine M. Carroll, R.N., B.S.N., M.B.A.

For Further Information

Chinyama, Catherine N. *Benign Breast Disease: Radiology, Pathology, Risk Assessment*. New York: Springer, 2004.

Ganschow, Pamela, et al., eds. *Breast Health and Common Breast Problems: A Practical Approach*. Philadelphia: American College of Physicans, 2004.

Love, Susan, and Karen Lindsey. *Dr. Susan Love's Breast Book*. 5th ed. Cambridge, Mass.: Da Capo Press, 2005.

Other Resources

American Cancer Society
http://www.cancer.org

Imaginins.com
http://www.imaginis.com

WebMd
Breast, Fibroadenoma
http://www.emedicine.com/radio/topic109.htm

See also: Adenocarcinomas; Breast cancer in men; Breast cancer in pregnant women; Breast cancers; Breast ultrasound; Caffeine; Calcifications of the breast; Estrogen-receptor-sensitive breast cancer; Fibrocystic breast changes; Lumps; Phyllodes tumors

▶ Fibrocystic breast changes

Category: Diseases, Symptoms, and Conditions
Also known as: Fibrocystic conditions of the breast

Related conditions: Cysts, mastaglia, trigger-zone breast pain, fibroadenoma, fibrosis, hyperplasia

Definition: Fibrocystic changes in the breast are benign (noncancerous) and related to normal hormonal fluctuations during a woman's menstrual cycle. The word refers to thickening of tissue (fibro) and fluid-filled sacs (cysts) in the breast. The term loosely groups several different benign conditions, some of which can cause physical symptoms of discomfort or pain, known as mastaglia; other conditions may be visible on mammograms but not noticeable physically.

In the past, the term "fibrocystic breast disease" was used, a misleading label, given that the majority of women experience some breast changes or have mammograms that reveal them.

Risk factors: Women in their childbearing years or postmenopausal women taking hormone replacement therapy may be prone to several types of fibrocystic changes. Because these changes are related to menstrual-cycle hormones, they usually cease after natural menopause.

Etiology and the disease process: Fibrocystic breast changes are not a disease. They include several different categories of benign changes in breast tissue caused by the fluctuations of hormones during a woman's menstrual cycle. Each month a woman's body prepares for pregnancy, and hormones stimulate milk-producing cells, creating as much as three to six teaspoons of fluid within each breast, which is then reabsorbed if pregnancy does not occur. The fluid can collect in sacs and form cysts.

Breast pain may be cyclical, appearing at the time of a woman's ovulation or just before or during her menstrual period. Cyclical breast pain may be related to the presence of cysts and the pressure they cause. However, the number of cysts or the amount of lumpiness a woman has does not necessarily relate to the amount of pain she experiences. Cyclical pain is usually most intense at the beginning and the end of the childbearing years, in a woman's teens and again in her forties.

Pain also may be noncyclical, with no apparent pattern related to the menstrual schedule. Often it is in a specific area of the breast and is known as trigger-zone pain. It can be constant or intermittent. The reasons for noncyclical breast pain are unclear. For some women, old trauma, like a blow to the breast or a biopsy, is sometimes a cause of noncyclical pain. There is some evidence that for some women, different levels of the hormone progesterone or a sensitivity to hormones produced by the thyroid may be the cause of the pain.

Other breast changes included under the term "fibrocystic changes" include fibrosis and hyperplasia. Fibrosis occurs in some women when the normal fatty tissue of the breast is replaced over time with fibrous tissue, which may feel firm or rubbery. Some women develop extra cells within the lobules of the breast, the tubes designed to move milk through the breast. These areas of extra cells are called hyperplasia and show up only on mammograms. They are not cause for concern unless the cells begin to change from their normal shape. This rare condition is called atypical hyperplasia. It does not cause cancer.

Incidence: Varying estimates indicate that anywhere from 40 to 90 percent of women have some form of fibrocystic changes, which supports the theory that the symptoms are mostly related to normal changes in the breasts.

Symptoms: Symptoms of fibrocystic changes vary according to the type of change a woman experiences. She may have feelings of heaviness, tenderness, or swelling of the breasts. Cysts are usually felt as smooth and are generally round and movable when prodded. If they are deep within the breast, they may feel hard because of the breast tissue overlaying them. Cysts may simply cause a feeling of lumpiness throughout the breast, or because of pressure on the breasts caused by collected fluid within the cysts, they may cause tenderness or actual pain. However, pain cannot always be attributed to cysts or other specific causes. The amount of pain may differ between a woman's right and left breast. The intensity of pain can vary from month to month for the same woman. Breast pain can sometimes be intense enough to interfere with a woman's normal life.

Some women experience no physical symptoms, but breast examinations or mammograms may reveal cysts or areas of fibrosis.

Screening and diagnosis: It is important for a woman to become familiar with the way her breasts feel at different times of the month so that she can identify any obvious changes. Annual breast examinations as part of a physical examination are also important to track any changes. Women over age forty should have routine annual mammograms. If breast examination reveals suspect lumps, mammograms may be needed at an earlier age. Women with hyperplasia may need more frequent breast examinations or follow-up mammograms.

A woman should bring any defined lumps or masses or persistent breast pain to her doctor's attention. A doctor may attempt to aspirate a suspect lump with a fine needle to determine whether it is a cyst or a solid lump. If it is a cyst, the doctor can puncture the cyst with the needle and draw the fluid out of the cyst. In this case, generally no further action is needed. However, the doctor may choose to have a pathologist check the fluid for cancer cells. If a lump yields no fluid and proves to be solid, a mammogram is generally done for further diagnosis. The technology of ultrasound has been improved for the creation of diagnostic images of the breast. Although it is generally not a good tool for screening, it is useful in the further diagnosis of areas of concern first identified on mammograms. Because it uses sound waves to create images of the breast, ultrasound is particularly useful for distinguishing between cysts and solid masses and between benign and cancerous lumps. For women with fibrocystic changes in the breast, which often cause the breast tissue to be particularly dense and may make mammograms difficult for radiologists to read, ultrasound is often a more accurate diagnostic tool.

Biopsy may be required to analyze cells to rule out cancer. This can be done by a needle core biopsy, where a doctor removes a sample of cells from the area of the breast. Alternatively, it can be done by surgical biopsy, in which case the whole lump or suspect area is cut out of the breast.

Treatment and therapy: Cysts generally need no treatment. If a cyst is very large and therefore creates a lot of pressure resulting in pain, a doctor may use a needle to aspirate it and remove the fluid in the cyst as described above. Once the fluid is gone, this deflates the cyst and resolves the pressure it caused.

Most cyclical changes in the breast do not cause enough discomfort to require any treatment. Breast pain generally can be relieved with anti-inflammatory drugs such as ibuprofen or naproxen. A bra with good support, like a sports bra, can relieve pressure and the related pain. Birth control pills can be used to treat more intense breast pain because they level out the fluctuations in hormonal levels.

Some women have found relief from symptoms by consuming fewer products that contain caffeine (such as coffee, tea, and chocolate) or using primrose oil or other herbal remedies. However, research has not provided convincing data that these make a difference for women overall. There is some evidence that a low-fat diet may reduce symptoms of cyclical breast pain.

Prognosis, prevention, and outcomes: About 54 percent of benign breast conditions go away by themselves over time. None cause cancer. Only one, atypical hyperplasia, is associated with any added risk of cancer. Women with atypical hyperplasia who also have a family history of breast cancer may have a slightly increased risk of cancer over their lifetimes.

Charlotte Crowder, M.P.H., ELS

For Further Information

Chinyama, Catherine N. *Benign Breast Diseases: Radiology, Pathology, Risk Assessment.* New York: Springer, 2004.

Love, Susan, and Karen Lindsey. *Dr. Susan Love's Breast Book.* 5th ed. Cambridge, Mass.: Da Capo Press, 2005.

Mansel, R. E., ed. *Recent Developments in the Study of Benign Breast Disease: The Proceedings of the Fifth International Benign Breast Symposium.* Park Ridge, N.J.: Parthenon, 1993.

Other Resources

MayoClinic.com

Fibrocystic Breast Disease: Any Link to Cancer? http://www.mayoclinic.com/health/fibrocystic-breast-changes/AN00715

Medline Plus

Fibrocystic Breast Disease http://www.nlm.nih.gov/medlineplus/ency/article/000912.htm

See also: Breast cancers; Caffeine; Estrogen-receptor-sensitive breast cancer; Fibroadenomas; Lumps

▶ Fibrosarcomas, soft-tissue

Category: Diseases, Symptoms, and Conditions

Related conditions: Angiosarcoma, alveolar soft part sarcoma, clear-cell sarcoma, dermatofibrosarcoma protuberans, desmoid tumors, desmoplastic small-cell tumor, elastofibroma, epithelioid hemangioendothelioma, epithelioid sarcoma, fibroma, fibrous histiocytoma, fibromatosis, gastrointestinal stromal tumor, glomangiosarcoma, leiomyosarcoma, liposarcoma, lymphangiosarcoma, Kaposi sarcoma, musculoaponeurotic fibromatosis, neurofibrosarcoma, rhabdomyosarcoma, superficial fibromatosis, synovial sarcoma, and malignant versions of fibrous histiocytoma, granular cell tumor, hemangiopercytoma, mesenchymoma, peripheral nerve sheath tumor, and schwannoma

Definition: Fibrosarcomas are soft-tissue sarcomas (malignant tumors) of the fibroblasts, the cells that produce the fibrous tissues that connect, support, or surround other organs and tissues in the body (such as those around the joints). They usually occur in the arms, legs, or torso area, most commonly in the legs. They are one of many types of soft-tissue sarcomas. They are called "soft tissue" to distinguish them from osteosarcomas, tumors that develop in the bone. Fibrosarcomas are often grouped together with the other soft-tissue sarcomas because these diseases share certain characteristics and have similar treatment options.

Risk factors: Most soft-tissue sarcomas have no known cause. However, there are several factors that may increase the risk of developing these types of cancer. Radiation therapy, usually for other types of cancer, is the best-documented risk factor for this disease, possibly because radiation may inactivate the lymph nodes. Surgical removal of the lymph nodes also seems to play a part in development of this disease.

Another risk factor for this type of disease is exposure to certain chemicals, usually at the workplace. Chemicals that may cause this type of cancer are arsenic, herbicides, vinyl chloride, and wood preservatives.

This disease is also associated with certain genetic mutations. People with alterations in the *FH* gene, the *NF1* gene, the *TP53* tumor-suppressor gene, or the *RB1* gene and who have the diseases associated with these genetic mutations (Li-Fraumeni syndrome and neurofibromatosis, also called von Recklinghausen disease) are much more likely to develop soft-tissue sarcomas, including fibrosarcoma.

Other diseases that seem to increase the risk for soft-tissue sarcomas are basal-cell nevus syndrome, Gardner syndrome, tuberous sclerosis, and Werner syndrome.

Etiology and the disease process: Fibrosarcomas begin in the cells that develop fibrous tissues. They start as a lump in these fibrous tissues, usually those that surround the joints in the arms, legs, and torso. The lump is usually painless; however, the tumor may grow, pressing against other tissues such as nerves and muscles, and cause pain. These tumors can spread throughout the body, most commonly to the lungs.

Incidence: Soft-tissue sarcomas are rare, and developing fibrosarcoma is even rarer. Only about 9,000 new cases of soft-tissue sarcoma are diagnosed in the United States each year. This type of cancer is most common in people between the ages of twenty and sixty, with most patients being age fifty or older. However, it can occur in people of any age, including infants.

Symptoms: This type of cancer is most likely to develop in the arms, legs, or torso. It usually appears as a lump or mass and is not usually painful or swollen. There are generally no other symptoms.

Screening and diagnosis: No screening test is available for fibrosarcoma. The only way to accurately diagnose this type of tumor is with a biopsy, surgical removal of part of the tumor. The tumor section is then examined under a microscope to determine whether the cells are cancerous. These cells may also be tested for the genetic mutations that are risk factors in this disease to determine the most effective treatment.

Doctors may use a computed tomography (CT) scan or magnetic resonance imaging (MRI) to help diagnose and stage this disease. These tests can help determine the size of the tumor and whether its location will allow for surgical removal. The stages of this disease depend on how abnormal the cells of the tumor appear, the size of the tumor, and how likely the tumor is to begin to spread and grow.

Staging of this disease follows the TNGM system. These letters represent the size of the primary tumor (T), whether the disease has spread to the lymph nodes (N), the grade of the tumor (G), and whether the tumor has spread or metastasized (M).

The size of the tumor (T) is assigned a number based on the size of the primary tumor as follows:

- T1: Tumor is 5 centimeters or less.
- T1a: Superficial (near the surface) tumor
- T1b: Deep tumor
- T2: Tumor is larger than 5 centimeters.
- T2a: Superficial tumor
- T2b: Deep tumor

Lymph node involvement (N) is assigned a number as follows:

- N0: No evidence of cancer is found in nearby lymph nodes.
- N1: Evidence of cancer is found in nearby lymph nodes.

Stage at Diagnosis and Five-Year Relative Survival Rates for Soft Tissue Cancer, Including Heart Cancer, 1996-2004

Stage	*Cases Diagnosed (%)*	*Survival Rate (%)*
Localized[a]	53	84.7
Regional[b]	25	60.0
Distant[c]	15	16.0
Unstaged	7	54.2

Source: Data from National Cancer Institute, Surveillance Epidemiology and End Results, Cancer Stat Fact Sheets, 2008

[a]Cancer still confined to primary site

[b]Cancer has spread to regional lymph nodes or directly beyond the primary site

[c]Cancer has metastasized

The grade of the tumor is assigned a number as follows:

- G0: Grade of tumor cannot be assessed.
- G1: The tumor is well defined without reaching into surrounding tissues.
- G2: The tumor has moderately reached into surrounding tissues.
- G3: The tumor has reached well into surrounding tissues.
- G4: The tumor cannot be distinguished from surrounding tissues.

The spread of the disease (M) is divided into two categories:

- M0: No disease is present elsewhere in the body.
- M1: Disease is present in a distant body area.

After the TNGM state of the cancer is determined, a stage is assigned.

- Stage I: Low grade and either superficial or deep (G1 or G2, any T or N, and M at 0)
- Stage II: High grade and either superficial or deep (G3 or G4, any T or N, and M at 0)
- Stage III: High grade, large, and deep (G3 or G4, T2b, N and M at 0)
- Stage IV: Any spread of disease to lymph nodes or other sites (any G, any T, and either N1 or M1)

Treatment and therapy: Treatment for fibrosarcoma usually starts with surgery to remove the tumor and some of the healthy tissue surrounding it. The surgeon must ensure that all edges of the tumor have been removed, and sometimes this involves removing a large amount of tissue. In about 10 to 15 percent of cases, this may even involve amputation of an arm or leg to ensure that the entire tumor is removed; however, surgeons often try to use limb-sparing techniques to avoid amputation. Some patients may need reconstructive surgery after removal of the tumor.

Radiation therapy (using high-energy rays to kill the cancerous cells or implanting a tumor with radioactive materials) also may be used with this type of cancer, especially if the cancer's location makes it difficult to remove the entire tumor or avoid damaging other body parts. Radiation therapy may be used along with surgery to ensure that any cancerous cells that may have been left behind are killed. It may also be used when limb-sparing techniques were used to avoid amputation to ensure that any remaining cancer cells are killed.

Chemotherapy (using drugs in the blood stream to kill cancer cells) may also be used with fibrosarcomas. If the cancer has certain gene mutations, it may be treated with drugs specifically developed to target that mutation. Chemotherapy could be used before surgery to try to shrink the tumor before removal.

MRIs or CT scans may be used after surgical removal to determine if the entire tumor was removed and to make sure the tumor is not growing back.

Prognosis, prevention, and outcomes: Prognosis depends on the patient's age, the size of the tumor, how deep or superficial the tumor is, and the likelihood of the tumor's spread at the time of diagnosis.

Patients with soft-tissue sarcomas such as fibrosarcoma need to receive follow-up care to ensure that there is no recurrence of the disease.

Outcomes are generally better for patients who are less than sixty years old or have tumors smaller than 5 centimeters.

Marianne M. Madsen, M.S.

For Further Information

Baker, Laurence H., ed. *Soft Tissue Sarcomas*. Boston: Martinus Nijhoff, 1983.

Montgomery, Elizabeth, and Alan D. Aaron, eds. *Clinical Pathology of Soft-Tissue Tumors*. London: Informa Healthcare, 2001.

Pollock, Raphael E., ed. *Soft Tissue Sarcomas*. Lewiston, N.Y.: BC Decker, 2002.

Other Resources

American Cancer Society
http://cancer.org

National Cancer Institute
Soft Tissue Sarcomas: Questions and Answers
http://www.cancer.gov/cancertopics/factsheet/Sites-Types/soft-tissue-sarcoma

See also: Amputation; Bone cancers; Dermatofibrosarcoma protuberans (DFSP); Limb salvage; Mediastinal tumors; Sarcomas, soft-tissue

▶ 5Q minus syndrome

Category: Diseases, Symptoms, and Conditions
Also known as: 5Q-syndrome, 5QMS

Related conditions: Myelodysplastic syndrome

Definition: 5Q minus syndrome is a rare genetic disorder in which a portion of the long arm (Q) of chromosome 5 is missing. Production of blood cells is affected, and this syndrome can lead to treatment-resistant anemia. 5Q minus syndrome is one in a series of blood disorders collectively called myelodysplastic syndromes (MDS's).

Risk factors: Risk factors are unknown. Gene mutation is probably spontaneous, although there is not enough data to suggest a familial pattern of transmission.

Etiology and the disease process: Chromosomes are numbered by size and position of the centromere (point of connection of identical halves). Chromosome 5 is a large chromosome. In 5Q minus syndrome, a portion of the deoxyribonucleic acid (DNA) in the long arm (Q) is absent, leading to lack of output from the missing genes. These genes define growth and differentiation of cells that manufacture most of the blood cells. Thus, bone marrow cells are often deformed and have abnormal growth and maturation. Other missing genes code for interleukins, chemical signals involved in immune protection.

Incidence: Although most forms of myelodysplastic syndromes are secondary and show up increasingly with age, 5Q minus syndrome is congenital and shows up early in life.

Symptoms: The primary symptoms are anemia, low total white cell count, and increased bone marrow blast cells. Patients with 5Q minus syndrome also have elevated platelet counts, something that distinguishes this group from other myelodysplastic syndromes. Because red blood cells are not manufactured properly, patients are anemic and require regular transfusions of red blood cells. In many cases, this anemia fails to respond to transfusions or other stimuli.

Screening and diagnosis: Total white blood cell count, monocyte and platelet count, and bone marrow biopsy are the best diagnostic tools. A definitive karyotype (analysis of chromosome count and pattern) helps to set 5Q minus syndrome apart from other myelodysplastic syndromes.

Treatment and therapy: There have been few breakthroughs in therapy. Hematopoietic growth factors and granulocyte-macrophage colony-stimulating factor have been tried with little success. Immunosuppressive drugs do not help most patients. One study involving the experimental leukemia drug lenalidomide showed substantial improvement to the point of being transfusion independent and going into cytogenic remission (the genetic abnormality was no longer displayed). Studies with bone marrow transplantation in patients with myelodysplastic syndromes have shown positive results, but no specific data on those patients with 5Q minus syndrome have been published.

Prognosis, prevention, and outcomes: Due to the rarity of this disease, prognosis is difficult to quantify. Progression to acute leukemia generally occurs, and long-term outcome is poor.

Kerry L. Cheesman, Ph.D.

See also: Acute Myelocytic Leukemia (AML); Anemia; Bone marrow aspiration and biopsy; Bone Marrow Transplantation (BMT); Chromosomes and cancer; Colony-Stimulating Factors (CSFs); Interleukins; Leukemias; Leukopenia; Myelodysplastic syndromes; Myelosuppression; Transfusion therapy

▶ Gallbladder cancer

Category: Diseases, Symptoms, and Conditions
Also known as: Gallbladder carcinoma

Related conditions: Bile duct cancer (cholangiocarcinoma)

Definition: Gallbladder cancer is a rare cancer that starts in the lining of the gallbladder. The gallbladder stores bile, a liquid necessary for the breakdown of fat. The vast majority of gallbladder cancers—more than 80 percent—are of a type known as adenocarcinoma. Other types of gallbladder cancer include squamous cell carcinoma and small-cell carcinoma.

Risk factors: Gallbladder cancer occurs more frequently in women than in men (a 4:1 ratio) and usually in people older than age fifty, with most patients in their mid- to late sixties. In the United States, Native Americans and Hispanics are at the highest risk for the disease. Worldwide, high incidence of the disease occurs in Chile, Bolivia, and parts of Asia. Obesity and a sedentary lifestyle have been identified as risk factors for gallbladder cancer.

About 80 percent of gallbladder cancer patients have gallstones. However, only 0.5 percent of patients with gallstones will go on to develop gallbladder cancer. Cysts in the bile ducts also raise the risk of gallbladder cancer. Calcification (hardening) in parts of the gallbladder increases the risk of gallbladder cancer. People with calcifications throughout the entire gallbladder wall have no higher risk than the general population.

Etiology and the disease process: There is strong circumstantial evidence that gallbladder cancer results from constant inflammation of the gallbladder. Gallstone disease causes repeated irritation and inflammation of the gallbladder. Most patients with gallbladder cancer have gallstones in addition to their cancer. Patients with large gallstones (greater than 3 centimeters, or cm) are at ten times the risk for developing gallbladder cancer. Also supporting the inflammation theory is the fact that repeated infections in the gallbladder seem to increase a person's risk of this cancer.

Gallbladder cancer spreads through the lymph nodes and lymph vessels as well as the blood vessels. Lymph vessels, which extend into every organ in the body, collect abnormal or foreign cells into the lymph nodes. This is why gallbladder cancer surgery often includes removal of the lymph nodes in the area of the gallbladder, liver, and pancreas.

Another route through which the cancer spreads is directly into the liver. Because there is no separation between the gallbladder and liver tissues, a gallbladder tumor can directly enter the liver.

Incidence: The disease is rare. There are approximately 7,000 new cases of gallbladder cancer each year in the United States. According to the American Cancer Society, the incidence of the disease decreased by 50 percent between 1973 and 2007. On average, there are 2.5 cases of the disease for every 100,000 people in the United States.

Symptoms: Unfortunately, symptoms of gallbladder cancer do not appear until the disease is advanced. When they do appear, they are not specific and are often identical to symptoms of other (benign) gallbladder or liver

problems. Symptoms of gallbladder cancer may include the following:
- Enlarged liver
- Fever
- Jaundice (yellowing of the skin and whites of the eyes)
- Loss of appetite
- Nausea or vomiting
- Pain in the upper right part of the abdomen
- Severe itching
- Swelling of the stomach due to fluid accumulation (ascites)
- Weight loss

Screening and diagnosis: There is no test to screen for gallbladder cancer. Because the symptoms are often the same as for other liver or biliary diseases, unless doctors find the cancer during surgery to remove gallstones, diagnosis is usually delayed until the cancer is advanced and symptoms appear.

Tests for suspected gallbladder cancer include the following:
- A complete physical examination
- Liver function tests
- Cancer antigen (CA) 19-9 assay (while this test identifies a marker that is not specific for gallbladder cancer, it may focus suspicion in combination with other test results)
- Endoscopic retrograde cholangiopancreatography (ERCP), an X ray of the bile ducts that uses a lighted tube (endoscope) passed from the mouth to the small intestine; a smaller tube inside the endoscope delivers a special dye into the bile ducts, and X rays of the dye can help diagnose blockage or narrowing of the ducts
- Blood tests, which may show abnormal amounts of certain chemicals in the blood
- Percutaneous transhepatic cholangiography (PTHC), an X ray of the liver and bile ducts during which a special dye is injected into the liver and X rays follow the dye through the bile ducts; PTHC helps diagnose blockage or narrowing of the bile ducts
- Biopsy, the examination of a tissue sample under a microscope
- Computed tomography (CT) scan and magnetic resonance imaging (MRI), usually the best diagnostic tools to verify gallbladder cancer

In the United States, staging of gallbladder cancer is done according to the criteria of the American Joint Commission on Cancer (AJCC). These criteria use the TNM (tumor/lymph nodes/metastasis) staging system, which looks at the tumor location, whether the cancer has invaded any near or distant lymph nodes, and whether the cancer has spread (metastasized) to other parts of the body. The TNM system for gallbladder cancer is as follows:
- TX: Primary tumor cannot be evaluated.
- T0: No evidence of primary tumor is found.
- Tis: The cancer is limited to the innermost layer of the gallbladder (mucosa).
- T1a: The tumor invades the lamina propria (the layer next to the mucosa).
- T1b: The tumor invades the muscle layer (the next layer).
- T2: The tumor invades the layer surrounding the muscle; it does not extend beyond the outer covering of the gallbladder (serosa) or into the liver.
- T3: The tumor goes through the serosa or into the liver or one other organ, such as the stomach, small intestine, or pancreas.
- T4: The tumor invades the main portal vein (connecting the digestive tract to the liver) or hepatic artery, or invades multiple organs outside the liver.
- NX: Regional lymph nodes cannot be assessed.
- N0: No regional lymph node spread is found.
- N1: Regional lymph node spread is found.
- MX: Distant metastasis cannot be assessed.
- M0: No distant metastasis is found.
- M1: Distant metastasis is found.

Staging is as follows:
- Stage 0: Tis, N0, M0
- Stage IA: T1, N0, M0
- Stage IB: T2, N0, M0
- Stage IIA: T3, N0, M0
- Stage IIB: T1, N1, M0; T2, N1, M0; or T3, N1, M0

Stage at Diagnosis and Five-Year Relative Survival Rates for Gallbladder Cancer, 1988-2001

Stage	*Cases Diagnosed (%)*	*Survival Rate (%)*
Localized[a]	21.5	41.7
Regional[b]	39.9	13.6
Distant[c]	35.9	1.2
Unstaged	2.7	13.1

Source: Data from L. A. G. Ries et al., eds., Cancer Survival Among Adults: U.S. SEER Program, 1988-2001—Patient and Tumor Characteristics, NIH Pub. No. 07-6215 (Bethesda, Md.: National Cancer Institute, 2007)

[a]Cancer still confined to primary site

[b]Cancer has spread to regional lymph nodes or directly beyond the primary site

[c]Cancer has metastasized

- Stage III: T4, any N, M0
- Stage IV: Any T, any N, M1

Treatment and therapy: Currently, the only realistic treatment option is surgery. Removal of the gallbladder can cure patients with Stage 0 or I cancer, and the cure rate is 80 to 100 percent.

There are several types of gallbladder removal surgery (cholecystectomy):

- Simple cholecystectomy: Removal of the gallbladder alone
- Extended cholecystectomy: Removal of the gallbladder, a small area of the liver right next to the gallbladder, and area lymph nodes
- Radical cholecystectomy: Removal of the gallbladder, a wedge-shaped part of the liver, the common bile duct, tissues between the liver and the small intestine, and the lymph nodes along the path between the liver and the small intestine

The type of surgery a patient will have depends on how the cancer was found and how advanced it is.

When surgery is not a treatment option, palliative surgery may help relieve symptoms. Palliative surgery is not intended to treat or control the disease.

Follow-up radiation after surgery helps prolong survival in some patients. Chemotherapy may be added to surgery and radiation. Two chemotherapy drugs that show some success in treating gallbladder cancer are 5-fluorouracil (5-FU) and gemcitabine. Radiation and chemotherapy (alone or in combination) can also be used before surgery to try to shrink a large tumor.

When surgery is no longer an option, patients should consider enrolling in clinical trials of new treatments.

Prognosis, prevention, and outcomes: Because the disease is often diagnosed at an advanced stage, the prognosis is usually poor. The median survival time from diagnosis is less than six months. The five-year survival rate is 5 percent. However, the prognosis depends on the stage of the cancer at diagnosis. When diagnosed early (usually during surgery to remove gallstones), patients can be completely cured.

Lifestyle modifications, such as weight loss and an exercise program, may help prevent gallbladder cancer.

Adi Ferrara, B.S.

For Further Information

Icon Health. *Gallbladder Cancer: A Medical Dictionary, Bibliography, and Annotated Research Guide to Internet References*. San Diego, Calif.: Author, 2004.

Ko, A., E. H. Rosenbaum, and M. Dollinger. *Everyone's Guide to Cancer Therapy: How Cancer Is Diagnosed, Treated, and Managed Day to Day*. 5th ed. Kansas City, Mo.: Andrews McMeel, 2007.

Sarg, M. J., and A. D. Gross. *The Cancer Dictionary*. 3d ed. New York: Facts On File, 2006.

Other Resources

American Cancer Society
Detailed Guide: Gallbladder Cancer
Http://www.cancer.org/docroot/CRI/CRI_2_3x.asp?rnav=cridg&dt=68

Clinical Trials Registry
http://clinicaltrials.gov/

National Cancer Institute
Gallbladder Cancer
http://www.cancer.gov/cancertopics/types/gallbladder/

See also: Bile duct cancer; CA 19-9 test; Cholecystectomy; Endoscopic Retrograde Cholangiopancreatography (ERCP); Endoscopy; Gastrointestinal cancers; Hepatic Arterial Infusion (HAI); Laparoscopy and laparoscopic surgery; Nuclear medicine scan; Obesity-associated cancers; Pancreatitis; Percutaneous Transhepatic Cholangiography (PTHC); Ultrasound tests

▶ Gardner syndrome

Category: Diseases, Symptoms, and Conditions
Also known as: Gardner's syndrome, familial adenomatous polyposis, familial polyposis coli, hereditary adenomatosis of the colon and rectum, bone tumor-epidermoid cyst-polyposis

Related conditions: Colon and rectal polyps, cancer

Definition: Familial adenomatous polyposis (FAP)PolypscolonColonpolypsGardner syndrome is a rare, genetically linked disorder that is classified as a variant form of familial adenomatous polyposis (FAP). FAP constitutes a group of disorders most commonly identified by the growth of numerous polyps in the large intestine or colon. In patients with Gardner syndrome, large amounts of benign tissue form in multiple organs. As with FAP, this includes colon polyps as well as skull tumors, cysts and fibrous tumors in the skin, extra teeth, and a congenital eye condition known as congenital hypertrophy of the retinal pigmented epithelium. Gardner syndrome significantly increases an affected patient's risk of developing colorectal cancer, small bowel cancer, pancreatic cancer, and papillary thyroid cancer. Early diagnosis of the disorder is essential, as colon polyps resulting from Gardner syndrome have a 100 percent chance of becoming cancerous.

Risk factors: Gardner syndrome is genetically linked, meaning that it is associated with a defect, or mutation, in one or more genes. A patient with immediate family members who have the disease or carry the defective gene is at high risk of developing this disorder. It is also estimated that 20 percent of patients do not have a family history of Gardner syndrome or FAP, which indicates a spontaneous mutation of the gene.

Etiology and the disease process: There are two forms of Gardner Syndrome affecting the same genes, one is autosomal dominant which would have a probability of 50% if one of the parents was affected. The second is an autosomal recessive mutation which would require both parents to carry the disease, resulting in a 25% probability of offspring inheriting the trait.

This disease is caused by a mutation in the *APC* (adenomatous polyposis coli) gene. The APC protein regulates levels of another protein called "β-catenin." β-Catenin controls the expression of a host of genes that stimulate cell growth and proliferation. Defective versions (or "alleles") of the APC gene increase cellular levels of β-catenin, which causes increased cellular proliferation. Uncontrolled growth of the colonic epithelial cells causes the cells to undergo the adenoma-to-carcinoma transition (or sequence) that drives cells in the colon to increase in number and form an adenomatous polyp that projects into the lumen of the colon. Most people who inherit this defective gene develop the disease. Although the development of Gardner syndrome varies from person to person, it always presents a high risk of developing polyps, tumors, and cancer, especially in the colon. Other physical changes (with their percentage of risk when known) include congenital hypertrophy of the retinal pigmented epithelium (55 to 88 percent), epidermoid cysts (53 percent), stomach and small intestine polyps (90 percent), thyroid cancer, desmoids (10 to 35 percent), dental abnormalities (70 percent), hepatoblastoma, and bone tumors.

Incidence: Gardner syndrome is rare, with only 1 case per 1 million people, while the incidence of FAP is much more common, with 1 case per 8,000 people. An increased risk for the development of thyroid cancer and desmoid tumors has been observed in women with Gardner syndrome. In many cases, diagnosis of the disease can be performed by dentists who treat children for the unique dental abnormalities associated with this disease. Most patients with Gardner syndrome have are diagnosed with polyps by the time they reach puberty. 80 to 90 percent of polyps are located in the left colon, including the splenic flexure and descending, sigmoid, and rectosigmoid colons. Cancers typically develop between ages twenty and thirty but can occur at any age.

Symptoms: Patients with Gardner syndrome may experience a wide variety of symptoms. The most common are gastrointestinal symptoms, including rectal bleeding, pain, diarrhea or constipation, nausea, and vomiting. Multiple cysts may be found on the patient's body, particularly on the face, scalp, and extremities; hey usually cause no symptoms but may become itchy or inflamed.

Screening and diagnosis: When a person has a family history of Gardner syndrome, a genetic analysis can detect mutations in the APC gene. A positive test result for an APC mutation is sufficient for diagnosis. Laboratory testing to determine the extent of the disease includes stool samples for occult blood, thyroid function studies, and liver function tests as well as basic chemistries, blood cell counts, and electrolyte levels. Imaging studies include upper and lower gastrointestinal series, esophagogastroduodenoscopy, colonoscopy, computed tomography (CT) scanning, magnetic resonance imaging (MRI), and ultrasonography to screen for polyps and tumors, as well as skull, facial, and dental X rays to evaluate oral abnormalities and screen for tumors. Most testing procedures should be performed on an annual basis after initial diagnosis.

Treatment and therapy: Extensive surgery is indicated when colon polyps are identified in a patient with Gardner syndrome because of the risk of colon cancer. Osteomas of the skull and dental abnormalities should be removed if they interfere with normal function or are deforming. Cysts on the skin may require removal if they are producing symptoms or are disfiguring. The necessity of surgery to remove other tumors is evaluated based on their location, type of tumor, patient's surgical risk, and potential risks of not removing them.

Chemotherapy, using doxorubicin with dacarbazine (imidazole carboxamide) or high-dose tamoxifen, has been shown to reduce polyps following colon surgery. Treatment with sulindac, a nonsteroidal anti-inflammatory drug, is recommended for every patient following a total colectomy; oral calcium has been shown to reduce the colon cancer risk; and sulindac, tamoxifen, or a combination of both is recommended for other manifestations of the disease. Research into other treatments, including gene therapy, is ongoing.

Prognosis, prevention, and outcomes: The five-year survival rate for patients older than forty-five who do not have surgery to remove the colon is 0 percent, but with surgery, it is nearly 100 percent. The recurrence rate after surgery ranges from 30 percent in twenty years to 45 percent in thirty years. There is no prevention for Gardner syndrome.

Annette O' Connor, Ph.D.

For Further Information

Butler, J., Healy, C., Toner, M., & Flint, S. (2005). Gardner syndrome: Review and report of a case. *Oral Oncology Extra,* 5(41), 89-92.

Hansmann, A., Adolph, C., Vogel, T., Unger, A., & Moeslein, G. (2004). High-dose tamoxifen and sulindac as first-line treatment for desmoid tumors. *Cancer,* 100(3), 612-620.

Pomery, Chris. (2004). DNA and family history. Toronto, Ontario: Dundurn Press Limited.

Half, E., Bercovich, D., & Rozen, P. (2009). Familial adenomatous polyposis. *Orphanet Journal of Rare Diseases,* 4, 22.

Other Resources

National Institutes of Health
https://rarediseases.info.nih.gov/gard/6482/gardner-syndrome/resources/1

The rare genetic disease center of the NIH provided this article that includes up to date information on diagnosis treatment and other current news and events
https://rarediseases.info.nih.gov/gard/6482/gardner-syndrome/resources/1

Medscape: Gardner's Syndrome
http://emedicine.medscape.com/article/190486-overview

A detailed discussion regarding various aspects of the genetics, manifestations, treatment and prognosis written for the lay person.

Medicine Net: Gardner Syndrome
http://www.medicinenet.com/gardner_syndrome/article.htm

This site answers a variety of questions for patients which includes information about current treatment protocols and has links to other information sources.

See also: Bone cancers; Colon polyps; Desmoid tumors; Fibrosarcomas, soft-tissue; Hereditary polyposis syndromes; Sarcomas, soft-tissue; Thyroid cancer; Turcot syndrome

▶ Gastric polyps

Category: Diseases, Symptoms, and Conditions
Also known as: Stomach polyps

Related conditions: Gastritis, familial adenomatous polyposis, Peutz-Jeghers syndrome, gastric carcinoid tumors

Definition: Gastric polyps are small tissue growths on the lining of the stomach.

Risk factors: Risk factors for gastric polyps are chronic inflammation and the long-term use of proton pump inhibitors.

Etiology and the disease process: The cause of gastric polyps is not completely understood. Hyperplastic polyps are thought to arise from irritation or chronic inflammation of the stomach lining. The nature of the causative agent has not been clearly established; suggested irritants include coffee, tea, and gastric acid. Long-term use of proton pump inhibitors is associated with development of hyperplastic and carcinoid polyps; this may be related to the decrease in stomach acid, which in turn causes an increase in gastrin, a hormone that supports cell growth. Familial cancer syndromes such as familial adenomatous polyposis and Peutz-Jeghers syndrome have been linked with gastric polyps, suggesting that genetic mutations have a role in polyp formation.

Incidence: The largest endoscopic study, of almost 13,000 patients during a four-year period, showed that gastric polyps were found in 157 patients (1.2 percent). About 66 percent of the gastric polyps were in patients over age sixty. The gastric polyps were hyperplastic (75.6 percent), inflammatory (17.8 percent), and adenomatous (6.6 percent). No correlation with stomach cancer and no gender preponderance were found with gastric polyps.

Symptoms: Patients usually have no symptoms. However, if they are symptomatic, they may develop bleeding from the stomach or obstruction (blockage of the digestive tract).

Screening and diagnosis: Most gastric polyps are discovered and diagnosed incidentally when endoscopy of the stomach is performed for an unrelated reason. Upper endoscopy is a procedure using an endoscope, a flexible tube with a small camera and an instrument for biopsy that is introduced through the upper digestive tract; it allows visual examination of the esophagus, stomach, and upper duodenum, the first part of the small intestine.

No staging is applicable for gastric polyps.

Treatment and therapy: Gastric polyps can be removed during endoscopy and examined in the laboratory. Multiple polyps may require removal of the largest polyp and sampling from the remaining polyps; there is no need to remove all polyps. Treatment will be based on the nature of these polyps.

Prognosis, prevention, and outcomes: The majority of gastric polyps are benign. Hyperplastic polyps are also generally benign. The polyps associated with familial adenomatous polyposis and Peutz-Jeghers syndrome can become adenomatous in nature. Adenomatous polyps have an increased risk for cancer transformation; therefore, regular surveillance with upper endoscopy is warranted for these familial conditions.

Miriam E. Schwartz, M.D., M.A., Ph.D., and Colm A. Ó'Moráin, M.A., M.D., M.Sc., D.Sc.

See also: Achlorhydria; Adenocarcinomas; Adenomatous polyps; Barium swallow; Gastrinomas; Gastrointestinal cancers; Gastrointestinal oncology; Gastrointestinal Stromal Tumors (GISTs); *Helicobacter pylori*; Krukenberg tumors; Small intestine cancer; Stomach cancers

▶ Gastrinomas

Category: Diseases, Symptoms, and Conditions
Also known as: Gastrin-secreting tumors, Zollinger-Ellison syndrome, nonislet cell pancreatic cancer

Related conditions: Peptic ulcers, gastroesophageal reflux disease (GERD), multiple endocrine neoplasia type 1 (MEN 1), liver cancer

Definition: Gastrinomas are slow-growing tumors that secrete large quantities of the peptide hormone gastrin. Gastrinomas most often arise in the wall of the duodenum, the pancreas, or the pancreatic lymph nodes.

Risk factors: Gastrinomas arise spontaneously or in association with the rare genetic disorder multiple endocrine neoplasia type 1 (MEN 1). Men have double the risk of developing gastrinoma relative to women. Approximately 60 percent of all MEN 1 patients will develop pancreatic gastrinomas.

Etiology and the disease process: The large amount of gastrin produced by gastrinomas causes the stomach to produce massive quantities of acid. The acid causes ulcers to form in the stomach and duodenum and can irritate and inflame the esophagus. The acid also produces water and ion imbalances in the small intestine, resulting in diarrhea. More than 50 percent of gastrinomas are malignant, usually metastasizing to nearby lymph nodes and the liver.

Incidence: Gastrinomas are exceedingly rare tumors, occurring in 1 to 3 people per million. Gastrinomas are usually diagnosed when people are in their forties but can occur at any age.

Symptoms: The most common symptom of gastrinoma is persistent upper abdominal pain due to severe or recurring ulcers. Chronic diarrhea is the second most frequent symptom, followed by heartburn. Other symptoms include nausea, vomiting, weight loss, and ulcer-related gastrointestinal bleeding.

Screening and diagnosis: Initial diagnosis is made by measuring gastrin levels in the blood and acid output by the stomach after an overnight fast. Elevated levels of both are a presumptive diagnosis of gastrinoma. Somatostatin receptor scintigraphy is the preferred imaging technology to locate the tumor and check for metastasis.

Treatment and therapy: Treatment of gastrinoma involves controlling acid production and surgical removal of tumors. Proton pump inhibitor medications are the most potent agents to block acid secretion. Chemotherapy with streptomycin, 5-fluorouracil, and doxorubicin can shrink tumors and control metastasis-associated symptoms but does not prolong survival time.

Prognosis, prevention, and outcomes: The five-year survival rate for patients with isolated, operable tumors is 86 percent, and surgery is curative in 20 to 30 percent of cases. For patients with liver metastasis or numerous, diffuse tumors, the five-year survival rate is 20 percent. Tumors that have spread to the liver are usually inoperable and are the main cause of death in gastrinoma patients. Tumor recurrence is monitored by regular screening of fasting gastrin levels. Lifelong treatment with medications to control acid production is often necessary.

Pamela S. Cooper, Ph.D.

See also: Cyclin-dependent kinase inhibitor-2A (*CDKN2A*); Endocrinology oncology; Gastrointestinal cancers; Islet cell tumors; Liver cancers; Multiple endocrine neoplasia type 1 (MEN 1); Neuroendocrine tumors; Pancreatic cancers; Small intestine cancer; Stomach cancers; Zollinger-Ellison syndrome

▶ Gastrointestinal cancers

Category: Diseases, Symptoms, and Conditions
Also known as: Abdominal and intestinal neoplasms

Related conditions: Cancer of the gallbladder and bile duct, pancreas, and liver; a *Helicobacter pylori* infection; pernicious anemia; acid reflux disease; gastric polyps; familial polyposis; ulcerative colitis; Crohn disease

Definition: Gastrointestinal cancers are malignant tumors in the various organs of the gastrointestinal tract—the esophagus, stomach, colon, small intestine, rectum, and anus—formed when normal cells enlarge and divide abnormally.

Risk factors: Major risk factors for developing gastrointestinal cancers are age, gender, race, tobacco use, exposure to carcinogens, family history, and diet. Esophageal cancer and cancer of the small intestine usually appear after a person reaches the age of sixty; stomach, over fifty-five; colorectal, over fifty; and anal, over forty.

Four times as many men as women develop esophageal cancer, and twice as many men as women get stomach cancer. More women are likely to have anal cancer of the inner part of the anus, while more men have outer involvement. African Americans are more likely to have gastric cancer than white Americans. Tobacco use may put people at risk for esophageal and gastric cancer.

Exposure to rubber, leather, or certain dyes increases the risk of esophageal cancer, while industrial dusts and fumes increase the risk for gastric cancer. Exposure to nitrosamine is a factor for cancer of the small intestine. A family history of polyps increases risk for gastric cancer. A history of some types of polyps; ulcerative colitis; cancer of the breast, ovary, or uterus; and cancer among first-degree relatives are risk factors for colon cancer.

Diet is a greater risk factor for gastric cancer in Japan, Korea, parts of Eastern Europe, and Latin America than in the United States, possibly because of diets high in dried, smoked, salted, and pickled foods. Diets high in fat and low in fruits, vegetables, and other high-fiber foods are risk factors for colorectal cancer.

Although cancer of the small intestine is unusual, certain inherited disorders may be risk factors. A history of genital warts, fistulas, fissures, genital herpes, gonorrhea, radiation dermatitis, homosexuality, symptomatic human immunodeficiency virus (HIV) disease, hemorrhoids, or anal degenerative skin changes increases the risk of anal cancer.

Etiology and the disease process: Although the causes of many gastrointestinal cancers are unknown, for some of these cancers, causative agents or factors have been found. Alcohol and tobacco abuse appear to be causes of esophageal cancer in North America; in other parts of the world, exposure to environmental carcinogens and diets deficient in riboflavin, magnesium, nicotinic acid, and zinc are causative factors. Chewing betel nuts and smoking bidi are major factors in India. The exact cause of stomach cancer is unknown, but carcinogens, notably nitrites found in smoked foods or used as preservatives, are suspect. Risk factors for colorectal cancer are diets high in saturated fat and low in fiber and calcium, a lack of exercise, and parasitic infestation of *Schistosomiasis japonicum*. Cancer of the small intestine is rare, and its causes are unknown. The primary cause of anal cancer is chronic irritation.

Incidence: Incidence rates vary by the affected digestive tract organ. Esophageal cancer occurs much more often in China, Singapore, Iran, Puerto Rico, Switzerland, and France than in North America. In the United States, three times as many men as women are stricken, and blacks outnumber whites 3.5 to 1. Stomach and colorectral cancer is most common in industrialized countries with high living standards; colorectal cancer is uncommon in Asian and Third World countries. Environmental and dietary factors in westernized countries probably account for the higher incidence. Cancer of the small intestine is almost twice as common in men as in women, and blacks are almost twice as likely to have it as whites. It is rare among American Indians and native Alaskans, and relatively rare among Hispanics and Asians and Pacific Islanders. Anal cancer accounts for only 1 percent or 2 percent of gastrointestinal cancers worldwide.

Symptoms: Symptoms vary depending on the part of the gastrointestinal tract that is affected. Esophageal cancer is marked by difficulty in swallowing; a feeling of fullness,

Estimated New Cases and Deaths from Gastrointestinal Cancers in 2008

Cancer	*Newly Diagnosed Cases*	*Deaths*
Esophagus	16,470	14,280
Stomach	21,500	10,880
Colon and rectum	148,810	49,960
Small intestine	6,110	1,100
Anus	5,070	680

Source: Data from National Cancer Institute, Surveillance Epidemiology and End Results, Cancer Stat Fact Sheets, 2008

pressure, or burning as food passes down the tract; indigestion; heartburn; vomiting; choking on food; weight loss; coughing and hoarseness; and pain behind the breastbone or in the throat. Stomach cancer may present no symptoms in the early stages; later, they are often vague and include indigestion or heartburn; abdominal pain or discomfort; nausea and vomiting; diarrhea or constipation; bloating after meals; loss of appetite; weakness and fatigue; and vomiting of blood or bloody stools. Colorectal cancer symptoms result from local obstruction or, in more advanced stages, from extension to adjacent organs. In early stages, symptoms are usually vague and vary according to the location of the tumor. In later stages, symptoms include pallor, cachexia, ascites, enlarged liver, and dilatation of lymphatic vessels. About 10 percent of people with cancer of the small intestine experience no symptoms, but most patients have abdominal pain or distension because of obstruction, as well as weight loss, nausea and vomiting, fever, change in bowel habits, and general malaise. Anal cancer may exhibit no symptoms in early stages; later, there may be bleeding, pressure, pain, itching, and a palpable mass.

Screening, diagnosis, and staging: Routine screening tests for gastrointestinal cancers are not generally performed, but a colonoscopy is used in people over the age of fifty to look for signs of polyps that might lead to colon cancer.

People should monitor digestive symptoms, particularly if these change or if they develop gastrointestinal reflux desease (acid reflux, or GERD), and immediately discuss such symptoms with their doctor. After symptoms have appeared, diagnosis usually begins with the physician performing a physical examination and taking a family medical history. Endoscopy, biopsy, and imaging tests such as a barium swallow, computed tomography (CT), and magnetic resonance imaging (MRI) are used for further study.

When symptoms of esophageal cancer appear, a thorough family medical history is done and a complete physical examination is performed. An X-ray study (barium swallow) or an esophagoscopy can find changes in the shape of the esophagus. The doctor can do a tissue biopsy through the endoscope and brush cells from the esophageal wall for examination by a pathologist. If cancer is found, additional tests to determine the extent of involvement include a CT scan, an MRI scan, a laryngoscopy, or a bronchoscopy. These tests will determine staging, or classification of the extent of the cancer. For esophageal cancer the stages are as follows:

- Stage I: Cancer is in only a small part of the esophagus; it has not spread to nearby tissues, lymph nodes, or other organs.
- Stage II: Cancer is in a large portion of the esophagus; it has spread to all sides of the esophagus but not to other tissues.
- Stage III: Cancer has spread to tissues or lymph nodes near the esophagus but not to other parts of the body.
- Stage IV: Cancer has spread to other parts of the body.

When symptoms of stomach cancer appear, the doctor will take a medical history, do a physical examination, and order additional tests: a fecal occult blood test, an upper gastrointestinal series (barium swallow), and an endoscopy. If cancer is identified, staging is as follows:

- Stage 0: Cancer is only in the innermost layer of the stomach wall.
- Stage I: Cancer is in the second or third layers of the stomach wall but has not spread to nearby lymph nodes, or it is in the second layer and nearby lymph nodes.
- Stage II: Cancer is in the second layer of the stomach wall and in more distant lymph nodes; in only the third (muscle) layer and the nearby lymph nodes; or in all four stomach wall layers but not in lymph nodes or other organs.
- Stage III: Cancer is in the third layer and more distal lymph nodes; in all four layers of the stomach wall and nearby or more distant lymph nodes; or in all four layers and nearby tissues, with or without nearby lymph node involvement.
- Stage IV: Cancer has spread to nearby tissues and to distant lymph nodes or to other parts of the body.

Although only tumor biopsy can verify colorectal cancer, several other tests that can aid in detection include digital examination, proctoscopy or sigmoidoscopy, colonoscopy, computed tomography scan, and barium X rays. The staging is as follows:

- Stage I: Cancer is present in the innermost and middle tissue layers of the colon.

- Stage II: Cancer has spread beyond the middle layers and into nearby tissues around the colon or rectum, or has spread through the peritoneum or to nearby organs.
- Stage III: Cancer has spread from the innermost layer to the middle layers and is in as many as three lymph nodes; or has spread to three lymph nodes and beyond the middle layers, to tissues nearby the colon or rectum, or into nearby organs or through the peritoneum; or to four or more lymph nodes and to or beyond the middle layers of the colon wall, to tissues nearby the colon or rectum, or to nearby organs or through the peritoneum.
- Stage IV: Cancer has spread to nearby lymph nodes and distant sites such as the lungs or liver.

Treatment for cancer of the small intestine is usually determined by cell type: adenocarcinomatous, lymphomatous, sarcomatous, or carcinoid. However, staging is done for lymphoma:

- Stage I: Cancer in only one lymph node area or one area or organ outside the lymph nodes
- Stage II: Cancer found either in two or more lymph nodes on the same side of the diaphragm or in only one area or organ outside the lymph nodes
- Stage III: Lymph node involvement on both sides of the diaphragm and possible spread to an area or organ near the lymph nodes

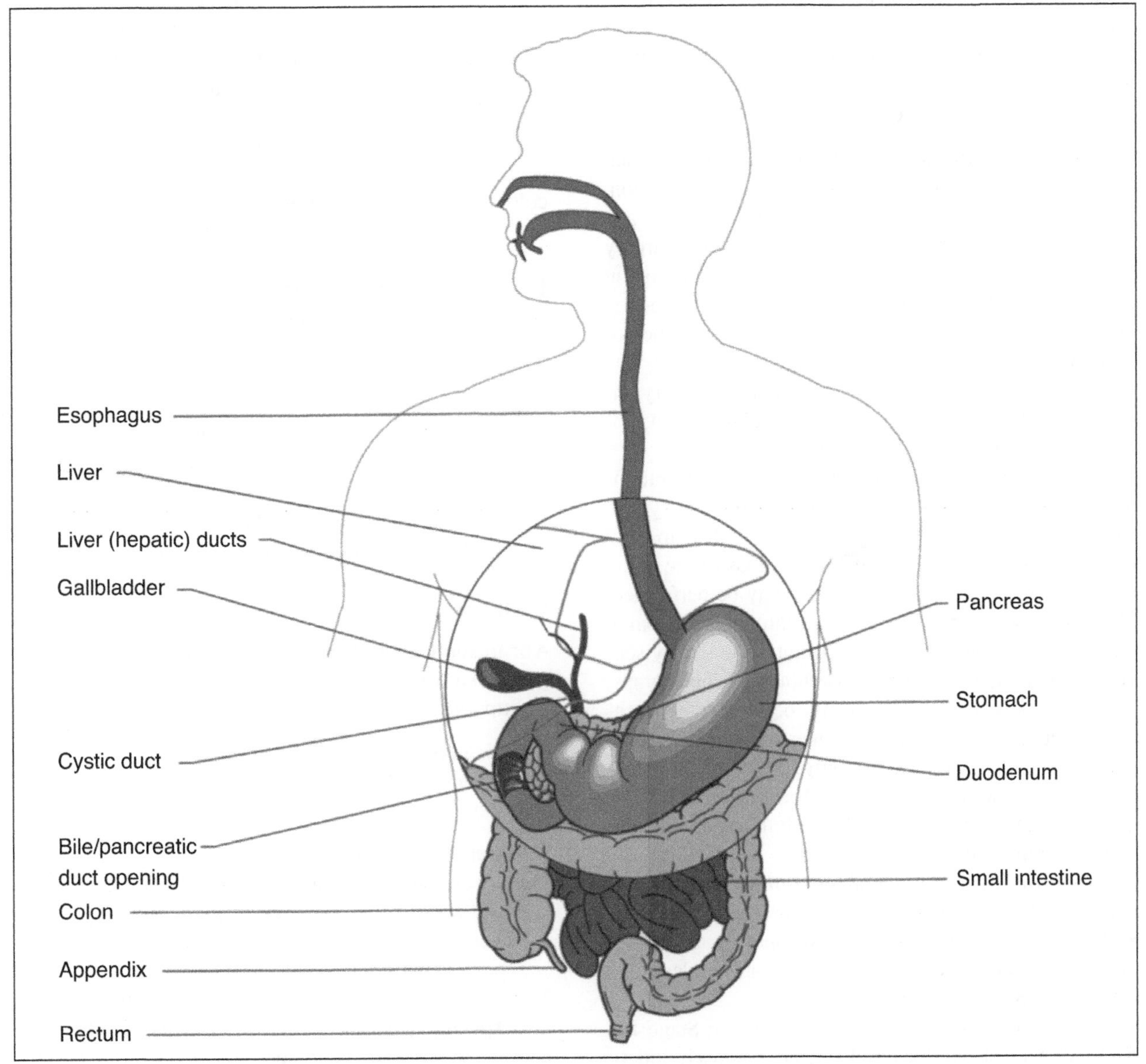

Cancer can affect most parts of the gastrointestinal system.

- Stage IV: Metastasis to one or more organs outside the lymph system or to only one organ outside the lymph system, but to lymph nodes far away from the organ involved

The following stages are used for anal cancer:

- Stage 0 (carcinoma in situ): Cancer is only in the top layer of anal tissue.
- Stage I: Cancer has spread beyond the top layer of anal tissue but involves less than an inch.
- Stage II: Cancer has spread beyond the top layer and is larger than an inch; no lymph node or organ is involved.
- Stage IIIA: Cancer involves lymph nodes around the rectum or has spread to nearby organs such as the vagina or bladder.
- Stage IIIB: Cancer has invaded lymph nodes in the middle of the abdomen or in the groin, or has spread to both nearby organs and lymph nodes around the rectum.
- Stage IV: Cancer has spread to distant lymph nodes within or outside the abdomen.

Treatment and therapy: Treatment of gastrointestinal cancers may vary depending on the tumor's location, size, extent, and cell type, as well as the patient's age and general health, but usual treatments include surgery to remove the tumor and nearby lymph nodes, radiation therapy to shrink the tumor before surgery or to destroy any cancerous cells remaining after surgery, and chemotherapy, alone or combined with radiation therapy. The ideal treatment for stomach cancer is radical surgery, involving a total or subtotal gastrectomy and the removal of a portion of tissue around the stomach.

Another treatment option is biological therapy (immunotherapy), designed to help the body's immune system attack and destroy the malignant cells With colorectal cancer, after surgery, if the healthy sections of the colon cannot be reconnected, a colostomy may be performed, allowing evacuation of body waste through an opening (stoma) in the abdomen. The small intestine is very sensitive to radiation, limiting the usefulness of this therapy, however. The size of the tumor may determine the method of treatment of anal cancer. Superficial in situ tumors (less than 1 inch) may require only local excision or radiotherapy alone. Tumors 1 to 2 inches are best treated by chemotherapy and radiation. Larger tumors may require chemotherapy, radiation, and surgery.

Prognosis, prevention, and outcomes: Five-year survival rates for gastrointestinal cancers are as follows:

- Esophageal cancer: Stage 0, excellent; Stage I, over 50 percent; Stage II, 10 to 15 percent; Stage III, less than 10 percent; Stage IV, unusual.
- Stomach cancer: Stage 0, over 90 percent; Stage I, a 52 to 85 percent rate for distal cancers (stomach outlet), but only 10 to 15 percent for proximal cancers (stomach entry); Stage II, 20 percent or less; Stage III, 17 percent for distal cancers, less for proximal tumors; Stage IV, less than 5 percent.
- Colorectal cancer: Stage I , 80 percent; Stage II, 50 percent; Stage III, about 25 percent; Stage IV, only 5 percent.
- Cancer of the small intestine: Adenocarcinoma type, 20 percent if it is resectable; sarcoma type, about 50 percent if surgical removal is possible; lymphoma type, 25 percent for diffuse lymphoma, but 50 percent or higher for nodular lymphoma; and for the carcinoid type, about 54 percent.
- Anal cancer: Stage 0 (in situ), 100 percent; Stage I, over 95 percent; Stage II, 75 percent; Stage IIIA, 60 percent; Stage IIIB, 10 percent; Stage IV, unusual.

Prevention of cancer involves trying to reduce risk; lifestyle, environment, and heredity help determine risk. To help prevent gastrointestinal cancers, people can stop or avoid smoking, reduce the amount of fat in the diet while increasing fruit and vegetable consumption, control acid refux and request testing if it persists, and undergo colon cancer screening after the age of fifty.

Victoria Price, Ph.D.

For Further Information

Bellenir, Karen, ed. *Cancer Sourcebook.* 4th ed. Detroit: Omnigraphics, 2003.

Cook, Allan R., ed. *The New Cancer Sourcebook.* Vol. 12. Detroit: Omnigraphics, 1996.

Dollinger, Malin, Ernest H. Rosenbaum, and Greg Cable. *Cancer Therapy.* Kansas City: Andrews and McMeel, 1994.

Kufe, Donald W., et al., eds. *Holland Frei Cancer Medicine 7.* 7th ed. Hamilton, Ont.: BC Decker, 2006.

Other Resources

Abramson Cancer Center of the University of Pennsylvania
http://www.oncolink.com

American Society of Clinical Oncology
Gastrointestinal Cancer
http://gicancers.asco.org

National Cancer Institute
Digestive/Gastrointestinal
http://www.cancer.gov/cancertopics/cancersbodylocation/page5

See also: Achlorhydria; Anal cancer; Appendix cancer; Appetite loss; Ascites; Barrett esophagus; Bile duct cancer; Cachexia; Carcinosarcomas; Colon polyps;

Colorectal cancer; Crohn disease; Desmoid tumors; Desmoplastic Small Round Cell Tumor (DSRCT); Diarrhea; Diverticulosis and diverticulitis; Duodenal carcinomas; Enteritis; Esophageal cancer; Esophagitis; Gallbladder cancer; Gardner syndrome; Gastric polyps; Gastrinomas; Gastrointestinal complications of cancer treatment; Gastrointestinal Stromal Tumors (GISTs); *Helicobacter pylori*; Hematemesis; Hemorrhoids; Hereditary diffuse gastric cancer; Hereditary mixed polyposis syndrome; Hereditary pancreatitis; Hereditary polyposis syndromes; Inflammatory bowel disease; Islet cell tumors; Juvenile polyposis syndrome; Krukenberg tumors; Leiomyomas; Leiomyosarcomas; Leptomeningeal carcinomas; Liver cancers; Nausea and vomiting; Obesity-associated cancers; Pancolitis; Pancreatic cancers; Pancreatitis; Peutz-Jeghers Syndrome (PJS); Polyps; Rectal cancer; Small intestine cancer; Stomach cancers; Taste alteration; Turcot syndrome; Weight loss; Yolk sac carcinomas; Zollinger-Ellison syndrome

▶ Gastrointestinal complications of cancer treatment

Category: Diseases, Symptoms, and Conditions
Also known as: Lower gastrointestinal complications, upper gastrointestinal complications

Related conditions: Nausea, vomiting, oral mucositis, diarrhea, constipation, impaction, bowel obstruction, radiation enteritis

Definition: Upper gastrointestinal complications of cancer treatment include nausea and vomiting, decreased appetite, mouth sores or inflammation (mucositis), and thrush (yeast infection of the mouth). Lower gastrointestinal complications of cancer treatment include diarrhea, constipation (infrequent passage of dry, hard stools), fecal impaction (accumulation of dry, hardened feces in the rectum or colon), bowel obstruction (blockage), and radiation enteritis (inflammation of the bowel lining due to radiation therapy).

Risk factors: Upper and lower gastrointestinal complications may occur as a result of cancer treatment, such as chemotherapy or other medications given to treat cancer, radiation therapy to the pelvis or abdomen, or surgery. These symptoms also may be the result of an underlying condition, including cancer, central nervous system disorders, bowel obstruction, diverticulitis (outpouchings of the colon), and hernia.

Upper gastrointestinal symptoms may occur as signs or symptoms of esophageal, laryngeal, and other cancers. Lower gastrointestinal symptoms may occur as signs or symptoms of gastric cancer, colon cancer, rectal cancer, bowel cancer, and other cancers. These symptoms also may occur upon the growth or spread of these types of cancer.

Anxiety about cancer or cancer treatment can contribute to the development of gastrointestinal symptoms. In addition, a history of lactose intolerance can increase the patient's risk of developing lower gastrointestinal complications associated with cancer treatment. Aging and declining health are other contributing factors.

Etiology and the disease process: Chemotherapy and radiation therapy can cause changes in the function of the intestines, including increased or decreased peristalsis (the wavelike contraction of the muscles to propel contents through the digestive tract). An increase in peristalsis can cause stool to move more quickly through the intestines, leading to diarrhea and cramping. A decrease in peristalsis can cause stool to move more slowly through the intestines, leading to constipation, difficulty passing stool, and, in severe cases, fecal impaction, a condition requiring emergency attention. Chemotherapy can also change the normal bacteria in the intestines, causing abdominal pain, cramping, or gas. Fungal, parasitic, or viral pathogens also may contribute to diarrhea.

Partial or complete intestinal or bowel obstructions may occur as the result of a tumor, postoperative adhesion, or a hernia.

Nausea is controlled by part of the central nervous system, and vomiting is a reflex controlled by the brain and stimulated by various triggers, including inflammation in the body. Chemotherapy drugs as well as radiation therapy directed to the gastrointestinal tract, liver, or brain can cause nausea and vomiting. Nausea can also be caused by constipation.

Incidence: Gastrointestinal complications are very common among patients undergoing cancer treatments. The rate of gastrointestinal complications is variable, depending on the type of cancer as well as the extent of the treatment. Side effects may not be the same for each patient or even for patients having the same treatments. In addition, a patient's side effects may change from one treatment session to the next. The National Cancer Institute reports that 70 to 80 percent of patients undergoing cancer treatment experience nausea and vomiting, and 25 percent of patients experience severe diarrhea.

Symptoms: Gastrointestinal symptoms range from moderate to severe and vary among patients. Symptoms can

Prescribed Techniques to Manage Gastrointestinal Complications

Symptom	*Medications*
Nausea, vomiting	serotonin-receptor antagonists such as granisetron, ondansetron, dexamethasone, and aprepitant (given intravenously before the administration of a chemotherapy agent) prochlorperazine metoclopramide promethazine dronabinol
Decreased appetite	dexamethasone prednisone megestrol
Diarrhea	loperamide and diphenoxylate/atropine (first-line treatment) octreotide subcutaneous injections (second-line treatment for persistent, chronic cases) antibiotics, may include fluoroquinolone
Constipation	bisacoyl lactulose

impede cancer treatment, resulting in a delay, dose reduction, or discontinuation of therapy.

Symptoms of nausea and vomiting may occur during chemotherapy treatment and last a few hours to a few days after treatment. If vomiting occurs for more than twenty-four hours, it is important for patients to notify their physician right away, especially if it is accompanied by abdominal pain or cramping.

Changes in stool frequency, consistency, or volume, or the presence of blood, mucus, or pus in the stool may indicate an underlying disease. If diarrhea occurs more than six times a day or does not resolve within twenty-four hours after taking prescribed antidiarrheal medications, patients should call their physician.

Screening and diagnosis: A thorough review of the patient's medical history and a physical exam are performed to diagnose gastrointestinal problems. Blood tests can be performed to identify neutropenia, electrolyte imbalances, and renal insufficiency. Stool tests can be performed to identify blood and bacterial, fungal, parasitic, or viral pathogens. Diagnostic tests include upper endoscopy, upper gastrointestinal series (barium swallow), abdominal X rays, sigmoidoscopy, and colonoscopy.

Treatment and therapy: Symptom management is critical to avoid an interruption in the delivery of cancer treatment. A registered dietitian can provide nutritional therapy to help patients develop eating plans that meet dietary requirements while reducing upper and lower gastrointestinal side effects, helping to make treatment more tolerable. In some cases, antinausea or antidiarrheal medications may be prescribed to help prevent or reduce these troublesome side effects. It is important for patients to ask their physician first before self-treating these side effects, as some over-the-counter remedies could interfere with cancer treatment.

Conservative self-management techniques can be used to manage gastrointestinal complications in many cases. Techniques to manage nausea, vomiting, and diarrhea include the following:

- Increasing fluid intake to prevent dehydration
- Eating bland foods in small amounts
- Following a clear liquid diet of juices and broth until symptoms subside
- Avoiding spicy, high-fat, and sugary foods
- Eating small, frequent meals
- Eating slowly and chewing food completely before swallowing
- Drinking cool beverages after meals
- Taking medication with food, unless advised otherwise
- Eating foods at room temperature

Many of these guidelines are also helpful in managing decreased appetite. Nutritional supplements may be recommended to ensure sufficient caloric and nutrient intake.

Additional tips for managing diarrhea include avoiding high-fiber foods, dairy products, caffeine, and alcoholic beverages and including high-potassium foods, as advised by the doctor.

Techniques for managing abdominal pain include avoiding aspirin and other nonsteroidal anti-inflammatory drugs, unless prescribed; avoiding alcohol and nicotine; and limiting caffeine. Techniques for managing constipation include exercising and increasing consumption of fluids and high-fiber foods.

In addition to these recommendations, relaxation techniques such as deep breathing and guided imagery may help. Patients should follow their physician's specific guidelines for managing treatment side effects and should call the doctor when symptoms are severe or persist for more than twenty-four hours.

Hospitalization is recommended for patients with dehydration, fever, neutropenia, bowel obstruction, fecal impaction, and nausea, vomiting, or diarrhea that results in the inability to maintain adequate hydration or nutrition. Hospitalization is also recommended for patients with chronic diarrhea that does not resolve within twenty-four hours after taking prescribed antidiarrheal medications. Intravenous fluids can be given, and the patient can be closely monitored in the hospital.

Treatment for a bowel obstruction includes surgical removal, a nasogastric tube to relieve a partial obstruction, or a gastrostomy tube to relieve fluid and air buildup. In some cases, an ileostomy or a colostomy may be recommended.

Prognosis, prevention, and outcomes: Gastrointestinal symptoms can be effectively managed with conservative treatments and medications, and they are generally relieved when cancer treatments are completed. There usually are no long-term effects of gastrointestinal symptoms that are properly managed, according to the American Cancer Society.

Left untreated, chronic gastrointestinal symptoms, particularly diarrhea and vomiting, can cause significant morbidity and mortality due to nutritional deficiencies and fluid and electrolyte imbalances that may result in life-threatening dehydration or impaired kidney function. Constipation can lead to fecal impaction, which can be a life-threatening condition requiring immediate medical attention.

Although cancer treatments can create gastrointestinal complications that are temporarily unpleasant to the patient, the potential side effects should be measured against the cancer-fighting benefits of a particular treatment.

Angela M. Costello, B.S.

For Further Information

American Society of Clinical Oncology. *Optimizing Cancer Care: The Importance of Symptom Management.* Dubuque, Iowa: Kendall/Hunt, 2001.

Moore, Katen, and Libby Schmais. *Living Well with Cancer: A Nurse Tells You Everything You Need to Know About Managing the Side Effects of Your Treatment.* New York: Putnam's, 2001.

National Cancer Institute. *Chemotherapy and You.* NIH Publication No. 07-7156. Bethesda, Md.: National Institutes of Health, U.S. Department of Health and Human Services, 2007.

Sharma, R., et al. "Management of Chemotherapy-Induced Nausea, Vomiting, Oral Mucositis, and Diarrhea." *Lancet Oncology* 6 (2005): 93-102.

Tyson, Leslie B., and Joanne Frankel Kelvin. *One Hundred Questions and Answers About Cancer Symptoms and Cancer Treatment Side Effects.* Sudbury, Mass.: Jones & Bartlett, 2005.

Other Resources

American Cancer Society
http://www.cancer.org

National Cancer Institute
http://www.cancer.gov

National Digestive Diseases Information Clearinghouse
http://digestive.niddk.nih.gov/index.htm

See also: Antidiarrheal agents; Antinausea medications; Ascites; Candidiasis; Chemotherapy; Colorectal cancer; Diarrhea; Drug resistance and multidrug resistance (MDR); Enteritis; Fatigue; Gastrointestinal cancers; Infection and sepsis; Inflammatory bowel disease; Living with cancer; Medical marijuana; Motion sickness devices; Mucositis; Nausea and vomiting; Overtreatment; Pain management medications; Side effects; Stress management; Taste alteration; Weight loss

▶ Gastrointestinal Stromal Tumors (GISTs)

Category: Diseases, Symptoms, and Conditions
Also known as: Gastrointestinal sarcomas

Related conditions: Soft-tissue sarcomas

Definition: Gastrointestinal stromal tumors (GISTs) are mesenchymal tumors, forming in the connective tissue of the gastrointestinal system. The most common forms of GISTs occur in the stomach, although tumors may also develop in the small intestine, the esophagus, and the colon or rectum. GISTs are differentiated from similar gastrointestinal tumors by an overexpression of the C-KIT protein, a tyrosine kinase receptor protein that, on activation, triggers protein-signaling pathways that initiate cell proliferation.

Risk factors: Currently, there are no well-defined risk factors for the development of gastrointestinal stromal tumors. Neurofibromatosis, a disease characterized by the formation of numerous benign tumors in nerves throughout the body, may be associated with the formation of GISTs. Most GISTs occur sporadically, but there have been a few reported cases of these tumors developing in members of the same family, perhaps due to inheritance of a mutation within the *C-KIT* gene. Additionally, familial gastrointestinal stromal tumor syndrome is an inherited disorder that predisposes individuals to the formation of GISTs. This rare condition is caused by mutations in the *C-KIT* gene. However, unlike people with sporadic GIST in which only the tumor expresses *C-KIT* mutations, individuals with gastrointestinal stromal tumor syndrome have *C-KIT* mutations in all the cells of their bodies.

Etiology and the disease process: Gastrointestinal stromal tumors arise because of activating mutations of one of two tyrosine kinase proteins important for triggering cell proliferation. The majority of GISTs occur subsequent to mutations within the gene encoding for the C-KIT protein, although mutations in the gene encoding the platelet-derived growth factor receptor (PDGFR) also may cause a GIST. The specific type of cell in which GISTs originate is what differentiates a GIST from similar gastrointestinal tumors. Most investigators believe that GISTs begin in specific cells within the connective tissue of the gastrointestinal tract, called interstitial cells of Cajal. Many GISTs are found not to be malignant and are instead benign growths within the gastrointestinal system.

Incidence: A gastrointestinal stromal tumor is considered to be a relatively rare cancer and is estimated to occur in 10 to 20 individuals per 1 million people. Each year, approximately 4,500 to 6,000 Americans have a GIST. Of these cases, 20 to 30 percent of the tumors are diagnosed as malignant. Most GISTs occur in people over the age of fifty, with the majority of tumors diagnosed between the ages of fifty-five and sixty-five. GISTs rarely occur in children or people younger than forty years. While GISTS are thought to affect both genders equally, some studies have suggested that there may be a slight prevalence of GIST development in men.

Symptoms: Depending on the size of the gastrointestinal stromal tumor, an individual may or may not experience any symptoms. As the tumor enlarges, patients often feel abdominal pain or develop intestinal bleeding. Upon examination, a GIST may be found to be the cause of these symptoms. Other symptoms that have been associated with GISTs include nausea, vomiting, and appetite or weight loss.

Screening and diagnosis: There are currently no effective screening tests to detect gastrointestinal stromal tumors. Some GISTs are diagnosed by chance, during abdominal surgery or a routine colonoscopy. Also, GISTs may be identified by radiological screening tests, such as a computed tomography (CT) scan, a barium X ray, or magnetic resonance imaging (MRI). In some cases, a doctor may perform a biopsy if a mass is detected. However, biopsies are often impractical, and instead surgery is performed to remove the mass, at which time a biopsy of the tumor tissue is removed to determine if it is malignant or benign. Using a biopsy sample, GISTs are histologically graded to determine the malignant potential of the tumor.

Treatment and therapy: The primary treatment for GIST is surgery, in which the goal is to remove as much of the tumor as possible. Surgery is more likely to be successful when the GIST is small. Most general anticancer chemotherapeutics previously used to treat GISTs were largely ineffective. The approval of the targeted therapy imatinib (Gleevec) has caused this drug to become part of the front-line therapy for the treatment of GISTs. Imatinib specifically inhibits both C-KIT and PDGFR, the two main proteins responsible for the development and survival of GIST cells. Although imatinib does not necessarily cure the GIST, it is often used to shrink the tumor size.

Prognosis, prevention, and outcomes: The prognosis for patients diagnosed with a GIST depends on several factors. These include the size and grade of the tumor, as well as the degree to which the tumor has spread, if at all. For people diagnosed and treated between 1992 and 2000, the overall five-year survival rate of patients with GIST was approximately 45 percent. This survival increases to 64 percent if the tumor has not spread but decreases to 13 percent if the tumor has spread to distant sites. However, because of the addition of new therapies to treat GIST, these survival rates have begun to increase.

Lisa M. Cockrell, B.S.

For Further Information

DeMatteo, R., et al. *One Hundred Questions and Answers About Gastrointestinal Stromal Tumor (GIST)*. Boston: Jones & Bartlett, 2006.

Kufe, Donald W., et al., eds. *Holland Frei Cancer Medicine 7*. 7th ed. Hamilton, Ont.: BC Decker, 2006.

Rubin, B. P., et al. "Gastrointestinal Stromal Tumor." *Lancet* 369 (2007): 1731-1741.

Other Resources

American Cancer Society
http://www.cancer.org

GIST Support International
http://www.gistsupport.org

See also: Angiogenesis inhibitors; Barium swallow; Duodenal carcinomas; Fibrosarcomas, soft-tissue; Gastrointestinal cancers; Gastrointestinal oncology; Leiomyosarcomas; Mesenchymomas; Small intestine cancer; Stomach cancers; Tyrosine kinase inhibitors

▶ Germ-cell tumors

Category: Diseases, Symptoms, and Conditions
Also known as: Seminoma, nonseminoma, embryonal cell cancer, teratoma, endothermal signal tumor, mature and immature teratomas

Related conditions: Testicular cancer, ovarian cancer

Definition: Germ-cell tumors (GCTs) are tumors of cancerous or noncancerous cells that arise from germ cells during embryonic development.

Risk factors: The only confirmed risk factors of germ-cell tumors involve birth defects. Male infants with undescended testis (chryptorchidism) are ten to forty times more likely to develop germ-cell tumors than male infants with normally descended testes. Children with the genetic disease Klinefelter syndrome are also at an increased risk for germ-cell tumors.

Etiology and the disease process: Germ cells are the cells that develop in the embryo and become the cells that make up the reproductive system in men and women. These germ cells follow a midline path through the body after development and descend into the pelvis as ovarian cells or into the scrotal sac as testicular cells. Most ovarian tumors and testicular tumors are of germ-cell origin. Germ-cell tumors can spread (metastasize) to other parts of the body. The most common sites for metastasis are the lungs, liver, lymph nodes, and central nervous system. Rarely, germ-cell tumors can spread to the bone, bone marrow, and other organs.

Types of germ-cell tumors include the seminoma (in testis), dysgerminoma (in ovary), teratoma, endodermal sinus tumor, embryonal, and choriocarcinoma.

Extragonadal germ-cell tumors form from developing sperm or egg cells that travel from the gonads to other parts of the body. Extragonadal germ-cell tumors can be benign (noncancerous) or malignant (cancerous). Benign extragonadal germ-cell tumors are called benign teratomas. These are more common than malignant extragonadal germ-cell tumors and often are very large. Teratomas can be further classified into mature (lining resembles that of skin) and immature (cancer cells look like cells from a developing fetus).

Incidence: Germ-cell tumors are diagnosed in about 900 children each year. Germ-cell tumors account for 16 percent of all cancers diagnosed in adolescents between the ages of fifteen and nineteen and nearly 4 percent of cancers diagnosed in children younger than fifteen. In women, germ-cell tumors account for 30 percent of ovarian tumors, but in patients under the age of twenty-one, 60 percent of ovarian tumors are of the germ-cell type. Most male adolescents are diagnosed with germ-cell tumors after puberty; these tumors are usually malignant. The incidence in whites is five times higher than in blacks.

For unknown reasons, worldwide incidence has more than doubled in the past forty years. The incidence of germ-cell tumors varies by geographic area. The highest incidence is in Scandinavia, Germany, and New Zealand; it is lower in the United States and lowest in Asia and Africa.

Symptoms: Patients with germ-cell tumors usually complain of a tumor, swelling, or mass that can be felt or seen, and abnormal shape, or irregularity in, testicular size. Additional symptoms can include elevated levels of alpha-fetoprotein (AFP), beta-human chorionic gonadotropin (β-hCG), and lactate dehydrogenase (LDH). Constipation, incontinence, and leg weakness can occur if the tumor is compressing structures in the sacrum (a segment of the vertebral column that forms the top part of the pelvis). Malignant extragonadal germ-cell tumors may cause symptoms such as chest pain or breathing problems.

Screening and diagnosis: Diagnostic procedures for germ-cell tumors may include biopsy of the tumor; blood tests, including a complete blood count (CBC) to determine the size, number, and maturity of different blood cells within the blood; and multiple imaging studies such as computed tomography (CT), magnetic resonance imaging (MRI), ultrasound, and X ray. Scientists have identified a tumor marker in the blood called lactate dehydrogenase isoenzyme 1 (LD1); increased levels of this enzyme indicate seminoma in more than 60 percent of patients.

Staging of the disease depends on its development in the ovary or testis.

Treatment and therapy: Specific treatment for germ-cell tumors is determined by the patient's age, overall health, medical history, and extent of the disease. The treatment plan will also rely heavily on whether the tumor is extragonadal and whether it is malignant. Treatments for germ-cell tumors are similar to those for ovarian tumors and testicular tumors, usually involving surgery to remove the tumors. If cells are malignant, patients may undergo chemotherapy or radiation to reduce the risk of recurrence of cancerous cells. In some cases, patients will require a bone marrow transplant or hormone replacement therapy.

Prognosis, prevention, and outcomes: Prognosis greatly depends on the extent of the disease, the size and location of the tumor, whether the cancer has spread, and the age and overall health of the patient. Prompt medical attention and aggressive therapy are important for the best prognosis. Continuous follow-up care is essential for a child diagnosed with a germ-cell tumor. Side effects of radiation and chemotherapy as well as second malignancies can occur in survivors of germ-cell tumors. New methods are continually being discovered to improve treatment and to decrease side effects.

Robert J. Amato, D.O.

For Further Information

Johanson, Paula. *Frequently Asked Questions About Testicular Cancer*. New York: Rosen, 2007.

Kurth, Karl H., Gerald H. Mickisch, and Fritz H. Schroder, eds. *Renal, Bladder, Prostate, and Testicular Cancer: An Update*. New York: Parthenon, 2001.

Parker, James N., and Philip M. Parker, eds. *The Official Patient's Sourcebook on Testicular Cancer: A Revised and Updated Directory for the Internet Age*. San Diego, Calif.: Icon Health, 2002.

Other Resources

CureSearch

Germ Cell Tumors

http://www.curesearch.org/for_parents_and_families/newlydiagnosed/article.aspx?ArticleId=3190&StageID=1&TopicId=1&Level=1

National Cancer Institute

Extragonadal Germ-Cell Tumors

http://www.cancer.gov/cancertopics/types/extragonadal-germ-cell/

See also: Brain and central nervous system cancers; Embryonal cell cancer; Klinefelter syndrome and cancer; Lactate Dehydrogenase (LDH) test; Mediastinal tumors; Ovarian cancers; Spermatocytomas; Teratocarcinomas; Teratomas; Testicular cancer; Thymomas; Yolk sac carcinomas; Young adult cancers

▶ Gestational Trophoblastic Tumors (GTTs)

Category: Diseases, Symptoms, and Conditions

Also known as: Gestational trophoblastic neoplasia (GTN), gestational trophoblastic disease (GTD), metastasizing mole, invasive mole, chorioadenoma destruens

Related conditions: Hydatidiform mole (H. mole), molar pregnancy, placental site trophoblastic tumor (PSTT), choriocarcinoma

Definition: Gestational trophoblastic tumors (GTTS) refer to a group of benign tumors and malignant cancers in the uterus originating from the trophoblast layer that begins to develop after conception and forms the embryonic placenta. GTTs can be classified as hydatidiform mole (complete or partial molar pregnancy), invasive mole (chorioadenoma destruens), choriocarcinoma, and placental site trophoblastic tumor (PSTT). Some 60 percent of gestational trophoblastic tumors are persisting hydatidiform moles. Although hydatidiform moles are classified as benign while invasive moles, choriocarcinoma, and PSTTs are classified as malignant, their behavior in real life may be similar, especially when aggressive benign tumors mimic malignant ones.

Risk factors: A number of factors may contribute to a woman's susceptibility to developing gestational trophoblastic tumors. All women of childbearing age are at risk, with women over age forty and under age twenty at highest risk for having a complete molar pregnancy. According to the American Cancer Society, women who have had a previous molar pregnancy, have blood type of A or AB (rather than B or O), used birth control pills, smoked or drank alcohol (although some studies failed to support this), had more than ten sexual partners, and are of lower socioeconomic status have a higher risk of developing a gestational trophoblastic tumor. The risk factor of being Asian or Native American is controversial. Conflicting figures preclude this as a solid risk factor, suggesting other factors (poor record keeping regarding numbers of births, diet) may falsely raise the incidence.

Etiology and the disease process: A hydatidiform mole arises from the fusion of an ovum and one or more sperm. The trophoblast, a layer of cells surrounding the embryo, produces finger-like villi that attach to the uterus. In a hydatidiform mole, the villi swell and grow in clusters to resemble bunches of grapes.

One of three scenarios is possible in the creation of a hydatidiform mole. The first involves the union of the ovum (unfertilized egg) with two sperm instead of one. The second scenario may involve a single sperm whose complement of 22 chromosomes and one sex chromosome (23 total) is duplicated. These moles contain fetal material and are known as partial moles. Only about 2 percent of partial moles become malignant. The third scenario involves the union of an ovum without a nucleus with one or two sperm. No fetal tissue is present in a complete molar pregnancy.

Invasive moles (chorioadenoma destruens) are hydatidiform moles, most commonly complete moles, that have invaded the myometrium (muscular wall of the uterus). Some 20 percent of women who have had a complete mole removed by scraping the uterus develop invasive moles. These moles usually must be treated with chemotherapy and sometimes spread to other organs such as the lungs or brain.

Choriocarcinoma are malignant tumors that usually develop from complete hydatidiform moles (50 percent), although they can result after a normal pregnancy (25 percent) or an abortion (25 percent). This type of cancer often spreads past the uterus.

Placental site trophoblastic tumor is a rare form of gestational trophoblastic tumor. It develops after a normal pregnancy or abortion in which the placenta attaches to the uterus. This type of tumor tends to be confined to the uterus and is usually removed by surgery, as it does not respond to chemotherapy.

Incidence: In the United States, hydatidiform moles occur in 1 out of every 2,000 deliveries, with progression to malignancy in 9 to 20 percent of women. It is estimated that 1 in 850 to 1 in 1,300 pregnancies are molar. A disproportionate number of complete moles is reported in nonwhite women. Complete moles were reported to arise in 1 in 400 Korean, Indonesian, or Native American women compared with 1 in 1,500 white women in the United States. However, data from multiple sources are conflicting. Choriocarcinomas are rare, occurring in 0.133 per 100,000 women in the United States and as many as 1 out of 50,000 live births in the United Kingdom.

Symptoms: Patients often complain of delayed menses, and gestational trophoblastic tumors can mimic a pregnancy. However, abnormalities such as painless uterine bleeding during the first trimester or the passing of grapelike material from deformed chorionic villi through the vagina suggest the presence of a gestational trophoblastic tumor. The condition may also mimic preeclampsia (elevated blood pressure, swelling, headache, blurring of vision) and persisting hyperemesis gravidarum (frequent bouts of nausea and vomiting initially associated with rapidly rising hormone levels). Hyperthyroidism symptoms (palpitations, diarrhea, heat intolerance, sweating, tremors, nervousness/irritability) from a molar analog of thyroid-stimulating hormone (human molar thyrotropin) or direct stimulation by beta-human chorionic gonadotropic hormone (β-HCG) can also occur.

Symptoms of spread to other parts of the body develop according to the involved organs. On physical examination, a disparity between gestational age and fundic height (length of uterus along its long axis) of four or more weeks is suggestive. A screening β-HCG of greater than 100,000 million international units per milliliter (mIU/ml) is highly suggestive of neoplasia.

Screening and diagnosis: No specific screening is recommended. The single most important laboratory test for diagnosis of GTT is a quantitative assay of HCG and all its subcomponents. Diagnosis is confirmed by pelvic ultrasound, where the grapelike vesicles may be seen, and partial moles may be found by the absence of a fetal heart and blood flow. A "snowstorm" appearance also may be described. Other imaging studies include a chest X ray and computed tomography (CT) scan or magnetic resonance imaging (MRI) of the head and abdominal and pelvic regions to find evidence of metastases. The criteria needed to diagnose gestational trophoblastic tumors are at least four values of persistently elevated HCG, a sequential rise of HCG for two weeks or longer, and lung metastases as seen on chest X ray.

The International Federation of Gynecology and Obstetrics (FIGO) has created the following staging system:

- Stage I: Gestational trophoblastic tumors strictly confined to the uterine corpus
- Stage II: Tumors extending to the adnexa or vagina but limited to the genital structures

- Stage III: Tumors extending to the lungs, with or without genital tract involvement
- Stage IV: All other metastases

The World Health Organization (WHO) created a prognostic scoring system which is used to further classify the stages used by FIGO into high and low risk. Point values are assigned to various factors present at the time of diagnosis. Prognostic factors include the following:

- Age: Being older than forty, 1 point
- Prior pregnancy: Hydatidiform mole, 0 points; abortion, 1 point; full-term pregnancy, 2 points
- Time from pregnancy to manifestation of the tumor: Less than four months, 0 points; four to six months, 1 point; seven to twelve months, 2 points; more than twelve months, 4 points
- HCG levels in blood (mIU/ml): Less than 1,000, 0 points; 1,000-9,999, 1 point; 10,000-100,000, 2 points, more than 100,000, 4 points
- Tumor size: Less than 3 centimeters (cm), 0 points; 3 to 5 cm, 1 point; more than 5 cm, 2 points
- Site of metastases: Lungs, 0 points; spleen, kidney, 1 point; gastrointestinal tract, 2 points; brain, liver, 4 points
- Number of metastases: One to four, 1 point; five to eight, 2 points; more than eight, 4 points
- Earlier failed chemotherapy: Single drug, 2 points; multiple drugs, 4 points

Low-risk patients have a WHO score of seven or less; high-risk patients have a score of eight or more. This stratification determines the best treatment course.

Metastasis to only the lungs with disease duration less than four months can be considered low risk.

Treatment and therapy: Treatment includes evacuation of the uterus by suction dilation and curettage, along with monitoring of HCG with the overall goal of achieving undetectable levels. A hysterectomy is avoided unless extensive invasion is present. Metastatic lesions are resected if possible. Evacuation is usually followed by chemotherapy according to risk stratification. Low-risk patients undergo any of several single-drug therapies, which may use methotrexate with or without leucovorin rescue or actinomycin-D given as intramuscular or intravenous injections at regular intervals. High-risk patients are given combination chemotherapy. The main regimen, known as the EMA-CO protocol, uses etoposide, methotrexate, and actinomycin D, given before cyclophosphamide and vincristine (Oncovin). Resistant disease utilizes the EMA-EP protocol in which EMA alternates with etoposide and cisplatin (EP). Other drugs used include pacliataxel (Taxol), 5-fluorouracil (FU), or vinblastine in various combinations with EP. Levels of HCG are monitored even after treatment, with two additional chemotherapy sessions after undetectable levels are seen. A minimum of twelve disease-free months is recommended prior to pregnancy, after which early monitoring is done.

Prognosis, prevention, and outcomes: Cure rate is excellent with surgery followed by chemotherapy, approaching 100 percent in low-risk patients and 75 percent for high-risk patients. Recurrence rates are low, at less than 1 percent. A second molar pregnancy may occur 1 to 2 percent of the time, but the likelihood of another molar pregnancy increases tenfold if the patient has had two molar pregnancies.

Aldo C. Dumlao, M.D.

For Further Information

Haas, Adelaide, and Susan L. Puretz. *The Woman's Guide to Hysterectomy: Expectations and Options*. Berkeley, Calif.: Celestial Arts, 2002.

Parker, James N., and Philip M. Parker, eds. *The Official Patient's Sourcebook on Gestational Trophoblastic Tumors*. San Diego, Calif.: Icon Health, 2002.

Rosenthal, Sara M. *The Gynecological Sourcebook*. 4th ed. New York: McGraw-Hill Professional, 2003.

Other Resources

American Cancer Society
Detailed Guide: Gestational Trophoblastic Disease
http://www.cancer.org/docroot/CRI/content/CRI_2_4_1X_What_are_gestational_trophoblastic_disease_49.asp?rnav=cri

American College of Obstetricians and Gynecologists
http://www.acog.org

National Cancer Institute
Gestational Trophoblastic Tumor
http://www.cancer.gov/cancertopics/types/gestationaltrophoblastic

WebMd
Gestational Trophoblastic Neoplasia
http://www.emedicine.com/med/TOPIC866.HTM

See also: Choriocarcinomas; Computed Tomography (CT) scan; Gynecologic cancers; Gynecologic oncology; Human Chorionic Gonadotropin (HCG); Hydatidiform mole; Ultrasound tests

▶ Giant Cell Tumors (GCTs)

Category: Diseases, Symptoms, and Conditions
Also known as: Osteoclastomas

Related conditions: Differential diagnosis includes other giant cell lesions, such as the brown tumor seen in hyperparathyroidism, giant cell reparative granuloma, chondroblastoma, pigmented villonodular synovitis, and giant cell tumor of the tendon sheath.

Definition: Giant cell tumors (GCTs) are relatively uncommon benign but locally aggressive bone neoplasms. The tumors are large, red-brown, and subject to frequent cystic degeneration. They are composed of uniform oval mononuclear cells with scattered osteoclast-type giant cells containing one hundred or more nuclei. The mononuclear cells are the proliferating component of the tumor. Necrosis, hemorrhage, hemosiderin (iron) deposition, and reactive bone formation are common secondary features.

Risk factors: There are no known predisposing factors that place a person at risk for having a giant cell tumor. Genetic changes (mutations) trigger the condition, but researchers do not know what conditions or factors might promote such mutations. Those diagnosed with this condition, however, will have an increased risk for joint collapse and degeneration and pathologic fractures. The incidence of metastasis is rare.

Etiology and the disease process: The tumor is located in the metaphysis or epiphysis of long bones, with 50 percent of the lesions occurring around the knee. The proximal humerus and distal radius are also common locations, as well as the pelvis and sacrum. Typically, the lesion presents as a painful, slowly enlarging mass. With proliferation of the mononuclear cells, tissue expansion creates a bone defect that is described as lytic (bringing about disintegration or dissolution), with sharply circumscribed margins. The lesion is often described as having an "eccentric soap bubble" pattern. There may be thinning of the cortex (outer ring of bone), and the lesion may extend into subchondral bone of the adjacent joint. Most tumors are solitary; however, multiple tumors do occur, especially in the distal extremities. Malignant degeneration is rare.

Basic science data strongly suggest a close molecular genetic relationship between the benign giant cell tumors of bone and the malignant osteosarcomas (bone cancer). Indeed, these two conditions have similar genetic alterations in the oncogenes (genetic material incorporated into chromosomes associated with various malignancies). Molecular genetic studies have found a higher incidence of p53 protein and alterations in the *MYC* gene in both tumors.

Incidence: Giant cell tumors usually arise in people from their early twenties to forties, with a slight female predominance. Giant cell tumors are exceedingly rare in patients younger than age thirteen, and only about 10 percent of cases occur in individuals older than sixty-five. The majority of giant cell tumors arise around the knee, but any bone may be involved, including the sacrum, pelvis, spine, and small bones of the hands and feet.

Symptoms: The location of these tumors in the ends of bones near joints frequently causes patients to complain of arthritic symptoms. Individuals may complain of pain, show signs of local swelling, or have a pathologic fracture through the lesion.

Screening and diagnosis: Diagnosis is based on X-ray evidence and confirmed by tissue biopsy. Magnetic resonance imaging (MRI) scans are often employed to define bone margins and soft-tissue involvement.

The current staging system is based on imaging studies. Stage I (latent-quiescent) delineates a lesion in cancerous bone with minimal cortical involvement. The most common stage is Stage II (active), which denotes extensive cortical thinning and creation of the "soap bubble" pattern. Stage III (aggressive) has a greater risk of recurrence. A more aggressive surgical approach is recommended for tumors in this stage.

Treatment and therapy: Watchful conservative care and treatment may be a reasonable approach if the lesion is small, localized, contained, and not painful. The use of radiation therapy is restricted to difficult lesions in the pelvis and spine, where an adequate surgical resection is not feasible because of anatomical considerations.

For a majority of Stage II and III lesions, surgical excision is the treatment of choice. This involves extensive exteriorization (removal of a large cortical window over the lesion), curettage with hand and power instruments, and chemical cauterization with phenol (a caustic chemical that destroys cells) or hydrogen peroxide, cryosurgery, or other methods of cavity sterilization. The large resulting defect is usually reconstructed with subchondral bone grafts and methylmethacrylate cement. Surgery with only limited curettage is associated with a 40 to 60 percent recurrence rate. Although benign, up to 4 percent of operative cases will metastasize to the lungs after surgery, suggesting dislodgement of tumor emboli. Lesions with significant extension into adjacent soft tissue require en bloc resection (complete removal of affected bone and surrounding tissue). In this more radical procedure, modified arthrodesis (fusion of a joint), allograft (replacement of bone segment with donor bone), or prosthetic reconstruction (artificial joint implant) is indicated. In the knee, this operation may require extensive bone resection, necessitating a total knee replacement.

Prognosis, prevention, and outcomes: Malignancy may occur in two forms: primary malignant giant cell tumor and secondary malignant giant cell tumor. Secondary tumors occur following radiation to a giant cell tumor or following multiple local recurrences. The most common scenario is associated with a patient who has a large aggressive giant cell tumor that is inoperable. These individuals receive irradiation for local control, but an osteosarcoma (bone cancer) may subsequently develop (15 percent incidence rate) in the irradiated field over an extended latency period of three to fifty years.

John L. Zeller, M.D., Ph.D.

For Further Information

Campanacci, M. *Bone and Soft Tissue Tumors.* New York: Springer, 1990.

Campanacci, M., et al. "Giant Cell Tumor of the Bone." *Journal of Bone Joint Surgery* 69A (1987): 106-114.

Manaster, B. J., and A. J. Doyle. "Giant Cell Tumors of the Bone." *Radiologic Clinics of North America* 31, no. 2 (1993): 299-323.

Pals, S. D., and R. M. Wilkins. "Giant Cell Tumor of the Bone Treated by Curettage, Cementation, and Bone Grafting." *Orthopedics* 15 (1992): 703-708.

Rooney, R. J., et al. "Giant Cell Tumor of the Bone: A Surgical Approach." *International Orthopaedics* 17, no. 2 (1993): 87-92.

Schajowicz, F. *Tumors and Tumorlike Lesions of the Bone: Pathology, Radiology, and Treatment.* Berlin: Springer-Verlag, 1994.

Other Resources

American Academy of Orthopedic Surgeons
http//www.aaos.org

Bonetumor.org
Giant Cell Tumor of Bone
http://bonetumor.org/tumors/pages/page106.html

See also: Bone cancers; Dermatofibrosarcoma Protuberans (DFSP); Malignant Fibrous Histiocytoma (MFH); Spinal axis tumors

▶ Glioblastomas

Category: Diseases, Symptoms, and Conditions

Related conditions: astrocytoma, brain tumor, central nervous system tumors, glioma, meningioma, oligodendroglioma

Definitions: Glioblastomas, also known as glioblastoma multiforme (GBM) or grade IV astrocytomas, are malignant primary brain tumors arising from malignant transformation of the glia, or support cells in the nervous system.

Risk factors: Advanced age is the main risk factor associated with glioblastomas, with the majority of incidence in patients over 50. Glioblastoma is slightly more common in males compared to females. Although many environmental factors have been studied, only exposure to ionizing radiation has been directly linked to an increased glioblastoma risk. Hereditary genetic factors have also been associated with increased risk for glioblastoma. Syndromes associated with increased glioblastoma risk, with associated gene in parentheses, are as follows: Neurofibromatosis 1 or 2 (NF1 or NF2), Turcot (APC gene), Gorlins (PTCH gene), Tuberous Sclerosis (TSC1 and TSC2 genes), Von Hippel-Lindau (VHL gene), and Li-Fraumeni syndrome (TP53 gene).

Etiology and the disease process: Glioblastoma occurs when abnormal neural cells grow in the brain. Glioblastoma is most associated with malignant transformation of astrocytes ("star-like" support cells), but recent research has also implicated oligodendrocytes (cells that insulate the "wires" of the brain) as well as neural progenitor or stem cells. Glioblastomas can arise spontaneously or evolve from lower-grade brain tumors. Glioblastoma cells divide rapidly and actively invade the surrounding normal brain, leading to "finger-like" projections of the tumor. Invading glioblastoma cells preclude complete surgical resection and effective adjuvant treatments, since such treatments lead to tumor re-growth in the areas immediately adjacent to the surgical cavity in greater than 90% of cases. Although it readily spreads throughout the brain, glioblastoma rarely metastasizes outside the central nervous system. Glioblastomas notoriously induce extensive angiogenesis (new blood vessel formation), often resulting in "leaky" immature vasculature and a reddish, hemorrhagic appearance compared to normal brain tissue. Abundant inflammation and the immature vasculature of glioblastomas cause fluid build-up in the surrounding brain (vasogenic edema), resulting in increased intracranial pressure and serious neurological symptoms and complications.

Incidence: Glioblastomas are relatively rare but are highly lethal and significantly reduce quality of life. According to the Central Brain Tumor Registry of the United States (CBTRUS), approximately 12,000 new glioblastomas will be diagnosed in 2016, composing about 15% of all primary nervous system tumors, but approximately 50% of all malignant brain tumors. Incidence rate for glioblastoma is about 3.4 per 100,000 adults (age 20+) and has remained fairly stable for many years. Glioblastoma accounts for about 0.6% of all cancer cases, but approximately 1.4% of cancer-related deaths.

Symptoms: Glioblastoma symptoms are most commonly due to increased intracranial pressure from unchecked cancer cell expansion and/or edema, and include headache, nausea, vomiting, and drowsiness. Severe neurological symptoms such as seizures, motor dysfunction, weakness or sensory impairment on one side of the body, or impairment of memory, vision, or language can occur with glioblastoma depending on tumor location. Subtle neurological symptoms such as personality changes, fatigue, and depression can also occur.

Screening and diagnosis: Currently, there exists no screening test for glioblastoma, and patients exhibiting symptoms of a suspected brain tumor are subjected to multiple diagnostic tests. A complete neurological exam is administered to detect any aberrations in senses, reflexes, motor balance and coordination, cognition, and others. The neurological exam determines if further diagnostic tests for a tumor are required and provides baselines of patient health to help determine treatment response during any future tumor therapies.

If a brain tumor is suspected, the patient undergoes magnetic resonance imaging (MRI), which uses a magnetic field and pulses of radio wave energy to noninvasively scan the brain. A malignant brain tumor is identified by changes in brain anatomy identified by MRI and location-specific enhancement by intravenously administered contrast agents such as gadolinium. Use of advanced MRI techniques or other imaging, such as computed tomography with X-rays or positron emission tomography to measure radiation emanating from injected molecular probes, can also provide complementary information for surgical planning or glioblastoma biology.

Final diagnosis of glioblastoma occurs after microscopic analysis of tissue obtained by biopsy or during surgery. Glioblastoma is diagnosed by abnormal looking glial cells (atypia), high cellular growth rate (mitotic index), dead cells in the center of the tumor (necrosis), and extensive induction of new blood vessels (vascular endothelial proliferation or angiogenesis). Although this method provides considerable information regarding outcome, significant variation exists within different patient glioblastomas, and integration of molecular diagnostics may complement traditional microscopic analysis in the future.

Treatment and therapy: Glioblastoma is treated aggressively using surgery, radiation, and chemotherapy. Surgery first removes as much glioblastoma as safely possible and is performed soon after diagnostic imaging reveals suspected brain tumor. Surgery additionally helps to alleviate symptoms associated with increased intracranial pressure. Greater amounts of tumor removed correlates with longer patient survival; however, glioblastoma location within or near a functional brain area controlling essential functions such as motor or language abilities would preclude maximal safe surgical resection.

Standard treatment after surgical removal is chemoradiation therapy. For glioblastoma, radiation is usually delivered externally on a daily basis, 5 times per week for 4 weeks, with patients concurrently receiving temozolomide (Temodar). Stereotactic radiosurgery (focused high dose radiation therapy) has a role in treating focal recurrent GBM, and is usually not used in the first phase of treating newly diagnosed GBM.

Chemotherapy for glioblastoma is started and continues after radiation treatments. As of 2005, the cellular DNA damaging agent temozolomide (Temodar) became the standard-of-care chemotherapy for glioblastoma. Temozolomide induces glioblastoma cell death and exhibits radio-sensitizing properties, and has largely replaced other DNA synthesis inhibitors or damaging agents due to its reduced toxic side effects and equivalent results compared to other cancer chemotherapeutics. Other approved treatments include sustained release of DNA damaging agents from polymer wafers, angiogenesis inhibiting agents, and tumor-treating electromagnetic fields, among others.

Prognosis, prevention, and outcomes: Glioblastoma accounts for approximately 7000 cancer deaths per year, or about 2.15 per 100,000 men and women. Two-year survival for glioblastoma is 15.2%, and 5-year survival rate for glioblastoma is about 5.1%. The most conclusive prognostic factors for glioblastoma are extent of tumor removal, age at diagnosis, and initial health and neurological performance (ie, Karnofsky) score. Molecularly, O^6-methylguanine-DNA-methyltransferase (MGMT) gene methylation, which presumably turns off expression of the MGMT enzyme that repairs DNA damage from alkylating agents such as temozolomide, predicts a favorable outcome for glioblastoma patients. There are no known preventative measures for glioblastoma, although those at familial risk could receive genetic counseling and possibly genetic testing.

Paul A. Clark, PhD
John S. Kuo, MD, PhD

For Further Information

Mehta, M.P., Chang, S.M., Guha, A., Newton, H.B., & Vogelbaum, M.A. (Ed.). (2011). *Principles and practice of neuro-oncology: A multidisciplinary approach*, New York, NY: Demos Medical Publishing.

Bernstein M., & Berger, M.S. (Ed.). (2014). *Neuro-Oncology: The essentials (3rd ed.).* New York, NY: Thieme Publishing Group.

Quinn, T., Ostrom, Q.T., Bauchet, L., Davis, F. G., Deltour, I., Fisher, J. L., … Barnholtz-Sloan, J. S. (2014). The epidemiology of glioma in adults: a "state of the science" review. *Neuro-Oncology*, 16(7): 896-913.

Other resources

American Brain Tumor Association
www.abta.org/
http://www.abta.org/brain-tumor-information/

American Association for Cancer Research
www.aacr.org

American Cancer Society
www.cancer.org

Society for Neuro-oncology (SNO)
http://www.soc-neuro-onc.org/

***See also*:** Astrocytomas, Meningiomas, American Cancer Society (ACS), Brain and central nervous system cancers

▶ Gliomas

Category: Diseases, Symptoms, and Conditions
Also known as: Malignant gliomas, brain tumors, astrocytomas, ependymomas, glioblastomas, oligodendrogliomas

Related conditions: Central nervous system tumors, primary brain tumors

Definition: A glioma is a brain tumor that develops from a neuroglia, commonly known as a glial cell. Glial cells are support cells for the neurons that send and receive signals in the nervous system. There are six types of glial cells—astrocytes, oligodendrocytes, and ependymal, Schwann, microglia, and satellite cells—that can grow into a glioma. Gliomas are categorized and named based on their glial cell of origin, are considered primary central nervous system tumors, and occur in both children and adults. A glioma is a primary brain tumor, meaning that the tumor started in the brain.

An astrocytoma is the most common glioma and occurs in children and adults. Brain stem gliomas form at the connection between the brain and the spinal cord and are most common in children between the ages of three and ten but do occur in adults. Glioblastoma multiformae is the most aggressive of gliomas and accounts for almost 25 percent of all primary brain tumors.

Risk factors: Most brain tumors have no known risk factors. Exposure to radiation or radiation of the brain may cause a brain tumor. There are no studies that prove brain tumors are caused by cell phone use, electric lines, injury or accidents, exposure to toxic fumes, hair dyes, or any food or food product. The National Cancer Institute reports that exposure to vinyl chloride, a gas used in making plastic, may increase the chance of developing glioma.

Etiology and the disease process: There is no known cause for glioma. Malignant gliomas are aggressive tumors that may spread quickly throughout the brain. Because the brain controls almost all body functions, a rapidly growing tumor may cause problems with breathing, sight, hearing, smell, balance, body temperature, and other functions, creating life-threatening conditions. As the glioma increases in size, the symptoms progress, leading to difficulty with activities of daily living. Gliomas are considered incurable, and once diagnosed, a survival time of less than one year is not unusual.

Incidence: Gliomas account for approximately 42 percent of all central nervous system (CNS) tumors and 77 percent of all malignant CNS tumors. Just over 9,000 gliomas are diagnosed each year in the United States. The average age at diagnosis for adults is fifty-four. Children with brain tumors are diagnosed evenly over the ages from birth to nineteen years.

Symptoms: Depending on the type and grade of the tumor, tumors may grow one to two years before symptoms develop. The brain can adjust to a slow-growing, low-grade tumor and may adapt over time, but symptoms eventually will occur. A high-grade or aggressive tumor

Five-Year Relative Survival Rate by Histologic Type for Adult Brain Cancers, 1988-2001

Histologic Type	*Survival Rate (%)*
Glioma[a]	45.2
Glioma, other[b]	36.3
Ependymoma	71.6
Astrocytoma	35.8
Glioblastoma	2.7
Oligodendroglioma	68.2
Medulloblastoma	66.4
Germ-cell neoplasms, other	50.3

Source: Data from L. A. G. Ries et al., eds., *Cancer Survival Among Adults: U.S. SEER Program, 1988-2001—Patient and Tumor Characteristics,* NIH Pub. No. 07-6215 (Bethesda, Md.: National Cancer Institute, 2007)

[a]Nasal glioma, subependymal glioma, missed gliomas

[b]Choroid plexus papilloma, malignant; primitive polar spongioblastoma; primitive neuroectodermal tumor

may cause dramatic symptoms that develop quickly. The most common symptoms are headache, seizures or convulsions, weakness or paralysis, nausea or vomiting, difficulty walking due to poor balance, behavior changes, confusion, and vision changes.

Screening and diagnosis: There are no screening tests for gliomas. Diagnosis begins when the patient complains of symptoms suggestive of a glioma. A physician with a specialty in neurology or neurosurgery should be involved in a comprehensive physical examination of the patient. Diagnostic radiology procedures such as computed tomography (CT) and magnetic resonance imaging (MRI) of the head are most commonly used when a patient exhibits symptoms. A positron emission tomography (PET) scan may be used as it can assist in determining if the tumor is malignant. A biopsy is generally not done for diagnosis because of inability to reach the tumor, but one is usually done at the time of surgery to determine the specific cell type. Staging is based on identifying the location of the primary tumor (T X-4), evidence of metastasis (M X-1), and grade (G I-IV).

Treatment and therapy: Treatment for gliomas is difficult and usually combines surgery (if the tumor can be reached) and radiation. Radiosurgery is an option if the tumor is inoperable. Chemotherapy has limited use because of the difficulty of getting the drugs into the brain in the proper amounts to kill cells. Carmustine (BCNU) is one drug that is able to penetrate into the brain and has shown some activity against gliomas. It does have toxicity that limits its use. Recommendations for treatment are consistently moving toward surgery, radiation, and systemic chemotherapy. Advances in the treatment of gliomas include a wafer with carmustine that is placed into the surgical site after removal of the tumor. Temozolomide (Temodar), an oral drug with few side effects, has shown activity when a glioma returns. Clinical studies are ongoing to determine other chemotherapy combinations that may be useful in treating gliomas.

Prognosis, prevention, and outcomes: The prognosis depends on the type of the glioma, the age of the patient, and the symptoms of the patient when diagnosed. Gliomas are difficult to treat, and survival time is often limited. Slower growing, low-grade tumors, even when treated successfully at first, have the potential to grow back and progress. Avoiding radiation to the head is the only documented prevention. If the tumor is treated successfully, which is rare, there may still be major physical limitations that exist from side effects of the tumor or its treatment.

Patricia Stanfill Edens, R.N., Ph.D., FACHE

For Further Information

Ashby, L. S., and T. C. Ryken. "Management of Malignant Glioma: Steady Progress with Multimodal Approaches." *Neurosurgical Focus* 20, no. 4 (2006): E6.

Barnett, Gene H., ed. *High-Grade Gliomas: Diagnosis and Treatment.* Totowa, N.J.: Humana, 2007.

Berger, Mitchel S., and Charles B. Wilson, eds. *The Gliomas.* Philadelphia: W. B. Saunders, 1999.

Other Resources

American Cancer Society
http://www.cancer.org

National Brain Tumor Foundation
http://www.braintumor.org

National Cancer Institute
http://www.cancer.gov

See also: Astrocytomas; Boron Neutron Capture Therapy (BNCT); *BRAF* gene; Brain and central nervous system cancers; Carcinomatous meningitis; Cell phones; Craniotomy; Cyclin-dependent kinase inhibitor-2A (*CDKN2A*); Ependymomas; Meningeal carcinomatosis; Mitochondrial DNA mutations; Neurofibromatosis type 1 (NF1); Neurologic oncology; Oligodendrogliomas; Orbit tumors; Pheochromocytomas; Spinal axis tumors; Spinal cord compression; Turcot syndrome; Von Hippel-Lindau (VHL) disease

▶ Glomus tumors

Category: Diseases, Symptoms, and Conditions
Also known as: Glomangiomas

Related conditions: Benign tumors of blood vessels and lymphatics (hemangiomas, lymphangiomas)

Definition: Glomus tumors are benign but often exquisitely painful tumors that are formed from nests of specialized cells from the glomus body, a specialized arteriovenous structure involved in thermoregulation (temperature control via the skin). They manifest as round, slightly elevated, firm nodules, and when visible, the lesion appears as a small reddish-blue discoloration of the skin. Solitary or multiple in number, they are generally less than 1 centimeter (cm) in diameter. Microscopically, a tumor consists of collections of uniform cells that appear epithelial in nature and lie along the outside of abundant, branching blood vessels. Smooth muscle fibers are seen as part of the connective tissue matrix along with nerve fibers. These nerve fibers are intermixed with thick-walled capillaries and are responsible for the lancinating pain.

Risk factors: There are no known risk factors for glomus tumors.

Etiology and the disease process: Although the initiating event is unknown, the disease process is clearly an abnormal proliferation of glomus cells. These cells are differentiated perivascular cells from the arterial portions of the glomus body (Sucquet-Hoyer canal), which is a common arteriovenous shunt located in the dermis. Most hereditary glomangiomas are associated with defects in the glomulin gene, located on chromosome 1.

Incidence: Although glomus tumors are more frequent in adults, the exact incidence is unknown. The skin and subcutaneous tissues of the hands and feet are usually affected, but a tumor may develop in any location in which a glomus body is found. These vascular tumors occur more often in the hand (75 percent) than elsewhere and are located beneath the fingernail (subungual) in 25 to 65 percent of patients. In the head and neck areas, glomus tumors account for 0.6 percent of all neoplasms.

Symptoms: Pain, cold sensitivity, and point tenderness are the characteristic symptoms of a glomus tumor. Direct pressure on the tumor can cause excruciating pain.

Screening and diagnosis: Because of this tumor's rarity and small size, a diagnosis may be problematic. In subungual tumors, X rays can demonstrate bony erosion in 14 to 60 percent of patients. Whereas bone scans and ultrasound scans have been helpful, high-resolution magnetic resonance imaging (MRI) remains the standard for imaging diagnostics.

Treatment and therapy: Nonoperative treatment is chosen if local measures such as nonsteroidal anti-inflammatory drugs (NSAIDs) and activity modification adequately control discomfort. For resistant tumors, surgery involves a meticulous and complete excision of the encapsulated lesion.

Prognosis, prevention, and outcomes: Wide excision is curative, although reoperation rates of 12 to 24 percent have been reported.

John L. Zeller, M.D., Ph.D.

See also: Benign tumors; Endotheliomas; Eye cancers; Hemangiosarcomas; Nuclear medicine scan; Orbit tumors; Spinal axis tumors

▶ Graft-Versus-Host Disease (GVHD)

Category: Diseases, Symptoms, and Conditions

Related conditions: Bone marrow transplantation, stem cell transplantation, allogeneic transplant

Definition: Following an allogeneic bone marrow transplant or umbilical cord blood transplant, graft-versus-host disease (GVHD) may develop. GVHD is a complication that occurs when white blood cells (or immune cells, also known as T cells) from the donor or cord blood, administered to the patient during the transplant, attack the patient's own cells as foreign. The donor cells are called the "graft" and the patient's body is considered the "host," hence the name graft-versus-host disease.

Risk factors: Those who have undergone an allogeneic bone marrow transplant or an umbilical cord blood transplant are at risk for this condition.

Etiology and the disease process: When patients have an allogeneic bone marrow transplant, they receive stem cells from a relative, usually a parent, sister, or brother. An unrelated person's stem cells may also be used if the donor's cells match the patient's. Umbilical cord blood, collected from the umbilical cord and placenta at the birth of a baby and stored in a cord blood bank, is rich in stem cells and may be used if a match to the patient is found. The transplant's success is often related to how well the proteins on the surface of the donated cells match the cells of the patient. These proteins are called human leukocyte-associated (HLA) antigens and are identified by a blood test. Acute GVHD can develop within a few weeks of the transplant but always within the first one hundred days after the transplant. Patients who get acute GVHD are more likely to develop chronic GVHD. Chronic GVHD develops well after the transplant, usually during or after the third month post transplant in patients who may or may not have developed acute GVHD. Chronic GVHD can last for years after the transplant and, like acute GVHD, can be mild to life-threatening.

Incidence: The incidence rate of acute GVHD varies from 33 percent in HLA identical siblings to 75 percent in unrelated, HLA matched, or related, partially matched transplants. Chronic GVHD may occur in one-third to two-thirds of transplant patients. Incidence rates vary with the initial use and aggressiveness of immunosuppressive therapy, and use of T-cell depleted stem cells. Incidence is generally thought to be lower in patients receiving matched cord blood.

Symptoms: Symptoms of GVHD depend on the part of the body affected by the disease. The skin, eyes, stomach, intestines, and liver are the most commonly affected organs in the body. In acute GVHD, skin symptoms include the development of a rash on the palms of the hands and soles of the feet. If GVHD is severe, blisters may appear. Cramping, nausea, and diarrhea may occur with digestive tract involvement, and jaundice (a yellowing of the skin) may occur with liver involvement. Chronic GVHD symptoms include skin changes, including rash, pain in the mouth, dry mouth and eyes, and digestive tract symptoms. Advanced chronic GVHD may cause a hardening or tightness in the skin, and joints may become stiff.

Screening and diagnosis: Screening and diagnosis are made based on symptoms occurring after transplant, including fever, rashes, and organ involvement. A definitive diagnosis is made by skin or organ biopsy. There are four stages of acute GVHD, with rankings based on skin, liver, and gastrointestinal changes. Five grades are given to the acute version, ranging from none to life-threatening. A higher stage and grade means a more aggressive, acute GVHD. Chronic GVHD is based on a grading related to skin involvement and liver function. An early diagnosis may provide a better chance for treatment.

Treatment and therapy: Because up to 75 percent of patients may develop acute GVHD, early diagnosis is critical so that treatment may begin promptly. The initial treatment is steroids for both acute and chronic GVHD. Prednisone and cyclosporine are the usual drugs of choice, along with symptom management. New agents are under study that may have a role in managing acute GVHD, including monoclonal antibodies and alemtuzumab (Campath). Chronic GVHD is usually treated with steroids every other day. Additional treatment manages the symptoms of GVHD, such as diarrhea and fever.

Prognosis, prevention, and outcomes: If steroids fail to control GVHD, the prognosis is poor, as there is no other proven therapy. Development of higher stage, acute GVHD is linked to increased morbidity and mortality. Chronic GVHD may be associated with longer term survival, as presence of chronic GVHD may protect a patient from relapse. Prevention includes drug prophylaxis with corticosteroids, and in some cases methotrexate and other drugs or agents; more accurate HLA typing with as strong a match as possible; and depletion of T cells prior to administration of the donor cells. Using umbilical cord blood may also be preventive for GVHD, as the stem cells are immature and less likely to cause GVHD. The disease can range from very mild to life-threatening.

Patricia Stanfill Edens, R.N., Ph.D., FACHE

For Further Information

Couriel, Daniel, et al. "Ancillary Therapy and Supportive Care of Chronic Graft-Versus-Host Disease: National Institutes of Health Consensus Development Project on Criteria for Clinical Trials in Chronic Graft-Versus-Host Disease—V. Ancillary Therapy and Supportive Care Working Group Report." *Biology of Blood and Marrow Transplantion* 12, no. 4 (2006): 375-396.

Lee, Stephanie J., Georgia Vogelsang, and Mary E. D. Flowers. "Chronic Graft-Versus-Host Disease." *Biology of Blood and Marrow Transplantion* 9, no. 4 (2003): 215-233.

Other Resources

Bone and Marrow Transplant Information Network
http://www.bmtinfonet.org

National Cancer Institute
Bone Marrow Transplantation and Peripheral Blood Stem Cell Transplantation: Questions and Answers
http://www.cancer.gov/cancertopics/factsheet/Therapy/bone-marrow-transplant

National Marrow Donor Program
Graft-Versus-Host Disease
http://www.marrow.org/PATIENT/Plan_Life_after_Tx/Managing_Long-Term_Effects_of_/Graft-Versus-Host_Disease/index.html

See also: Bone Marrow Transplantation (BMT); Cyclosporin A; Pheresis; Stem cell transplantation; Transfusion therapy; Umbilical cord blood transplantation

▶ Granulosa cell tumors

Category: Diseases, Symptoms, and Conditions

Related conditions: Endocrine imbalances, endometrial hyperplasia, endometrial adenocarcinoma

Definition: Granulosa cell tumors are slow-growing tumors almost always found in the ovaries. They have a low potential for becoming malignant. These tumors usually secrete large amounts of estrogen, although occasionally they secrete androgens (male hormones).

Risk factors: Granulosa cell tumors are evenly distributed among women of all races and ethnicities. Most tumors occur in postmenopausal women and are diagnosed between the ages of fifty and fifty-five. Only 5 percent are found in women under age thirty.

Etiology and the disease process: Researchers are unclear about how these malignancies arise. One theory is that they are related to chromosomal abnormalities. Another is that they are caused by a defect in hormonal regulation. These tumors grow slowly.

Incidence: Granulosa cell tumors make up about 5 to 8 percent of malignant tumors of the ovaries. Between 1,500 and 2,000 cases are diagnosed each year in the United States.

Symptoms: Granulosa cell tumors usually secrete estrogen. In children this tends to cause abnormally early signs of puberty. In reproductive-age women, it disrupts the menstrual cycle, and in postmenopausal women, the most common symptom is uterine bleeding. Other symptoms include an increase in the size of the abdomen and abdominal or pelvic pain.

Screening and diagnosis: Most women seek medical attention because of the side effects of increased estrogen. On physical examination, the physician can feel the tumor in more than 90 percent of women. Average diameter of the tumor at diagnosis is 4.7 inches (12 centimeters). Physical findings are confirmed with blood tests, imaging tests, and biopsy.

Some 90 percent of tumors are diagnosed in Stage I with malignancy confined to only one ovary. In Stage II, the tumor has begun to extend into the tissues near the ovary. In Stage III, it has metastasized to the abdomen, and in Stage IV to distant sites.

Treatment and therapy: Treatment is always surgical removal of the affected ovary. Postmenopausal women may also have a hysterectomy. Chemotherapy and radiation treatment are used in the 10 percent of women whose cancer has advanced beyond Stage I.

Prognosis, prevention, and outcomes: Prognosis is excellent for tumors in Stage I, with ten-year survival rates of 90 to 96 percent. The ten-year survival rate for more advanced cancers is about half this rate. Tumors diagnosed in women under age thirty tend to recur within three years, but in postmenopausal women years or even decades may pass before recurrence.

Martiscia Davidson, A.M.

See also: Dilation and Curettage (D&C); Endometrial cancer; Endometrial hyperplasia; Hormone Replacement Therapy (HRT); Ovarian cancers; Ovarian cysts

▶ Gynecologic cancers

Category: Diseases, Symptoms, and Conditions
Also known as: Cervical cancer, uterine cancer, ovarian cancer, gestational trophoblastic disease, and cancers of the vulva, vagina, and Fallopian tubes

Related conditions: Cancer of the colon and rectum, cancer of the bladder, peritoneal carcinomatosis

Definition: Gynecologic cancers are cancers that arise in one of the anatomic structures of the female reproductive tract: the Fallopian tubes, the ovaries, the uterus, the cervix, the vagina, and the vulva. Historically, cancer of the breast has not been considered to be a gynecologic cancer.

Risk factors: Risk factors have been identified for many of the gynecologic cancers. For cervical cancer, they include a woman's having her first sexual encounter at less than age fifteen, multiple sexual partners, promiscuous male partners, a history of sexually transmitted diseases, an impaired immune system, and cigarette smoking.

Age Groups with the Highest Incidence of Specific Gynecologic Cancers

Type of Cancer	*Age at Diagnosis*	*Women Diagnosed (%)*
Gestational trophoblastic	20-29	43.9
Cervical	40-49	27.0
Uterine	50-59	27.9
Ovarian	50-59	23.1
Fallopian tube	60-69	28.7
Vulva	70-79	29.7

Source: Data from L. A. G. Ries et al., eds., *Cancer Survival Among Adults: U.S. SEER Program, 1988-2001—Patient and Tumor Characteristics,* NIH Pub. No. 07-6215 (Bethesda, Md.: National Cancer Institute, 2007)

Risk factors for uterine cancer are use of medications containing estrogen without the addition of progesterone (the so-called unopposed estrogen effect), use of the medication tamoxifen for more than two years, onset of late menopause (at greater than age fifty-two), obesity, never having had children (nulliparity), diabetes, high blood pressure, and increased dietary fat intake as well as having had estrogen-secreting ovarian tumors, polycystic ovarian syndrome, or radiation therapy to the pelvis.

Risk factors for ovarian cancer are not having been pregnant, incessant ovulation (ovulation not interrupted by use of oral contraceptives or by pregnancy), a family history of ovarian cancer, breast cancer, Western lifestyle, and exposure to talc.

A risk factor for cancer of the vulva is exposure to the human papillomavirus (HPV).

Risk factors for cancer of the vagina include age, HPV infection, exposure to diethylstilbestrol (DES), a history of cervical cancer, vaginal adenosis, uterine prolapse, cigarette smoking, chronic vaginal irritation, low socioeconomic status, hysterectomy at an early age, and vaginal trauma.

The major risk factors for cancer of the Fallopian tube are chronic inflammation in the form of endometriosis or pelvic infections, a history of infertility, and low parity (no children or only one or two).

The primary risk factors for gestational trophoblastic disease are being over age forty or less than age twenty and having a history of a prior molar pregnancy.

Etiology and the disease process: What is known about the etiology of gynecological cancers varies. Cancer of the Fallopian tube and ovary share abnormalities of the cancer genes *TP53* and *ERBB-2*, suggesting similar genetic risks and environmental factors. HPV causes cervical cancer and is believed to cause changes that progress to cancer of the vulva. If left untreated, up to one-third of women infected with HPV will develop cervical cancer. Women who have long-term unopposed estrogen stimulation undergo benign changes in the endometrium that can precede the development of uterine cancer.

Most vaginal cancers are metastatic, originating from cancers of the cervix or vulva and spreading to the vagina, although metastases have been reported to occur from the uterus, ovaries, colon, rectum, breast, and even the kidney.

Gestational trophoblastic disease, which can mimic a normal pregnancy, progresses rapidly and is fatal if not treated but has a good prognosis with treatment. Ovarian cancer is an insidious disease, and with the lack of screening and the associated vague symptoms, most cases are advanced at the time of diagnosis.

Incidence: Cancer of the uterus is the most frequent cancer involving the female reproductive tract in the United States, and the fourth most frequent cancer affecting women, behind breast, lung, and colorectal cancer. There are approximately 41,000 new cases of uterine cancer each year, with about 7,300 deaths. An individual woman's lifetime risk of cancer of the uterus is about 1 in 50. Ovarian cancer is the second most common cancer involving the female reproductive tract and is the leading cause of death of all gynecologic cancers. There are approximately 26,000 new cases diagnosed each year and 16,000 deaths. The lifetime risk for ovarian cancer is 1 in 70. The third most common gynecologic cancer is cervical cancer, with 12,800 new cases per year and 4,600 deaths.

Less common cancers are those of the vagina, with about 2,000 new cases each year, and cancer of the vulva, with 1,000 to 1,500 new cases per year. About 5 percent of all gynecologic cancers are vulvar, and 1 to 2 percent of malignancies involving the female reproductive tract are vaginal cancer. Fallopian tube cancer is the rarest cancer involving the female genital tract, accounting for approximately 1 percent of all gynecologic malignancies. There are approximately 300 cases diagnosed in the United States each year. Gestational trophoblastic disease occurs in 1 in 850 to 1,300 pregnancies and 1 in 2,000 deliveries.

Symptoms: Many gynecologic cancers share symptoms such as abnormal bleeding; however, some are much harder to detect. Abnormal bleeding through the vagina is the most common symptom associated with cancer of the uterus, occurring in approximately 90 percent of cases. For premenopausal women, this may take the form of so-called breakthrough bleeding, prolonged bleeding, or heavy bleeding, all of which generally reflect an underlying hormonal imbalance and can be treated as such. For postmenopausal women, any bleeding should be considered abnormal and should be evaluated by a gynecologist. Abnormal uterine bleeding is the most frequent symptom of gestational trophoblastic disease. The most common symptoms associated with cancers of the vagina are abnormal bleeding or an excessive, nonodorous, watery discharge; less frequent symptoms include pelvic pain, an increased frequency of urination or pain with urination, and constipation. Cancer of the Fallopian tube, for the most part, is a disease without specific symptoms. Symptoms that are associated with cancer of the Fallopian tube include an abnormal, watery vaginal discharge or excessive bleeding. Pain and a palpable pelvic mass are infrequently associated with Fallopian tube cancer. For cancer of the vulva, irritation and itching are the most common symptoms.

Cervical and ovarian cancer are harder to detect through symptoms. An abnormal Pap smear is the earliest "symptom" of cervical cancer, as most patients with cervical cancer are physically asymptomatic. In more advanced cases of cervical cancer, bleeding after intercourse (postcoital bleeding), intermenstrual bleeding, or postmenopausal bleeding may occur. The symptoms of ovarian cancer are nonspecific, and because of this, the diagnosis is often delayed. The most common symptoms include bloating, abdominal fullness (necessitating an increase in clothing size), early fullness after eating, heartburn, and abdominal pain.

Screening and diagnosis: Screening for gynecologic cancers ranges from the common Pap smear to visual inspection to no screening for rarer cancers. Pap smears are used to screen for cervical cancer. The diagnosis of cervical cancer is established by consistent findings on an abnormal Pap smear with a large biopsy of the cervix (conization), performed as an outpatient in the hospital. Stage I cervical cancer is confined to the cervix, Stage II involves spread to the upper two-thirds of the vagina, Stage III involves spread to the lower one-third of the vagina, and Stage IV involves cancer that has spread to the bladder or rectum, or outside the pelvis.

No routine screening test exists for cancer of the uterus, but those at high risk for the cancer can be screened by endometrial sampling and measurement of the endometrial thickness (or lining). Endometrial sampling is an office-based procedure in which a small, flexible plastic catheter is inserted into the uterus and the cells lining the uterus (endometrial cells) are drawn into the catheter. Endometrial sampling can also serve as the diagnostic test for endometrial cancer. In some cases, if the diagnosis of uterine cancer is in question based on endometrial sampling, a dilation and curettage (D&C) can be performed as an outpatient procedure in which more extensive sampling of the uterine cavity can be performed. Measurement of the endometrial thickness is also an office-based procedure, but in some cases is done by a radiologist. Using an ultrasound probe through the vagina (transvaginal ultrasound), the thickness of the lining of the uterus is measured. Stage I cancer is limited to the uterus, Stage II involves extension from the body of the uterus to the cervix, Stage III occurs when the tumor protrudes through the uterus or metastasizes to the vagina, pelvis, or lymph nodes adjacent to the aorta, and Stage IV cancer exists when metastases involve the bladder, the bowel, or organs outside the pelvis in the abdomen.

Other than an annual well-woman examination with palpation of the ovaries, no specific screening is recommended for ovarian cancer. However, for women at high risk or those specifically concerned about ovarian cancer, a transvaginal ultrasonogram (in which the volume of the ovaries is determined), combined with a cancer antigen (CA) 125 blood test, can be performed. The diagnosis of ovarian cancer is made at the time of surgery, although abdominal ultrasonography and computed tomography (CT) scans of the pelvis generally are obtained first. Ovarian cancer is staged as follows: Stage I involves a tumor limited to one or both ovaries, Stage II ovarian cancer exists when the tumor has extended to the pelvis, Stage III cancer involves a tumor outside the pelvis, and Stage IV cancer is characterized by distant metastases (lungs or liver).

For cancer of the vulva, no screening is recommended other than visual inspection during an annual well-woman examination. The diagnosis is made by biopsy of any suspicious lesion. Stage I cancer is less than 2 centimeters (cm) in diameter and confined to the vulva, Stage II cancer is greater than 2 cm in diameter and confined to the vulva, Stage III cancer extends to the anus or urethra or lymph nodes on one side, and Stage IV involves spread to the bladder, rectum, bones of the pelvis, or lymph nodes on both sides.

Screening for vaginal cancer should be performed in the context of the annual well-woman examination. Stage 0 vaginal cancer is referred to as carcinoma in situ, referring to cancer that is localized without apparent spread.

Stage I vaginal cancer is limited to the vaginal wall. Stage II vaginal cancer has extended to the subvaginal tissues but not to the pelvic wall. Stage III vaginal cancer involves the pelvic wall. Stage IV vaginal cancer has spread beyond the pelvis or has extended to the bladder or rectum.

No screening exists for cancer of the Fallopian tube. Stage 0 is cancer limited to the lining of the Fallopian tube. Stage I is cancer limited to one tube with extension into the muscular layer of the tube but not to the external surface of the tube. Stage II cancer involves one or both tubes with extension beyond the Fallopian tube. Stage III cancer involves one or both tubes with spread beyond the pelvic cavity. Stage IV cancer involves one or both Fallopian tubes with distant metastases, for example, the lungs.

Specific screening is not recommended for gestational trophoblastic disease. With the advent of obstetric ultrasonography, few cases of gestational trophoblastic disease are diagnosed in advanced stages when symptoms occur. The diagnosis is made when the pregnancy blood test shows that the level of beta-human chorionic gonadotropin (β-HCG) is elevated beyond what is expected and the ultrasound shows no fetus (exhibits a snowstorm pattern). Gestational trophoblastic disease is staged as follows: Stage I is limited to the uterus, Stage II involves the female reproductive tract, Stage III has spread to the lungs, and Stage IV has spread elsewhere.

Treatment and therapy: Most gynecologic cancers are treated first with surgery and then by radiation therapy or chemotherapy; however, uterine cancer is treated primarily by surgery. Cervical cancer and cancer of the vulva are treated by surgery with or without radiation therapy. Cancer of the vagina is treated by surgery or radiation or a combination of the two, depending on the type of tumor. Ovarian cancer is treated by surgery with chemotherapy, and cancer of the Fallopian tube is treated by surgery, with or without chemotherapy. Gestational trophoblastic disease is treated by evacuation of the uterus with chemotherapy.

Prognosis, prevention, and outcomes: Gynecologic cancers range from cancers with excellent prognoses, such as low-risk gestational trophoblastic disease, to those with less favorable prognoses, such as ovarian cancer, which is usually detected in an advanced state. The prognosis of gestational trophoblastic disease is based on the woman's age, pregnancy history, β-HCG level, tumor size, metastases, and response to chemotherapy. For those at low risk, the cure rate is 100 percent; for those at high risk, the cure rate is 75 percent.

Prognostic factors for uterine cancer include the woman's age at the time of diagnosis, race, tumor stage, type of tumor, size of the uterus at the time of diagnosis, depth of invasion of the tumor into the layer of uterine muscle, presence of tumor in the blood vessels supplying the uterus, and spread of the tumor outside the uterus to other organs or lymph nodes. The overall five-year survival rates for cancer of the uterus are 87, 72, 51, and 9 percent for stages I, II, III, and IV, respectively.

The prognosis for cervical cancer depends on tumor stage, size of tumor, depth of invasion, and lymph node spread. The availability of a vaccine against HPV has provided a means for the prevention of cervical cancer. Five-year survival rates for Stages I to IV are 80 to 95, 64, 38, and 14 percent, respectively.

Prognosis of cancer of the vulva is related to the tumor stage, size of the lesion, and lymph node involvement. Five-year survival rates for Stages I to IV are 71, 61, 44, and 8 percent, respectively.

The prognosis for vaginal cancer is directly related to the stage at the time of diagnosis. The five-year survival rates for Stages I to IV are 68, 54. 35, and 20 percent, respectively. The overall five-year survival for cancer of the vagina is approximately 45 percent.

The five-year survival rate for all stages of Fallopian tube cancer combined is approximately 40 to 50 percent. Women with Stage I Fallopian tube cancer have five-year survival rates of 65 percent, Stage II disease is 50 to 60 percent, and Stages III and IV are 10 to 20 percent.

Prognosis of ovarian cancer is related to tumor stage as well as the amount of residual tumor after surgery. Because most patients are diagnosed in advanced stages, the five-year survival rate is approximately 50 percent.

D. Scott Cunningham, M.D., Ph.D.

For Further Information

Grimes, D. A. "Economy KE: Primary Prevention of Gynecologic Cancers." *American Journal of Obstetrics and Gynecology* 172 (1995): 227.

Hartmann, Lynn C., and Charles L. Loprinzi, eds. *Mayo Clinic Guide to Women's Cancers.* Rochester, Minn.: Mayo Clinic, 2005.

Krychman, Michael L. *One Hundred Questions and Answers for Women Living with Cancer: A Practical Guide for Survivorship.* Sudbury, Mass.: Jones and Bartlett, 2007.

Sutton, Amy, ed. *Cancer Sourcebook for Women.* 3d ed. Detroit: Omnigraphics, 2006.

Other Resources

American Association for Cancer Research
Support and Advocacy Groups: Gynecologic Cancers
http://www.aacr.org/home/survivors—advocates/cancer-resources—organizations,-agencies-and-web-sites/support-and-advocacy-groups/us-and-canadian-groups-by-focus/gynecologic-cancers.aspx

American Society of Clinical Oncology
Gynecologic Cancers
http://gyncancers.asco.org

Eyes on the Prize.org
http://www.eyesontheprize.org/links/gynca.html

See also: Amenorrhea; Breast cancer in pregnant women; Cervical cancer; Childbirth and cancer; Choriocarcinomas; Colposcopy; Dilation and Curettage (D&C); Endocrine cancers; Endocrinology oncology; Endometrial cancer; Endometrial hyperplasia; Fallopian tube cancer; Fertility drugs and cancer; Fertility issues; Gestational Trophoblastic Tumors (GTTs); Gynecologic oncology; Hormone Replacement Therapy (HRT); Hysterectomy; Hysterography; Hystero-oophorectomy; Hysteroscopy; Infertility and cancer; Oophorectomy; Ovarian cancers; Ovarian cysts; Ovarian epithelial cancer; Pap test; Pelvic examination; Placental Alkaline Phosphatase (PALP); Pregnancy and cancer; Salpingectomy and salpingo-oophorectomy; Sterility; Transvaginal ultrasound; Uterine cancer; Vaginal cancer; Vulvar cancer

▶ Hairy cell leukemia

Category: Diseases, Symptoms, and Conditions
Also known as: Leukemic reticuloendotheliosis

Related conditions: Anemia, thrombocytopenia (excessive bleeding and bruising)

Definition: Hairy cell leukemia is a rare, chronic, slow-progressing cancer of the blood and bone marrow that is most often found in people over age forty and does not occur in children.

Risk factors: Although there is some debate about the role of risk factors in hairy cell leukemia, the following appear to increase the likelihood of developing this cancer: a family history of blood cancers, Ashkenazi Jewish heritage, a previous diagnosis of cancer, and exposure to radiation, sawdust, and toxins, especially those in agricultural chemicals and petrochemicals.

Etiology and the disease process: Researchers have not yet determined exactly what changes in deoxyribonucleic acid (DNA) cause the development of hairy cell leukemia. They do know that hairy cell leukemia begins in the bone marrow. The bone marrow makes stem cells that develop into three types of blood cells: red blood cells, white blood cells, and platelets. Hairy cell leukemia is a defect in white blood cell production.

White blood cells are part of the immune system. Their function is to produce antibodies (proteins) and fight infection. Hairy cell leukemia affects the type of white blood cells called lymphocytes. There are three kinds of lymphocytes. In response to foreign organisms (bacteria, viruses, fungi), B lymphocytes produce antibodies that help destroy these foreign organisms. They are helped by two other types of lymphocytes, T lymphocytes and natural killer (NK) cells. All three types of lymphocytes must function properly to control infections.

In people with hairy cell leukemia, too many stem cells turn into B lymphocytes. These B lymphocytes develop abnormal threadlike projections that make them look "hairy." Hairy lymphocytes are defective and do not function correctly in fighting infections. Because an abnormally large number of stem cells turn into hairy B lymphocytes, the number of other blood cells is smaller than usual. A decrease in red blood cells leads to anemia. A decrease in platelets makes it difficult for the blood to clot. The increase in hairy B lymphocytes occurs gradually and at first produces no obvious signs. Nevertheless, as the bone marrow produces more and more defective B lymphocytes, these cells collect in the spleen (an organ in the abdomen) and sometimes in the liver. The spleen begins to swell and become tender.

Incidence: About 600 to 800 people in the United States are newly diagnosed with hairy cell leukemia each year. Five times more men than women develop this cancer. Most are diagnosed in their early fifties.

Symptoms: Hairy cell leukemia usually produces gradual, very general symptoms that initially are not very noticeable. A decrease in the number of red blood cells causes anemia, which results in unusual tiredness, weakness, and shortness of breath. A decrease in platelets causes easy bruising and difficulty getting blood to clot. Defective B lymphocytes lead to increased infections and sometimes a low-grade fever associated with chronic infection. The individual may feel bloating or tenderness below the ribs. This is caused by swelling of the spleen (splenomegaly) as masses of hairy B lymphocytes collect there and sometimes in the liver. Individuals may lose weight for no obvious reason.

Screening and diagnosis: Hairy cell leukemia is rare, so there are no routine screening tests for this cancer. Most people first see a physician for symptoms related to anemia or because of repeated infections due to malfunctioning B lymphocytes. Hairy cell leukemia is usually discovered during testing to determine the cause of these symptoms.

Diagnosis of hairy cell leukemia begins with a physical examination. About 80 percent of people with hairy cell leukemia have a spleen so enlarged that the physician can feel it by pressing on (palpating) the abdomen. However, an imaging scan (computed tomography, ultrasound) may be done to determine the size of the spleen, especially if the individual complains of bloating and tenderness. A complete blood count (CBC) determines the number and type of blood cells. If the lymphocyte count is high, a peripheral blood smear is done. This test looks at a thin layer of blood under a microscope to check for abnormal or "hairy" cells. About 20 percent of people with hairy cell anemia show abnormalities on liver function tests.

Diagnosis continues with a bone and bone marrow biopsy. Under local anesthetic, a small piece of bone and marrow is removed from the hip bone and examined in the laboratory for cancer cells. Definitive diagnosis of hairy cell leukemia comes from examining under the microscope the pattern of proteins on the surface of B lymphocytes. This is called immunophenotyping, and it helps distinguish between hairy cell leukemia and other blood cancers.

Since hairy cell leukemia is a chronic, slow-growing cancer, it is not staged using the standard TNM (tumor/lumph node/metastasis) system. The staging of hairy cell leukemia is as follows:

- Untreated or newly diagnosed hairy cell leukemia: Hairy B lymphocytes are found in the blood and bone marrow. Other blood cell levels may be decreased, and the spleen is enlarged.
- Progressive hairy cell leukemia: The cancer has been treated with chemotherapy or removal of the spleen (splenectomy). There is an increased number of hairy cells, or other blood cell levels are below normal.
- Relapsed or refractory hairy cell leukemia: Hairy cell leukemia has returned after treatment (relapsed) or has not responded to treatment (refractory).

Treatment and therapy: Because hairy cell leukemia progresses very slowly and sometimes not at all, the patient and physician may decide to wait and monitor the blood to see if conditions worsen. Early treatment—although imperative for most other cancers—does not improve the chance for remission, survival, or cure, so if symptoms are not too burdensome, waiting does not harm the patient. Eventually most people need treatment, but some individuals go ten or more years before treatment becomes necessary.

One course of chemotherapy puts as much as 80 percent of hairy cell leukemia cases into complete remission and the remainder in partial remission. Remission is a condition in which symptoms disappear, but the cancer is still present in the body and can reoccur. The chemotherapy drug of choice is cladribine (Leustatin), and the alternative is pentostatin (Nipent).

About 10 percent of patients do not improve with chemotherapy, and others have health conditions that prohibit chemotherapy treatments. These individuals may receive biological therapy (immunotherapy). The goal of biological therapy is to boost the immune system and make cancer cells more recognizable to healthy immune system cells so that they will be destroyed. Interferon alpha and rituximab (a monoclonal antibody made in the laboratory) are the standard biological therapies for hairy cell leukemia. Biological therapy is frequently successful in bringing about remission.

Surgery to remove the spleen may also be done when the spleen is so enlarged that it may burst. This does not cure hairy cell leukemia but does restore the blood count to normal, which helps the body fight infection.

Clinical trials are under way to test new treatments for hairy cell leukemia. There is no cost to the patient to participate in a clinical trial.

Prognosis, prevention, and outcomes: Hairy cell leukemia rarely is cured but usually can be put into remission through treatment. Remission can last many years before symptoms recur. Recurring symptoms are often successfully treated. Overall survival rate at twelve years is about 87 percent, with more than half of individuals showing no progression of symptoms. About 17 percent of people with hairy cell leukemia eventually go on to develop other types of cancer.

Martiscia Davidson, A.M.

For Further Information

Icon Health. *Hairy Cell Leukemia: A Medical Dictionary, Bibliography, and Annotated Research Guide to Internet References*. San Diego, Calif.: Author, 2004.

Parker, James N., and Phillip M. Parker, eds. *The Official Patient's Sourcebook on Hairy Cell Leukemia*. San Diego, Calif.: Icon Health, 2002.

Ravandi, F., and S. O'Brien. "Chronic Lymphoid Leukemias Other than Chronic Lymphocytic Leukemia: Diagnosis and Treatment." *Mayo Clinic Proceedings* 80, no. 12 (December, 2005): 1660-1674.

Other Resources

Hairy Cell Leukemia Research Foundation
http://www.hairycellleukemia.org

The Leukemia and Lymphoma Society
http://www.leukemia-lymphoma.org

MayoClinic.com
Hairy Cell Leukemia
http://www.mayoclinic.com/health/hairy-cell-leukemia/DS00673

National Cancer Institute
Hairy Cell Leukemia Treatment
http://www.cancer.gov/cancertopics/pdq/treatment/hairy-cell-leukemia/Patient

See also: Aleukemia; Biological therapy; Blood cancers; Cytokines; Leukemias; Lymphocytosis; Oncogenic viruses; Splenectomy; Staging of cancer; Watchful waiting

▶ Hand-Foot Syndrome (HFS)

Category: Diseases, Symptoms, and Conditions
Also known as: Palmar-plantar erythrodysesthesia (PPE), hand-to-foot syndrome, Burgdorf's reaction, chemotherapy-induced acral erythema

Related conditions: Hand-foot skin reaction (HSFR)

Definition: Hand-foot syndrome (HFS) is a chemotherapy-induced skin reaction characterized by swelling, tingling, redness, tenderness, pain, and possibly peeling and blistering of the palms of the hands and soles of the feet. Occurrence of HFS in patients receiving chemotherapy may result in lowering of dosage levels and interruption or discontinuation of treatment.

Risk factors: HFS is a common side effect of high-dosage treatment of certain traditional cancer chemotherapeutic agents, including 5-fluorouracil (5-FU), capecitabine, liposomal doxorubicin, and docetaxel. HFS typically occurs within the first few weeks of chemotherapy but may also occur after several weeks or months of treatment.

Etiology and the disease process: The cause of HFS is not completely understood. The most widely accepted theory is that capillaries in the palms and soles break because of several factors including overuse, pressure, or increased temperature. Breakage of the blood vessels may release small amounts of the chemotherapeutic agent into the surrounding tissue, resulting in an inflammatory reaction in the affected areas. Another theory is that the drugs pass from the body through sweat secretion, and the hands and feet are more susceptible to HFS due to the large number of sweat glands present in those areas. The hands tend to be more commonly affected than the feet; in some patients, they may be the only areas affected. HFS may also occur elsewhere on the skin, such as the neck and chest, but it is much less common. HFS is distinct from hand-foot skin reaction (HSFR), a condition reported with the use of various targeted kinase inhibitors (such as sunitinib) that is characterized by more localized, thicker, callus-like lesions.

Incidence: The occurrence of HFS is known to depend on agent, dose, and administration of the chemotherapeutic drug responsible. For example, in early phase II studies of capecitabine monotherapy for metastatic colorectal and breast cancer patients, HFS occurred in approximately 50 percent of patients; severe HFS was noted in approximately 10 percent of these patients.

Symptoms: HFS typically begins as a feeling of numbness or tingling in the palms or soles. These symptoms may rapidly progress in three to four days to swelling, redness, tenderness, and burning pain in the affected areas. If treatment with the chemotherapeutic agent is not promptly interrupted or the dose of the agent reduced, blisters may develop, causing increased pain and interfering with general activities of daily living such as walking and handling objects.

Screening and diagnosis: Histological examination of affected tissue does not discern from normal inflammation processes, preventing a true diagnostic marker for HFS. The National Cancer Institute has a general system for classifying HFS and HFSR based on three grade levels of severity:

- Grade 1: Skin changes or dermatitis without pain, for example, erythema, peeling
- Grade 2: Skin changes with pain, not interfering with function
- Grade 3: Skin changes with pain, interfering with function

Treatment and therapy: Control of symptomatic pain may occur through the use of cold compresses, particularly those that conform to the shape of the hands and feet (such as ice packs or bags of frozen corn or peas). Frequent but gentle application of highly moisturizing lotions and creams is also recommended. Elevation of the hands and feet may reduce swelling, and pain may be controlled through the use of pain relievers such as acetaminophen. Systemic corticosteroids, vitamin B6 (pyridoxine), and dimethyl-sulfoxide (DMSO) has been proposed to reduce or relieve symptoms, but conclusive evidence for these treatments has yet to be demonstrated. The only proven means to reverse the signs and symptoms of HFS is through interruption or dose reduction of chemotherapeutic therapy.

Prognosis, prevention, and outcomes: Patient education in the early phases of treatment is vital to prevent complications brought on by HFS. Patients should be instructed to contact their doctor immediately if symptoms develop, as a quick reaction can often prevent development of more severe effects. Patients receiving agents known to cause HFS are instructed to avoid wearing tight-fitting clothes (gloves, socks, stockings) and shoes as well as to avoid excessive sun exposure, hot baths and showers, steam rooms, and excessive rubbing of the soles and palms. Comfortable slippers, sandals, or shock-absorbing shoe liners should be worn to relieve painful pressure points. Moisturizing creams and lotions should be applied liberally but gently to the hands and feet. However, creams or lotions containing alcohol, perfumes, or glycerin should be avoided. Sunscreen (SPF 30 or higher) and long-sleeved shirts and pants should be worn during prolonged exposure to the sun. Strenuous physical activity and long-term alcohol use should be avoided. Once actions to interrupt or reduce the dose of chemotherapy are undertaken, reversal of symptoms is typically rapid and without long-term consequences. Chemotherapeutic treatment can typically resume at a lower dose once symptoms improve.

Scott A. Boerner, M.S.

For Further Information

Chu, Edward, and Vincent T. DeVita. *Physicians' Cancer Chemotherapy Drug Manual 2007.* Sudbury, Mass.: Jones and Bartlett, 2007.

Lassere, Yvonne, and Paulo Hoff. "Management of Hand-Foot Syndrome in Patients Treated with Capecitabine (Xeloda)." *European Journal of Oncology Nursing* 8 (2004): S31-S40.

Nagore, Eduardo, Amelia Insa, and Onofre Sanmartín. "Antineoplastic Therapy-Induced Palmar Plantar Erythrodysesthesia ('Hand-Foot') Syndrome: Incidence, Recognition, and Management." *American Journal of Clinical Dermatology* 1, no. 4 (2000): 225-234.

Yarbro, Connie H., Michelle Goodman, and Margaret H. Frogge, eds. *Cancer Symptom Management.* 3d ed. Sudbury, Mass.: Jones and Bartlett, 2004.

Other Resources

American Cancer Society
http://www.cancer.org

Cancer.Net
http://www.cancer.net/portal/site/patient

See also: Chemotherapy; Side effects

▶ Head and neck cancers

Category: Diseases, Symptoms, and Conditions
Also known as: Cancers of the mouth, sinuses, nose, salivary glands, throat, lymph nodes in neck

Related conditions: Squamous cell carcinoma, adenocarcinoma, oral cancer, laryngeal cancer, nasal cavity cancer, parasinus cancer, nasopharyngeal cancer, oropharyngeal cancer, hypopharyngeal cancer, salivary gland cancer

Definition: Head and neck cancers refers to a wide variety of cancers occurring in the head and neck region, including cancers of the throat, mouth, voice box (larynx), salivary glands, lips, nose, and sinus cavities. Cancers of the scalp, skin, bones, muscles, brain, eye, and thyroid are not usually referred to as head and neck cancers.

Risk factors: Smoking or using chewing tobacco is the greatest risk factor for head and neck cancers; in fact, tobacco use can be linked to 85 percent of these cancers. Cigarette smokers have a markedly increased chance of developing these cancers, up to a 25 percent greater risk than nonsmokers. Smoking cigars or marijuana also increases one's risk of getting these cancers. Alcohol use increases risk, and using alcohol and tobacco in combination increases risk even further. Use of betel (a seed chewed as a stimulant, mainly in Southeast Asia) or maté (a beverage consumed like tea, generally in South America) also increases the risk of head and neck cancer. These substances damage the squamous cells that form a lining of many structures in the head and neck.

Diet may also increase the risk of head and neck cancers. Processed meats, red meat, and salted fish have all been linked to increased risk of cancers of the head and neck.

White patches or spots in the mouth, called leukoplakia, are also a risk factor. About one-third of the time, these spots will turn into cancer.

Other risk factors include sun exposure, radiation to the head and neck, and environmental exposure to wood dust, paint fumes, asbestos, nickel refining, textile fibers, and chemicals used by the petroleum industry. Poor oral hygiene, poor nutrition (especially low levels of vitamins A and B), a weakened immune system, gastroesophageal reflux disease (GERD), and exposure to secondhand smoke may also play a role.

Medical experts are currently exploring the relationship between oral cancers and certain strains of human papillomavirus (HPV) infection. Epstein-Barr virus has also been associated with higher risk of cancer of the nose and throat.

Etiology and the disease process: Most head and neck cancers are squamous cell carcinomas, cancers that begin in the cells lining the mucosal tissues in the mouth and throat. If the cancer is limited to these cells, it is called carcinoma in situ. If it has spread into deeper tissues or to other sites in the body, it is called invasive squamous cell carcinoma.

Other head and neck cancers begin in the glands and are called adenocarcinomas. These types of cancer are much rarer than squamous cell carcinomas. Any tumors in these glands are usually benign and occur in people in their sixties and seventies. Another very rare type of head and neck cancer can begin in connective tissues.

Incidence: Head and neck cancers account for 3 to 5 percent of all types of cancer in the United States. Experts estimate that about 45,000 people per year in the United States will develop these types of cancer, and these cancers will cause more than 11,000 deaths. (These numbers do not include skin cancers that occur in the head and neck, which account for many more cases and deaths.) In the United States, cancers involving the mouth and throat are the most common type.

These cancers are more common in people over age fifty. They are slightly more common in men than in women and somewhat more common in African Americans than in those of other genetic backgrounds. Men are more than twice as likely as women to die of these cancers.

Symptoms: Symptoms of these types of cancers include a sore throat, neck pain, trouble swallowing, pain when swallowing, a red or white patch in the oral cavity, bad breath, swelling of the jaw, hoarseness or a change in voice, bloody sputum, bleeding from the mouth, unexplained weight loss, fatigue, sinus congestion that does not go away, loose teeth or dentures that no longer fit properly, or a lump or sore that does not heal. Cancer of the nasal cavity or throat area may involve nosebleeds or ear pain. A less common symptom is numbness of facial muscles.

Age-Adjusted Incidence Rates for Invasive Head and Neck Cancers by Site

Site	*Rate per 100,000 Adults*
Lip	0.7
Tongue	2.8
Salivary gland	1.2
Floor of mouth	0.7
Gum and other mouth	1.5
Nasopharynx	0.5
Tonsil	1.6
Orophaynx	0.4
Hypopharynx	0.8
Other oral cavity and pharynx	0.2
Nose, nasal cavity, and middle ear	0.7
Larynx	4.1

Source: U.S. Cancer Statistics Working Group, *United States Cancer Statistics: 1999-2004 Incidence and Mortality Web-Based Report* (Atlanta: U.S. Department of Health and Human Services, Centers for Disease Control and Prevention and National Cancer Institute, 2007)

Screening and diagnosis: Many of the symptoms of head and neck cancers can be caused by other conditions, so people who use alcohol and tobacco should be screened at least yearly for head and neck cancers. Some types of tests that doctors or dentists may use to screen for these cancers are a visual inspection of the oral or nasal cavity using a small mirror and light, a physical examination for lumps, an endoscopy of the nasal or oral cavities, laboratory tests, X rays, ultrasounds, computed tomography (CT) scans, magnetic resonance imaging (MRI), positron emission tomography (PET) scans, fine-needle aspirations, or biopsies of tissue. Surgery may be required to see if cancer has spread to lymph nodes in the neck.

Microscopic examination of a tissue sample is required to confirm a diagnosis. After diagnosis is confirmed and the extent of the tumor or cancer has been assessed, a stage is assigned to the cancer.

Staging of head and neck cancers is rather complicated. Basically, the staging system uses the extent of the tumor's spread as the primary basis of assigning a stage, but information on how large the tumor is and whether and to what extent lymph nodes are involved is also used. A commonly used staging division is the TNM system. This system uses letters and numbers to describe the size of the tumor (T), how many lymph nodes are involved (N), and whether the cancer has spread or metastasized (M).

The tumor (T) is most often assigned a number based on the size of the primary tumor. In some cases (for example, in a tumor in the sinus cavity), a number is assigned based on the extent to which the tumor has invaded and destroyed tissues. Designations based on the size of the tumor are as follows:

- T1: Tumor is 2 centimeters (cm) or less.
- T2: Tumor is larger than 2 cm but smaller than 4 cm.
- T3: Tumor is larger than 4 cm or multiple smaller tumors have spread to a single lymph node.
- T4: Tumors larger than 4 cm have spread to distant areas of the body.

Lymph node involvement (N) is assigned a number as follows:

- N0: No evidence of cancer exists in nearby lymph nodes.
- N1: A tumor measuring 3 cm or less is found in one lymph node on the same side as the primary tumor.
- N2: Either a tumor measuring between 3 and 6 cm is found in a lymph node on the same side as the primary tumor, tumors are in multiple lymph nodes on the same side but measure less than 6 cm, or tumors are found in lymph nodes on both sides, with the largest tumor measuring less than 6 cm.
- N3: Tumor greater than 6 cm is found in any lymph node.

The spread of the disease (M) is divided into two categories:

- M0: No disease is present elsewhere in the body.
- M1: Disease is present in a distant body area.

After determining the TNM state of the cancer, a stage is assigned.

- Stage 0: The cancer is only in the layer of cells lining the lips, mouth, or throat.
- Stage I: T1 N0 M0 tumors
- Stage II: T2 N0 M0 tumors
- Stage III: T3 N0 M0 or T1-3 N1 M0 tumors
- Stage IV: Any T4 tumor, any N2 or N3 tumor, and any M1 tumor

This staging process is complex and certainly not foolproof. For example, a small primary tumor that has spread to a lymph node on the opposite side and a large tumor that has not spread at all may be assigned the same disease stage. However, assigning a stage to the cancer can help determine treatment options.

Treatment and therapy: Treatments for head and neck cancers depend on the type of cancer, location of tumors, severity of symptoms, age and general health of the patient, stage of the cancer, and preference of the patient. These treatments often include surgery and may also involve radiation therapy or chemotherapy.

Some types of head and neck cancer may require surgery to remove the cancer and perhaps surrounding tissue or lymph nodes; in fact, surgery is the type of treatment most often used for these cancers. In some cases, nerves, muscles, glands, and veins in the neck must be removed. These removals can significantly affect a patient's quality of life. Any surgical treatment plan should consider how surgery and removal of tissues will affect how a person breathes, eats, talks, or looks.

If it is possible that the cancer has spread, radiation treatment may also be necessary following surgery. Radiation therapy can involve either a beam of radiation or implantation of tiny radioactive "seeds" to destroy the cancerous tissues. Chemotherapy may also be used depending on where the cancer is located and whether it has spread. Sometimes chemotherapy is used to enhance radiation therapy.

Rehabilitation or occupational therapy can be an important part of treatment for patients who are recovering from surgery or other types of treatment for these cancers. Patients may need to relearn how to chew, swallow, or speak. Reconstructive surgery to improve the patient's physical appearance, ability to function, or quality of life may also be part of a patient's rehabilitation. Physical therapy may also be involved in a follow-up treatment plan, and education for patients and families, especially education about smoking cessation and any necessary diet changes, is helpful in recovery and future prevention efforts.

Prognosis, prevention, and outcomes: Even though some people with no risk factors develop head and neck cancers, most of these cancers are caused by smoking and can be prevented. When found early, these cancers are often curable. However, up to 50 percent of patients with head and neck cancers have advanced cancers by the time they are discovered. For example, more than 70 percent of throat cancers are at an advanced stage when discovered. An advanced stage on discovery reduces the chances of a cure or the ability to halt the progression of the disease.

A person who has had a cancer of the head or neck is at increased risk for developing a new cancer in the head, neck, esophagus, or lungs. Usually, a recurrence or secondary cancer will happen in the first two to three years following diagnosis of the first cancer, but a cancer may recur even up to twenty years later. These secondary tumors are a major cause of death even after a successful course of therapy has eliminated the primary tumor. Medical professionals are currently investigating a vitamin-like substance called isotretinoin and whether it can reduce the risk of tumors recurring in the head and neck.

The most effective way to reduce the chance of another head and neck cancer occurring is to stop tobacco use. Other prevention tactics include using sunscreen and eating a diet low in fat, moderate in alcohol, and high in whole grains, fruits and vegetables.

Caring properly for dentures can also help. Dentures that do not fit properly can trap cancer-causing substances and keep those substances in the mouth for a long time, increasing the chances that tissues will be damaged by those substances.

Marianne M. Madsen, M.S.

For Further Information

Carper, Elise. *One Hundred Questions and Answers About Head and Neck Cancer*. Sudbury, Mass.: Jones and Bartlett, 2007.

Myers, Eugene N., Michael R. Smith, Jeffrey Myers, and Ehab Hanna. *Cancer of the Head and Neck*. Philadelphia: Saunders, 2003.

Ward, Elizabeth C., and Corina J. Van As-Broosk, eds. *Head and Neck Cancer: Treatment, Rehabilitation, and Outcomes*. San Diego, Calif.: Plural, 2006.

Other Resources

National Cancer Institute
Head and Neck Cancer
http://www.cancer.gov/cancertopics/types/head-and-neck

Oral Cancer Foundation
http://www.oralcancerfoundation.org

Support for People with Oral and Head and Neck Cancer
http://www.spohnc.org

Yul Brynner Head and Neck Cancer Foundation
http://www.headandneck.org

See also: Epidermoid cancers of mucous membranes; Glossectomy; Hypopharyngeal cancer; Lip cancers; Lymphedema; Metastatic squamous neck cancer with occult primary; Nasal cavity and paranasal sinus cancers; Oral and oropharyngeal cancers; Otolaryngology; Parathyroid cancer; TP53 protein

▶ Hemangioblastomas

Category: Diseases, Symptoms, and Conditions
Also known as: Lindau tumors

Related conditions: Von Hippel-Lindau disease

Definition: Hemangioblastomas are benign tumors of the nervous system. These tumors form a knot of blood vessels and may be surrounded by a hollow cyst containing a yellowish fluid. The most common location for hemangioblastomas is the cerebellum. The cerebellum is the part of the brain located at the base of the back of the head. Its primary function is to coordinate voluntary movement. The second most common location for hemangioblastomas is on the spinal cord. Only rarely are hemangioblastomas found on other nerves. Although hemangioblastomas are not usually cancerous, their growth can increase pressure in the brain and interfere with brain and spinal cord functions.

Risk factors: Men develop hemangioblastomas at twice the rate of women. Most hemangioblastomas are diagnosed in people between the ages of twenty and fifty.

Etiology and the disease process: Genetic abnormalities are thought to be the underlying cause of hemangioblastomas. About 25 percent of people who develop these tumors have von Hippel-Lindau (VHL) disease. VHL is a hereditary disorder in which hemangioblastomas form along with other tumors of the adrenal gland, pancreas, and kidney.

Incidence: Hemangioblastomas are rare. They make up only about 2.5 percent of all abnormal growths (neoplasms) on the brain and spinal cord.

Symptoms: Symptoms depend on the location of the tumor. In the cerebellum, hemangioblastomas can cause lack of coordination, problems with balance, dizziness, and headache. On the spinal cord, they can cause pain and progressive dysfunction.

Screening and diagnosis: There is no routine screening for hemangioblastomas. These tumors are diagnosed by magnetic resonance imaging (MRI) studies. If a hemangioblastoma is suspected, imaging studies such as a computed tomography (CT) scan, angiography, and ultrasound are done to provide additional information before surgery. There is no staging for hemangioblastomas.

Treatment and therapy: Hemangioblastoms are surgically removed unless the risks of the operation are greater than the expected benefits. Damage to surrounding brain tissue may occur during surgery depending on the location of the tumor. After surgery, regular follow-up visits are needed to check for recurrent tumors.

Prognosis, prevention, and outcomes: The outcome of surgery depends largely on the location of the hemangioblastoma but is usually good. About 25 percent of patients develop additional hemangioblastomas. The recurrence rate is higher in younger individuals and in those with VHL disease.

Martiscia Davidson, A.M.

See also: Benign tumors; Brain and central nervous system cancers; Brain scan; Pheochromocytomas; Spinal axis tumors; Von Hippel-Lindau (VHL) disease

▶ Hemangiopericytomas

Category: Diseases, Symptoms, and Conditions
Also known as: Solitary Fibrous Tumor, Perithelioma, myopericytoma

Related conditions: Soft-tissue sarcomas

Definition: Hemangiopericytomas are soft-tissue sarcomas derived from pericytes (cells of the connective tissue surrounding capillaries and other small blood vessels). Malignancy is variable and unpredictable, and the disease is most commonly encountered in adults.

Risk factors: There are no readily identifiable risk factors particular to hemangiopericytoma, although several risk factors associated with soft-tissue sarcomas in general have been identified. These include exposure to chlorophenols in wood preservatives and phenoxyacetic acid in herbicides, exposure to ionizing radiation, and very rare genetic predispositions in some families.

Etiology and the disease process: Tumor cells are derived from multipotent mesenchymal stem cells found in the lining of the blood vessels. Connections with diet, smoking, alcohol, or preexisting conditions have not been established.

Incidence: Less than 1 percent of newly diagnosed cancers are soft-tissue sarcomas, and only 1-2 percent of these are hemangiopericytomas. They typically arise in the fifth or sixth decade of life (median age is 45-50 years), and only 5 to 10 percent of the cases are found in children. A distinct rare infantile form is known in children less than one year in age.

Symptoms: Tumors usually develop as a deep soft-tissue mass, most commonly in the legs, pelvis, and retroperitoneum (back of the abdominal cavity), although one study reports that 16 to 25 percent of new cases manifest as lesions in the head and neck. Detection is often first noted as a painless swelling of the soft tissue, although growing abdominal tumors may cause painful intestinal or urinary symptoms. An occasional symptom is pronounced hypoglycemia resulting from tumor secretion of insulin-like growth factors. The disease typically spreads through the bloodstream, and only rarely through the lymphatic system. The cause of death is usually metastatic disease.

Screening and diagnosis: The existence of hemangiopericytoma as a distinct class of sarcomas is controversial, because other related neoplasms show a very similar vascular growth pattern. Diagnosis is always based on direct histological examination of tumor tissue. Open incisional biopsies are required in most cases; only if the mass is unusually accessible is a core needle biopsy a practical alternative. Given the histological similarities between hemangiopericytoma cells and synovial sarcoma cells, cytogenetic studies are often used to make the distinction, since almost all synovial sarcomas demonstrate a characteristic chromosomal translocation. No screening tests exist, and hemangiopericytoma is sufficiently rare and unpredictable that uniform staging criteria have yet to be developed.

Treatment and therapy: In adults, complete surgical removal and resection is favored whenever possible. Radiotherapy has proven effective and is particularly recommended for patients with incomplete resection or large invasive tumors. Chemotherapy has not proved to be effective in most cases and is not generally recommended.

Prognosis, prevention, and outcomes: Malignant hemangiopericytoma is prone both to local recurrence and to metastasis to distant sites, most commonly the lungs and bones. Tumors of the head, neck, and trunk seem far more likely to recur locally than do tumors of the extremities. One study reported a five year survival rate of 89-100 percent and a ten-year survival rate of 70 percent, but local and distant recurrences are known to occur after a prolonged disease-free interval.

Jeffrey A. Knight, Ph.D.

See also: Nasal cavity and paranasal sinus cancers; Sarcomas, soft-tissue

▶ Hemangiosarcomas

Category: Diseases, Symptoms, and Conditions
Also known as: Angiosarcomas, malignant hemangiotheliomas, hemangiomas

Related conditions: Soft-tissue sarcomas

Definition: Hemangiosarcomas are rare soft-tissue sarcomas affecting the endothelial cells that line blood vessels. These tumors can develop anywhere, but they most commonly are associated with the skin of the head and neck (50% of all cases). Visceral hemangiosarcomas of the liver, heart, spleen, bowel, and bone marrow are also known.

Risk factors: There are no well-established risk factors for most hemangiosarcomas, although several rare genetic disorders that predispose subjects to these rare cancers are known. Hemanagiosarcoma of the liver is known to be associated with exposure to genotoxic compounds such as vinyl chloride, vinyl fluoride, vinyl bromide, thorium dioxide, and arsenic. External irradiation for another malignancy has been shown to predispose rare hemangiosarcomas of the bowel.

Etiology and the disease process: The mechanisms giving rise to these tumors are poorly understood, although activated mutations in known oncogenes have been detected in some cases. Once initiated in the lining of the blood vessels, the tumor spreads rapidly and builds its own blood vessel network. The tumor itself is often filled with blood, since the blood vessels grow directly into it. Recent reports suggest that hemangiosarcomas are most likely derived from hematopoietic stem cells, and there is no evidence that hemangiosarcomas arise from the far more common hemangiomas.

Incidence: Less than 1 percent of newly diagnosed cancers are soft-tissue sarcomas, and only about 2 percent of these are classified as hemangiosarcomas. An incidence rate of 0.21 cases per 100,000 people (0.00021 percent) has been reported.

Symptoms: Dermal hemangiosarcomas usually appear as a rosy red or purple growth on the skin, which is often raised. When the tumors arise as a deep soft-tissue mass, a painless swelling is often the first indication. Hemangiosarcomas of the heart, liver, bowel, and pulmonary aorta may become quite large before organ function is compromised and symptoms develop.

Screening and diagnosis: Diagnosis is based on surgical biopsy and direct histological examination of tumor tissue. The characteristic network of blood vessels usually provides an unambiguous identification. Screening tests for industrial workers exposed to vinyl chloride are available, but hemangiosarcomas are sufficiently rare and unpredictable that uniform staging criteria are unavailable.

Treatment and therapy: Treatment varies considerably depending on tumor location, although surgical removal is always recommended whenever possible. Immunotherapy with recombinant interleukin-2 and chemotherapy (doxorubicin-based or paclitaxel regimens) have proven effective in some cases, and some research supports the efficacy of adding dacarbazine to doxorubicin-based treatments. Recent evidence suggests that beta adrenergic signaling drives several important cellular pathways that promote tumor progression, and a variety of beta blocker pharmaceuticals are now in clinical trials.

Prognosis, prevention, and outcomes: Patients with excised dermal hemangiosarcomas have an excellent prognosis if the cancer is detected early. The prognosis for patients with deep tissue or visceral tumors is relatively poor. One study reports a five-year survival rate at 30%. A frequent cause of death is tumor rupture, which can cause the victim to rapidly bleed to death.

Jeffrey A. Knight, Ph.D.

See also: Endotheliomas; Lymphangiosarcomas; Sarcomas, soft-tissue; Veterinary oncology

▶ Hematemesis

Category: Diseases, Symptoms, and Conditions
Also known as: Vomiting of blood

Related conditions: Esophageal, stomach (gastric), and duodenal ulcers, esophagitis; gastritis; esophageal and stomach varices; melena; Mallory-Weiss tears; Dieulafoy's lesion; blood-clotting problems; cirrhosis; portal hypertension

Definition: Hematemesis is vomiting of blood or material that resembles coffee grounds from the upper gastrointestinal (UGI) tract, which includes the mouth, part of the throat, the esophagus, the stomach, and the first part of the small intestine (called the duodenum) up to the ligament of Treitz, a tough fibrous-muscle band tissue supporting the duodenum.

Risk factors: Risk factors for hematemesis include prolonged vomiting, bleeding ulcers, *Helicobacter pylori* infection, nosebleeds, and use of nonsteroidal anti-inflammatory drugs, alcohol, and tobacco.

Etiology and the disease process: Hematemesis and melena (black, tarry stools) are common symptoms of upper gastrointestinal bleeding (UGIB). The most common causes of UGIB include esophagitis, gastritis, peptic ulcer disease, esophagogastric varices, arteriovenous malformations (abnormal blood vessels in the digestive tract), Mallory-Weiss tears (lacerations on the lining of the junction of the esophagus and stomach), tumors (cancers), and nonspecific abnormalities of the upper gastrointestinal lining.

Incidence: Approximately 100 cases of upper gastrointestinal bleeding occur per 100,000 hospitalizations annually; this bleeding causes hematemesis.

Symptoms: Vomiting of blood is the result of upper gastrointestinal bleeding. Although not all cases can cause a major medical problem, it is necessary to seek medical help immediately. If large quantities of blood are lost, the patient could develop low blood pressure, increased heart rate, and shock.

Screening and diagnosis: A flexible tube extending from the nose or mouth to the stomach and into the duodenum will be inserted to remove blood and prevent blood going into the lungs. Blood tests will include blood-clotting factors, liver function tests, and a complete blood count, which evaluates how much blood was lost. Upper endoscopy will be performed to visualize the upper gastrointestinal tract and to treat the bleeding. If endoscopy fails to identify the site of bleeding, other methods such as angiography (radiographic visualization of blood vessels) and radioactive scan of tagged red blood cells can be employed.

Treatment and therapy: Endoscopic treatments to stop bleeding include injection methods with absolute alcohol, salt solution, or epinephrine, or mechanical methods such as applying heat directly and placing hemoclips (metal clips for grasping blood vessels or surrounding tissues). A combination of injection followed by mechanical methods is another treatment modality. If *H. pylori* infection is present, the bacteria will be eradicated with antimicrobials, proton pump inhibitors, and acid suppressors. Aspirin and nonsteroidal anti-inflammatory drugs will be stopped. If large volumes of blood are lost, emergency measures may include intravenous fluids, blood transfusions, and medications such as proton pump inhibitors and acid suppressors. Consultations will include a gastroenterologist and a surgeon, who may operate if bleeding does not stop.

Prognosis, prevention, and outcomes: Repeated hematemesis due to upper gastrointestinal tract bleeding increases the mortality rate. Associated factors that increase the mortality rate include age, poor nutrition, and having other medical problems and blood-clotting disorders. Related medical conditions such as ulcers should be appropriately treated and risk factors addressed for prevention.

Miriam E. Schwartz, M.D., M.A., Ph.D., and Colm A. Ó'Moráin, M.A., M.D., M.Sc., D.Sc.

See also: Coughing; Esophageal cancer; Esophagitis

▶ Hematuria

Category: Diseases, Symptoms, and Conditions
Also known as: Blood in the urine

Related conditions: Cancers of the bladder, kidney, prostate, or urethra

Definition: The American Urological Association defines hematuria as three or more red blood cells per high-power field in two of three specimens. Hematuria can originate from any site along the urinary tract.

Risk factors: The presence of heme or red blood cells in microscopic or gross amounts in the urine is a sign requiring interpretation within the context of the patient's presenting symptoms to rule out kidney or urinary tract disease.

Etiology and the disease process: The cause of hematuria may range from transitory and insignificant to increasingly serious diagnoses. The blood may be from excessive or strenuous exercise, menstrual bleeding, hemorrhoids, trauma, infection, stones or calculi, obstruction, drugs, poisoning, or tumors. Hematuria is among the most common and earliest indications of cancers of the bladder, kidney, prostate, or urethra.

Incidence: The American Urological Association reports that the prevalence of asymptomatic microscopic hematuria varies from less than 1 to 21 percent.

Symptoms: Hematuria manifests in urine that is smoky, pink, bright red, or dark red (although urine may appear clear and still result in a diagnosis of hematuria).

Screening and diagnosis: Blood in urine is detected in the form of intact red blood cells under the microscope or as the heme subunit of the hemoglobin molecule in a routine chemical evaluation of urine. Screening involves a routine urinalysis in each of the three distinct testing phases:

- Physical examination (the urine sample may appear in color and clarity from clear to smoky, pink, bright red, or dark red.

- Microscopic examination (identifies and counts the blood cells per high-power field)
- Biochemical examination (to determine the presence or absence of blood in the urine; relies on the peroxidase activity of the heme moiety, which leaks from the red blood cell or from muscle tissue in the form of myoglobin into the urine)

Because hematuria can originate from a wide variety of causes, the presence of red blood cells in the urine is not a useful screening tool to detect tumors of the urinary tract. Once hematuria has been detected, the clinician must find the cause. Often the diagnosis of cancer begins with ruling out all other possible sources of blood in the urine.

Definitive diagnosis may require one or more exploratory and confirmatory procedures: urine cytology; intravenous urography (IVU), a radiology procedure that uses an injected dye to show the kidneys, ureters, and bladder; ultrasonography; computed tomography (CT); magnetic resonance imaging (MRI); or a cystoscopy with biopsy.

Treatment and therapy: Treatment depends on the underlying cause.

Prognosis, prevention, and outcomes: Hematuria requires evaluation within the context of the patient's history and physical examination. Asymptomatic, microscopic hematuria may range from insignificant to life-threatening. Risk factors for significant disease in patients with microscopic hematuria include smoking, occupational exposure to chemicals, analgesic abuse, urinary tract infection, and a history of urologic disorders.

Jane Adrian, M.P.H., Ed.M., M.T. (ASCP)

See also: 4-Aminobiphenyl; Bladder cancer; Cyclophosphamide; Hereditary Leiomyomatosis and Renal Cell Cancer (HLRCC); Hereditary non-VHL clear cell renal cell carcinomas; Hereditary papillary renal cell carcinomas; Kidney cancer; Malignant rhabdoid tumor of the kidney; Transitional cell carcinomas; Urinalysis; Urinary system cancers

▶ Hemochromatosis

Category: Diseases, Symptoms, and Conditions
Also known as: Hematochromatosis; bronze diabetes; hereditary, familial, or type 1 hemochromatosis; iron overload

Related conditions: Liver cancer, heart disease, impotence, infertility, premature menopause, diabetes, arthritis, cirrhosis of the liver, bronze skin

Definition: Hemochromatosis is a metabolic disorder in which iron accumulates in the liver, heart, skin, pancreas, and other organs. Once iron is absorbed, the only way the body can excrete the excess iron is through bleeding.

Hemochromatosis may be either genetic or nongenetic in origin. Nongenetic sources include excess deposition of iron in the tissues due to multiple transfusions, chronic hepatitis, excessive iron intake, or megadoses of vitamin C, which promotes iron absorption. Genetic hemochromatosis is inherited in an autosomal recessive pattern, as with homozygous mutations in the *HFE* gene region. The most common *HFE* gene mutation is C282Y, followed by H63D.

Risk factors: Hereditary hemochromatosis is most prevalent among persons of European descent. Not everyone who demonstrates the *HFE* mutation will develop hemochromatosis.

Etiology and the disease process: Normally the *HFE* gene codes for the intestinal transmembrane glycoprotein that regulates dietary iron absorption. A mutation causes the system to deposit more iron in the organs than is needed, leading to increased absorption and creating an overload of unbound iron molecules circulating within the system.

Once the body exceeds its natural limit of iron storage of ferritin molecules, the excess unbound iron molecules promote free-radical formation, resulting in peroxidation of the lipid membrane and cellular injury. People who are predisposed to hemochromatosis may accumulate 0.5 to 1.0 gram of iron per year.

Incidence: The Centers for Disease Control and Prevention estimate that 1 million people in the United States have hemochromatosis.

Symptoms: Early symptoms of hemochromatosis include fatigue, weakness, weight loss, joint pain, or abdominal pain. These symptoms typically appear after the age of forty in men and after fifty in women.

Screening and diagnosis: A series of fasting serum blood tests—ferritin, iron, total iron binding capacity (TIBC), unsaturated iron binding capacity (UIBC), or transferring saturation (TS)—assist in the diagnosis of hemochromatosis. The TS may be calculated or measured directly by immunoassay. Genotyping may confirm if the *HFE* mutation is present. A liver biopsy may establish a prognosis of risk of advancing fibrosis.

Treatment and therapy: Therapeutic phlebotomy to decrease the excess iron stores is especially effective before symptoms of complications appear.

Prognosis, prevention, and outcomes: Early detection and therapeutic phlebotomy to maintain iron levels within established limits results in the prevention of tissue and organ complications associated with hemochromatosis. For individuals who have already experienced organ compromise, while earlier damage may not be reversed, further damage can be slowed with therapeutic phlebotomy.

Jane Adrian, M.P.H., Ed.M., M.T. (ASCP)

See also: Genetic testing; Hematologic oncology; Hepatomegaly; Liver cancers

▶ Hemolytic anemia

Category: Diseases, Symptoms, and Conditions
Also known as: Autoimmune hemolytic anemia

Related conditions: Lymphoproliferative disorders such as chronic lymphocytic leukemia, lymphoma, multiple myeloma, and thymoma. May be seen in patients with carcinoma of the breast or stomach as well as cancers of the colon, prostate, lung, cervix, and pancreas. Also seen in patients with hepatitis, cytomegalovirus, or streptococcus.

Definition: Hemolytic anemia occurs when there are too few red blood cells in the body as a result of premature destruction of red blood cells. Destruction occurs more quickly than the bone marrow can produce new cells.

Risk factors: Patients receiving chemotherapy or radiation for the treatment of a lymphoproliferative disease or solid tumors of the breast, stomach, colon, prostate, lung, cervix, or pancreas are at risk for developing hemolytic anemia. Also at risk are people suffering with an infection, such as hepatitis, cytomegalovirus, or streptococcus, or those taking penicillin, sulfa drugs, or large quantities of acetaminophen. People diagnosed with autoimmune disorders, lupus, rheumatoid arthritis, or ulcerative colitis can also be at risk.

Etiology and the disease process: This destruction of red blood cells, or hemolysis, falls into two groups: intrinsic and extrinsic. Intrinsic refers to the destruction of the red blood cells due to a defect within the cells themselves. Intrinsic hemolysis is caused by an inherited condition such as sickle cell anemia or thalassemia, which cause red blood cells to have a shorter life span than normal. Extrinsic refers to red blood cells that develop in a healthful manner but then are destroyed by infection or drugs. Extrinsic hemolysis can be temporary and resolve over several months.

Incidence: Some 20 percent of hemolytic anemias are caused by lymphocytic leukemia, 10 percent are the result of an autoimmune disease, and all others are related to medications. Women are twice as likely to contract hemolytic anemia as are men. One in 80,000 cases of anemia is hemolytic anemia.

Symptoms: Symptoms of hemolytic anemia include pale skin, a yellowing of the skin or eyes, dark urine, fever, weakness, dizziness, confusion, inability to tolerate physical activity, an enlarged spleen and liver, rapid heart rate, or heart murmur.

Screening and diagnosis: Hemolytic anemia is found when a patient visits the physician's office with complaints of tiring easily, dizziness, or paleness of the skin. The physician will order laboratory tests to monitor the patient's red blood cell count. Laboratory tests include tests for hemoglobin levels, reticulocyte counts, liver function tests, and, in more serious conditions, a bone marrow aspiration and biopsy. A urine sample may be needed to evaluate for increased proteins or hemoglobin.

Treatment and therapy: Treatment is based on the patient's overall condition and type of anemia. The patient's age, medical history, cause of disease, and ability to tolerate treatment are considered. Treatment includes blood transfusions, steroid medications, and infusions of immune globulins to strengthen the immune system. More severe cases are treated with surgical removal of the spleen or immunosuppressive therapy.

Prognosis, prevention, and outcomes: There is no known prevention for intrinsic hemolytic anemia. Extrinsic hemolytic anemia can be prevented by avoiding the use of medications that may cause anemia. Mild cases may not need treatment, whereas severe cases can be life-threatening. An inherited form of anemia will require lifelong treatment.

Katrina Green, R.N., B.S.N., O.C.N.

See also: Anemia; Transfusion therapy

▶ Hemoptysis

Category: Diseases, Symptoms, and Conditions
Also known as: Coughing up of blood or blood-stained sputum

Related conditions: Tuberculosis, bronchitis, bronchiectasis, aspergilloma, coccidioidomycosis, pulmonary embolism, pneumonia, pneumonic plague, lung cancer (especially bronchogenic carcinoma)

Definition: Hemoptysis is the coughing up of blood or blood-stained sputum that originates in the bronchi, lungs, trachea, or some other part of the respiratory tract.

Etiology and the disease process: There are many potential causes for hemoptysis, but it is most often caused by an underlying condition. The most common worldwide cause of hemoptysis is *Mycobacterium tuberculosis* infection. The most common causes of hemoptysis in industrialized nations are bronchitis, bronchiectasis, and bronchogenic carcinoma. Other pulmonary conditions, such as aspergilloma, coccidioidomycosis, pulmonary embolism, pneumonia, and pneumonic plague may also cause hemoptysis. Hemoptysis can also be caused by the presence of a foreign object in the respiratory tract, although this is much more common in children than in adults.

Incidence: Some form of lung cancer causes hemoptysis in 23 percent of cases in the United States. One form in particular, bronchogenic carcinoma, causes hemoptysis in 5 to 44 percent of cancer-related cases.

Symptoms: Hemoptysis, itself the symptom of an underlying disorder, is marked by the color of the blood in sputum, normally bright red and foamy as opposed to dark red.

Screening and diagnosis: In most cases, hemoptysis is diagnosed with a physical examination. One of the most important things in the examination is determining if the blood being coughed up is really hemoptysis. Blood that is coughed up can also originate from the gastrointestinal tract. The origin of blood can be determined by its color. Bright red, foamy blood originates from the respiratory tract, while dark red blood originates from the gastrointestinal tract.

Sometimes a chest radiograph will be used to diagnose hemoptysis. In more complicated cases, advanced tests may be employed. The most common set of advanced tests includes fiber-optic bronchoscopy and high-resolution computed tomography. This set of tests is often used when the cause of hemoptysis is suspected to be a malignant cancer.

Treatment and therapy: Goals in treating hemoptysis are stopping the bleeding, clearing the airways, and treating the underlying condition. Patients who are not high risk and have chest radiographs that appear to be normal may be treated as outpatients with close monitoring and antibiotics to treat any underlying infection that could be causing the hemoptysis.

If the patient is diagnosed with life-threatening, massive hemoptysis, the situation becomes much more urgent. Massive hemoptysis is defined by the rate of bleeding rather than the volume of blood coughed up. The risk of death from massive hemoptysis is not from the loss of blood but from possible asphyxiation from blockage of the airways. Massive hemoptyis is defined as more than 200 milliliters of blood coughed up per day. Massive hemoptysis is a medical emergency and must be treated immediately. The most common treatments for massive hemoptysis are bronchial angiography with embolization or surgical removal of the bleeding site.

Prognosis, prevention, and outcomes: Outcomes depend on the type of cancer or other disorder for which hemoptysis is a symptom.

Jeremy W. Dugosh, Ph.D.

See also: Bronchial adenomas; Bronchoalveolar lung cancer; Bronchography; Coughing; Kaposi sarcoma; Lung cancers; Mediastinal tumors; Mustard gas; Superior vena cava syndrome

▶ Hepatomegaly

Category: Diseases, Symptoms, and Conditions
Also known as: Fatty liver, enlarged liver

Related conditions: Hepatitis, alcoholic cirrhosis, hepatocellular carcinoma (HCC)

Definition: Hepatomegaly is a potentially reversible symptom of an underlying disease or condition in which the size of the liver (about 9 centimeters, or cm, in women and less than 12 cm in men) is abnormally increased as estimated by the amount of the liver's edge below the lower edge of the ribs (coastal margin).

Risk factors: Hepatomegaly, commonly known as an enlarged liver, can be caused by alcoholism (early stages), hepatocellular carcinoma (HCC, or primary liver cancer), nonalcoholic fatty liver disease, cirrhosis of the liver, chronic heart failure, infection with hepatitis (A, B, or C), a protein deficiency, diabetes, obesity, starvation, endocrine disorders (Cushing syndrome), and many chronic diseases with nutrition or absorption problems. Other risk factors include corticosteroid use and exposure to aflatoxins, parasites, antibiotics (tetracyclines), contraceptive steroids, halothane, arsenic, thorium, and yellow phosphorus.

Etiology and the disease process: Liver cells perform some of the most important biochemical functions, such as detoxication of ammonia and foreign chemicals and degradation and synthesis of carbohydrates, proteins, amino acids, hormones, fatty acids, glycerides, cholesterol, bile salts, heme, and porphyrin. A problem with one or more of the metabolic functions can lead to both structural and functional abnormalities.

Liver cells respond in various ways to etiologic agents to become enlarged. Pathophysiologic mechanisms include inflammation, excessive storage, infiltrations, congestion, and obstruction. Examples include dilated hepatic sinusoids (due to heart failure), persistently high venous pressure causing liver congestion (in chronic obstructive pancreatitis), dysfunction and enlargement of hepatocytes (during hepatitis), fatty infiltration of parenchymal cells causing fibrosis (in cirrhosis), distension of liver cells (in alcoholism), fatty degeneration and infiltration of hepatocytes (diabetes mellitus, alcoholism, amyloid or glycogen storage), hyperplasia (cirrhoses or hepatomas) leading to sarcoma (metastic carcinoma), and tenderness (congestive heart failure and infectious hepatitis).

Incidence: The major causes of hepatomegaly depend on the age, geographical location, and metabolic-nutritional status of the patient. Hepatomegaly can be found in countries where there are hepatitis epidemics, children suffering from malnutrition, food contaminated with chlorinated hydrocarbons, and grains and oils contaminated with *Aspergillus* fungi. Some 15 to 20 percent of the general population in the United States are estimated to have fatty liver. An enlarged liver is caused primarily by alcoholism in the United States and Europe and by protein malnutrition in infancy and early childhood in tropical countries. Uncontrolled diabetes and obesity often cause people to have fatty livers.

Symptoms: Hepatomegaly often produces no symptoms, although the liver may be tender to the touch and the patient may experience some abdominal pain or a feeling of fullness. Asymptomatic cases are usually related to congenital cystic disease, metastasis, or alcoholism. On palpitation, an alcoholic liver is enlarged and firm. In alcoholic hepatitis, hepatomegaly may be associated with jaundice, anorexia, and vomiting. In alcoholic cirrhosis, the enlarged liver is tender and may be associated with hepatitis, usually asymptomatic but occasionally with abdominal pain, jaundice, and gastrointestinal complaints and ascites. In cardiac cirrhosis, the liver may be slightly enlarged and tender. In nodular cirrhosis, the liver is palpable and firm with a blunt edge.

Hepatomegaly with fever and tenderness may be due to acute viral hepatitis (A and B), mononucleosis, and ascending cholangitis (infection of the bile duct). In hepatocytic adenomas (in women age thirty to forty), typically there are solitary tumors of up to 10 centimeters in diameter in the right lobe, usually the result of the use of hormones and corticosteroids. Hepatomegaly with gross or occult blood in the stool would suggest metastatic neoplasm of the gastrointestinal tract.

In hepatocellular carcinoma, symptoms may be vague and include loss of appetite and body weight, nausea, weakness, and sometimes fever with chills. If the tumor blocks the bile duct (cholangiocarcinoma), then

Disorders That Can Lead to Hepatomegaly in Adults

Type of Disorder	*Disorder*
Autoimmune	Autoimmune liver disease
Biliary	Extrahepatic obstruction, primary liver cirrhosis, primary sclerosing cholangitis
Cardiovascular	Congestive heart failure, right ventricular failure, constrictive pericarditis, Budd-Chiari syndrome
Drug-related	Alcoholic liver disease, acute alcoholic hepatitis, alcoholic fatty liver, hepatitis induced by statins, tetracyclines, phenylbutazone, vinyl chloride, carbon tetrachloride, arsenic, thorium, yellow phosphorus, macrolide, amiodarone, paracetamol
Hematological	Sickle cell disease, hemolytic anemia, myeloma, leukemia, lymphoma
Infectious	Viral hepatitis, Epstein-Barr virus (EBV), cytomegalovirus (CMV), malaria, pyrogenic abscess, amoebic abscess
Metabolic	Hemochromatosis, Wilson disease, glycogen storage diseases, porphyria, nonalcoholic fatty liver disease
Tumor-related	Metastatic carcinoma, hepatocellular carcinoma, granulomatous hepatitis, amyloidosis

symptoms may include jaundice, black-colored urine, pale stool, and ascites.

Screening and diagnosis: The procedure for diagnosis depends on the suspected cause of hepatomegaly. The physician conducts a physical examination and takes the patient's history. Through skillful palpitation, the physician can determine whether the mass or swelling in the liver area is indeed an enlarged liver. Then, the physician can use the symptoms reported by the patient to begin to distinguish between the many causes of hepatomegaly.

Further diagnosis is aided by tests of liver function. The initial workup involves a complete blood count, urinalysis, sedimentation rate study, chemistry panel, amylase and lipase level testing, and an X ray of the abdomen, followed by ultrasound, computed tomography (CT) scans, and magnetic resonance imaging (MRI).

Additional tests are conducted based on the suspected condition. Patients who are likely to have hepatocellular carcinoma undergo a CT scan of the abdomen, followed by biopsy and histopathology to confirm the diagnosis. If chronic heart failure is suspected, a circulation time test and spirometry can confirm the diagnosis. A chest X ray and electroencephalograph (EEG) are also needed. If obstructive jaundice is suspected, endoscopic retrograde cholangiopancreatography may be done following a CT scan of the abdomen. The infectious diseases associated with hepatomegaly are diagnosed by antibody titers, blood smears, or skin tests.

Treatment and therapy: Treatment for chronic enlarged liver depends on the underlying cause and the degree of liver damage, especially in the case of cancer. In nonalcoholic fatty liver cases, where any liver damage is minimal, the patient is directed to lose weight, exercise, and avoid alcohol. In advanced stages of hepatomegaly, the liver may undergo necrosis (due to hepatitis, alcoholism, or drug and toxin exposure) and fibrosis (due to alcoholic cirrhosis, chemical carcinogenesis, liver cancer). In patients with metastatic tumors, chemotherapy and nuclear medicine may prolong life. The treatments for hepatocellular carcinoma include liver transplant, chemotherapy, and radiation; however, death generally occurs within six to twenty months.

Prognosis, prevention, and outcomes: Hepatomegaly is a symptom of liver diseases and other conditions. If the underlying condition causing the enlarged liver can be successfully treated, the prognosis is good. Ways to prevent hepatomegaly include exercising and eating healthfully, avoiding contact with others' blood and bodily fluids to minimize the risk of hepatitis, limiting contact with toxins, drinking alcohol in moderation, not mixing medications such as acetaminophen with alcohol, and avoiding overuse of medications and supplements that can affect the liver.

M. A. Q. Khan, M.D., Ph.D., and
A. K. Khan, M.D., M.R.C.P.

For Further Information

Kasper, D. L., et al. *Harrison's Principles of Internal Medicine*. 16th ed. New York: McGraw-Hill, 2005.

Khan, M. A. Q., and R. H. Stanton. *Toxicology of Halogenated Hydrocarbons*. New York: Pergamon Press, 1980.

Klaassen, C. D., M. O. Amdur, and J. Doull. *Toxicology: The Basic Science of Poisons*. New York: Macmillan, 1986.

Kumar, V., N. Fausto, and A. Abbas. *Robbins and Cobran Pathological Basis of Disease*. 7th ed. Philadelphia: Saunders, 2003.

Other Resources

Liver Cancer Network
http://www.livercancer.com

MayoClinic.com
Enlarged Liver
http://www.mayoclinic.com/health/enlarged-liver/DS00638

National Cancer Institute
http://www.cancer.gov

See also: Aflatoxins; Alcohol, alcoholism, and cancer; Amyloidosis; Liver cancers

▶ Hereditary diffuse gastric cancer

Category: Diseases, Symptoms, and Conditions
Also known as: HDGC syndrome

Related conditions: Lobular breast cancer, colon cancer

Definition: Hereditary diffuse gastric cancer is a rare cancer that affects many parts of the stomach simultaneously rather than forming localized tumors.

Risk factors: Hereditary diffuse gastric cancer has a strong inherited component and is highly likely to occur in people who have a mutation on the *CDH1* gene. However, other genes are also thought to be involved because

30 percent of people with hereditary diffuse gastric cancer do not have the *CDH1* mutation. The average age at diagnosis is thirty-eight (the age range for diagnosis is fourteen to sixty-nine). Lifetime risk of having the syndrome is 67 percent for men and 83 percent for women.

Etiology and the disease process: The *CDH1* gene is an autosomal dominant gene, meaning that the individual needs to inherit a mutation in this gene from only one parent to be at risk for hereditary diffuse gastric cancer. Children who have one parent with the mutated gene have a 50 percent chance of inheriting the condition. Cancer develops when individual cancer cells invade the stomach wall in many places, causing cancerous patches. This cancer does not form discrete tumors.

Incidence: The rate of gastric cancers is highest in Japan, China, Russia, and other Southeast Asian countries (about 40 cases per 100,000 population). It is lowest in Western Europe and North America (about 4 cases per 100,000). Hereditary diffuse gastric cancer accounts for between 35 and 50 percent of all gastric cancers.

Symptoms: Most people do not show symptoms until hereditary diffuse gastric cancer is advanced. Advanced cases of the disease cause stomach pain, nausea, vomiting, and bloating, often accompanied by weight loss.

Screening and diagnosis: Although their value in screening remains statistically unproven, endoscopies are recommended for people who have a family history of hereditary diffuse gastric cancer. Colon cancer screening and breast cancer screening are also recommended, as these cancers commonly co-occur in people with hereditary diffuse gastric cancer. Genetic testing for the *CDH1* mutation is available, and genetic counseling may be helpful. Diagnosis is most often made on a family history of hereditary diffuse gastric cancer or early gastric cancer and a biopsy.

Treatment and therapy: Because cancer occurs throughout the stomach, complete surgical removal (gastrectomy) is the standard treatment. TNM (tumor/lymph node/metastasis) staging of hereditary diffuse gastric cancer has not been standardized because of the nature of the cancer and its rarity.

Prognosis, prevention, and outcomes: If diagnosed and treated with gastrectomy early (an uncommon event), the five-year survival rate is about 90 percent. When diagnosed in a late stage (most common), the five-year survival rate is less than 20 percent. Because of its strong inherited component, there is no known way to prevent hereditary diffuse gastric cancer.

Martiscia Davidson, A.M.

See also: Colorectal cancer; Family history and risk assessment; Gastric polyps; Gastrinomas; Gastrointestinal cancers; Invasive lobular carcinomas; Lobular Carcinoma In Situ (LCIS); Stomach cancers

▶ Hereditary Leiomyomatosis and Renal Cell Cancer (HLRCC)

Category: Diseases, Symptoms, and Conditions
Also known as: Hereditary renal carcinoma

Related conditions: Uterine fibroids, von Hippel-Lindau (VHL) disease, hereditary papillary renal carcinoma, Birt-Hogg-Dubé syndrome (BHDS)

Definition: Hereditary leiomyomatosis and renal cell carcinoma (HLRCC) is an inherited condition characterized by the development of one or more skin lesions called leiomyomas (tumors of smooth muscle tissue), uterine fibroids in women, and a form of renal cell carcinoma called papillary renal cancer.

Risk factors: The only known risk factor for HLRCC is having a parent with the disease. If a parent has this condition, there is a 50 percent chance that it will be passed on to his or her children. Although this disease is hereditary, it can be caused by a genetic mutation.

Etiology and the disease process: HLRCC is a dominant genetic trait. The affected gene is the one that produces the enzyme fumarate hydratase. This enzyme assists in the conversion of fumarate into L-malate in the Krebs cycle (involved in the metabolism of carbohydrates by the cells). As a result, fumarate accumulates in the cells. It is theorized that the high levels of fumarate interfere with the availability of oxygen for activation of several genes involved in angiogenesis (the formation of new blood vessels), cell metabolism, and cell growth and reproduction. This is called pseudohypoxia. It is thought that fumarate hydratase plays a role in the suppression of tumor formation in the body.

Incidence: HLRCC is an extremely rare condition. Less than 1,000 cases have been documented.

Symptoms: The major symptom of HLRCC is the presence of one or more leiomyomas on the skin. The leiomyomas are painful nodules that range from flesh colored to light brown. About 75 percent of persons with HLRCC develop leiomyomas. Almost all women with HLRCC will develop uterine fibroids. They cause pelvic pain and heavy menstrual periods. Patients with renal cell cancer may not exhibit any symptoms initially but later will exhibit hematuria (blood in the urine), lower back pain, and a palpable mass. Renal cell carcinoma develops in only 10 to 16 percent of persons with HLRCC.

Screening and diagnosis: There is no routine screening for HLRCC. If the patient has a family history of HLRCC, genetic testing is performed on all family members. Once HLRCC has been diagnosed, the patient should have annual skin examinations for leiomyomas and regular screenings for renal cell cancer. Female patients should have annual pelvic examinations or uterine or transvaginal ultrasounds to screen for uterine fibroids.

HLRCC is suspected when a person seeks treatment for painful leiomyomas. A biopsy of a leiomyoma is taken, and the cells are examined for the activity of fumerate hydratase. In a person with HLRCC, there would be a significant reduction in activity of this enzyme.

Uterine fibroids are not accepted as an indicator of HLRCC because of the high prevalence of uterine fibroids in the general female population. While most uterine fibroids are benign, occasionally a leiomyosarcoma (cancer of the uterus) is discovered in a woman with HLRCC.

Once a diagnosis of HLRCC is made, the patient is screened for renal cell cancer, by abdominal computed tomography (CT) scan or magnetic resonance imaging (MRI). The renal cell cancer related to HLRCC is particularly aggressive and grows and spreads faster than other renal cell cancers.

Because HLRCC is not a cancer, there is no staging for the condition. If a person with HLRCC develops renal cell cancer, then this cancer is staged like other renal cell cancers.

Treatment and therapy: There is no cure for HLRCC; it can only be managed. The leiomyomas of the skin can be removed by surgical excision, cryoablation (freezing), or laser surgery. If there are many leiomyomas, removal may not be possible. There are a number of medications that are effective in treating the pain caused by the skin leiomyomas. They are calcium-channel blockers, alpha-blockers, nitroglycerine, antidepressants, and some antiepileptic (antiseizure) medications.

Uterine fibroids can be removed surgically by myomectomy (removal of the fibroids) or hysterectomy. To preserve the uterus and shrink the fibroids, embolization of the arteries feeding the fibroids can be performed. Medications for treating uterine fibroids include gonadotropin-releasing hormone agonists, antihormonal medications, and pain relievers.

Once a renal cell cancer is discovered in a person with HLRCC, the tumor is surgically removed. The tumor can be removed by direct surgical radical nephrectomy (removal of the kidney and adrenal gland), by a partial nephrectomy, or by one of several laparoscopic nephrectomy procedures.

Prognosis, prevention, and outcomes: HLRCC is a chronic condition. However, with careful monitoring, a person with this disease can live a fairly normal life. Because HLRCC is caused by a genetic mutation, there is no way to prevent it. An important part of the management of HLRCC is genetic testing of all related family members and genetic counseling. Even siblings of an affected person should be screened for HLRCC because of the possibility of their having additional unpaired genes. Should two persons with the gene for HLRCC wish to have a child, their child would possess both HLRCC genes. This genetic combination is marked by severe encephalopathy (brain damage).

Christine M. Carroll, R.N., B.S.N., M.B.A.

For Further Information

Kiuru, M., and V. Launonen. "Hereditary Leiomyomatosis and Renal Cell Cancer (HLRCC)." *Current Molecular Medicine* 4, no. 8 (December, 2004): 869-875.

Sudarshan, Sunil, Peter A. Pinto, Len Neckers, and W. Marston Linehan. "Mechanisms of Disease: Hereditary Leiomyomatosis and Renal Cell Cancer—A Distinct Form of Hereditary Kidney Cancer." *Nature Clinical Practice—Urology* 4, no. 2 (February, 2007): 104-110.

Other Resources

American Cancer Society
http://www.cancer.org

National Cancer Institute
http://www.cancer.gov

See also: Birt-Hogg-Dubé Syndrome (BHDS); Family history and risk assessment; Hereditary non-VHL clear cell renal cell carcinomas; Hereditary papillary renal cell carcinomas; Hysterectomy; Kidney cancer; Leiomyomas; Renal pelvis tumors; Urinary system cancers; Von Hippel-Lindau (VHL) disease

▶ Hereditary mixed polyposis syndrome

Category: Diseases, Symptoms, and Conditions
Also known as: Colorectal adenoma and carcinoma 1 (CRAC1), HMPS

Related condition: Juvenile polyposis

Definition: Hereditary mixed polyposis syndrome is a dominantly inherited condition that predisposes an individual to the development of polyps in the gastrointestinal tract. Patients with this syndrome exhibit multiple polyp types—including atypical juvenile polyps, hyperplastic polyps, colonic adenomas, and colonic adenocarcinomas—as well as polyps that show mixed or hybrid characteristics. The syndrome predisposes patients to developing colorectal cancer.

Risk factors: Hereditary mixed polyposis syndrome is a genetic disorder that is transmitted in a dominant fashion. This means that only one of the two copies of a gene needs to be affected to develop the condition. Therefore, if one parent has the disease, then there is a 50 percent chance that his or her child will have it.

Etiology and the disease process: Hereditary mixed polyposis syndrome is a genetic disorder. Although the specific gene that is mutated has not been identified, numerous genetic studies have shown that the disease is linked to regions on chromosome 6, chromosome 10, and chromosome 15. The disease begins by the formation of polyps, or growths of tissue originating from a mucous membrane. Although polyps are usually benign, they can develop into tumors if they are not removed.

Symptoms: Symptoms of hereditary mixed polyposis syndrome are associated with polyp formation and can include anemia, blood loss, the passage of bright red, bloody stool, or bowel obstruction.

Incidence: Hereditary mixed polyposis syndrome is a rare disease that has been described in only a few families.

Screening and diagnosis: Patients with a family history of hereditary mixed polyposis syndrome should undergo frequent colonoscopies to screen for polyp formation because polyps that are left untreated can develop into cancer. Screening by colonoscopy should begin by age twenty-five and be repeated every two years. Patients with hereditary mixed polyposis syndrome usually have less than fifteen polyps during colonoscopy. Diagnosis is made based on the presence of multiple types of polyps or polyps with mixed characteristics in histological examination as well as a family history of the disease.

Treatment and therapy: Colonoscopy with polyp removal is usually sufficient to control the symptoms.

Prognosis, prevention, and outcomes: The median age of diagnosis for hereditary mixed polyposis syndrome is forty years. The median age of cancer diagnosis is forty-seven years. The lifetime risk for developing colorectal cancer is 30 percent. Prevention is based on identifying at-risk individuals based on a family history of hereditary mixed polyposis syndrome.

Lindsay Lewellyn, B.S.

See also: Adenomatous polyps; *APC* gene testing; Ashkenazi Jews and cancer; Bethesda criteria; Colon polyps; Colorectal cancer; Colorectal cancer screening; Cyclooxygenase 2 (COX-2) inhibitors; Desmoid tumors; *DPC4* gene testing; Duodenal carcinomas; Endometrial cancer; Endometrial hyperplasia; Enterostomal therapy; Ethnicity and cancer; Family history and risk assessment; Gardner syndrome; Gastric polyps; Gastrointestinal cancers; Genetics of cancer; Hereditary cancer syndromes; Hereditary polyposis syndromes; Juvenile polyposis syndrome; *MLH1* gene; *MSH* genes; Pancreatic cancers; Peutz-Jeghers Syndrome (PJS); *PMS* genes; Premalignancies; Sarcomas, soft-tissue; Small intestine cancer; Turcot syndrome

▶ Hereditary Non-Polyposis Colorectal Cancer (HNPCC)

Category: Diseases, symptoms and conditions
Also known as: Lynch syndrome (LS) after Dr. Henry Lynch, "the father of hereditary cancers," who pioneered the link between cancer and genetics. HNPCC is divided into Lynch syndrome I (familial colon cancer) and Lynch syndrome II (HNPCC related to other cancers of the gastrointestinal or reproductive system).

Definition: A hereditary condition that causes predisposition to many cancers, especially cancers of the large bowel and rectum (colorectal) and cancers of the endometrium (uterus lining) and ovaries in women.

Related conditions: Cancers of the large and small intestine/colon/bowel, rectum, stomach, pancreas, hepatobiliary system (liver/gallbladder/bile ducts), urinary tract (kidneys/ureters/bladder/urethra), skin, sebaceous oil glands, brain (gliomas/astrocytomas), and prostate. Cancers in women (endometrium/uterine lining, ovaries and breasts); Muir-Torre syndrome; Turcot syndrome.

Etiology and the disease process: Patients with Lynch syndrome (HNPCC) have a gene defect of the DNA mismatch repair (MMR) genes (*MLH1*, *MSH2*, *MSH6*, and *PMS2*) or the *EPCAM* gene which inactivates its neighboring *MSH2* gene; these gene defects cause errors in DNA repair. DNA (deoxyribonucleic acid) stores genetic information in the cells of living organisms in units of heredity called genes. DNA repair is needed at different times such as during DNA replication when errors can occur. The MMR gene products (proteins) repair these errors made during DNA replication, a process that occurs before cell division. When these repair genes are defective, the DNA errors are perpetuated, and can lead to uncontrolled cell division and possibly cancer. The hallmark characteristic of defective MMR genes is the presence of many mutations (alterations) in specific DNA areas called microsatellites; this is referred to as microsatellite instability (MSI). Patients with HNPCC have increased risks of developing colorectal cancer (80% increase), endometrial cancer (60% increase) and other cancers. HNPCC is inherited in an autosomal dominant manner. The genes affected are located on autosomal (non-sex determining) chromosomes. For an autosomal dominant inheritance, one copy of a defective gene from a parent is enough to cause the presence of HNPCC-related diseases, even though the other parent has a normal gene for this trait.

Incidence: HNPCC is the most common cause of hereditary colorectal cancer (2% to 3% of colorectal cancers). Women with HNPCC represent 2% to 5% of endometrial cancers and they have a lifetime risk of 27% to 71% for endometrial cancer, compared to 3% in the general women population. They also have an increased lifetime risk of 3% to14% for ovarian cancer, compared to 1.5% in the general women population. Women with HNPCC develop gynecological cancers at a younger age (endometrial cancer ranging from 46 to 54 years old and ovarian cancer ranging from 43 to 50 years old), compared to the mean age of 60 with other women in the general population. Prevalence of HNPCC is estimated at 1 in 440 Americans, and the majority of cases are undiagnosed.

Symptoms: Colorectal cancer (CRC) patients present with any of the following: diarrhea, constipation, nausea, vomiting, narrower stools than usual, blood in the stool, change in bowel habits, feeling of incomplete bowel movement, non-intentional weight loss, fatigue, feeling bloated/full and experiencing frequent abdominal gas, pain or cramps. Endometrial/Uterine cancer patients present with any of the following: unusual vaginal bleeding or discharge, bleeding after menopause, problem with urinating, pain during intercourse, or pelvic pain. Ovarian cancer patients present with any of the following: pain, swelling, lump or feeling of pressure in the abdomen or pelvis; heavy or irregular vaginal bleeding or discharge, especially after menopause; urinary frequency or urgency; and abdominal discomfort such as constipation, feeling bloated/full and experiencing frequent abdominal gas.

Muir-Torre syndrome is a variant of HNPCC in which patients present with cancers associated with HNPCC and skin problems; an example is uncontrolled growth of cells near the hair units such as sebaceous (oil) glands or keratoacanthomas (small, round, red or skin-colored bumps, dome-shaped with a central plug that when removed shows a mini-volcano shape).

Turcot syndrome is a rare condition, and considered a variant of HNPCC and another form of inherited colorectal cancer (familial adenomatous polyposis or FAP). Patients with Turcot syndrome present with colon polyps with an increased risk of CRC and brain tumors (most common: glioblastomas/astrocytomas, which are supportive cells of the brain, in HNPCC, and medulloblastoma in FAP).

Screening and diagnosis: Individuals who present to their clinical providers are evaluated with a thorough medical history and physical examination.

Different methods to identify patients with HNPCC include: obtaining a comprehensive family history of cancers, using medical criteria and utilizing prediction models (eg, MMRpredict model, MMRpro model, PREMM model, and Leiden model) that incorporate various data and assist providers in deciding whether to pursue genetic testing for the presence of MMR gene mutations.

Identification of patients who are at risk for HNPCC utilize the Amsterdam criteria I later modified to Amsterdam criteria II to include other cancers in addition to CRC. The Amsterdam criteria can be easily remembered with the "3-2-1" rule: three or more relatives with proven HNPCC cancers, at least two generations affected, and at least one cancer diagnosed before age 50 years. The Revised Bethesda Criteria were developed to identify patients who should have gene testing for microsatellite instability (MSI) by using the polymerase chain reaction (PCR) which amplifies DNA sequences; the MSI is reflected by the loss or mutations of MMR genes. Another diagnostic test used is immunohistochemistry (IHC) which uses dye or radioactive tracer-tagged antibodies against MMR proteins, and looks for the MMR proteins in a tissue biopsy sample. The loss or absence of MMR proteins reflects the presence of MMR gene mutations. Gastroenterology experts agree in recommending genetic evaluation of all CRC patients with MSI for gene mutations or IHC for gene products (proteins). If *MLH1* protein is missing, further testing for other gene mutations (*BRAF* gene and *MLH1* gene alteration) is needed to distinguish hereditary from sporadic cases of HNPCC. A *BRAF* mutation essentially excludes HNPCC, and *MLH1* gene mutation causes endometrial cancer similar to that of HNPCC.

Other recommendations include genetic evaluation for: individuals who score >5% probability in the prediction models, first-degree relatives of those with known MMR/*EPCAM* gene mutation, patients with family cancer history meeting Amsterdam I or II criteria or revised Bethesda guidelines, and women with endometrial cancer before the age of 50.

For the evaluation of colorectal (CRC), endometrium/uterine and ovarian cancers, please see the specific sections on these topics.

Treatment and therapy: Total abdominal colectomy (surgical removal of the large colon from the end of the small colon to the rectum and connecting these ends) is the recommended management of patients with HNPCC who have CRC or with benign growths (adenoma) that are difficult to remove. Colonoscopy surveillance of the remaining rectum is recommended every 1 to 2 years. Surgical removal of affected parts of the colon (segmental colectomy) combined with regular colonoscopy surveillance can be done for patients who are unsuitable for total colectomy.

Surgical treatment of low risk localized endometrial cancer is usually curative. The surgery, with its associated staging of endometrial cancer, is called total abdominal hysterectomy with bilateral salpingo-oophorectomy (TAH/BSO) and dissection of pelvic and para-aortic lymph nodes. This surgery involves removal of the uterus, fallopian tubes, ovaries, and sampling of lymph nodes in the pelvis and nearby abdominal aorta. These tissues are examined microscopically, and the extent of cancer spread is determined. Other options for this abdominal surgery include the vaginal approach, laparoscopy (surgery that uses a thin lighted tube inserted through small cuts in the abdomen), and robotic-assisted approaches. Ovarian cancer management and staging also often requires surgery such as TAH/BSO noted above and omentectomy, which is removal of the omentum (tissue lining the abdomen and covering the organs there).

The stages of colorectal, endometrium and ovarian cancers will determine other treatment modalities such as radiation, chemotherapy, or different surgeries. The specific sections for these cancers discuss further details of these options.

Screening and early detection are the keys to manage patients with HNPCC or Lynch Syndrome; colonoscopy every two years is recommended for first-degree family members.

Prognosis, prevention, and outcomes: The most important prognostic indicator of outcome after surgical treatment of CRC is the stage of the disease at presentation. The earlier stages will have more favorable prognosis and outcomes. Interestingly, patients with localized CRC and tumors that have high levels of DNA MSI have higher survival rates; the reason for this is currently unknown.

The majority of women with HNPCC and endometrial cancers are diagnosed in the early stages of the cancers; they have favorable prognosis when treated with surgery and other appropriate modalities early on. Women with HNPCC and ovarian cancers have similar survival rates as the patients with sporadic or non-heritable ovarian cancer, depending on the stage of the disease at the time of presentation and treatment.

Prophylactic TAH/BSO surgery should be offered to women who are known HNPCC mutation carriers and who have finished child bearing (optimally at age 40 to 45 years) because this management largely prevents the development of endometrial and ovarian cancers. If colon surgery is scheduled, the option of prophylactic gynecological surgery at the same time should be considered. The risks/benefits of this management should be discussed in detail.

Although the value of screening for endometrial cancers is still unknown, experts agree that screening for endometrial cancer and ovarian cancer should be offered to women at risk for or affected with HNPCC by a gynecological examination, endometrial biopsy and transvaginal ultrasound annually, starting at age 30 to 35 years before undergoing surgery or if surgery is deferred. Screening from the age of 35 to 40 years may lead to finding premalignant disease and early cancers.

For patients who are at risk and affected with HNPCC, the recommendations are: (1) a baseline endoscopy with stomach biopsy at age 30 to 35 years (a procedure that uses a flexible tube with a light and camera at its tip to look at the esophagus, stomach and duodenum, upper part of the small bowel) and (2) treatment of *Helicobacter pylori* infection if present. The benefits of this regular screening have limited data but it is suggested that screening is done every 3 to 5 years if there is family history of stomach cancer.

The American College of Gastroenterology does not recommend screening for other cancers unless the patient has family history of the specific cancers. The benefits for screening cancers other than CRC are still unknown.

The American Gastroenterological Association suggests that aspirin be offered for cancer prevention in patients with HNPCC. The European Mallorca Group suggests that the optimal dose of aspirin is unknown at this time; they recommend smoking prevention and maintenance of normal weight.

Miriam E. Schwartz, MD, MA, PhD
Colm A. Ó'Moráin, MA, MD, MSc, DSc

For Further Information

Ahnen, Dennis J., & Axell, Lisen. (2015). Lynch syndrome (hereditary nonpolyposis colorectal cancer): Clinical manifestations and diagnosis. In J. Thomas Lamont and Shilpa Grover (Eds.), *UpToDate*. Retrieved at: www.uptodate.com .

Lu, K. H., & Schmeler, K. M. (2015). Endometrial and ovarian cancer screening and prevention in women with Lynch syndrome (hereditary nonpolyposis colorectal cancer). In Barbara Goff and Sandy J. Falk (Eds.), *UpToDate*. Retrieved at: www.uptodate.com.

Munoz, Juan Carlos, & Lambiase, Louis R. (2015). Hereditary Colorectal Cancer. In Francisco Talavera and BS Anand (Eds.), *Medscape* (April, 2015). Retrieved from http://emedicine.medscape.com/article/188613-overview

Rubenstein, Joel H., Enns, Robert, Heidelbaugh, Joel, Barkun, Alan & the Clinical Guidelines Committee. (2015). American gastroenterological association institute guideline on the diagnosis and management of lynch syndrome. *Gastroenterology*, 149(3): 777–782. Guideline for clinicians who treat patients with Lynch Syndrome or HNPCC. It contains the official recommendations of the American Gastroenterological Association (AGA) Institute on the diagnosis and management of Lynch syndrome or HNPCC. This article is freely available at http://www.gastrojournal.org/article/S0016-5085%2815%2901031-8/abstract?referrer=http%3A%2F%2Fwww.ncbi.nlm.nih.gov%2Fpubmed%2F%3Fterm%3DRubenstein%252C%2BJoel%2BH.%252C%2BEnns%252C%2BRobert%252C

Syngal, S., Brand, R. E., Church, J. M., Giardiello , F. M., Hampel, H. L., & Burt, R. W. (2015). American college of gastroenterology (ACG) clinical guideline: Genetic testing and management of hereditary gastrointestinal cancer syndromes. *American Journal of Gastroenterology*, 110(2): 223-262. Recommendations of the American College of Gastroenterology for the management of patients with hereditary gastrointestinal cancer syndromes. This article is freely available at http://www.ncbi.nlm.nih.gov/pmc/articles/PMC4695986/

Vasen, H. F. A., Blanco, I., Aktan-Collan, K., Gopie, J. P., Alonso, A., Aretz, S., ... the Mallorca Group. (2013). Revised guidelines for the clinical management of Lynch syndrome (HNPCC): Recommendations by a group of European experts. *Gut*, 62(6): 812-823. The Mallorca Group is a group of European experts who got together and developed this revised guidelines for the clinical management of Lynch syndrome (HNPCC). This article is freely available at http://gut.bmj.com/content/62/6/812.full

Other Resources:

American College of Gastroenterology.
http://patients.gi.org/topics/colorectal-cancer/

American Gastroenterological Association.
http://www.gastro.org/guidelines/2015/10/19/diagnosis-and-management-of-lynch-syndrome

American Gastroenterological Association.
http://www.gastro.org/info_for_patients/2015/8/11/a-patient-guide-understanding-lynch-syndrome

American Society of Clinical Oncology (ASCO)
http://www.cancer.net/cancer-types/lynch-syndrome

Centers for Disease Control (CDC) and Prevention
http://www.cdc.gov/features/lynchsyndrome

Genetics Home Reference—Your Guide to Understanding Genetic Conditions. A service of the U.S. National Library of Medicine
http://ghr.nlm.nih.gov/condition/lynch-syndrome

Lynch Syndrome Blog
http://www.ihavelynchsyndrome.com/lynch-syndrome

Lynch Syndrome International
http://lynchcancers.com

Lynch Syndrome Ireland
http://lynchsyndromeireland.com/

Macmillan Cancer Support —United Kingdom
http://www.macmillan.org.uk/information-and-support/diagnosing/causes-and-risk-factors/genetic-testing-and-counselling/lynch-syndrome.html

National Cancer Institute
http://www.cancer.gov/types

National Cancer Institute—Surveillance, Epidemiology and End Results Program
http://seer.cancer.gov/statfacts

U.S. National Library of Medicine—Colorectal Cancer
https://www.nlm.nih.gov/medlineplus/colorectalcancer.html

U.S. National Library of Medicine—Endometrial/Uterine Cancer
https://www.nlm.nih.gov/medlineplus/uterinecancer.html

See also: Endometrial Cancer; Uterine Cancer

▶ Hereditary non-VHL clear cell renal cell carcinomas

Category: Diseases, Symptoms, and Conditions
Also known as: Hereditary non-VHL CCRCC

Related condition: Clear cell renal cell cancer (CCRCC)

Definition: Hereditary non-VHL clear cell renal cell carcinoma is a cancer that develops in the nephrons, the filtering parts of the kidney. Its cells are characterized by clear cytoplasm. The *VHL* (von Hippel-Lindau) gene, which is a more common cause of clear cell renal cell carcinoma, is absent.

Risk factors: The primary risk factor is a family history of clear cell renal cell carcinoma in the absence of the *VHL* gene.

Etiology and the disease process: Hereditary non-VHL clear cell renal cell carcinoma arises from a single cell of the tubular epithelium of the nephron. It spreads through the lymph nodes and the bloodstream. The most common sites of metastases are the other kidney, the lung, the adrenal gland, the bones, or the liver.

Incidence: Hereditary non-VHL clear cell renal cell carcinoma is very rare.

Symptoms: Typically, this type of kidney cancer appears as a single tumor. There are no symptoms until the tumor has become quite large or has metastasized. The symptoms are hematuria (blood in the urine), abdominal mass, back or flank pain, weight loss, recurrent fever, and fatigue.

Screening and diagnosis: There is no routine screening for hereditary non-VHL clear cell renal cell carcinoma. However, if a person has a family member with the disease, that person and other family members would be screened annually. Both screening and diagnosis are performed by abdominal computed tomography (CT) scan, ultrasound, or magnetic resonance imaging (MRI). A biopsy is done to determine the type of cancer. It may be performed by inserting a core needle through the skin into the kidney or by ureteroscopy.

Hereditary non-VHL clear cell renal cell carcinoma is staged in the same way as other kidney cancers, using numeric groupings from I to IV and the TNM (tumor/lymph node/metastasis) staging system.

Treatment and therapy: Usually, the affected kidney is removed, although sometimes only part of the kidney is removed. Research is investigating the use of radioablation (destroying the tumor with radiation), cryoablation (freezing), and arterial embolization.

Kidney cancers, including hereditary non-VHL clear cell renal cell carcinoma, are not treated with chemotherapy or radiation therapy, unless they are Stages III or IV, as these therapies produce a low survival rate.

Prognosis, prevention, and outcomes: The prognosis depends on the stage of the tumor. With Stages I and II, surgical intervention is likely to cure the cancer. With Stage III and IV kidney cancer, the prognosis is guarded and depends on the patient's response to chemotherapy. Hereditary non-VHL clear cell renal cell carcinoma cannot be prevented.

Christine M. Carroll, R.N., B.S.N., M.B.A.

See also: Birt-Hogg-Dubé Syndrome (BHDS); Family history and risk assessment; Giant Cell Tumors (GCTs); Hereditary Leiomyomatosis and Renal Cell Cancer (HLRCC); Hereditary papillary renal cell carcinomas; Kidney cancer; Ovarian epithelial cancer; Renal pelvis tumors; Salivary gland cancer; Urinary system cancers; Uterine cancer; Vaginal cancer; Von Hippel-Lindau (VHL) disease; Wilms' tumor

▶ Hereditary pancreatitis

Category: Diseases, Symptoms, and Conditions
Also known as: HP

Related conditions: Diabetes mellitus, malabsorption, pancreatic cancer

Definition: Hereditary pancreatitis is an inherited disease characterized by recurrent acute (short and severe) episodes of pancreatitis (inflammation of the pancreas) that often progress to chronic (persistent) pancreatitis. Most people develop symptoms before the age of twenty. A person with hereditary pancreatitis has a 40 percent chance of developing pancreatic cancer by the age of seventy.

Risk factors: Because hereditary pancreatitis is inherited, the main risk factor is having a family history of this disease. Each child born to a person with hereditary pancreatitis has a 50 percent chance of inheriting the disease. Alcohol may worsen pain and other symptoms, and smoking increases the risk of developing pancreatic cancer.

Etiology and the disease process: The underlying genetic cause of most cases of hereditary pancreatitis is a mutation, or a genetic change, in the *PRSS1* gene. Normally, the protein made by *PRSS1*—called cationic trypsinogen—is changed into trypsin, which is an enzyme that helps digest protein. In people with hereditary pancreatitis, an excess of trypsin damages the pancreas by autodigestion (the trypsin destroys cells of the pancreas). The process by which pancreatitis causes pancreatic cancer is not well understood.

Usually, each person has two normal copies of the *PRSS1* gene. A mutation in one copy of the gene is sufficient to cause hereditary pancreatitis. A person with hereditary pancreatitis has a *PRSS1* gene mutation from the time of conception. About 20 percent of people with a *PRSS1* mutation do not develop pancreatitis.

Incidence: It is estimated that at least 1,000 people in the United States are affected with hereditary pancreatitis.

Symptoms: Symptoms include abdominal pain, nausea, vomiting, malnutrition (not getting enough nutrients from food), and diabetes mellitus.

Screening and diagnosis: Generally, imaging studies of the pancreas, a detailed family history, and blood tests help diagnose this disease. Because most cases of hereditary pancreatitis are caused by mutations in the *PRSS1* gene, genetic testing may assist in confirming a suspected diagnosis.

Treatment and therapy: The main focus of treatment is to reduce the symptoms by giving pancreatic enzyme supplements to treat malnutrition, insulin to treat diabetes, and medication to treat pain. Occasionally surgery removing part or all of the pancreas is performed to treat complications. Treatment for pancreatic cancer may include surgery, radiation therapy, and chemotherapy.

Prognosis, prevention, and outcomes: Because hereditary pancreatitis is a genetic condition, it cannot be prevented. To reduce the risk of pancreatic cancer and to prevent the worsening of pancreatitis, the patient should avoid smoking and alcohol. Imaging of the pancreas may be done to detect cancer at an early stage. The medical team caring for the patient decides the age at which monitoring should start.

Abbie L. Abboud, M.S., C.G.C.

See also: Antidiarrheal agents; Antiviral therapies; CA 19-9 test; Endoscopic Retrograde Cholangiopancreatography (ERCP); Family history and risk assessment; Hepatomegaly; Hypercalcemia; Pancreatic cancers; Pancreatitis; Paracentesis; Thoracentesis; Ultrasound tests

▶ Hereditary papillary renal cell carcinomas

Category: Diseases, Symptoms, and Conditions
Also known as: HPRCC

Related condition: Papillary renal cell carcinomas

Definition: Hereditary papillary renal cell carcinoma develops in the nephrons, the filtering parts of the kidney. Papillary tumors are characterized by fingerlike projections from the tumor. There are two types of papillary renal cell cancers, and HPRCC is type 1.

Risk factors: The primary risk factor is a family history of hereditary papillary renal cell carcinoma.

Etiology and the disease process: Hereditary papillary renal cell carcinoma is characterized by multifocal sites of papillary tumor development within one or both kidneys. These sites develop concurrently rather than spreading from an initial site. The sites often vary in size. Research demonstrates that hereditary papillary renal cell carcinoma is caused by a mutation in the *MET* gene. However, hereditary papillary renal cell carcinoma is less aggressive than other renal cell cancers and is less likely to metastasize.

Incidence: Hereditary papillary renal cell carcinoma is quite rare. It is much more common in men and in African Americans than in the population as a whole.

Symptoms: There are no symptoms until the tumors have become large enough to interfere with kidney function. The symptoms are hematuria (blood in the urine), abdominal mass, back or flank pain, weight loss, recurrent fever, and fatigue.

Screening and diagnosis: There is no routine screening for hereditary papillary renal cell carcinoma, unless a person has a family member who develops it. In this case, family members would be screened annually. Both screening and diagnosis are performed by abdominal computed tomography (CT) scan, ultrasound, or magnetic resonance imaging (MRI). A biopsy is required to determine the type of cancer. It may be performed by inserting a core needle through the skin into the kidney or by ureteroscopy.

Hereditary papillary renal cell carcinoma is staged in the same manner as other kidney cancers, using numeric groupings from I to IV, and the TNM (tumor/lymph node/metastasis) staging system.

Treatment and therapy: Hereditary papillary renal cell carcinoma is usually treated by partial nephrectomy or by destruction of the tumor sites only. This can be performed by radioablation (destroying the tumor with radiation), cryoablation (freezing), or arterial embolization.

The presence of many sites of hereditary papillary renal cell carcinoma makes it likely that all stages of this cancer are treated with chemotherapy, immunotherapy, and radiation. Here, the goal is to maintain some kidney function.

Prognosis, prevention, and outcomes: Hereditary papillary renal cell carcinoma is more likely to be a chronic condition because it rarely metastasizes. However, a patient with Stage III or IV hereditary papillary renal cell carcinoma could require dialysis because of a lack of kidney function. Hereditary papillary renal cell carcinoma cannot be prevented.

Christine M. Carroll, R.N., B.S.N., M.B.A.

See also: African Americans and cancer; Family history and risk assessment; Hereditary Leiomyomatosis and Renal Cell Cancer (HLRCC); Hereditary non-VHL clear cell renal cell carcinomas; Kidney cancer; Renal pelvis tumors; Urinary system cancers

▶ Hereditary polyposis syndromes

Category: Diseases, Symptoms, and Conditions
Also known as: Familial adenomatous polyposis (FAP), Peutz-Jeghers Syndrome (PJS), juvenile polyposis syndrome, Gardner syndrome, hereditary mixed polyposis syndrome, harmatomas, adenomas, juvenile polyps

Related conditions: Colorectal cancer, bowel obstruction, rectal bleeding desmoid tumors, osteomas, soft-tissue tumors, pigmented lesions, intestinal polyps

Definition: Hereditary polyposis syndromes are several disorders caused by a genetic predisposition for the growth of large numbers of polyps in the small and large intestine: familial adenomatous polyposis, Gardner syndrome, Peutz-Jeghers syndrome, juvenile polyposis syndrome, and hereditary mixed polyposis syndrome.

Individuals diagnosed with familial adenomatous polyposis (FAP) have an *APC* gene alteration on chromosome 5q21 and are likely to grow large numbers (more than one hundred) of intestinal polyps.

Gardner syndrome is a variant of FAP that causes intestinal polyps, skin and soft-tissue tumors, desmoid tumors, and multiple osteomas. The intestinal polyps have an almost 100 percent chance of becoming malignant. This condition can begin in puberty, but the average age for diagnosis of malignancy is thirty-nine years. Nonmalignant soft-tissue growths and osteomas can appear earlier.

Peutz-Jeghers syndrome is caused by an *STK11/LKB1* mutation and produces multiple polyplike growths called hamartomas that grow in the small intestine rather than the large intestine. They have a low potential for becoming malignant but can become quite large and cause symptoms requiring surgery.

Juvenile polyposis syndrome is a rare childhood-onset, autosomal dominant disease. It produces hamartomous polyposis rather than adenomatous polyposis.

Hereditary mixed polyposis syndrome, a rare syndrome seen in families, causes a variety of colon polyp types.

Polyps are initially benign but can easily become malignant because of the genetic abnormalities. The term "adenomatous polyp" refers to a nonmalignant polyp with a high predisposition to become malignant.

Risk factors: The hereditary polyposis syndromes all involve some sort of genetic error that is autosomal dominant. That means that if one parent carries the genetic mutation, there is a 50 percent chance that his or her child will have the disease. The sex of the child does not matter. Although genetic alterations can occur for unknown reasons, people who do not carry the mutated gene have an extremely small chance of randomly developing one of these syndromes and cannot transfer it to their offspring. Familial adenomatous polyposis (FAP) and its variant, Gardner syndrome, involve an error in the gene *APC* on chromosome 5, which is autosomal dominant. The gene responsible for Peutz-Jeghers is *STK11/LKB1*. Two genes, *BMPR1A* and *SMAD4,* have been identified as causing juvenile polyposis syndrome. Hereditary mixed polyposis syndrome is believed to arise from a gene error on chromosome 15.

Etiology and the disease process: Polyps can begin at any age; however, polyps caused by FAP rarely occur before age ten, and juvenile polyposis syndrome is a very rare disease. The chromosome abnormalities in hereditary polyposis syndromes are responsible for cellular changes in the mucosal lining of the intestine that initiate the formation of polyps. The chromosomal abnormality drastically increases the possibility of a polyp becoming malignant. Individuals with FAP and Gardner syndrome will develop multiple polyps, so many, in fact, that surgical removal of the colon is sometimes the only option. Surveillance and screening are the best methods for prevention and early detection of intestinal polyps.

Nonfamilial causes of polyps are not well understood but seem to be responsible for isolated polyp formation. Some of these polyps will become malignant if left untreated. Colorectal cancer screening without genetic predisposition for familial polyposis or cancer usually begins at age fifty.

Incidence: FAP affects 1 in 30,000 people, with 800 to 1,000 new cases per year. It is more common in Western countries. A person with a family history of adenomatous polyps has between a 15 and 20 percent risk of developing polyps and is at a much higher risk of developing colorectal cancer than the general population. Without intervention, 90 percent of those with FAP will develop colorectal cancer by their fourth or fifth decade of life.

Gardner syndrome occurs in 1 in 1 million people. There is an almost 100 percent chance that polyps due to this syndrome will become malignant.

Peutz-Jeghers syndrome occurs in 1 in 7,000 live births.

Symptoms: Patients with familial adenomatous polyposis initially do not exhibit symptoms. However, polyps can cause blood to be passed in the stool, which can be detected through a fecal occult blood test (FOBT). As polyps get larger, patients experience symptoms such as diarrhea, constipation, and abdominal pain. Gardner syndrome causes osteomas, or bone cysts, in the jaw, skull, and teeth. Epidermoid cysts can be present on the face, scalp, arms, and legs. Juvenile polyposis syndrome can cause diarrhea, constipation, gastrointestinal hemorrhage, and protein-losing abnormalities.

Screening and diagnosis: People with a family history of polyps should have genetic testing to see if they are carriers of hereditary polyposis syndromes. Also, all of their primary relatives (parents, siblings, and children) should receive genetic testing. Earlier colorectal cancer screening is indicated if genetic testing is positive.

Symptoms of hereditary polyposis syndromes, such as fecal blood or gastrointestinal problems, indicate the need for diagnostic tests such as sigmoidoscopy, barium-contrast X rays, or colonoscopy. All of these tests can find polyps, but only a colonoscopy allows a biopsy to be performed. Biopsies are taken to determine the type of tissue: adenomatous, harmatomous, or cancerous. In cases of familial adenomatous polyposis, more than one hundred polyps can be present, making total polyp removal impossible. In addition to the presence of polyps, Gardner syndrome can be diagnosed from the presence of osteomas, or bone tumors (usually in the jaw, skull, and teeth), and epidermoid cysts.

Treatment and therapy: Patients with familial adenomatous polyposis often have so many polyps that individual polyp removal during colonoscopy is not an option. In these cases, surgical removal of part or all of the large intestine and the rectum is the main treatment. In a colectomy with ileorectal anastomosis (IRA), the entire colon is removed. The last part of the small intestine (ileum) is attached (anastomosed) to the top of the rectum. Total proctocolectomy with permanent ileostomy involves the removal of the entire colon, rectum, and anus. A small opening is made through the abdominal wall (ostomy), where a bag can be attached to collect fecal material.

The rationale for these seemingly radical procedures is that there is no way to prevent the formation of numerous polyps that have a high probability of becoming malignant. Removing the colon prevents the formation of the adenomatous polyps, lowers the chance of developing colorectal cancer, and saves lives.

Recovery from colectomy takes approximately six to eight weeks. Patients may have to avoid certain foods that upset the bowel, adapt to more frequent bowel movements, and find out what foods and drink work best for them. Adjusting to a colostomy can be difficult and life-altering. Issues related to self-image, general well-being, and sexuality need to be addressed. Counseling and family support are important components of physical and mental health.

Epidermoid cysts and osteomas from Gardner syndrome can be removed if painful or disfiguring, but they are unlikely to become malignant.

In Peutz-Jeghers syndrome and juvenile polyposis syndrome, the polyps are harmatomas, which usually appear in the small intestine and are fewer in number. Individual polyps can be removed if the patient develops symptoms and there is the chance of obstruction.

Prognosis, prevention, and outcomes: People who have the gene alteration that causes a hereditary polyposis syndrome will develop the disease. Therefore, it is important for these people to see specialists in gastroenterology and genetics who can manage routine health, screening, and illness when indicated. It is recommended that patients with Gardner syndrome have a fecal occult blood test (FOBT), sigmoidoscopy or colonoscopy, and upper gastrointestinal tract testing every one to two years until age fifty.

There is some evidence that a class of drugs called COX-2 (cyclooxygenase 2) inhibitors can prevent the growth of some intestinal polyps and limit the size of the ones that do form. This does not mean, however, that COX-2 inhibitors are effective for those with hereditary polyposis syndromes.

Surgical removal of the colon alters patients' lifestyles but can be lifesaving. Routine medical visits are still necessary, but the surgery significantly reduces the risk of developing colorectal cancer.

Janet R. Green, M.S.P.H.

For Further Information

Fisher, Stephen. *Colon Cancer and the Polyps Connection*. Tuscon, Ariz.: Fisher Books, 1995.

Gardner, E. J. "A Genetic and Clinical Study of Intestinal Polyposis, a Predisposing Factor for Carcinoma of the Colon and Rectum." *American Journal of Human Genetics* 3, no. 2 (June, 1951): 167-176.

Herrera, Lemuel, ed. *Familial Adenomatous Polyposis*. New York: A. R. Liss, 1990.

Other Resources

American Cancer Society
http://www.cancer.org

American Gastroenterology Association
http://www.gastro.org

National Cancer Institute
http://www.cancer.gov

National Institute of Diabetes and Digestive and Kidney Diseases
http://www2.niddk.nih.gov

See also: Adenomatous polyps; *APC* gene testing; Ashkenazi Jews and cancer; Bethesda criteria; Colon polyps; Colorectal cancer; Colorectal cancer screening; Cyclooxygenase 2 (COX-2) inhibitors; Desmoid tumors; *DPC4* gene testing; Duodenal carcinomas; Endometrial cancer; Endometrial hyperplasia; Enterostomal therapy; Ethnicity and cancer; Family history and risk assessment; Gardner syndrome; Gastric polyps; Gastrointestinal cancers; Genetics of cancer; Hereditary cancer syndromes; Hereditary mixed polyposis syndrome; Juvenile polyposis syndrome; *MLH1* gene; *MSH* genes; Pancreatic cancers; Peutz-Jeghers Syndrome (PJS); *PMS* genes; Premalignancies; Sarcomas, soft-tissue; Small intestine cancer; Turcot syndrome

▶ Histiocytosis X

Category: Diseases, Symptoms, and Conditions
Also known as: Langerhans cell histiocytosis, eosinophilic granuloma, pulmonary histiocytosis X (PHX), eosinophilic granulomatosis, pulmonary Langerhans cell histiocytosis X (PLCH), Langerhans cell granulomatosis

Related conditions: Non-Langerhans cell histiocytosis, T-cell lymphoma (malignant histiocytosis syndrome)

Definition: Histiocytosis X, now generally called Langerhans cell granulomatosis (LCG) or Langerhans cell histiocytosis (LCH), is characterized by granulomatous lesions containing Langerhans cells. Histiocytosis X is a group of diseases that exhibit an increase in histiocytes. Variants of the condition may be localized or systemic. Once considered cancerous, these diseases are now classified as autoimmune diseases.

Histiocytes are cells critical to the immune response and arise from the mononuclear phagocytic system in the bone marrow. These precursor cells have the potential to transform into macrophage or Langerhans cell lineages. Langerhans cells engulf antigens such as foreign microbes and then alert the immune system to their presence.

Histiocytosis X now includes Letterer-Siwe disease and Hand-Schüller-Christian disease. These conditions, seen in children, were once considered separate diseases. When children are afflicted, the disease erupts in many organs, while in adults the condition affects primarily the lung and more rarely the bones (about 4 to 20 percent of cases) and, even less likely, the skin.

Risk factors: Risk factors include smoking and possibly genetic factors, but the exact etiology is unknown.

Etiology and the disease process: The defining pathology is an accumulation of Langerhans cells in epithelial cells lining the lung tissue. These lung-tissue cells first undergo an increase in their numbers (hyperplasia) following some chronic insult, such as persistent smoking, then begin an uncontrolled immune response. The result and hallmark of this disease are discrete granulomatous lesions scattered through the upper and middle portions of the lung. These lesions are composed, in the early stages, mostly of Langerhans cells surrounded by eosinophils, lymphocytes, macrophages, and plasma cells.

Granulomatous lesions are similar in the pediatric version of the disease but are scattered through the viscera, skin, and bones. Although the disease process in children includes the classic lung pathology, it also results in skin and bone lesions and, typically, an enlarged liver and spleen. There are also severe dental consequences such as inflamed gums, loss of teeth, and mandibular hyperplasia.

Incidence: In the United States, the condition afflicts 1 in 250,000 children and 1 in 1 million adults. Langerhans cell granulomatosis represents approximately 1 percent of all interstitial lung disease. Most adult patients are between twenty and forty years old and have a history of smoking, while the childhood disease is most prevalent between ages one and three. Most cases of the disease occur before age seventeen.

Symptoms: Adults may first complain of a persistent cough, lethargy, and labored breathing. Less frequently there is an associated weight loss, fever, and a vague feeling of illness, but, surprisingly, about 25 percent of cases are symptom free. The classic finding is pneumothorax, a collection of air in the plural cavity, which may eventually cause the lung to collapse. This occurs in as many as 10 to 20 percent of cases. Typical symptoms may include cough, chest pain, fever, weight loss, bone pain, and skin rash.

In young children, symptoms may vary with the severity of organ compromise. In the form called Letterer-Siwe disease, there is a generalized involvement of the viscera with potentially fatal consequences. Skin lesions range from small papules to hemorrhagic nodules. Oral symptoms include ulcerations, bruising, gum inflammation, and tooth loss. Fetid breath odor is a conspicuous result. Other symptoms reflect organ and tissue damage in the liver, spleen, and bones. Typical symptoms may include weight loss, fever, abdominal pain, jaundice, dermatitis, mental deficits, short stature, abdominal pain, ear drainage, and enlarged lymph nodes.

Another childhood variation, Hand-Schüller-Christian disease, manifests itself in three ways: diabetes insipidus, lytic bone lesions, and a bulging of the eyes called proptosis. This condition also results in a dental pathology similar to Letterer-Siwe disease.

Screening and diagnosis: In the adult form of the disease, the symptoms are nonspecific and reflect interstitial lung disease, which may be common to other conditions. Chest imaging including high-resolution computed tomography (CT) scans is useful in revealing nodules, and pulmonary function tests may uncover obstructive irregularities. Additionally, the results of bronchoalveolar lavage and a history of smoking may prove useful indicators, but they are not definitive. Only lung tissue biopsy will confirm the diagnosis.

In children, bone radiographs, tissue and bone marrow biopsy, and general laboratory work are instructive, but biopsies containing clusters of Langerhans cells are required for a diagnosis.

Treatment and therapy: The cardinal treatment is smoking cessation in the adult. Corticosteroid therapy is case dependent and is used only in patients with notable lung function deficits. In the childhood form of the disease, there has been notable success using immune-signaling molecules such as interleukins, and research is investigating their potential in the adult form of the disease. Other treatment options are palliative, such as infection control, supplemental oxygen, and bronchodilator therapy. Asymptomatic patients having only mild impairment are treated conservatively.

Prognosis, prevention, and outcomes: Smoking cessation may halt the progression of the disease and possibly initiate its reversal. For the very young and the elderly, the prognosis is poor. This is also the case for those who have been treated with corticosteroids over an extended period, in patients suffering from multiorgan involvement, and when there are an extensive number of cysts revealed radiographically. When the disease involves only the lung and smoking is stopped, 50 percent of patients will improve (or at least get no worse), while 50 percent will suffer permanent pulmonary function loss. The outcome in children ranges from poor to excellent depending on the extent of the disease.

Richard S. Spira, D.V.M.

For Further Information

Andersson, B. U., E. Tani, U. Andersson, and J. I. Henter. "Tumor Necrosis Factor, Interleukin 11, and Leukemia Inhibitory Factor Produced by Langerhans Cells in Langerhans Cell Histiocytosis." *Journal of Pediatric Hematology Oncology* 26, no. 11 (2004): 706-711.

Broadbent, V., H. Gadner, D. M. Komp, and S. Ladisch. "Histiocytosis Syndromes in Children: II. Approach to the Clinical and Laboratory Evaluation of Children with Langerhans Cell Histiocytosis." *Medical and Pediatric Oncology* 17, no. (1989): 492-495.

Friedman, P. J., A. A. Liebow, and J. Sokoloff. "Eosinophilic Granuloma of Lung: Clinical Aspects of Primary Pulmonary Histiocytosis in the Adult." *Medicine* 60 (1981): 385.

Travis, W. D., et al. "Pulmonary Langerhans Cell Granulomatosis (Histiocytosis X): A Clinicopathologic Study of Forty-eight Cases." *American Journal of Surgical Pathology* 17 (1993): 971.

Other Resources

MedlinePlus
Histiocytosis
http://www.nlm.nih.gov/medlineplus/ency/article/000068.htm

University of Maryland Medical Center
Histiocytosis
http://www.umm.edu/ency/article/000068.htm

See also: Fibrosarcomas, soft-tissue; Pediatric oncology and hematology; Primary central nervous system lymphomas

▶ Hodgkin disease

Category: Diseases, Symptoms, and Conditions
Also known as: Hodgkin's disease, Hodgkin lymphoma, HD

Related condition: Mononucleosis

Definition: Hodgkin disease is the malignant growth of abnormal immune cells called lymphocytes in the lymphatic system—a critical part of the body's immune system. There are two main types of lymphocytes, B and T. The malignant cells in Hodgkin disease are usually (in 98 percent of the cases) the B lymphocytes.

There are five types of Hodgkin disease: nodular lymphocyte-predominant Hodgkin lymphoma and four classic types:

- Nodular sclerosing Hodgkin lymphoma
- Mixed-cellularity Hodgkin lymphoma
- Lymphocyte-depletion Hodgkin lymphoma
- Lymphocyte-rich Hodgkin lymphoma

These five types differ mostly in how they look under a microscope. However, nodular lymphocyte-predominant Hodgkin lymphoma also behaves differently from the classic types.

Risk factors: The risk for Hodgkin disease depends on gender, age, race, medical condition, and family history. The disease is more common in men, and the difference is particularly evident in children younger than age ten, with the number of boys with the disease up to four times the number of girls with the disease. With the exception of nodular lymphocyte-predominant Hodgkin lymphoma, the risk of developing the disease is highest in young adulthood and in later life. The risk for nodular lymphocyte-predominant Hodgkin lymphoma is highest in a person's thirties and forties. Hodgkin disease is more common in whites, and infection with the Epstein-Barr virus (EBV), which causes infectious mononucleosis, increases a person's risk of developing Hodgkin disease up to four times that of a person who has not had Epstein-Barr. Having a first-degree relative with Hodgkin disease increases the risk for the disease. The identical twin of a Hodgkin patient has one hundred times the risk of developing this cancer compared with the general population.

Etiology and the disease process: The causes of Hodgkin disease are unclear. There are no known chemicals or environmental factors that increase the risk of Hodgkin. However, in some cases, a good argument can be made for a combination of genetics and infection with the Epstein-Barr virus as causing the disease. EBV infects the majority of the world's population—estimates put the infection rates at 90 percent of adults worldwide. Not all infected people develop signs of EBV infection. The virus infects B lymphocytes and is thought to cause other types of cancer as well, including Burkitt lymphoma, another type of immune system cancer. Malignant cells of Hodgkin disease patients often carry EBV deoxyribonucleic acid (DNA).

At the heart of Hodgkin disease are two types of large, abnormal cells. One type is the Reed-Sternberg cell, and the other is the Hodgkin lymphoma cell. Hodgkin disease patients usually have tumors made up of these cells and inflammatory immune cells that surround them. The exception is nodular lymphocyte-predominant Hodgkin lymphoma, in which there are hardly any Reed-Sternberg cells. Instead, this type of Hodgkin disease has typical abnormal cells known as "L and H" or "popcorn cells."

The abnormal cells, surrounded by inflammatory cells, create tumors that usually start in lymph nodes in the chest or neck. These tumors cause the swollen glands that are usually the first sign of the disease.

Hodgkin disease spreads through the lymphatic system and, in advanced disease, blood vessels. It invades the lungs, bones, bone marrow, and liver. The presence of Hodgkin anywhere else usually means the patient has an HIV infection, which makes Hodgkin disease behave differently.

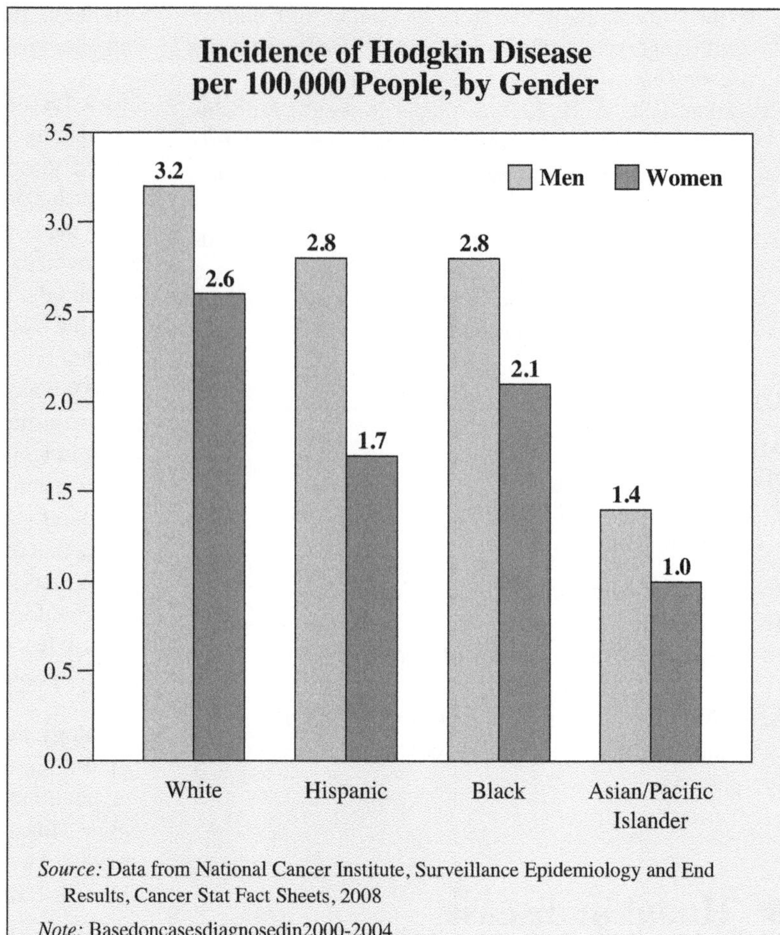

Source: Data from National Cancer Institute, Surveillance Epidemiology and End Results, Cancer Stat Fact Sheets, 2008

Note: Basedoncasesdiagnosedin2000-2004

Incidence: New cases of Hodgkin disease occur in roughly 8,000 people each year. The incidence rate has been decreasing slightly over the past several decades. Hodgkin disease makes up 5 percent of childhood cancers and approximately 1 percent of adult cancers.

Symptoms: Swollen lymph nodes are often the first sign of Hodgkin disease. In most cases, the swollen nodes will be above the diaphragm, in the chest or neck. Sometimes there are no symptoms, but people may feel pain in the affected nodes after drinking alcohol. The tumors in Hodgkin can get fairly large and may cause symptoms such as difficulty swallowing and breathing. Itching, sometimes severe, can precede the development of Hodgkin disease by several years.

Systemic symptoms that indicate a disease that is more serious are as follows:

- Persistent fever higher than 38 degrees Celsius (100.4 degrees Fahrenheit)
- Weight loss of more than 10 percent of the total body weight in six months
- Drenching night sweats

Screening and diagnosis: Diagnosing Hodgkin disease requires a complete medical history and a number of tests. These tests include a complete blood count (CBC) to look at the different cells in the blood and their levels; an erythrocyte sedimentation rate (ESR) test to see how fast blood cells settle to the bottom of a test tube and thereby detect possible infection, cancer, or a bone marrow problem; a bone marrow biopsy; a fine-needle or surgical biopsy of the affected nodes; plus X-ray, computed tomography (CT), and positron emission tomography (PET) scans. Though surgery to determine the stage of the cancer is no longer standard, some patients may still need it if the affected areas are hard to reach or hard to see or sample with nonsurgical techniques.

Staging of Hodgkin disease is done according to criteria established in Ann Arbor, Michigan, and modified in Cotswolds, England. The staging system is known as either the modified Ann Arbor system or the Cotswolds classification system. The stages are as follows:

- Stage I: The cancer affects only one lymph node or one area of the body but no lymph nodes. If an area outside the lymph node is affected, with no lymph node involvement, the letter E is added to the stage designation. Stage I may also be the presence of cancer in one lymphatic organ, such as the spleen or thymus, without the involvement of lymph nodes or other areas in the body.
- Stage II: The cancer is in two or more lymph node areas on the same side of the diaphragm (above or below). Alternatively, one lymph node area and the part of the body with which it is associated are affected (IIE). A subscript next to the stage number indicates the number of lymph node regions involved (for example, Stage II_3).

- Stage III: The cancer has invaded lymph node areas on both sides of the diaphragm (above and below). In addition, the areas of the body connected to the affected nodes may also be affected (IIIE), the spleen may be affected (IIIS), or both conditions may occur (IIIE + S). Two subdivisions of Stage III exist, denoting the extent of the disease in the abdominal area and the spleen.
- Stage IV: There are several tumors in one or more areas of the body outside the lymph nodes. The associated lymph nodes may or may not have cancer in them. Alternatively, there may be cancer in one area of the body and a nonrelated (distant) lymph node region.

A designation of A or B is added to each stage; a B designation means the patient has systemic symptoms.

Treatment and therapy: Oncologists decide on treatment for Hodgkin disease according to the predicted behavior of the disease. This predicted behavior depends not only on the stage of the cancer but also on several risk factors. The presence of these risk factors usually means the disease will be harder to control, and patients are likely to relapse unless they receive more intense or longer treatment. Therefore, even in early-stage Hodgkin, some patients may require treatments similar to those given to patients with advanced disease.

Risk factors for early-stage (Stages I and II) adult Hodgkin disease include the following:

- The presence of a tumor larger than 10 centimeters (cm; 3.9 inches) in size
- The presence of systemic symptoms
- An ESR value greater than 50
- Cancer outside the lymph nodes
- Cancer in three or more lymph nodes

For advanced disease in adults (Stage III and IV), the risk factors are as follows:

- Age older than forty-five years
- Male gender
- Serum albumin levels lower than 4 grams/deciliter (this is a measure of the levels of the most important protein in the blood)
- Hemoglobin levels below 10.5 grams/deciliter
- High white cell count
- Low lymphocyte count
- Stage IV disease

Four categories determine treatment:

- Early-stage favorable: Stage I or II disease with no risk factors
- Early-stage unfavorable: Stage I or II with one or more early-stage risk factors
- Advanced favorable: Stage III or IV with up to three advanced-stage risk factors
- Advanced unfavorable: Stage III or IV with four or more advanced-stage risk factors

Treatment for early-stage favorable disease consists of short-duration chemotherapy with radiation to the affected areas or a longer duration of chemotherapy without radiation. The current standard chemotherapy regimen, known as ABVD, uses a combination of four drugs: doxorubicin (Adriamycin), bleomycin, vinblastine, and dacarbazine. Another common regimen, though less effective and more likely to cause infertility, is MOPP: mechlorethamine, vincristine (Oncovin), procarbazine, and prednisone. Other combinations of chemotherapy drugs are also available.

Treatment of early-stage unfavorable disease consists of radiation to the affected site and four to eight cycles of chemotherapy.

Advanced disease is treated with chemotherapy combinations.

Patients who do not respond to treatment, or respond and relapse, can still be cured by high-dose chemotherapy treatment followed by a transplant of their own stem cells. Harvesting of stem cells is done before beginning the high-dose chemotherapy. The stem cells are then transplanted back to produce healthy red and white blood cells.

Risk factors in children are the same as those of the adult early-stage risk factors. Treatments in children are different in intensity of radiation and the drug combinations used in chemotherapy. For example, in drug protocols for boys, etoposide is substituted for procarbazine because procarbazine induces sterility.

Because Hodgkin disease often strikes during the childbearing years, the question of treatment during pregnancy may arise. Treatment decisions for pregnant patients are individualized and depend on the stage of the disease, the stage of the pregnancy, and the mother's preferences. In many cases, treatment of Hodgkin can be delayed until the end of the pregnancy, unless life-threatening symptoms occur. Early labor might be induced to allow for earlier start of treatments. Case reports also show that women receiving radiation treatments to the upper body, with heavy shielding of the fetus, deliver healthy babies with no apparent abnormalities. However, there is possibly a danger of future cancer in the child, resulting from stray radiation that may have penetrated the shield. Chemotherapy treatments with vinblastine during the second part of the pregnancy are safe and effective, as is the ABVD combination treatment. The ABVD regimen during the first trimester may harm the fetus.

Prognosis, prevention, and outcomes: Hodgkin disease has a high cure rate. The total cure rate is approximately 75 percent in adults, and nearly 95 percent in children.

Because Hodgkin is highly curable, more and more patients find themselves facing late complications of treatment years after their disease had disappeared. Late complications include infertility, hypothyroidism, and lowered immunity. A particularly worrisome late complication is the development of secondary cancers, including leukemia as well as breast, skin, and lung cancers.

Death in the first fifteen years following a Hodgkin diagnosis is usually due to the primary cancer. After fifteen years, death is more often due to secondary cancers.

Adi Ferrara, B.S.

For Further Information

Dores, G. M., T. R. Coté, and L. B. Travis. "New Malignancies Following Hodgkin Lymphoma, Non-Hodgkin Lymphoma, and Myeloma." In *New Malignancies Among Cancer Survivors: SEER Cancer Registries, 1973-2000*, edited by R. E. Curtis et al. NIH Publication 05-5302. Bethesda, Md.: National Cancer Institute, 2006.

Holman, Peter, Jodi Garrett, and William Jansen. *One Hundred Questions and Answers About Lymphoma.* Sudbury, Mass.: Jones and Bartlett, 2004.

Ko, A., E. H. Rosenbaum, and M. Dollinger. *Everyone's Guide to Cancer Therapy: How Cancer Is Diagnosed, Treated, and Managed Day to Day.* 5th ed. Kansas City, Mo.: Andrews McMeel, 2007.

Parker, James N., and Philip M. Parker, eds. *The Official Patient's Sourcebook on Adult Hodgkin's Disease: A Revised and Updated Directory for the Internet Age.* San Diego, Calif.: Icon Health, 2002.

Other Resources

American Cancer Society
Learn About Hodgkin Disease
http://www.cancer.org/docroot/lrn/lrn_0.asp

National Cancer Institute
Hodgkin Lymphoma
http://www.cancer.gov/cancertopics/types/hodgkinslymphoma

See also: Agent Orange; Blood cancers; Childhood cancers; Eye cancers; Fever; Hematologic oncology; HIV/AIDS-related cancers; Imaging tests; Infertility and cancer; Lymphomas; Mantle Cell Lymphoma (MCL); Mediastinal tumors; Mediastinoscopy; Non-Hodgkin lymphoma; Oncogenic viruses; Pericardial effusion; Pheresis; Pregnancy and cancer; Protein electrophoresis; Splenectomy; Surgical biopsies; Thymus cancer; Viral oncology; Young adult cancers

▶ Horner syndrome

Category: Diseases, Symptoms, and Conditions
Also known as: Horner's syndrome

Related conditions: Neuroblastoma, Pancoast tumor of the lung

Definition: Horner syndrome is not a disease but a collection of symptoms that are caused by damage to a nerve that controls the muscles of the eye. Horner syndrome has many causes, some of which are related to tumor growth.

Risk factors: Risk factors for developing Horner syndrome vary and are related to the risk factors for developing the underlying disease that causes Horner syndrome symptoms.

Etiology and the disease process: Horner syndrome is a disorder of the eye named for William Edmonds Horner, a Virginia physician who developed an operation to correct some of the symptoms associated with the syndrome. To understand the syndrome and how it is related to cancer, it is necessary to understand some information about the nervous system.

The nervous system has two divisions. The voluntary nervous system consists of nerves that are under conscious control. These nerves control actions such as turning the head or raising the arm. The involuntary, or autonomic, nervous system controls muscle movements that are not under conscious control. The autonomic nervous system regulates activities such as breathing, digesting food, and the contraction and dilation (expansion) of the pupil of the eye.

The autonomic nervous system has two divisions, the sympathetic and the parasympathetic nervous systems. Stimulation of the sympathetic nerves prepares the body for action by doing things such as moving more blood to the skeletal muscles. Stimulation of the parasympathetic nervous system calms the body by doing things such as allowing muscles to relax.

The eye contains both sympathetic and parasympathetic nerves. Normally these two nervous systems balance each other. In Horner syndrome, the sympathetic nerve to the eye is damaged. As a result, there is only parasympathetic stimulation; the upper eyelid droops and the lower eyelid swells, and the pupil remains small and does not dilate. These changes occur only in one eye.

The sympathetic nerve that is damaged in people with Horner syndrome does not go directly from the brain to the eye. It has a three-step path, and in each stage, different events can cause Horner syndrome. In the first step, the nerve starts in the brain and goes down the spinal cord to the chest. Damage to this part of the pathway (called first-neuron Horner syndrome) can be caused by brain tumors, by a tumor of the pituitary gland (an organ at the base of the brain), or by brief interruption in blood flow to the brain (a transient ischemic attack, or TIA).

The next part of the pathway takes the nerve from the chest over the top of the lungs and up along the carotid artery in the side of the neck. Damage to the nerve in this part of the pathway (called second-neuron Horner syndrome) can be caused by a tumor in the upper part of the lung (a Pancoast tumor) or a tumor in the chest cavity (thoracic tumor). Noncancerous causes include trauma to the chest cavity or neck (either from surgery or an accident), an enlarged thyroid gland, and spinal cord injury or disease.

In the final part of the pathway, the nerve goes from the neck through the middle ear and into the eye. Damage to the nerve in this part of the pathway (called third-neuron Horner syndrome) has noncancerous causes such as injury to the skull, middle-ear infections, and migraine or cluster headaches.

Symptoms similar to Horner syndrome can also be caused by various drugs, including some antipsychotics, anesthetics, and drugs used for treating Parkinson's disease.

Incidence: The incidence of Horner syndrome is not known, but the syndrome is uncommon.

Symptoms: Symptoms include a drooping upper eyelid and a puffy lower eyelid. The eyeball may appear sunken. The pupil of the affected eye is smaller than the pupil of the healthy eye. Children with congenital Horner syndrome (caused by nerve-cell tumors) often have eyes that are different colors. People who have third-neuron Horner syndrome do not sweat from the affected side of the face.

Screening and diagnosis: An ophthalmologist (eye specialist) usually diagnoses Horner syndrome. A few drops of a solution containing a small amount of cocaine are put in the affected eye. If the sympathetic nerve to the eye is undamaged, then the pupil will dilate (enlarge). If there is damage, pupil size remains unchanged. Other drugs such as apraclonidine or hydroxyamphetamine help confirm the diagnosis. Following diagnosis, imaging scans (magnetic resonance imaging, computed tomography, ultrasound) are done to locate tumors that may be the source of the damage.

Treatment and therapy: Treatment varies depending on the underlying cause of the symptoms.

Prognosis, prevention, and outcomes: Prognosis and outcome depend on the cause of the syndrome.

Martiscia Davidson, A.M.

For Further Information

Icon Health. *Horner's Syndrome: A Medical Dictionary, Bibliography, and Annotated Research Guide to Internet References*. San Diego, Calif.: Author, 2004.

Lee, J. H., et al. "Neuroimaging Strategies for Three Types of Horner Syndrome with Emphasis on Anatomic Location." *American Journal of Roentgenology* 188, no. 1 (January, 2007): W74-W81.

Rabady, D. Z. "Pediatric Horner Syndrome: Etiologies and Roles of Imaging and Urine Studies to Detect Neuroblastoma and Other Responsible Mass Lesions." *American Journal of Ophthalmology* 144, no. 3 (September, 2007): 481-482.

Other Resources

MedlinePlus
Horner Syndrome
http://www.nlm.nih.gov/medlineplus/ency/article/000708.htm

National Organization for Rare Diseases
http://www.rarediseases.org

See also: Eye cancers; Lung cancers

▶ Hydatidiform mole

Category: Diseases, Symptoms, and Conditions
Also known as: Molar pregnancy, gestational trophoblastic disease

Related conditions: Choriocarcinoma

Definition: A hydatidiform mole is a growth that forms in the uterus during early pregnancy. About 20 to 25 percent of hydatidiform moles form a choriocarcinoma, a rare type of uterine cancer.

Risk factors: Pregnancy in the early teen years or after age thirty-five increases the risk for a hydatidiform mole. A previous hydatidiform mole very slightly increases the chance of a future one.

Etiology and the disease process: A hydatidiform mole arises from an abnormally fertilized egg. The early placental tissue grows into a mass containing cysts that look like a cluster of grapes. There is usually no embryo present; however, in about 1 percent of cases, a normal fetus and hydatidiform mole develop together.

There are two types of hydatidiform moles: A complete mole does not contain tissue from the embryo, and a partial mole often contains embryonic tissue.

If the abnormal tissue continues to grow after treatment, it is considered persistent gestational trophoblastic disease (GTD). Choriocarcinoma, a cancerous form of gestational trophoblastic disease, may develop in rare cases.

Incidence: In the United States, a hydatidiform mole occurs in about 1 of every 1,000 to 1,500 pregnancies. The rate is higher in Asian countries.

Symptoms: The most common symptom is vaginal bleeding around the tenth week of pregnancy. Other symptoms may include nausea, vomiting, and signs of an overactive thyroid, such as a rapid heartbeat, sweating, and tremor. The woman may have a larger-than-normal uterus and signs of preeclampsia, including high blood pressure, protein in the urine, and swelling of the lower legs and feet.

Screening and diagnosis: Ultrasound allows most moles to be diagnosed in the first trimester, before symptoms develop. A blood test that shows higher-than-normal levels of human chorionic gonadotropin (HCG) may indicate a complete mole.

Treatment and therapy: A hydatidiform mole is a medical emergency. Treatment involves a dilation and curettage (D&C), a surgical procedure that gently scrapes the lining of the uterus to remove all molar tissue, including a developing embryo, if present. Levels of HCG are checked for up to a year after surgery to make sure no molar tissue remains. If a woman has an HCG level of zero after surgery, no further treatment is needed.

Prognosis, prevention, and outcomes: There is no known prevention. Women who have had a hydatidiform mole should avoid pregnancy for six to twelve months, as pregnancy can interfere with HCG monitoring. Untreated, a hydatidiform mole can cause significant bleeding and, in some cases, may progress to cancer.

Kelli Miller Stacy, ELS

See also: Choriocarcinomas; Dilation and Curettage (D&C); Gestational Trophoblastic Tumors (GTTs); Gynecologic oncology; Human Chorionic Gonadotropin (HCG); Moles; Pregnancy and cancer; Salpingectomy and salpingo-oophorectomy

▶ Hypercalcemia

Category: Diseases, Symptoms, and Conditions
Also known as: High levels of calcium in the blood

Related conditions: Primary hyperparathyroidism, hyperthyroidism

Definition: Hypercalcemia is a condition in which the calcium level in the blood is above normal limits (greater than 10.4 milligrams/deciliter, or mg/dl). Serum-ionized calcium and intracellular calcium concentrations play a major role in many biologic activities, including bone formation, hormone secretion, neurotransmitter release, muscle contraction, and enzyme activities. Two hormones serve as primary regulators of calcium: parathyroid hormone (PTH) and calcitonin. Parathyroid hormone stimulates the bones to release calcium into the blood, while the thyroid gland produces calcitonin, a hormone that slows the release of calcium. A condition of hypercalcemia reflects a significant disturbance in this delicate balance.

Risk factors: Two fundamental types of genetic defects have been identified in parathyroid gland tumors: the overactivity of oncogenes and the loss of function of tumor-suppressor genes.

Etiology and the disease process: Causes of hypercalcemia can include the following:

- Primary hyperparathyroidism (excessive secretion of PTH)
- Malignancy (with and without bony metastasis)
- Cancers that produce blood dyscrasias: lymphoma, multiple myeloma, leukemia
- Multiple endocrine neoplasias (MEN): hormone-producing tumors
- Granulomatous diseases: sarcoidosis, tuberculosis
- Hyperthyroidism
- Vitamin D and vitamin A intoxication
- Medications: lithium therapy, corticosteroids, thiazide diuretics
- Milk-alkali syndrome
- Severe, generalized immobilization
- Other conditions: Addison disease, peptic ulcer disease, hypophosphatasia, familial hypercalcemia

Primary hyperparathyroidism and malignancy account for nearly 90 percent of all cases of hypercalcemia.

Incidence: The annual incidence of hypercalcemia is estimated to be 0.2 percent in patients over the age of sixty, with an estimated prevalence of greater than 1 percent of the general population. It is estimated to affect 10 to 20 percent of people with cancer. The condition may manifest in subtle ways and have a benign course for many years or for a lifetime. It is more common in women than men by a ratio of 3:1.

Symptoms: In mild hypercalcemia, many patients do not exhibit symptoms. Patients with moderate hypercalcemia can complain of a constellation of symptoms involving the skeletal system (bones and muscles), the gastrointestinal tract, the kidneys, and the central nervous system. Severe symptoms (these associated with calcium levels of 13 to 15 mg/dl) include the following:

- Nausea and vomiting
- Anorexia
- Polydipsia (excessive thirst)
- Polyuria (frequent urination)
- Recurrent nephrolithiasis (formation of kidney stones)
- Profound muscle weakness (fatigue)
- Severe abdominal pain (constipation, peptic ulcer disease, pancreatitis)
- Muscle and joint ache
- Depression
- Delirium (mental confusion) and psychosis
- Coma
- Cardiac arrhythmias (irregular heartbeat leading to cardiac arrest)

Screening and diagnosis: The current consensus is that simple medical surveillance is appropriate for patients over fifty years of age when bone and renal statuses are satisfactory. Differential diagnosis of hypercalcemia is best achieved by using clinical criteria (assessment of symptoms, dietary history, the use of vitamin supplements, drugs, and physical examination), but the immunoassay for parathyroid hormone (PTH) is especially useful, reliable, and accurate in distinguishing major causes.

Diagnostic tests to confirm a diagnosis of hypercalcemia include PTH immunoassays (checking circulating levels of parathyroid hormone); serum calcium and creatinine tests, along with a twenty-four-hour urinary calcium test; and creatinine clearance tests. Selective imaging may employ the evaluation of bone density (X ray, computed tomography, or dual energy X-ray absorptiometry, or DEXA scans). Identification of soft-tissue masses is usually demonstrated by magnetic resonance imaging (MRI).

Treatment and therapy: In cases of severe hypercalcemia, individuals may need to be hospitalized to reduce calcium to a safe level. Treatment protocols include the following:

- Intravenous fluids
- Loop diuretic medications (furosemide-lasix) to flush excess calcium from the body and keep the kidneys functioning
- Intravenous bisphosphonates (drugs that inhibit bone breakdown)
- Calcitonin, a hormone produced by the thyroid gland to reduce bone resorption and slow bone loss
- Glucocorticoids to help counter the effects of vitamin D toxicity
- Cinacalet, a drug used to lower blood calcium levels by reducing production of PTH
- Mobilization to prevent bone resorption
- Hemodialysis (filtering of the blood to remove excess calcium)
- Surgery

The critical management question is whether the disease should be treated surgically. A 30 percent reduction in creatinine clearance, a twenty-four-hour urinary calcium of greater than 400 mg, and an elevated serum calcium level are persuasive factors. Traditionally, surgery (for hyperparathyroidism) has involved an extensive cervical incision and general anesthesia. A newer technique (radioguided parathyroidectomy) is now available. In this procedure, a radioisotope scan is performed preoperatively to locate the abnormal parathyroid gland. The operation is performed in less than an hour through a 1-inch incision. All surgery poses some risks. A small percentage of people undergoing this intervention can experience damage to the nerves controlling the vocal cords, and some develop a chronically low calcium level requiring lifelong supplements of calcium and vitamin D.

Prognosis, prevention, and outcomes: Calcium metabolism is carefully and strictly regulated within a narrow range (8.5 to 10.2 mg/dl). Too much calcium, for whatever reason, can interfere with essential life processes. Conservative care is indicated for mild to moderate electrolyte disturbances, but surgery is a viable treatment option and should be considered in conditions related to hyperparathyroidism and malignancy.

John L. Zeller, M.D., Ph.D.

For Further Information

Bilezikian, J. "Management of Acute Hypercalcemia." *New England Journal of Medicine* 326 (1992): 1196-1203.

Fauci, A., et al., eds. *Harrison's Principles of Internal Medicine*. New York: McGraw-Hill Health, 1998.

Kovacs, C., S. MacDonald, C. Chik, and E. Bruera. "Hypercalcemia of Malignancy: A Treatment Strategy." *Journal of Pain and Symptom Management* 10 (1995): 224-232.

Kumar, V., A. Abbas, N. Fausto, and R. Mitchell, eds. *Robbins Basic Pathology*. Philadelphia: Elsevier/Saunders, 2007.

Rankin, W., V. Grill, and T. Martin. "Parathyroid Hormone-Related Protein and Hypercalcemia." *Cancer* 80, no. 8 (1997): 1564-1571.

Other Resources

American College of Physicians
http://www.acponline.org

American College of Surgeons
http://www.facs.org

National Cancer Institute
Hypercalcemia
http://www.cancer.gov/cancertopics/pdq/supportivecare/hypercalcemia/patient

See also: Androgen drugs; Bisphosphonates; Calcium; Mediastinal tumors; Parathyroid cancer; Side effects; Zollinger-Ellison syndrome

▶ Hypercoagulation disorders

Category: Diseases, Symptoms, and Conditions
Also known as: Hypercoagulable states, blood-clotting disorders, thrombophilia or thrombotic disorders

Related conditions: Blood clots, deep vein thrombosis, pulmonary embolism

Definition: Hypercoagulation disorders are inherited or acquired conditions that increase the tendency to develop excessive or abnormal blood clots in the arteries or veins. These disorders increase the risk of blood clots even in the absence of injury.

A thrombus is a blood clot that forms and remains in a certain location, such as a blood vessel or the heart. An embolus is a blood clot that travels through the bloodstream to another location. People with hypercoagulation disorders have an increased risk of a deep vein thrombosis (blood clot in the deep leg vein) or a pulmonary embolism (blockage in a lung artery caused by a traveling blood clot), two conditions collectively termed "venous thromboembolism."

The majority of hypercoagulation disorders are acquired, with cancer as the primary cause. A malignancy is the underlying cause in about 10 percent of patients with venous thromboembolism.

Factor V Leiden is the most common inherited hypercoagulation disorder. Other inherited disorders include prothrombin gene mutation, elevated or abnormal fibrinogen levels, antithrombin deficiency, and protein C and S deficiencies.

Risk factors: Risk factors for acquired disorders include cancer, recent trauma or surgery, pregnancy, hormone replacement therapy, oral contraceptive use, heparin-induced thrombocytopenia, antiphospholipid antibody syndrome, deep vein thrombosis, pulmonary embolism, myeloproliferative disorders (including polycythemia vera or essential thrombocytosis), elevated homocysteine levels (hyperhomocysteinemia), diabetes, prolonged bed rest with immobility or inactivity, advanced age, and smoking.

Risk factors for hereditary disorders include a family history of blood-clotting disorders or venous thromboembolism. Hereditary defects in one or more of the clotting factors may also increase a person's risk.

Etiology and the disease process: Hemostasis is the body's natural mechanism to stop bleeding upon injury. Blood clot formation is part of this process and involves a variety of blood cells, platelets, blood proteins, and coagulation (clotting) factors. If there is an inherited or acquired imbalance or malfunction in any of these substances, the process of clot formation becomes abnormal.

Certain chemotherapy drugs, such as asparaginase, can increase the risk of clotting. Estrogen in hormone replacement therapy or oral contraceptives can also increase the risk of excessive clot formation.

Incidence: The precise number of people affected by hypercoagulation disorders is unknown. According to the Centers for Disease Control and Prevention, about five to eight percent of the U.S. population have one of several genetic risk factors for inherited hypercoagulation disorders. Additionally, an estimated 60,000 to 100,000 Americans die each year from a venous thromboembolism.

Symptoms: There are no specific signs or symptoms of hypercoagulation disorders.

Screening and diagnosis: Laboratory tests to measure blood-clotting time include the prothrombin time test (used to calculate the International Normalized Ratio (PT-INR)), activated partial thromboplastin (APTT)

fibrinogen level, and thrombin time. Genetic blood tests may be performed to identify certain gene mutations when an inherited hypercoagulation disorder is suspected.

Complete medical history and physical evaluations are used for diagnosis including a complete blood count; liver function test; urinalysis; chemistry panel including electrolytes, calcium, and creatine; and chest X ray. When an abnormality is indicated, further tests should be performed to determine the underlying cause of the disorder. Further screening is also recommended for patients with recurrent venous thromboembolism to detect a malignancy.

Treatment and therapy: Treatment for hypercoagulation disorders varies depending on the type of disorder. Generally, treatment includes anticoagulant medications to decrease the blood's clotting ability and reduce the risk of clot formation.

Anticoagulants, given in pill or injection form, include warfarin (Coumadin), anisindione, heparin, low molecular-weight heparin, aspirin, clopidogrel (Plavix), prasugrel (Effient), tricagrelor (Brilinta), dipyridamole (Persantine), cilostazol (Pletal), aggrastat (Tirofiban), eptifibatide (Integrilin), abciximab (ReoPro), and fondaparinux sodium (Arixtra). Several other anticoagulants directly inhibit thrombin, including Lepirudin (Refludan), bivalirudin (Angiomax), argatroban (Novastan), and dabibatran (Pradaxa). There are also two new oral anticoagulants: rivaroxaban (Xarelto) and apixiban (Eliquis) inhibit Factor Xa. These two important proteins help induce clotting.

The use of anticoagulants in patients with a known malignancy increases the risk of complications, particularly when the malignancy is advanced. Therefore, the potential benefits of each anticoagulant therapy should be weighed against the risks. Some studies have suggested a reduced mortality risk with the use of heparin injections instead of oral anticoagulants. With the use of all anticoagulants, close monitoring is required to evaluate the patient's response to the medication and to adjust dosages as needed.

Thrombolytic (fibrinolytic) drugs include streptokinase (Kabikinase, Streptase) and tissue plasminogen activator (tPA) agents such as alteplase (Activase), reteplase (Retavase), or tenecteplase (TNKase). These drugs are injections that may be given to dissolve a blood clot in select patients. They are administered in a hospital setting and are effective only when given within six hours after the onset of a clot-induced stroke or heart attack.

Prognosis, prevention, and outcomes: The outcomes of patients with hypercoagulation disorders depend on the rates of venous thromboembolism recurrence associated with the different disorders. Patients with inherited hypercoagulation disorders do not have a reduced survival rate, according to published data.

Patients with cancer and venous thromboembolism have an increased risk of recurrent thromboembolic events and major bleeding. Thrombosis can potentially complicate the course of cancer treatment by increasing the rate of hospital readmission as well as morbidity and mortality.

Angela M. Costello, B.S.

For Further Information

Barras, M. A., Hughes, D., & Ullner, M. (2016). Direct oral anticoagulants: New drugs with practical problems. How can nurses help prevent patient harm? *Nursing and Health Sciences,* doi: 10.1111/nhs.12263.

Couturaud, F., Leroyer, C., Julian, J. A., Kahn, S. R., Ginsberg, J. S., Wells, P. S., ... Kearon, C. (2009). Factors that Predict Risk of Thrombosis in Relatives of Patients with Unprovoked Venous Thromboembolism. *Chest,* 136(6): 1537-1545.

Perez, A., & Merli, G. J. (2013). Novel Anticoagulant Use for Venous Thromboembolism: A 2013 Update. *Current Treatment Options in Cardiovascular Medicine,* 15(2): 164-172.

Other Resources

National Blood Clot Alliance
http://www.nattinfo.org

National Heart, Lung and Blood Institute, National Institutes of Health
http://www.nhlbi.nih.gov

Society for Vascular Surgery
VascularWeb.org. http://vascularweb.org

See also: Amputation; Crohn's disease; Disseminated Intravascular Coagulation (DIC); Fever; Hematemesis; Myeloproliferative disorders; Thrombocytopenia

▶ Hypopharyngeal cancer

Category: Diseases, Symptoms, and Conditions
Also known as: Throat cancer

Related conditions: Head and neck cancers

Definition: Hypopharyngeal cancer is a cancer of the throat (pharynx).

Risk factors: Tobacco use (smoking and chewing), heavy alcohol use, and eating a very poor diet increase the risk of developing hypopharyngeal cancer. In the United States, hypopharyngeal cancer is three times more common in men than in women.

Etiology and the disease process: Hypopharyngeal cancer develops in squamous epithelial cells lining the throat. Primary tumors may occur in more than one area. This is an aggressive cancer that spreads quickly.

Incidence: This cancer is uncommon, with only about 2,500 new cases diagnosed in the United States each year. It is most often found in people from the ages of fifty to sixty and is rare in people under age thirty.

Symptoms: Symptoms are general, making early diagnosis difficult. The most common symptoms are a sore throat (usually on one side only) that does not respond to antibiotics, a lump on the neck (swollen lymph node), hoarseness, difficulty swallowing, and ear pain.

Screening and diagnosis: There is no routine screening for hypopharyngeal cancer. Diagnosis is made by a physical examination of the neck and throat, followed by imaging studies (X rays, magnetic resonance imaging, or computed tomography scans). An endoscopy (lighted tube passed down the throat) and biopsy (tissue sample) confirm the diagnosis.

The same procedures used in diagnosis are used for staging the cancer:

- Stage 0: Cancer is on only the lining of the throat (carcinoma in situ).
- Stage I: One tumor smaller than 2 centimeters (cm) in diameter is present.
- Stage II: The tumor is 2 to 4 cm in diameter and has not spread to the larynx (voice box) but may be in more than one area of the pharynx.
- Stage III: The tumors are less than 4 cm in diameter, but cancer has spread to at least one lymph node.
- Stage IV: The tumor has spread to surrounding tissues and lymph nodes or to other parts of the body.

Treatment and therapy: The tumor and surrounding tissue are surgically removed. This may cause permanent voice loss. Radiation treatments usually follow surgery. Chemotherapy may be used in very aggressive or inoperative cases.

Prognosis, prevention, and outcomes: Most hypopharyngeal cancer is diagnosed in Stage III or IV. The five-year survival rate for cancers found in Stages I and II is 50 to 60 percent, and for those found in Stages III and IV, it falls to 15 to 30 percent. Recurrence may occur, usually within the first two years following surgery. Eating a good diet, avoiding tobacco products, and restricting alcohol help prevent this cancer.

Martiscia Davidson, A.M.

See also: Barium swallow; Chewing tobacco; Cigarettes and cigars; Epidermoid cancers of mucous membranes; Esophageal cancer; Head and neck cancers; Oral and oropharyngeal cancers; Throat cancer; Tobacco-related cancers

▶ Infection and sepsis

Category: Diseases, Symptoms, and Conditions

Related conditions: Any type of infection is a risk for a cancer patient. Pneumonia is especially common in certain types of blood cancer.

Definition: An infection is the growth of a parasitic organism in the body, and sepsis is a widespread infection resulting from the presence of infectious organisms in the bloodstream. Sepsis overwhelms many parts of the body at once. Cancer patients are at risk for sepsis and various more limited infections as a result of their disease and the treatments they receive. Bacteria cause most infections in cancer patients, but serious fungal and viral infections are also common. Infection and sepsis are common causes of death in cancer patients.

Risk factors: All cancer patients are at risk for infection and sepsis. Their risk may be higher or lower depending on the type of cancer they have and their body's reaction to treatment. Patients at highest risk are those receiving bone marrow or stem cell transplants and patients with acute leukemias. Cancer patients with certain preexisting conditions are also at higher risk for infection.

Etiology and the disease process: Cancer can make the body more vulnerable to infection in several ways. The destruction of tissues resulting from invading tumors may allow infectious organisms access to places they do not normally enter. An example would be *Staphylococcus aureus*, a type of bacteria that normally lives on the skin. A break in the skin as the result of a malignancy (such as squamous cell carcinoma) may allow *S. aureus* to invade the inside of the body, causing a dangerous infection.

Common Sources of Infections in People with Cancer

Bacteria
- *Clostridium difficile*
- Enterococcus
- Escherichia coli
- Klebsiella pneumonia
- Pneumococcus
- Pseudomonas aeruginosa
- Salmonella
- Staphylococcus aureus
- Staphylococcus epidemidis

Fungi
- Aspergillus
- Candida
- Coccidioides
- Cryptococcus
- Histoplasma
- Phycomycetes

Protozoa
- Cryptosporidium
- Pneumocystis carinii
- Toxoplasma gondii

Viruses
- Cytomegalovirus (CMV)
- Herpes simplex virus (HSV)
- Varicella-zoster virus (VZV)

Source: American Cancer Society

Tumors may block ducts or other structures in the body. The blockage may trap infectious organisms that the body might have otherwise cleared out. An example is a tumor that blocks a bile duct. Trapped bacteria in the duct can multiply and reach the bloodstream, the liver, or the abdominal cavity, causing infection.

Immunity depends on the normal production and growth of white blood cells. The bone marrow produces these cells, and they mature and take on specialized immune functions in the bloodstream. Cancers that affect the blood or bone marrow—the leukemias, lymphomas, and multiple myeloma—severely cripple the immune system. Individuals with these types of cancer are at very high risk of death from infection or sepsis.

Cancer treatments also increase the risk of infection and sepsis. Chemotherapy drugs, especially at high doses, cause a condition known as neutropenia, an abnormally low level of neutrophils. Neutrophils are the most common white blood cells, constituents of the immune system. A low neutrophil count (level) means low immunity.

Catheters implanted in cancer patients—for the ease of medication delivery and blood draws—are a potential gateway through which infectious organisms can enter the body.

Chemotherapy drugs often cause ulceration of the mucous membranes in the mouth and the digestive tract. These ulcerations are a gateway for infectious organisms that may invade areas not normally accessible to them.

Treatment of certain cancers, such as lymphoma, sometimes requires the removal of the patient's spleen. The spleen is an extremely important part of the body's immune system. Patients who have had their spleens removed are vulnerable to severe infections for up to twenty-five years following the surgery.

Common sites of infection in cancer patients include the lungs, the skin, and the digestive tract, beginning with the mouth.

Incidence: Incidence depends on the type of cancer or other condition.

Symptoms: Symptoms of sepsis include fever, chills, skin rash, rapid breathing, rapid heart beat, decreased urination, and confusion, hallucination, or agitation. Many early symptoms of sepsis are similar to symptoms of more limited infections. Additional symptoms of nonseptic infection vary by the location of infection and may include any of the following: red streaks on the skin; diarrhea; abdominal pain; nausea or vomiting; ulcerations (open sores) on the skin or in the mouth; difficulty swallowing; sore throat; discharge from the wounds, nose, or any opening in the body (such as the vagina or penis); swelling and tenderness; headache; stiff neck; cough; and difficulty breathing.

Screening and diagnosis: At times, it may be very hard to determine whether symptoms are the result of an infection or a side effect of cancer treatment. Tests that look for the type and cause of infection vary by the location of the suspected infection. Such tests may include biopsy (obtaining a sample of infected tissue and testing it in the laboratory); X rays; blood counts, especially a neutrophil count; liver function tests; and cultures (attempts to grow an infectious organism) grown from samples from stool, sputum, blood, and any oozing from a sore.

Treatment and therapy: Because the vast majority of cancer patients develop bacterial infections, when symptoms of infection develop, doctors immediately start treatment with a broad-spectrum antibiotic. This type of antibiotic is effective against many different bacteria. There are many broad-spectrum antibiotics available. There is no standard initial antibiotic treatment that shows more benefits than others do. If needed, treatment can be modified when tests determine which bacteria cause the patient's infection.

If antibiotic treatment fails to make the patient better, antifungal medicine is added to the treatment. The most-often used antifungal medicines are amphotericin B and voriconazole.

In cases where the infection centers around the catheter, it may be necessary to remove the catheter to eliminate the infection.

Viral infections, especially with the human herpesvirus family, are also a major problem in cancer patients. The most common treatment is acyclovir, though newer antiviral medications are available. Patients with a history of herpes simplex infection may get acyclovir as a prophylaxis (preventative).

Viral respiratory infections, especially the flu and respiratory syncytial virus (RSV), also present major risks for people with cancer. Treatments for these infections include oseltamivir and zanamivir against influenza, and ribavirin for RSV and hepatitis viruses.

The American Society of Clinical Oncology now recommends the use of granulocyte colony-stimulating factor (G-CSF, filgrastim) for high-risk patients beginning chemotherapy. G-CSF accelerates the production of white blood cells. Studies that looked at a total of more than three thousand patients showed those receiving G-CSF before complications occurred were almost 50 percent less likely to develop neutropenia and infections.

Prognosis, prevention, and outcomes: The outcome of infections in cancer patients varies. It depends on the type of infection, the patient's overall condition, and the state of the patient's immune system.

Doctors sometimes give severely immune-compromised patients a prophylactic broad-spectrum antibiotic. Such patients may also get prophylactic antifungal medicine. This method is not recommended for all patients, because resistant bacteria or fungi can develop and cause worse infections. Doctors use prophylactic antibiotic and antifungal treatment in patients after bone marrow transplants or in those whom the doctors expect to stay immune compromised for lengthy periods.

Cancer patients should receive certain vaccinations:

- Annual influenza ("flu") vaccine
- Pneumonia vaccine (known as a pneumococcal vaccine or 23-valent pneumococcal vaccine)
- Bacterial meningitis vaccine (known as a meningococcal vaccine or 4-valent meningococcal vaccine)

Doctors may recommend other vaccines depending on the patient's particular disease, treatment, and overall health. People with cancer should never receive vaccination without consulting with their oncologist (cancer specialist).

It is important to remember that while a person is immune compromised, even a mild cold can become life-threatening. Children who receive vaccination with a live virus (for example, chicken pox or live polio vaccines) may pass the live virus to others. These viruses can cause a serious illness in the immune-compromised patient. People receiving treatments for cancer should avoid contact with those who have recently had a live-virus vaccine.

Patients can prevent some infections through the use of certain precautions. These precautions include the following:

- Frequent hand washing (on the part of patient, visitors, and other household members)
- Avoiding undercooked or raw foods
- Letting someone else clean up after pets, especially cat litter boxes and birdcages
- Practicing good oral hygiene
- Thoroughly cleaning any breaks in the skin
- Keeping surgical and catheter sites clean
- Avoiding people with contagious diseases
- Avoiding sexual practices that can result in skin breaks
- Avoiding contact with those who have recently had a live-virus vaccine

Adi Ferrara, B.S.

For Further Information

Kelvin, Joanne F., and Leslie Tyson. *One Hundred Questions and Answers About Cancer Symptoms and Cancer Treatment Side Effects*. Sudbury, Mass.: Jones and Bartlett, 2005.

Ko, A., E. H. Rosenbaum, and M. Dollinger. *Everyone's Guide to Cancer Therapy: How Cancer Is Diagnosed, Treated, and Managed Day to Day*. 5th ed. Kansas City, Mo.: Andrews McMeel, 2007.

Thiboldeaux, Kim, and Mitch Golant. *The Total Cancer Wellness Guide: Reclaiming Your Life After Diagnosis*. Dallas: BenBella Books, 2007.

Other Resources

American Cancer Society
http://www.cancer.org

Cancer.Net
http://www.cancer.net/portal/site/patient

See also: Antifungal therapies; Antiviral therapies; Blood cancers; Candidiasis; Chemotherapy; Culdoscopy; Disseminated Intravascular Coagulation (DIC); Fever; Infectious cancers; Infusion therapies; Mucositis; Overtreatment; Penile cancer; Pneumonectomy; Thrombocytopenia

▶ Infectious cancers

Category: Diseases, Symptoms, and Conditions
Also known as: Viral cancer, bacterial cancer, parasitic cancer

Related conditions: Oncogenic infections (bacterial, viral, parasitic), hepatitis, herpes, infection with human immunodeficiency virus (HIV), acquired immunodeficiency syndrome (AIDS), mononucleosis, schistosomiasis

Definition: Infectious cancers are malignant tumors that result from disruptions and diseases caused by invasion and multiplication of microorganisms and parasites in body tissues and cells and that therefore could be transmitted from person to person.

Risk factors: Some human infections of ribonucleic acid (RNA) and deoxyribonucleic (DNA) viruses, bacteria, and parasitic worms cause diseases, inflammation, and suppression of the immune system, leading to a higher risk of mutations and cancer. Long-term infection with *Helicobacter pylori* (*H. Pylori*) bacteria increases the risk of developing stomach cancer and lymphoma, which is also influenced by diet and smoking.

Two RNA viruses and the linked cancers are HIV, which induces sarcoma, and human T-cell lymphotropic virus (HTLV), which causes leukemia. HIV infection promotes viral cancers such as Kaposi sarcoma, cancers linked to human herpesvirus 8 (HHV-8) and human papillomavirus (HPV), invasive cervical cancer, lymphomas, invasive anal cancer, Hodgkin disease, lung cancer, cancer of the mouth and throat, cancer of the testicles, and skin cancers.

DNA viruses cause cancers of the nasopharynx and Burkitt lymphoma (Epstein-Barr virus, or EBV), liver (hepatitis B virus, or HBV), and cervix (HPV).

The risk of developing cancer is increased by certain tropical parasitic worm infections, such as infections with liver flukes and blood flukes (*Schistosoma haematobium*), which are linked to bile duct cancer.

Etiology and the disease process: Infectious cancer is induced by three main mechanisms: agents that increase cancer risk indirectly by interfering with the immune system (HIV); infectious agents that create tissue destruction and chronic inflammation (*H. pylori*), and agents that act as direct triggers for the proliferation of infected cells (viruses and a few bacteria). Many oncogenic viruses remain latent in cells until activation by toxic chemicals, hormones, radiation, or other viruses. People infected with human T-cell lymphotropic virus type 1 (HTLV-1) develop adult T-cell leukemia/lymphoma (ATL) after a latent period of twenty years or more.

Hepatitis C virus triggers long-term chronic infections, 5 percent of which result in liver cancer after several decades. HIV infection stimulates Kaposi sarcoma about two years after the virus is first detected. HIV infects and destroys white blood cells (helper T cells) and weakens the body's immune system, allowing viruses such as HPV to attack and trigger cancer development. *H. pylori* bacterial infections secrete toxins that cause chronic inflammation followed by abnormal cells that become cancerous, especially in the lower part of the stomach.

The Epstein-Barr virus causes infectious mononucleosis, cancers of the throat (nasopharyngeal carcinoma) and stomach, Hodgkin disease, and lymphomas (cancers in the lymphatic system including the spleen, tonsils, and thymus), particularly in people with organ transplants. The hepatitis B virus (HBV) and hepatitis C virus (HCV) can cause chronic infections that lead to most liver cancers. Some human papillomaviruses (HPV) initiate cervical cancer, promoted by hormones in oral contraceptives and *Chlamydia trachomatis* infection of the reproductive system. HPVs also cause some cancers of the penis, anus, vagina, and vulva, and are possibly linked with mouth, throat, head, and neck cancers.

Blood flukes create chronic inflammation in the blood vessels of the intestine or bladder, which occasionally causes bladder and bile duct cancers.

Incidence: Roughly 15 percent of all cancers worldwide are linked to viral (11 percent), bacterial (4 percent), or parasitic infections (0.1 percent). In the United States and other developed countries, fewer than 10 percent of cancers are linked to infectious agents, but they account for 20 percent of cancers in developing countries.

Cancers from Epstein-Barr virus infections are few but are more common in Africa and parts of Southeast Asia. HBV infections (causing liver cancer) are prevalent in China, Southeast Asia, northern Canada, Africa, Alaska, and Amazonia. In the United States, 30 percent of liver cancers are related to hepatitis B or C virus infections.

Infectious Agents That Are Risk Factors for Cancer

Viruses
- Epstein-Barr virus (EBV)
- Hepatitis B virus (HBV)
- Hepatitis C virus (HCV)
- Human herpesvirus 8 (HHV-8)
- Human immunodeficiency virus (HIV)
- Human papillomavirus (HPV)
- Human T-lymphotropic virus type 1 (HTLV-I)

Bacteria
- *Chlamydia trachomatis*
- *Helicobacter pylori (H. pylori)*

Parasites
- *Clonorchis sinensiare (liver fluke)*
- *Opisthorchi viverrini (liver fluke)*
- *Schistosoma haematobium*

Source: American Cancer Society

Kaposi sarcoma was the most common cancer among the 40 million worldwide HIV infections recorded in 2004. HPV causes 70 percent of cervical cancers and is the second most common cancer among women worldwide. HTLV-1 infections, mostly in southern Japan, the Caribbean, Central Africa, parts of South America, and among immigrants in the southeastern United States, create up to a 5 percent chance of developing adult T-cell leukemia/lymphoma.

More than half of the worldwide cases of stomach cancer (the fourth most common cancer) are linked to *H. pylori* infection.

About 10,000 parasitic infection cancer cases are reported annually. Parasitic bile duct cancer is localized in East Asia, while blood-fluke-induced bladder cancer is localized in Africa and Asia.

Symptoms: Patients with infectious cancers exhibit symptoms of the viral, bacterial, or parasitic worm diseases associated with the particular infectious cancer, plus other general cancer symptoms such as a swelling (indicating a tumor), incessant pain, fever, constipation, weakness, fatigue, loss of appetite, anemia, nausea, vomiting, bone fractures, weakness or numbness in legs, weight loss, repeated infections, and urination problems.

For example, symptoms of infectious mononucleosis (caused by the Epstein-Barr virus) are fever, sore throat, swollen lymph glands, and occasionally a swollen spleen or liver. Kaposi sarcoma (associated with HIV infection) appears as reddish-purple or blue-brown tumors just underneath the skin. Patients infected with the hepatitis B virus have symptoms such as a flulike illness and a yellowing of the eyes and skin (jaundice of the liver). The hepatitis C virus normally has no symptoms but causes chronic infections that lead to liver damage.

Screening and diagnosis: Screening of all donated blood in the United States has greatly reduced the chance of infection through transfusion, which has helped to control the spread of HIV, HTLV-1, and many other forms of infection. Epidemiological studies, combined with molecular analysis, enhance the diagnosis, screening, and analysis of stages in carcinogenesis and development of infectious cancers. Such studies have shown, for example, that infections of *H. pylori* are present before the appearance of stomach cancer.

Using modern technology, viral infections can be monitored by polymerase chain reaction methods. Biochemical markers are useful for carcinogen exposure determinations, such as urine biochemical studies confirming a synergism between aflatoxin fungal and hepatitis B viral infections.

Treatment and therapy: Antibiotics and other medicines effectively destroy carcinogenic infectious microorganisms such as *H. pylori*. Immunotherapy is a modern method of treating infectious cancers. Antigens expressed by virus-induced cancers generate host antibodies capable of killing the cancer cells. Vaccines against the types of HPV that cause cancer have been developed: One vaccine (Cervarix) protects against infection from two types of HPV; the other (Gardasil, which has U.S. Food and Drug Administration approval) protects against four types. The vaccine is recommended for girls and young women from ages nine through twenty-six.

Few drugs can treat hepatitis B or C, but a vaccine is available to prevent hepatitis B virus infection. In the United States, it is recommended for all children and for adults who are at risk, such as health care workers and intravenous drug users. Hepatitis C virus has no preventive vaccine at present. Anti-HIV drugs reduce the risk of Kaposi sarcoma and cervical cancer in those infected with HIV.

Prognosis, prevention, and outcomes: Epidemiological studies plus descriptive and clinical studies provide information on carcinogenic microorganisms and the effectiveness of cancer prevention and treatment. Antimicrobial drugs that kill or suppress growth of infectious cancer-causing agents can be administered as a preventive measure against infectious cancers or after surgery that removes suspected abnormal cells. Stomach cancers

from *H. pylori* infection, for example, have been effectively eliminated with antibiotics after removal of superficial cancerous areas.

Exposure to carcinogenic infectious agents can be avoided or reduced through lifestyle changes, including diet management and healthy sexual practices (avoiding multiple partners and regulating contraception). Condoms reduce the risk of viral infection but do not protect exposed areas. Pap tests detect precancerous cervical cells for treatment and prevention of HPV-induced cancer. Screening of donated blood greatly reduces the chance of infection through transfusion. The Kaposi sarcoma rate has dropped in the United States because of better treatment of HIV infections.

Investigations of carcinogenic infections continue, alongside the exploration of novel cancer treatments with minimum side effects, such as gene therapy, immunotherapy, and proton radiotherapy.

Samuel V. A. Kisseadoo, Ph.D.

For Further Information

American Cancer Society. "Cancers Linked to Infectious Disease." In *Cancer Facts and Figures*. Atlanta: Author, 2005.

Armstrong, G. L., et al. "The Prevalence of Hepatitis C Virus Infection in the United States, 1999 Through 2002." *Annals of Internal Medicine* 144 (2006): 705-714.

Bonnet, F., et al. "Malignancy-Related Causes of Death in Human Immunodeficiency Virus-Infected Patients in the Era of Highly Active Antiretroviral Therapy." *Cancer* 101 (July 15, 2004): 317-324.

Kleinsmith, L. J. *Principles of Cancer Biology*. New York: Pearson, Benjamin Cummings, 2006.

Lambert, P. F., and B. Sugden. "Viruses and Human Cancer." In *Clinical Oncology*, edited by M. D. Abeloff et al. 3d ed. Philadelphia: Elsevier Churchill Livingstone, 2004.

Other Resources

American Cancer Society
Infectious Agents and Cancer
http://www.cancer.org/docroot/PED/content/PED_1_3X_Infectious_Agents_and_Cancer.asp

Center for Immunotherapy of Cancer and Infectious Diseases
http://immunotherapy.uchc.edu/

National Cancer Institute
http://www.cancer.gov

See also: Aflatoxins; Bacteria as causes of cancer; Epidemiology of cancer; Epstein-Barr Virus; Hepatitis B virus (HBV); Hepatitis C virus (HCV); Herpes simplex virus; Herpes zoster virus; HIV/AIDS-related cancers; Infection and sepsis; Vaccines, preventive; Viral oncology; Virus-related cancers

▶ Infertility and cancer

Category: Diseases, Symptoms, and Conditions
Also known as: Subfertility, subfecundity

Related conditions: Sterility, premature menopause

Definition: Infertility is the inability to achieve pregnancy after one year of intercourse without contraception. Infertility, as it relates to cancer, refers to the loss of fertility due to cancer or its treatment and can be temporary or permanent. Infertility in men is caused by an absence of or a decrease in sperm production; a deficiency in the sperm quality affected by changes in sperm morphology, motility, or DNA integrity; or an inability to deliver sperm through ejaculation. Female infertility is caused when an egg cannot be successfully fertilized, a fertilized egg cannot implant in the uterus, or a pregnancy cannot be maintained.

Risk factors: The risk of infertility depends on the type of cancer and its location; the cancer treatment, including the type, dose, location, and method of administration; and the use of any fertility preservation or sparing procedures before or during treatment. The risk of infertility is also affected by the person's age, general health, and pretreatment fertility status. Testicular cancer and Hodgkin disease are associated with both pretreatment and posttreatment infertility in men.

Etiology and the disease process: Cancer-related infertility is usually caused by the effects of treatment rather than the actual disease. Chemotherapy can damage the stem cells that make sperm or immature eggs (oocytes) and mature eggs. The effects of chemotherapy are drug specific and dose dependent, with alkylating agents causing the most damage.

The effect of radiation on fertility depends on the dose and the location. Patients receiving very high doses delivered through total body irradiation or radiation focused to the abdomen, pelvis, or cranium are at highest risk for infertility. Radiation can kill sperm stem cells or oocytes, damage reproductive structures, or alter the pituitary gland.

Techniques for Preserving Fertility Before or During Cancer Treatment

For Women
- Embryo freezing
- Egg freezing
- Ovarian tissue freezing
- Ovarian transposition (moving ovaries to avoid radiation)
- Radical trachlectomy (removing the cervix but not the uterus and ovaries)
- Fertility-sparing procedure (removing only the affected ovary in cases of ovarian cancer)

For Men
- Sperm banking
- Sperm extraction
- Testicular tissue freezing
- Radiation shielding

Source: American Cancer Society

Surgery to remove reproductive structures may cause intractable infertility (sterility) or require the use of assisted reproductive technologies to assist in conception. Unintended side effects of surgery, such as nerve damage, scarring, or vascular changes, can also cause infertility.

Incidence: The occurrence of infertility is highly variable based on patient- and cancer-related factors. Data quantifying infertility in all cancer patients are scant.

Symptoms: Infertility is not often detected until a person attempts to conceive. After cancer treatment, men may be unable to ejaculate (anejaculation) or may experience retrograde ejaculation, in which little or no semen is produced. Women may have an absence or cessation of menstruation, have irregular menstrual cycles, or experience painful intercourse.

Screening and diagnosis: Screening for infertility occurs if there is difficulty conceiving or high- to medium-risk cancer treatments were used. Male infertility is diagnosed primarily through semen analysis to assess the number and quality of the sperm. Infertility in women can be diagnosed by assessing hormone levels, an ultrasound examination for ovulation, or visualization of reproductive structures through an ultrasound, a hysterosalpingogram, or laparoscopic surgery. The cause of infertility is sometimes indeterminable.

Treatment and therapy: The underlying cause of infertility often cannot be treated; however, many cancer survivors are candidates for assisted reproductive technologies to enable conception of a child biologically related to both parents. Men with low sperm count or low sperm motility may be able to father a child through intrauterine insemination (IUI), in vitro fertilization (IVF), or in vitro fertilization using intracytoplasmic sperm injection (IVF-ICSI). If there are no sperm in the ejaculate, surgical sperm extraction techniques may be used to retrieve sperm from the testicles or epididymis for use in IVF-ISCI. Anejaculation or retrograde ejaculation may be addressed through surgery, medications, or use of mechanical or electrical stimulators. Women are often given fertility medications to induce ovulation. The eggs can be fertilized through sexual intercourse, IUI, or IVF. Scarring or vascular changes affecting female reproductive structures may be treatable by surgery. A surrogate mother may be used in instances in which a woman's eggs can be fertilized but the pregnancy cannot be maintained.

Prognosis, prevention, and outcomes: It is advised that cancer patients discuss options to preserve or spare fertility with their oncologists before treatment and consult a fertility specialist. Before treatment, sperm can be frozen for use at a later time in IUI, IVF, or IVF-ISCI procedures; however, this may not be an option for men with testicular cancer or Hodgkin disease, whose sperm is already compromised. Researchers are investigating whether sperm production can be restored by freezing testicular tissue and later grafting the tissue onto the testicle or using it to isolate stem cells.

Women can have their eggs collected and fertilized with partner or donor sperm. The resulting embryos are frozen for future implantation. Unfertilized eggs or ovarian tissue may also be frozen for later use in IVF procedures or transplantation back into the body, respectively; however, these techniques are experimental.

Patients may benefit from options sparing fertility during treatment. These include protecting or shielding reproductive organs from radiation, conservative surgery when possible, and experimental hormonal therapy.

Amanda McQuade, Ph.D.

For Further Information

Lee, S. J., et al. "American Society of Clinical Oncology Recommendations on Fertility Preservation in Cancer Patients." *Journal of Clinical Oncology* 24, no. 18 (2006): 2917-2931.

Oktay, K. H., L. Beck, and J. D. Reinecke. *One Hundred Questions and Answers About Cancer and Fertility*. Sudbury, Mass.: Jones and Bartlett, 2008.

Potter, D. A., and J. S. Hanin. *What to Do When You Can't Get Pregnant: The Complete Guide to All the Technologies for Couples Facing Fertility Problems*. New York: Marlowe, 2005.

Other Resources

Cancer.Net
http://www.cancer.net/portal/site/patient

Fertile Hope
http://www.fertilehope.org

InterNational Council on Infertility Information Dissemination
http://www.inciid.org/

Lance Armstrong Foundation
http://www.livestrong.org

See also: Amenorrhea; Antiestrogens; Birth control pills and cancer; Breast cancer in pregnant women; Childbirth and cancer; Diethylstilbestrol (DES); Endocrine cancers; Endometrial cancer; Fallopian tube cancer; Fertility drugs and cancer; Fertility issues; Gynecologic cancers; Gynecologic oncology; Hormone replacement therapy (HRT); Hysterectomy; Ovarian cancers; Placental alkaline phosphatase (PALP); Pregnancy and cancer; Sterility; Uterine cancer; Vaginal cancer

▶ Inflammatory bowel disease

Category: Diseases, Symptoms, and Conditions
Also known as: IBD, Crohn disease, ulcerative colitis

Related conditions: Colon cancer, irritable bowel syndrome (IBS)

Definition: Inflammatory bowel disease is a chronic inflammation of the intestinal tissue. The two main conditions are Crohn disease and ulcerative colitis.

Risk factors: Inflammatory bowel disease may be at least partially inherited, as studies have shown that 20 to 25 percent of IBD patients have a close relative with the disease. Race and ethnicity may also be important determinants in the formation of inflammatory bowel disease, and American Jews of European descent are particularly prone to developing Crohn disease. For unknown reasons, higher socioeconomic status seems to predispose for IBD.

Etiology and the disease process: The development of inflammatory bowel disease is still undetermined, but it is thought to be the result of an abnormal immune response to an unknown antigen. In genetically susceptible individuals, this immune activation is prolonged, resulting in an inflammatory response that leads to intestinal tissue damage.

Incidence: Nearly 1 million Americans are estimated to be affected by inflammatory bowel disease, with an equal prevalence of ulcerative colitis and Crohn disease. Men and women are equally affected.

Symptoms: The symptoms of inflammatory bowel disease depend on the severity of the disease. Ulcerative colitis and Crohn disease patients may both complain of diarrhea, although bloody diarrhea is more characteristic of ulcerative colitis. Weight loss, nausea, vomiting, and fever are also common symptoms.

Screening and diagnosis: Because the symptoms associated with inflammatory bowel disease are common to many other gastrointestinal disorders, a colonoscopy is used both to confirm a diagnosis of inflammatory bowel disease and to differentiate between ulcerative colitis and Crohn disease.

Treatment and therapy: Treatment of inflammatory bowel disease depends entirely on the severity of the disease. The chronic nature of inflammatory bowel disease causes patients to experience extended periods of symptom-free living, interrupted by inflammatory "flares." These flares are treated with a variety of agents, including anti-inflammatory drugs, steroids, and immunosuppressants. Some biological therapies have proven effective in inflammatory bowel disease. Most of these biological therapies are antibodies that inhibit proinflammatory molecules within the intestine. The goal of therapy is to induce and maintain remission.

Prognosis, prevention, and outcomes: The quality of life of patients with inflammatory bowel disease depends on the severity of their disease. Severe gastrointestinal symptoms can cause patients to restrict their lifestyles. Patients with inflammatory bowel disease are at an increased risk for developing colon cancer, although more than 90 percent of inflammatory bowel disease patients never develop intestinal cancers. Inflammatory bowel disesase is rarely fatal, but death can occur if serious complications are not properly treated.

Lisa M. Cockrell, B.S.

See also: Azathioprine; Coloanal anastomosis; Colon polyps; Colonoscopy and virtual colonoscopy; Colorectal cancer; Crohn disease; Enterostomal therapy; Fecal occult blood test (FOBT); Ileostomy; Immunoelectrophoresis (IEP); Pancolitis; Premalignancies; Risks for cancer

▶ Invasive cancer

Category: Diseases, Symptoms, and Conditions

Related conditions: Cancer in situ, metastatic cancer

Definition: Invasive cancer describes the dispersion and invasion of cancer cells into surrounding normal cells and tissues. It is preceded by cancer in situ (CIS) and precedes metastasis.

Risk factors: Once cancer in situ has developed, the risk of invasive cancer increases with increasing tumor vascularity, loss of cell adhesion molecules, and expression of proteolytic enzymes.

Etiology and the disease process: Invasiveness is a stage of cancer development that is preceded by dysplasia and then by cancer in situ (CIS). Several related changes occur for the transition from CIS to invasive cancer. Normal cell adhesion molecules must be disrupted, and invasive tumor cells show alterations in the integrin and cell adhesion families of proteins. In addition, invasive tumor cells secrete proteolytic enzymes that digest the surrounding extracellular matrix. Invasive tumor cells also secrete motility factors that prompt migration into adjacent tissues. Invasion can be into adjacent organs, blood vessels, or lymphatic vessels. Even though the efficiency with which invasive cancer cells establish metastatic lesions is low, about 60 percent of patients with invasive cancer have overt or occult metastases at diagnosis.

Incidence: At diagnosis, the ratio of localized (preinvasive) cancer to invasive cancer varies from organ to organ. In prostate cancer, for example, 83 percent of new cases are confined to the prostate, but only 8 percent of pancreatic cancers are localized at diagnosis.

Symptoms: Symptoms of invasive cancer are usually nonspecific and related to infiltration of adjacent structures. They depend highly on the identity, vascularization, and innervation of the invaded structures.

Screening and staging: Determination of a tumor's invasiveness is done in the operating room and the laboratory. At surgery, invasiveness may be present as grossly apparent tumor growth into and around surrounding structures. Microscopic invasiveness is less apparent but contributes to the adherence of tumor cells to surrounding tissue. Diagnosis of invasiveness can also be made by screening blood for the presence of circulating tumor cells.

Treatment and therapy: Therapeutic options directed at inhibiting tumor invasiveness include biologic agents that block growth factor receptors and antibodies that target the integrin family of extracellular adhesion molecules. For example, blockade of the vitronectin receptor (an integrin) reduces the vascularization of tumor masses and may improve patient outcomes.

Prognosis, prevention, and outcomes: Tumor invasion complicates complete surgical removal of a tumor and is a precondition for metastases, significantly worsening prognosis. Prevention of invasive cancer requires early detection and removal of cancerous in situ lesions.

John B. Welsh, M.D., Ph.D.

See also: Breast cancer in men; Cancer biology; Carcinomatosis; Gestational Trophoblastic Tumors (GTTs); Invasive ductal carcinomas; Invasive lobular carcinomas; Malignant tumors; Metastasis

▶ Invasive ductal carcinomas

Category: Diseases, Symptoms, and Conditions
Also known as: Breast cancer, infiltrating ductal carcinomas

Related conditions: Inflammatory breast cancer

Definition: Invasive ductal carcinoma originates in the ducts of the milk-secreting glands and has invaded to other tissues of the breast.

Risk factors: Risk factors include never having a full-term pregnancy, first becoming pregnant after age thirty, starting menarche early, and entering menopause late. Risk increases with age, family history, carrying the breast cancer susceptibility genes *BRCA1* and *BRCA2*, and the use of synthetic hormones.

Etiology and the disease process: Invasive ductal carcinoma invades the surrounding breast tissue and lymph nodes and can spread throughout the body.

Incidence: About 12.7 percent of women will be diagnosed with breast cancer, making it the most common type of cancer in women other than skin cancer. Some 80 percent of breast cancers are invasive ductal carcinomas.

Symptoms: Any change in the size or shape of the breast or in the look or feel of the breast or nipple, or any lumps or thickening in or near the breast or underarm area, may be a symptom of breast cancer. Other more obvious changes include nipple discharge, tenderness, an inverted nipple, and ridges or pitting of the breast (when the skin looks like that of an orange).

Screening and diagnosis: Monthly breast self-exams after the age of twenty, yearly checkups, and regular mammograms after the age of forty are crucial to early detection. Biopsies of a suspicious lesion are taken to obtain a diagnosis.

Staging of breast cancer is based on the TNM (tumor/lymph node/metastasis) system:

- Stage I: Has not spread beyond the breast
- Stage II: May or may not have spread to lymph nodes under the arm
- Stage III: Has spread to nearby lymph nodes but not spread beyond the breast
- Stage IV: Has spread to other parts of the body

Treatment and therapy: Treatments, which vary from case to case, include surgery, radiation treatment, and chemotherapy. A lumpectomy or mastectomy followed by radiation is the standard treatment and is followed by whole-body treatments, including hormonal therapies, chemotherapies, and biological therapies.

Prognosis, prevention, and outcomes: Early detection and treatment increase overall survival rates. Invasive ductal carcinoma has a five-year disease-free survival rate of 83.5 percent. Physical activity, multiple pregnancies, breast-feeding, and early removal of both ovaries may lower the risk of getting this disease.

Terry J. Shackleford, Ph.D.

See also: Breast cancer in children and adolescents; Breast cancer in men; Breast cancers; Comedo carcinomas; Ductal Carcinoma In Situ (DCIS); Ductal lavage; Ductogram; Lobular Carcinoma In Situ (LCIS); Medullary carcinoma of the breast; Mucinous carcinomas; Progesterone receptor assay; Tubular carcinomas

▶ Invasive lobular carcinomas

Category: Diseases, Symptoms, and Conditions
Also known as: Stage I-IV breast cancer, infiltrating lobular carcinomas

Related conditions: Breast cancer

Definition: Invasive lobular carcinoma originates in the lobules (milk-producing glands) and has invaded other tissues of the breast.

Risk factors: Risk factors include reproductive factors such as never having had a full-term pregnancy, first becoming pregnant after age thirty, starting menstruation early, and entering menopause late. Using synthetic hormones, having a family history of breast cancer, carrying the breast cancer susceptibility genes *BRCA1* and *BRCA2*, and advancing age also increase a woman's risk.

Etiology and the disease process: In invasive lobular carcinoma, the cancer starts in the lobules, invades the surrounding breast tissue and lymph nodes, and can spread throughout the body.

Incidence: About 12.7 percent of women will be diagnosed with breast cancer, making it the most common type of cancer in women other than skin cancer. Only 10 to 15 percent of breast cancer cases are diagnosed as invasive lobular carcinoma.

Symptoms: Any change in the look, size, or shape of the breast, and any lumps or thickening in or near the breast or underarm area, may be a symptom of breast cancer. Symptoms also include any change in the feel of the breast or nipple, such as nipple discharge, tenderness, a nipple turned in toward the breast, and ridges or pitting of the breast (when the skin looks like the skin of an orange).

Screening and diagnosis: Women should undergo monthly self-exams after the age of twenty, yearly checkups, and regular mammograms after the age of forty. Once breast cancer is detected, biopsies of the tumor are taken to obtain a diagnosis.

Staging of breast cancer is based on the TNM (tumor/lymph node/metastasis) system:

- Stage I: Has not spread beyond the breast
- Stage II: May or may not have spread to lymph nodes under the arm
- Stage III: Has spread to nearby lymph nodes but has not spread beyond the breast
- Stage IV: Has spread to other parts of the body

Treatment and therapy: Treatments include surgery, radiation treatment, and chemotherapy, with the extent of treatment depending on the stage and hormone-receptor status. Surgery followed by radiation is the standard treatment and may involve a lumpectomy or mastectomy. Other treatments include hormonal therapies, chemotherapy, and biological therapies.

Prognosis, prevention, and outcomes: Invasive lobular carcinoma has a five-year disease-free survival rate of 85.7 percent. Factors that reduce the risk of breast cancer include physical activity, multiple pregnancies, breast-feeding, and early removal of both ovaries.

Terry J. Shackleford, Ph.D.

See also: Breast cancers; Lobular Carcinoma In Situ (LCIS); Tubular carcinomas

▶ Islet cell tumors

Category: Diseases, Symptoms, and Conditions
Also known as: Neuroendocrine tumors of the pancreas, Pancreatic NETs, islets of Langerhans tumors

Related conditions: Multiple endocrine neoplasms, von Hippel-Lindau disease, Zollinger-Ellison syndrome

Definition: Islet cell tumors are abnormal cell masses that develop in the islet cells (islets of Langerhans) of the pancreas. These tumors can be either malignant (cancerous) or benign.

Risk factors: About 15 to 25 percent of islet cell tumors are associated with the inherited disorder multiple endocrine neoplasia type 1 (MEN 1), but most arise spontaneously with no known risk factors.

Etiology and the disease process: The pancreas is a digestive organ located on the right side of the abdomen near where the stomach joins the small intestine. It is composed of two cell types. About 95 percent of pancreas cells (the exocrine pancreas) secrete digestive juices that flow into ducts that empty into the small intestine. The remaining cells (the endocrine pancreas) release the hormones insulin, glucagon, gastrin, vasoactive intestinal peptide (VIP), and somatostatin directly into the bloodstream. Insulin and glucagon regulate the use of glucose (sugar) in the body. Gastrin regulates the secretion of acid in the stomach. VIP stimulates the intestinal cells to release water and salts into the intestines. Somatostatin helps maintain a balance of glucose and salt in the bloodstream when the levels of other pancreatic hormones are excessively high.

When islet cell tumors develop, about 75 percent of the tumors produce excess amounts of hormones. These are called functioning tumors. The remaining 25 percent do not produce excess hormones and are called nonfunctioning tumors. Either type of tumor can be malignant or benign. Nonfunctioning tumors are more likely to be malignant than functioning tumors.

Islet cell tumors arise from different types of islet cells and are named for the main hormone that they secrete. Insulinomas produce insulin, which decreases the amount of glucose in the blood and increases the amount of glucose stored in the body. Insulinomas make up about three-quarters of all islet cell tumors. Glucagonomas produce glucagon, which releases stored glucose and increases the level of glucose in the blood, causing high blood sugar (hyperglycemia). Gastrinomas produce gastrin, which causes the stomach to secrete acid. Excess acid leads to stomach and intestinal ulcers. Vasoactive intestinal peptide tumors (VIPomas) produce vasoactive intestinal peptide, which relaxes smooth muscles in the digestive system and increases the amount of water in stool, causing severe diarrhea. Somatostatinomas produce extreme amounts of somatostatin, which reduces insulin secretion, diminishes glucose use, and drives overproduction of glucose by the liver.

Although islet cell tumors can occur in people of any age, most are diagnosed in young to middle-aged individuals. In most, especially those who do not have MEN 1, these tumors tend to develop slowly.

Incidence: Tumors of the islet cells are rare. They constitute less than 2 percent of all pancreatic cancers. Only about 2,500 cases are diagnosed in the United States each year, although autopsies of people dying from other causes find much higher rates of these tumors.

Symptoms: Nonfunctioning tumors produce few symptoms. Symptoms of functioning tumors depend on the type of hormone secreted. Insulinomas cause low blood sugar (hypoglycemia), hunger, weight gain, sweating, and nausea. Glucagonomas cause high blood sugar or mild diabetes accompanied by severe skin inflammation (dermatitis). Gastronomas cause stomach pain and ulcers. VIPomas cause severe watery diarrhea. Somatostatinomas cause weight loss and diarrhea.

Screening and diagnosis: Diagnosis of a suspected islet cell tumor is difficult. Various blood and urine tests are used to determine the level of specific hormones in the body. Once a tumor is suspected, an array of imaging studies, including magnetic resonance imaging (MRI), computed tomography (CT) scans, ultrasound, and arteriography, are used to locate the tumor. Certain biochemical tests are being developed to pinpoint the type of islet cells involved.

There is no specific staging for islet cell cancers. The staging in use as of 2014 is the same as for exocrine pancreatic cancer and is as follows:

- Stage I: The primary tumor is 2 centimeters (cm) or smaller at its widest part, and cancer has not spread to the lymph nodes or to other parts of the body.
- Stage IIA and IIB: The tumor is larger than 2 cm and has not spread to the lymph nodes or other parts of the body.
- Stage IIC: The tumor has spread to nearby bone, muscle, connective tissue, or cartilage but not to the lymph nodes or distant parts of the body.
- Stage III: The cancer has spread to the lymph nodes and may have spread to nearby bone, muscle, connective tissue, or cartilage.
- Stage IV: The tumor has spread to distant parts of the body, such as the liver, lung, bone, or brain.

Treatment and therapy: Treatment involves removing the tumor and sometimes the surrounding tissue. This is often followed by chemotherapy. When surgery is not an option, chemotherapy is often given, followed by hormone therapy to slow the growth of the cancer. Clinical trials are under way to develop better ways to treat islet cell cancer. A searchable list of current clinical trials can be found at http://www.clinicaltrials.gov.

Prognosis, prevention, and outcomes: The prognosis and outcome of islet cell cancer are highly variable because of the different tumors involved. Large, nonfunctioning tumors produce the worst outcome. In functioning tumors, tumor size is not related to outcome. Many tumors grow slowly and people survive for years. Islet cell cancer most often metastasizes to the liver and lymph nodes. If metastasis occurs, the outcome is poor. There is no known way to prevent this cancer.

Tish Davidson, A.M.

For Further Information

Pattou, François, & Proye, Charles. (2001). Endocrine tumors of the pancreas. In R. G. Holzheimer, & J. A. Mannick (Eds.), *Surgical treatment: Evidence-based and problem-oriented.* Munich: Zuckschwerdt. Retrieved from http://www.ncbi.nlm.nih.gov/books/NBK6889. An extended discussion of treatment strategies for endocrine tumors of the pancreas.

Pea, A., Hruban, R. H., & Wood, L. D. (2015). Genetics of pancreatic neuroendocrine Tumors: Implications for the Clinic." *Expert Review of Gastroenterology & Hepatology.* 9(11), 1-13. Advances in the genetics of pancreatic neuroendocrine tumors and the potential to use this information in diagnosis and treatment.

Reid, M. D., Balci, S., Saka, B., & Adsay, N. V. (2014). Neuroendocrine tumors of the pancreas: Current concepts and controversies. *Endocrine Pathology,* 25(1), 65-79. A review of staging and prognostic indicators for islet cell tumors.

Other Resources

American Cancer Society
What is Pancreatic Cancer?
http://www.cancer.org/cancer/pancreaticcancer/detailedguide/pancreatic-cancer-what-is-pancreatic-cancer

National Cancer Institute
Pancreatic Neuroendocrine Tumors (Islet Cell Tumors) Treatment
http://www.cancer.gov/types/pancreatic/patient/pnet-treatment-pdq

Pancreatica
Neuroendocrine, Islet Cell and Carcinoid Tumors
http://pancreatica.org/faq/carcinoid-neuroendocrine-islet-cell-tumors

Memorial Sloan Kettering Cancer Center. "Pancreatic Neuroendocrine Tumors." 2015.
https://www.mskcc.org/cancer-care/types/gastrointestinal-neuroendocrine/pancreatic-neuroendocrine-tumors

See also: Endocrine cancers; Endocrinology oncology; Gastrinomas; Histiocytosis X; Multiple endocrine neoplasia; Neuroendocrine tumors; Pancreatic cancers

▶ Juvenile polyposis syndrome

Category: Diseases, Symptoms, and Conditions
Also known as: JPS, multiple polyposis coli

Related conditions: Hereditary colon cancer syndromes, colorectal carcinoma

Definition: Juvenile polyposis syndrome is a hereditary disease in which patches of overproliferative inner intestinal tissue (polyps) occur, which can progress to colon cancer.

Risk factors: A family history is an important risk factor in juvenile polyposis syndrome, particularly the diffuse type. Risk factors for subsequent development of colon cancer include increasing age and duration of disease.

Etiology and the disease process: Juvenile polyposis syndrome is an autosomal dominant disease caused by mutations in two genes: *SMAD4/DPC4* on chromosome 18q21 and *BMPR1A* on chromosome 10q21-22. These mutations predispose proliferating intestinal glandular tissue to developing into cancerous cells.

Incidence: Juvenile polyposis syndrome is rare compared with other causes of colon cancer in spite of its inheritance pattern. The name "juvenile" is a misnomer; the incidental discovery of a polyp can occur as early as infancy. In addition, juvenile polyposis syndrome peaks during two age groups: late childhood (average age of nine years) and young adulthood (average age of twenty-five). The incidence of detected colon cancer peaks at around age sixty.

Symptoms: The first symptom in a child is usually bleeding from the rectum, owing to spontaneous amputation of a polyp. The bleeding often stops without further intervention. However, several instance of bleeding over time may predispose the patient to iron deficiency anemia in more extreme cases, seen as slowing growth, fatigue, and pallor. Persistent, intermittent abdominal pain can result from telescoping of the intestine into itself (intussusception), with a polyp as the lead point. In adults, similar symptoms may be observed.

Screening and diagnosis: The diagnosis of juvenile polyposis syndrome is suggested by a patient with three to five polyps or a family history in conjunction with the physical finding of a polyp. Isolated polyps that are removed or that avulse (tear away) and bleed spontaneously require no further intervention, and once they have been removed, they no longer put the patient at risk for colon cancer later in life. Screening colonoscopies are done earlier in individuals with afflicted first-degree relatives, starting at the age of twelve and performed every three years.

Treatment and therapy: Removal of polyps (polypectomy), whether through colonoscopy or surgical removal of the entire colon, is warranted. There are no effective chemotherapies in use at present.

Prognosis, prevention, and outcomes: Prognosis generally improves with removal of all polyps that are detected by regular colonic surveillance. Patients who have this done also have a significant decrease in the risk of developing colon cancer.

Aldo C. Dumlao, M.D.

See also: Adenomatous polyps; Colon polyps; Colorectal cancer; Colorectal cancer screening; *DPC4* gene testing; Family history and risk assessment; Hereditary mixed polyposis syndrome; Hereditary polyposis syndromes; Premalignancies; Turcot syndrome; Young adult cancers

▶ Kaposi sarcoma

Category: Diseases, Symptoms, and Conditions
Also known as: KS, classic Kaposi sarcoma, AIDS-related or epidemic Kaposi sarcoma, endemic Kaposi sarcoma, acquired Kaposi sarcoma

Related conditions: Human herpesvirus 8 (HHV-8), acquired immunodeficiency syndrome (AIDS), organ transplant

Definition: Kaposi sarcoma is a cancer of connective tissue named for dermatologist Moritz Kaposi, who first described endothelial raised lesions that develop in connective tissues and mucosal membranes. Four types of Kaposi sarcoma affect varying populations: Classic Kaposi sarcoma afflicts Eastern European Jewish or Mediterranean Italian men from the ages of fifty to seventy years; endemic Kaposi sarcoma develops in people of equatorial Africa; acquired Kaposi sarcoma develops in posttransplant patients; and AIDS-related or epidemic Kaposi sarcoma afflicts people with human immunodeficiency virus (HIV) and AIDS. Epidemic Kaposi sarcoma is the most clinically aggressive and most prevalent form of the disease.

Risk factors: Risk factors differ for each type of Kaposi sarcoma but include ethnicity, age, and disease state; HIV is a distinct risk factor for epidemic Kaposi sarcoma. Human herpesvirus 8 (HHV-8), a deoxyribonucleic (DNA) virus, is a risk factor for all types of Kaposi sarcoma.

Etiology and the disease process: Kaposi sarcoma develops from excessive spindle cell proliferation. HHV-8 is likely causative. Exact mechanisms are unclear; abnormal cytokine development that incites cell proliferation may contribute. HHV-8 DNA seroconversion typically precedes lesion development, and antibodies in blood and saliva indicate Kaposi sarcoma even before lesions appear. Neutralizing antibodies appear to prevent clinical Kaposi sarcoma.

Lesions initially develop as raised, colored blotches under the skin or mucous membranes. Swelling may impair nearby organ function, especially in the lungs, liver, and gastrointestinal (GI) tract.

Classic, endemic, and transplant-associated Kaposi sarcoma lesions usually occur on the skin and only occasionally spread into the lymph or gastrointestinal systems. However, aggressive endemic Kaposi sarcoma tumors do penetrate bone or manifest in lymph nodes and organs.

AIDS-related Kaposi sarcoma lesions are nodular, widespread, and rapidly multiplying. They develop in the skin, mouth, lymph, and organs, especially in the gastrointestinal tract, lung, liver, and spleen. Untreated, AIDS-related Kaposi sarcoma spreads extensively through organs.

Incidence: Classic Kaposi sarcoma is rare but has increased in women, although it still occurs in a 4:1 ratio of men to women. Endemic Kaposi sarcoma accounts for 9 percent of cancers in Ugandan men and occurs in prepubescent boys three times more often than in girls. People who have received organ transplants are 150 to 200 times more likely to develop Kaposi sarcoma than the general population.

Epidemic Kaposi sarcoma occurs as the AIDS-defining illness in 10 to 15 percent of homosexual, HIV-infected

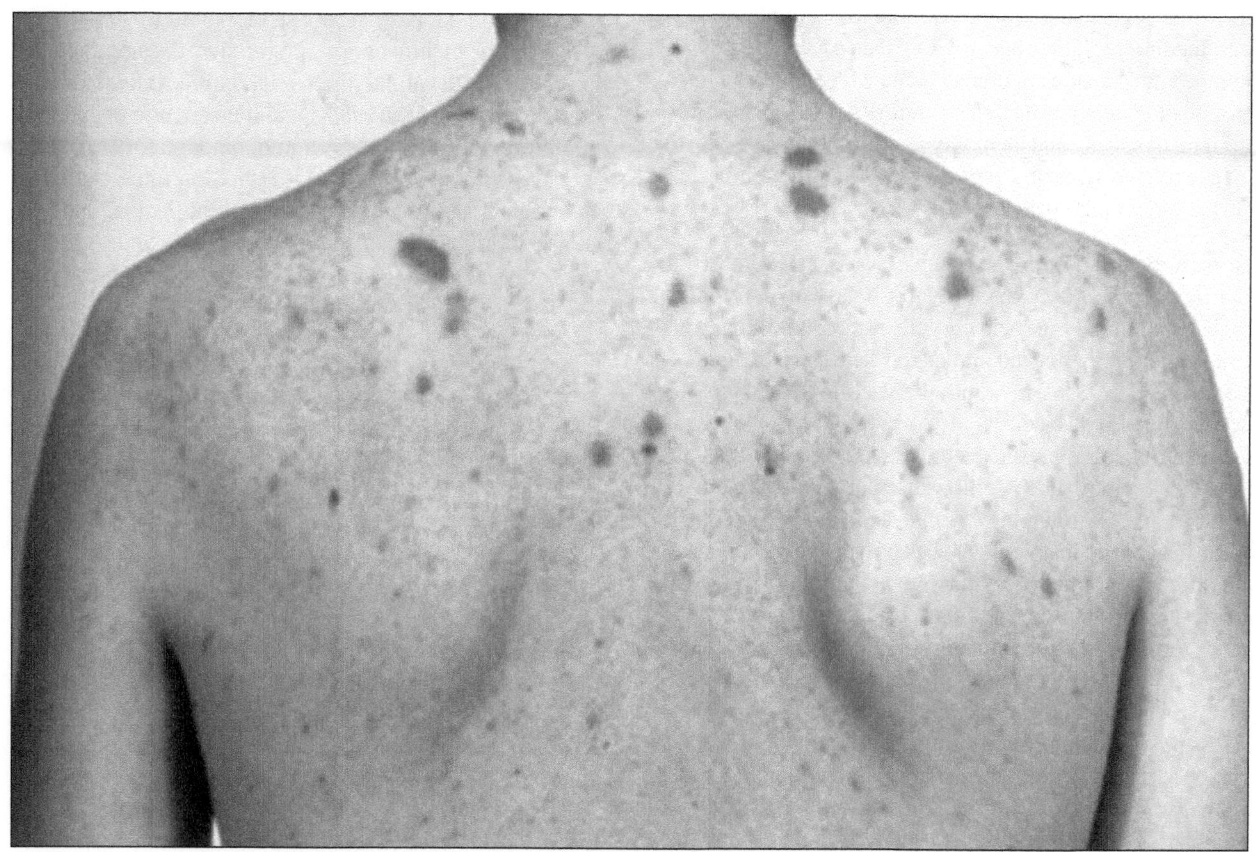

Kaposi sarcoma lesions on the back of a patient. (National Institutes of Health)

Stages of HIV-Related Kaposi Sarcoma

Stage	*Tumor*	*Immune System*	*Systemic Illness*	*Prognosis*
0, Early	Skin, lymph, minimal oral involvement	CD4 count greater than 200 cells/cubic millimeter	No opportunistic infections, thrush, or other infections; weight loss not greater than 10 percent	Good
1, Late	Pulmonary or gastrointestinal involvement, extensive oral involvement, edema, or ulceration	CD4 count is less than 200 cells/cubic millimeter	History of opportunistic infection, thrush, or other disease; weight loss greater than 10 percent	Poor

men and is the most common AIDS-related cancer in the United States. The overall incidence of HIV-related Kaposi sarcoma once was as high as 20 percent, but it has decreased steadily with the use of antiretroviral regimens.

Symptoms: Lesions are often disfiguring, palpable, and painful when swollen. Tumors bleed easily, causing ulceration, necrosis, and tissue discoloration. Symptoms are directly related to lesion location; for example, speech and feeding problems occur with palate tumors. Common symptoms of lesions in organs include bleeding from gastrointestinal lesions, nausea, vomiting, bowel obstruction, cough, dyspnea, and hemoptysis. Symptoms unique to AIDS-related Kaposi sarcoma are swollen lymph nodes, fever, and weight loss.

Screening and diagnosis: Much of Kaposi sarcoma evaluation focuses on epidemic Kaposi sarcoma. Although HHV-8 is directly associated with Kaposi sarcoma, routine screening is not recommended. Ultrasounds, endoscopies, and chest X rays may be used to screen for KS lesions but are unspecific.

Identifiable diagnostic features are purple nodules along skin tension lines, green-yellow discoloration secondary to hemorrhage, surrounding edema, and lesion dissemination. Diagnostic histology shows an intact epidermis, new blood vessel formation with extravasated red blood cells, hemosiderin deposits, infiltrates of spindle-shaped cells, and lymphocytic inflammatory infiltrate. Lesion biopsies are definitive but carry a bleeding risk. Detection of HHV-8 in tumor tissue can confirm an uncertain diagnosis.

Kaposi sarcoma lesions are hard to measure and cannot be staged by traditional cancer classification methods. However, the AIDS Clinical Trials Group has developed staging for HIV-related Kaposi sarcoma that accounts for lesion size and presence and for HIV stability.

Treatment and therapy: Kaposi sarcoma treatment involves local, systemic, and antiretroviral treatments or any combination of these. Surgical treatment is limited to diagnostic biopsies and often requires concomitant radiation to prevent spreading.

Local treatment with radiation, cryotherapy, or topical retinoids is best for palliation, for cosmetically unacceptable lesions, or for refractory disease. Radiation, the primary method, has a response rate of 80 to 90 percent.

Systemic treatment for progressive disease includes interferon (INF)-alpha, liposomal anthracyclines or paclitaxel, and investigational signal transduction or cytokine inhibitors. INF-alpha is an immunomodulatory agent associated with 45 to 70 percent remission rates. Palliative chemotherapeutics may eradicate some lesions and decrease morbidity. Ganciclovir, foscarnet, and cidofovir antivirals are active against HHV-8 and are being studied to reduce lesion size or progression.

First-line treatment of HIV-related Kaposi sarcoma is highly active antiretroviral therapy (HAART), which decreases HIV replication and thereby decreases the frequency of Kaposi sarcoma lesion development. In addition, protease inhibitors such as saquinavir, indinavir, and ritonavir have direct antitumor and antiproliferative effects that can improve Kaposi sarcoma even without an observed increase in the CD4 count. Additional treatments are reserved for visceral disease progression despite HAART.

Prognosis, prevention, and outcomes: Kaposi sarcoma may resolve spontaneously or with treatment. However, prepubescent patients with aggressive endemic Kaposi sarcoma face mortality within three years, and approximately 30 percent of patients with classic Kaposi sarcoma risk development of secondary tumors. Although AIDS-related Kaposi sarcoma with respiratory failure was once associated with fatality within weeks,

HIV-suppressive therapy has made stabilization, complete remission, and prevention of new lesions possible.

Nicole M. Van Hoey, Pharm.D.

For Further Information

Boshoff, C., and R. A. Weiss, eds. "Kaposi Sarcoma Herpesvirus: New Perspectives." *Current Topics in Microbiology and Immunology* 312 (2007).

Clayton, G., A. Omasta-Martin, and M. Bower. "The Effects of HAART on AIDS-Related Kaposi's Sarcoma and Non-Hodgkin's Lymphoma." *Journal of HIV Therapy* 11, no. 3 (September, 2006): 51-53.

Di Lorenzo, G., et al. "Management of AIDS-Related Kaposi's Sarcoma." *Lancet Oncology* 8, no. 2 (February, 2007): 167-176.

Konstantinopoulos, P. A., R. J. Sullivan, M. V. Karamouzis, and B. J. Dezube. "Investigational Agents for Treatment of AIDS-Related Kaposi's Sarcoma." *Expert Opinion on Investigational Drugs* 16, no. 4 (April, 2007): 495-504.

Other Resources

American Cancer Society
Detailed Guide: Kaposi Sarcoma
http://www.cancer.org/docroot/CRI/content/CRI_2_4_1X_What_is_Kaposis_Sarcoma_21.asp

The Body
Kaposi's Sarcoma
http://www.thebody.com/index/treat/kaposis.html

See also: African Americans and cancer; Africans and cancer; Biological therapy; Carcinoma of Unknown Primary origin (CUP); Cytokines; Dermatology oncology; Developing nations and cancer; Electroporation therapy; Fibrosarcomas, soft-tissue; HIV/AIDS-related cancers; Infectious cancers; Itching; Lymphangiosarcomas; Oncogenic viruses; Organ transplantation and cancer; Sarcomas, soft-tissue; Viral oncology; Virus-related cancers; Young adult cancers

▶ Keratosis

Category: Diseases, Symptoms, and Conditions
Also known as: Actinic (solar) keratosis, seborrheic keratosis, keratosis pilaris (chicken skin)

Related conditions: Actinic keratosis, seborrheic keratosis, keratosis pilaris

Definition: Keratosis is a benign growth of keratin on the skin. There are three main kinds of keratosis: actinic keratosis, seborrheic keratosis, and keratosis pilaris.

Risk factors: Risk factors are sun exposure, fair skin, and genetic factors.

Etiology and the disease process: Actinic keratosis is a premalignant condition of the skin, presenting as thick, scaly, or crusty patches. Frequent sun exposure and fair skin may increase the risk of developing actinic keratosis. A seborrheic keratosis is a benign skin growth on the top layers of the epidermis. It has been associated with a mutation in the growth factor receptor (*FGFR3*) gene. Keratosis pilaris is a follicular condition that runs in families. It is often worse in winter than in the summer, but it often improves with age. There are several different types of keratosis pilaris, including keratosis pilaris rubra (inflamed and red bumps), alba (bumpy skin without irritation), and rubra faceii (reddish rash on the cheeks).

Incidence: Seborrheic keratosis is most common among people over forty years of age. Keratosis pilaris affects an estimated 50 to 80 percent of adolescents and 40 to 50 percent of the adult population. It is more common in women than in men.

Symptoms: In actinic keratosis, the affected area of the skin may be the same color, darker, or lighter than the skin. It is often accompanied by solar damage on consistently sun-exposed areas. Seborrheic keratosis growths resemble warts and may exhibit a variety of colors, from yellow through black. Keratosis pilaris is excess keratin in the skin that accumulates within the hair follicles. Keratosis pilaris appears as rough bumps on the skin, most often on the backs and outer sides of the upper arms. It may also appear on the lower arms or on the thighs, or any body part except on glabrous (hairless) skin.

Screening and diagnosis: People with mild keratosis pilaris often are not aware of the condition. Diagnosis is generally made by visually examining the skin. Skin biopsies are sometimes done in seborrheic and actinic keratosis.

Treatment and therapy: Actinic keratosis is often treated with cryosurgery. Other therapies involve the application of 5-fluorouracil, a chemotherapy agent, photodynamic therapy, electrocautery (burning off the area with electricity), and topical immunotherapy.

Prognosis, prevention, and outcomes: Preventive measures for actinic keratosis are similar to those for skin cancer, such as limiting sun exposure and applying sunscreens. Because seborrheic keratosis tumors are a benign and not painful condition, treatment is often not necessary. There is no cure for keratosis pilaris, but there are treatments to alleviate symptoms.

Anita Nagypál, Ph.D.

See also: Aplastic anemia; Leukoplakia; Moles; Premalignancies; Skin cancers

▶ Kidney cancer

Category: Diseases, Symptoms, and Conditions
Also known as: Renal cancer, renal cell cancer, transitional cell cancer, clear cell renal cancer, papillary renal cancer, chromophil renal cancer, chromophobe renal cancer, renal oncocytoma, collecting duct renal cancer, medullary renal cancer, sarcomatoid renal cancer, Wilms' tumor

Related conditions: Kidney cysts

Definition: The two main types of kidney cancer are renal cell cancer, which arises from the filtering part of the kidney, the nephrons, and transitional cell cancer, which arises from the renal pelvis, where the urine passes from the nephrons to the ureter and then to the bladder. It more closely resembles bladder cancer than renal cell cancer.

Renal cell cancer falls into these subtypes: clear cell, papillary, chromophobe, renal oncocytoma, collecting duct, medullary, sarcomatoid, Wilms' tumor, and unclassified. Clear cell cancer is the most common type and represents 66 to 75 percent of all cases of kidney cancer. Its name derives from the clear cytoplasm within its cells. A majority of clear cell renal cancer cases have the von Hippel-Lindau (VHL) genetic mutation. The two types of papillary renal cancer (characterized by fingerlike projections) are differentiated by the type of cells found in the tumor. Type I tends to be more common in African Americans and to involve both kidneys. Type II is associated with hereditary leiomyomatosis and can be difficult to treat once it has metastasized (spread to other organs). It is the second most common renal cell cancer and represents about 10 to 15 percent of cases. Sometimes papillary renal cancer is called chromophil renal cancer. About 5 percent of renal cell cancers are chromophobe. The cells of this type of cancer are similar to those in renal oncocytoma, but they are resistant to some stains used to analyze cancer cells. Chromophobe renal cancer is often related to Birt-Hogg-Dubé syndrome, a dominant hereditary trait that is marked by renal tumors, lung cysts, fibrofolliculomas (benign tumors of hair follicles), and spontaneous pneumothorax (collapse of the lung). It is the third most common type of kidney cancer. Renal oncocytoma is a benign kidney tumor that is also related to Birt-Hogg-Dubé syndrome. This type of tumor does not metastasize, although it can grow quite large. Its cells are similar to those of chromophobe renal cancer.

Collecting duct renal cancer is rare but quite aggressive. Often it has metastasized before being discovered. Its name comes from the fact that the tumor cells often form a tube. Medullary renal cancer is also rare and quite aggressive. It is related to the sickle cell trait. Sarcomatoid renal cancer is thought to arise from the blood vessels of the kidney. It also is quite rare and quite aggressive. Its name comes from the fact that its cells appear like those of a sarcoma (cancer of the soft tissues). Wilms' tumor is found predominantly in infants and young children, under the age of five. It is relatively rare and tends to spread locally into the lymph nodes, renal vein, and vena cava. Wilms' tumor is an embryonal adenomyosarcoma. Unclassified renal cell cancer has cells that do not appear like those of other types of kidney cancer.

Risk factors: The most common risk factor for kidney cancer is smoking cigarettes. Kidney cancer also appears to be more common in persons who are obese or who have high blood pressure. There are three hereditary syndromes that put a person at a higher risk of developing kidney cancer. They are von Hippel-Lindau disease, hereditary leiomyomatosis, and Birt-Hogg-Dubé syndrome. These syndromes may be caused by spontaneous mutations. Some occupations put a person at higher risk for developing kidney cancer. These include occupations in which a person is exposed to certain toxic chemicals or substances, such as petroleum-based products, asbestos, lead, or cadmium. Also, persons who are on long-term dialysis therapy for kidney failure are at higher risk of developing kidney cancer.

Etiology and the disease process: Kidney cancer arises from a single cell that grows wildly. For renal cell cancer, this is a cell of the tubular epithelium of the nephron, the part of the kidney that filters the blood of waste products and produces urine for excreting these wastes. Transitional cell renal cancer manifests itself in the renal pelvis, where urine is delivered by the nephrons. The types of renal cancer vary in their aggressiveness and in how

Stage at Diagnosis and Five-Year Relative Survival Rates for Cancer of the Kidney and Renal Pelvis, 1996-2004

Stage	*Cases Diagnosed (%)*	*Survival Rate (%)*
Localized[a]	55	89.6
Regional[b]	19	60.8
Distant[c]	20	9.5
Unstaged	5	35.2

Source: Data from National Cancer Institute, Surveillance Epidemiology and End Results, Cancer Stat Fact Sheets, 2008

[a]Cancer still confined to primary site

[b]Cancer has spread to regional lymph nodes or directly beyond the primary site

[c]Cancer has metastasized

quickly they metastasize. Some will metastasize from a small tumor in the kidney, and other types do not metastasize until they have engulfed the kidney. Kidney cancer spreads through the lymph nodes and the bloodstream. Common sites for metastases are the other kidney, the lung, the adrenal gland, the bones, and the liver.

Incidence: Kidney cancer strikes about 51,000 people a year in the United States. It is twice as common in men as in women. However, kidney cancer is actually relatively rare compared with other cancers. It represents about 3 percent of all cases of cancer in the United States. About 12,000 people die of kidney cancer each year.

Symptoms: The symptoms of kidney cancer do not appear until the tumor is fairly large or has metastasized. The symptoms are blood in the urine (hematuria), abdominal mass, back or flank pain, weight loss, recurrent fever, and fatigue. Blood tests may demonstrate a high serum calcium and either anemia or high red blood cell counts. A urine analysis test may show microscopic hematuria that is not visible to the eye. Kidney cancer can also cause hypertension, although this symptom is not particularly helpful in diagnosing kidney cancer because it is so common.

Screening and diagnosis: There is no routine screening performed for kidney cancer. However, kidney cancer may be found incidentally on a chest, abdominal, or pelvic ultrasound; computed tomography (CT) scan; or magnetic resonance imaging (MRI) performed for another reason.

Kidney cancer is usually diagnosed by a renal ultrasound, an abdominal CT scan, an MRI, or a positron emission tomography (PET) scan. Occasionally, an intravenous pyelogram (IVP) is performed, although this diagnostic test has largely been replaced by ultrasounds, CT scans, and MRIs. Once a kidney tumor is discovered, it needs to be biopsied to identify the type of cells in the tumor. Kidney cancers may be biopsied by fine needle through the skin below the rib cage on the back or by ureteroscopy (the passing of a ureteroscope through the urethra, the bladder, one of the ureters, and the renal pelvis, and then into the body of the kidney). Both procedures require fluoroscopy to localize the tumor.

Kidney cancer is usually staged with a combination of the American Joint Committee on Cancer (AJCC) TNM staging system and a numeric grouping. "T" refers to the size of the tumor, "N" refers to lymph node involvement, and "M" refers to whether there are metastases. The stages are as follows:

- Stage I, T1a-T1b, N0, M0: The tumor is less than 7 centimeters (cm) with no lymph node involvement and no metastases.
- Stage II, T2, N0, M0: The tumor is greater than 7 cm with no spread outside the kidney.
- Stage III, T1a-T3b, N1, M0 or T3a-3c, N0, M0: The tumor has spread to a single lymph node but not metastasized, or has spread to adjacent tissue or structures, such as the adrenal glands, to fatty tissue around the kidney, or into the vena cava.
- Stage IV, T4, N0-N1, M0; any T, N2, M0; or any T, any N, M1: The tumor extends beyond the kidney locally and has spread into the lymph system. It is present in more than one lymph node. There may also be metastases to other organs.

Treatment and therapy: For many years, the only treatment for kidney cancer was to remove the affected kidney. This was done unless the cancer was so far advanced that there was little hope for the patient. Kidney cancer did not respond well to either radiation therapy or chemotherapy. Consequently, these treatments were used only to treat metastatic kidney cancer, to relieve the symptoms, and to prolong the patient's life. However, in the mid-2000's, the treatment options for kidney cancer proliferated. Research to develop additional new drugs that are effective for treating kidney cancer is ongoing.

Kidney cancer surgery includes a total radical nephrectomy, laparoscopic radical nephrectomy, partial nephrectomy, radioablation (destroying the tumor with radiation therapy), cryoablation (freezing), and arterial embolization (blocking the artery feeding the tumor with material). The original total radical nephrectomy procedure, in which an 18-inch incision is made from below the mediastinum (breast bone) to the middle of the back, is no longer the sole surgical option. Several laparoscopic radical nephrectomy procedures are available. These laparoscopic procedures require a 3- to 4-inch incision and 3.5-inch incisions. Recovery time for the patient is four weeks rather than the twelve weeks of recovery required for the original procedure.

Kidney cancer still does not respond well to radiation therapy. Advances in the development of chemotherapy drugs have benefited the treatment of kidney cancer. However, it is still not routine to prevent the recurrence of a kidney cancer with chemotherapy, as is done with other cancers. The focus of chemotherapy treatment for kidney cancer is to prolong the life of the patient. As a result, chemotherapy is reserved for treating advanced renal cancers with metastases. Kidney cancer may be treated with angiogenesis inhibitors (drugs that inhibit the growth of blood vessels feeding the tumors), such as sorafenib tosylate (Nexavar) and sunitinib malate (Sutent). In May of 2007, the drug temsirolimus (Torisel) was approved by the Food and Drug Administration for treating kidney cancer. Temsirolimus is an enzyme inhibitor that interferes with cell growth, development, and survival.

Other drugs now being used to treat advanced kidney cancer are bevacizumab, interleukin-2, and interferon. Avastin is a monoclonal antibody that interferes with the growth and development of new blood vessels within a tumor. Interleukin-2 and interferon are referred to as biological therapy, because these substances are normally produced by the body in small amounts. Their role in kidney cancer treatment is to stimulate the body's normal immune defenses. Like other chemotherapy drugs, these drugs have many severe side effects.

Prognosis, prevention, and outcomes: With kidney cancer, the prognosis depends on the stage of the cancer at diagnosis. With Stages I and II, surgical intervention is likely to cure the kidney cancer. With Stages III and IV, the prognosis is guarded and depends on the patient's response to treatments, particularly drug therapy. In Stages III and IV, treatment may be aimed at extending the patient's life and providing a reasonable quality of life.

It is not possible to prevent kidney cancer. Certainly, not smoking cigarettes will decrease a person's likelihood of developing kidney cancer. Other lifestyle choices, such as occupation, might also decrease the likelihood of developing kidney cancer, but many of the substances thought to cause kidney cancer are fairly pervasive in the environment. Some kidney cancers develop in people with no apparent risk factors for the disease.

Christine M. Carroll, R.N., B.S.N., M.B.A.

For Further Information

Diaz, José I., Linda B. Mora, and Ardeshir Hakam. "The Mainz Classification of Renal Cell Tumors." *Cancer Control: Journal of the Moffitt Cancer Center* 6 (November/December, 1999): 571-579.

Nuñez, Kevin R., ed. *Trends in Kidney Cancer Research.* New York: Nova Biomedical Books, 2006.

Patel, Uday, ed. *Carcinoma of the Kidney.* New York: Cambridge University Press, 2008.

Rodriquez, Alejandro, and Wade J. Sexton. "Management of Locally Advanced Renal Cell Carcinoma." *Cancer Control: Journal of the Moffitt Cancer Center* 13 (July, 2006): 199-210.

Other Resources

American Cancer Society

Detailed Guide: Kidney Cancer
http://www.cancer.org/docroot/cri/content/cri_2_4_1x_what_is_kidney_cancer_22.asp

Kidney Cancer Association

http://www.kidneycancer.org

National Cancer Institute

http://www.cancer.gov/cancertopics/types/kidney

National Kidney Foundation

http://www.kidney.org

See also: Adenocarcinomas; Adrenal gland cancers; Angiogenesis inhibitors; Biological therapy; Birt-Hogg-Dubé Syndrome (BHDS); Bladder cancer; Denys-Drash syndrome and cancer; Diethanolamine (DEA); Endocrine cancers; Fanconi anemia; Hematuria; Hereditary Leiomyomatosis and Renal Cell Cancer (HLRCC); Hereditary non-VHL clear cell renal cell carcinomas; Hereditary papillary renal cell carcinomas; Malignant rhabdoid tumor of the kidney; Nephroblastomas; Nephrostomy; Organ transplantation and cancer; Renal pelvis tumors; Syndrome of Inappropriate Antidiuretic Hormone production (SIADH); Transitional cell carcinomas; Urinalysis; Urinary system cancers; Urography; Urologic oncology; Von Hippel-Lindau (VHL) disease; Wilms' tumor; Wilms' Tumor Aniridia-Genitourinary anomalies-mental Retardation (WAGR) syndrome and cancer

▶ Klinefelter syndrome and cancer

Category: Diseases, Symptoms, and Conditions
Also known as: Klinefelter's syndrome, XXY syndrome, 47,XXY syndrome

Related conditions: Breast, prostate, and lung cancer; non-Hodgkin lymphoma; extragonadal (often mediastinal) germ-cell tumors; testicular tumors (such as germinoma)

Definition: Klinefelter syndrome is a condition caused by an extra sex chromosome (usually 47,XXY) that results in a phenotypic man with several characteristic manifestations.

Risk factors: The risks of certain cancers are increased in Klinefelter syndrome. Klinefelter patients given testosterone hormone replacement therapy increase their risk of prostate cancer.

Etiology and the disease process: The XXY chromosome arrangement disrupts normal testicular development, leading to impaired sex hormone production. This is the etiology of many symptoms of Klinefelter syndrome. Klinefelter patients are sterile because of seminiferous tubule dysgenesis. Genes not related to sex on the X chromosome may cause other manifestations.

Incidence: Klinefelter syndrome occurs in 1 in 500 to 1 in 1,000 newborn male children. The overall incidence of all malignancies in patients with Klinefelter syndrome is not significantly different from the incidence among men with normal male chromosomes. However, certain types of cancer are more common among Klinefelter patients than 46,XY (so-called normal) men. These include male breast cancer, non-Hodgkin lymphoma, extragonadal (often mediastinal) teratomas, germ-cell tumors of the testes, and possibly lung cancer, gallbladder cancer, and extrahepatic bile duct tumors. Prostate cancer risk is very low unless hormone therapy with testosterone is initiated; then, the risk for adenocarcinoma of the prostate is increased.

Symptoms: Klinefelter patients typically have small, atrophic testes (microorchidism), infertility, a small penis, gynecomastia (enlarged breasts), tall stature, truncal obesity, autoimmune disorders, diabetes, and an increased risk of behavioral, emotional, and intellectual difficulties. Life expectancy is normal. Hypogonadism results from abnormally low male sex hormone production and abnormally high female hormone levels.

Precocious puberty may result from germ-cell tumor production of male sex hormones in children with Klinefelter.

Screening and diagnosis: Cytogenetic analysis is necessary to diagnose Klinefelter syndrome. Klinefelter is often discovered coincidentally during cytogenetic testing for cancer, infertility, or prenatal birth defects (amniocentesis). Doctors may notice clinical signs of Klinefelter syndrome and request cytogenetic testing.

Treatment and therapy: Hormone replacement therapy is given to some patients to reduce symptoms and improve masculinization; however, testosterone therapy will increase the risk of prostate cancer. It is not necessary to treat Klinefelter syndrome. Assisted reproductive technologies have been used to overcome sterility.

Prognosis, prevention, and outcomes: The long-term prognosis for Klinefelter syndrome is good because the condition is not life-threatening. Surveillance for cancers that are more common in men with Klinefelter syndrome should be instituted.

Christopher Pung, B.S., C.L.Sp. (CG)

See also: Breast cancer in men; Childhood cancers; Cryptorchidism; Germ-cell tumors; Prostate cancer; Teratocarcinomas; Testicular cancer; Testicular Self-Examination (TSE)

▶ Krukenberg tumors

Category: Diseases, Symptoms, and Conditions
Also known as: Metastatic stomach cancer

Related conditions: Stomach cancer

Definition: Krukenberg tumors are bilateral ovarian tumors resulting from the spread of primary stomach cancer. Other possible sources of primary malignancy include the breast, colon, and biliary tract. Friedrich Ernst Krukenberg of Germany first described this tumor in 1896.

Risk factors: Women between the ages of forty and fifty are most frequently affected. The tumor occurs more in Asian women because stomach cancer is a common malignancy of adult women in this geographic region. A history of stomach cancer in a middle-aged female patient should alert the physician to the possible risk of developing a Krukenberg tumor.

Etiology and the disease process: The mechanism of tumor spread to the ovaries has not yet been determined. Blood and lymph fluid flow may be responsible for stomach tumor cell metastasis to the ovaries.

Incidence: Krukenberg tumors make up 5 to 6 percent of all malignant ovarian tumors. Japan, China, and Korea have a particularly high incidence of Krukenberg tumors.

Symptoms: Most patients complain of pain and abdominal distension, ascribed to both ovarian enlargement and ascites (fluid accumulation in the abdominal cavity). Abnormal menstruation, pain during sexual intercourse, and vaginal bleeding are other notable symptoms. A small number of patients remain asymptomatic or complain of gastrointestinal symptoms related to the primary cancer.

Screening and diagnosis: A laparotomy (a surgical incision of the abdominal wall) is important in diagnosing a Krukenberg tumor. Chest X rays, abdominal computed tomography (CT) scans, and pelvic ultrasound are useful in determining the extent of tissue involvement. A biopsy of the ovary will confirm the diagnosis: Microscopically, Krukenberg tumors are characterized by cancer cells with a "signet-ring" appearance, that is, identical to tumor cells in stomach cancer tissue. The presence of a Krukenberg tumor signifies that the primary stomach cancer is in an advanced stage (Stage IV, distant metastasis).

Treatment and therapy: In cases in which the tumor is confined to the ovaries and the stomach, surgical removal of both the ovarian tumor and the primary cancer is recommended. Chemotherapy and radiotherapy may be required in cases in which cancer has spread beyond the ovaries and the stomach.

Prognosis, prevention, and outcomes: The prognosis is poor for patients diagnosed with a Krukenberg tumor. Prophylactic surgical removal of both ovaries during gastric cancer surgery may be the only way of preventing tumor growth. Because the tumor is a sign of advanced gastric cancer, the outcome is poor for patients with Krukenberg tumors.

Ophelia Panganiban, B.S.

See also: Asian Americans and cancer; Ovarian cancers; Ovarian cysts; Stomach cancers

▶ Lacrimal gland tumors

Category: Diseases, Symptoms, and Conditions
Also known as: Orbital tumors

Related conditions: Lymphomas

Definition: Lacrimal gland tumors are rare neoplasms of tear-secreting glands located above the outer corner of each eye. The most common benign and malignant lacrimal gland tumors are called pleomorphic adenomas and adenoid cystic carcinomas, respectively.

Risk factors: Benign tumors are commonly diagnosed in adults between the ages of forty and fifty years, while malignant neoplasms typically occur during the third decade and the teenage years. Individuals previously diagnosed with lymphoma are at risk for developing orbital lymphoma.

Etiology and the disease process: The etiology of lacrimal gland tumors is unknown. Benign tumors arise from epithelial or mesenchymal cells, while malignant lesions originate from duct cells.

Incidence: In the United States, 2 percent of orbital tumors are malignant epithelial tumors of the lacrimal gland. There are only a few reports of this tumor in the literature because of its rarity.

Symptoms: Some patients may be asymptomatic, while some may complain of a mild fullness in the affected eyelid. Occasionally, patients may have gross bulging of the affected eye (proptosis), blurry or double vision, and a visible mass on the eyelid. Eye pain may or may not be present.

Screening and diagnosis: A tissue biopsy is the definitive tool for diagnosing lacrimal gland tumors. Imaging tests such as a computed tomography (CT) scan, magnetic resonance imaging (MRI), bone scans, and positron emission tomography (PET) scanning are useful for determining adjacent tissue involvement. The TNM (tumor/lymph node/metastasis) system is used for staging lacrimal gland tumors.

Tumor size and location are described as Tx (primary tumor not evaluable), T0 (no tumor), T1 (tumor is 2.5 centimeters, or cm, or less and limited to the lacrimal gland), T2 (tumor is 2.5 to 5 cm and limited to the lacrimal gland), T3a (tumor extends to periosteum but is 5 cm or less), T3b (tumor extends to periosteum and is greater than 5 cm), and T4 (tumor invasion of surrounding structures such as the orbital structures or brain). Node involvement is classified as Nx (regional lymph nodes not evaluable), N0 (no metastasis to regional nodes), and N1 (metastasis to regional nodes). Metastasis is assessed as Mx (distant metastasis not evaluable), M0 (no distant metastasis), or M1 (distant metastasis present).

Treatment and therapy: Treatment depends on the type of tumor. Benign lacrimal gland tumors are treated by complete excisional biopsy. Adenoid cystic carcinoma is treated by surgically removing all orbital structures and bone (exenteration).

Prognosis, prevention, and outcomes: An incompletely excised benign tumor of the lacrimal gland has a 10 to 20 percent chance of becoming malignant. Because of bone and nerve involvement, malignant lacrimal gland tumors have a poor prognosis.

Ophelia Panganiban, B.S.

See also: Adenoid Cystic Carcinoma (ACC); Eye cancers; Eyelid cancer; Orbit tumors; Rhabdomyosarcomas

▶ Lambert-Eaton Myasthenic Syndrome (LEMS)

Category: Diseases, Symptoms, and Conditions
Also known as: Lambert-Eaton syndrome, Eaton-Lambert syndrome

Related conditions: Small-cell lung cancer (SCLC), non-Hodgkin lymphoma, thymoma, carcinoma of the breast and colon, autoimmune disorders

Definition: Lambert-Eaton myasthenic syndrome (LEMS) is a rare disorder of the neuromuscular junction, the point where nerve endings meet muscle fibers. LEMS affects muscles and nerves, causing progressive muscle weakness and decreased reflexes. Commonly, the first symptom noticed by an individual with the syndrome is an exceptionally dry mouth, which stems from the disorder's effect on the autonomic nervous system. LEMS is frequently an early indication of cancer, allowing for early detection and treatment of the disease. It most often is associated with small-cell lung cancer (SCLC) and also has been linked to non-Hodgkin lymphoma, thymoma, and carcinoma of the breast and colon.

Risk factors: People with various types of cancer, especially small-cell lung cancer, are at increased risk for developing Lambert-Eaton myasthenic syndrome. Additional risk factors include advanced age and smoking.

Etiology and the disease process: Lambert-Eaton myasthenic syndrome is an autoimmune disease caused by antibodies acting at the neuromuscular junction. These antibodies target the area of the nerve fiber responsible for releasing acetylcholine, a chemical needed to stimulate normal muscle contraction. The antibodies cause too little acetylcholine to be released, and muscle contractions are weakened. When patients have cancer (about half of LEMS cases), antibodies are thought to be released in response to cancer cell growth, affecting the muscles and autonomic nervous system as secondary reactions. When patients do not have cancer, what triggers the antibody release is unknown.

Typically, patients seek care well before the cancer is diagnosed because antibody release occurs at a very early stage in a tumor's development. Symptoms of LEMS may begin two or more years before detection of a tumor. Because LEMS is a progressive disease, increasing weakness usually limits patients' ability to perform normal daily activities. Although LEMS can cause respiratory difficulties, successful cancer treatment or death usually occurs before LEMS progresses to a life-threatening stage.

Incidence: The exact incidence rate of Lambert-Eaton myasthenic syndrome is unknown because it is not common; however, it is estimated to occur at a rate of 1 per 100,000 people in the United States. The highest incidence occurs in people who are middle-aged and older, but it has also occurred in children. Between 50 and 70 percent of cases of LEMS are associated with small-cell lung cancer, but only about 3 percent of people with small-cell lung cancer develop LEMS. All patients with LEMS and small-cell lung cancer have a long-term history of smoking.

Symptoms: The symptoms of Lambert-Eaton myasthenic syndrome usually begin slowly, developing over a period of months or years. The most common symptom is progressive weakness of the arms and legs that typically occurs in the muscles closest to the body, with the thighs and hips being the most frequently affected. Reflexes in the affected extremities are usually absent or reduced. People with LEMS often have trouble climbing stairs, getting up from a seated or reclining position, and walking. As the disorder affects the autonomic nervous system, patients may complain of mouth dryness, dizziness after standing up, and impotence. Additional symptoms found in people with LEMS include double vision, constipation, excessive sweating, and difficulty talking, chewing, and swallowing.

Screening and diagnosis: There are no screening tests for Lambert-Eaton myasthenic syndrome. The disorder is typically diagnosed by clinical history, physical examination, and laboratory testing. If it is advanced and related to a malignancy, symptoms of the underlying cancer may be present; however, LEMS is usually diagnosed before the cancer produces discernible symptoms. Diagnostic tests include basic blood tests, such as complete blood count and chemistry; testing for voltage-gated calcium channel antibodies, which are present in 50 to 100 percent of patients with LEMS; chest X rays and a computed tomography (CT) scan if malignancy is suspected; electromyography and nerve conduction studies; bronchoscopy; and positron emission tomography (PET) scanning. A Tensilon (edrophonium chloride) test, which is commonly used to differentiate LEMS from myasthenia gravis, may produce a noticeable short-term increase in strength. Staging would be determined by the associated cancer.

Treatment and therapy: When Lambert-Eaton myasthenic syndrome has been diagnosed with an underlying cancer, successful treatment of the cancer usually results in improvement of LEMS. When no cancer has been diagnosed, continued monitoring and testing are recommended because the typical time interval between the onset of LEMS and the diagnosis of cancer can be prolonged.

Immunosuppression therapy with corticosteroids or gamma globulin has proven to provide short-term relief of LEMS but should be used only if symptoms do not resolve after effective treatment of an underlying cancer or if no cancer is present, as it may reduce immunologic suppression of tumor growth. Several drugs, including guanidine and 3,4-diaminopyridine, increase the release of acetylcholine and have been shown to significantly decrease symptoms.

Physical therapy and a regular exercise routine can help patients maintain muscle tone and strength.

Prognosis, prevention, and outcomes: The prognosis of Lambert-Eaton myasthenic syndrome varies and is dependent on the prognosis for the associated cancer. There is no known prevention for LEMS; however, patients should be made aware that certain medications, such as neuromuscular blocking agents, aminoglycosides, magnesium, and calcium channel blockers, can make their condition worse. Patients should also be advised that exposure to hot environments and fever during illness can increase the weakness in their extremities.

Dorothy P. Terry, R.N.

For Further Information

Pascuzzi, Robert M. "Myasthenia Gravis and Lambert-Eaton Syndrome." *Therapeutic Apheresis and Dialysis* 6, no. 1 (February, 2002): 57-68.

Schiff, David, and Patrick Y. Wen, eds. *Cancer Neurology in Clinical Practice*. Totowa, N.J.: Humana Press, 2002.

Verschuuren, J. J., et al. "Available Treatment Options for the Management of Lambert-Eaton Myasthenic Syndrome." *Expert Opinion on Pharmacotherapy* 7, no. 10 (July, 2006): 1323-1336.

Other Resources

Merck Manuals

Neuromuscular Junction Disorders
http://www.merck.com/mmhe/sec06/ch095/ch095c.html

WebMd

Lambert-Eaton Myasthenic Syndrome
http://www.webmd.com/cancer/lambert-eaton-myasthenic-syndrome

See also: Dry mouth; Lung cancers; Paraneoplastic syndromes; Side effects

▶ Laryngeal cancer

Category: Diseases, Symptoms, and Conditions
Also known as: Cancer of the larynx, voice box cancer

Related conditions: Cancer of the lymph nodes, throat cancer, lung cancer, bone cancer, liver cancer

Definition: Laryngeal cancer is a cancer of the larynx, or voice box. The larynx is situated between the pharynx, the passage that connects the back of the mouth and nose to the esophagus, and the trachea. It is a muscular passage through which food passes from the back of the mouth toward the stomach.

The larynx has three divisions. The first, called the supraglottic larynx, contains the false vocal cords, the epiglottis or small flap that keeps food from entering the lungs, and other structures high in the throat toward the base of the tongue. The glottis, situated below the supraglottic larynx, contains the true vocal cords. The subglottis lies below the glottis and continues down the throat to the first ring of cartilage that surrounds the trachea.

Risk factors: The major risk factors in laryngeal cancer are heavy tobacco smoking and the regular consumption,

Age at Diagnosis for Laryngeal Cancer, 2001-2005

Age Group	*Cases Diagnosed (%)*
Under 20	0.0
20-34	0.5
35-44	3.9
45-54	15.6
55-64	28.5
65-74	29.7
75-84	17.8
85 and older	4.0

Source: Data from National Cancer Institute, Surveillance Epidemiology and End Results, Cancer Stat Fact Sheets, 2008

Note: The median age of diagnosis from 2001 to 2005 was sixty-five, with an age-adjusted incidence rate of 3.6 per 100,000 men and women per year.

over an extended period, of excessive quantities of alcoholic beverages, generally construed as being more than three ounces a day. This cancer affects men, especially those over the age of sixty, more often than it does women. In the late 1990's, ten men were afflicted by this disease for every woman who suffered from it, although an increase in the number of women with the disease has been observed since then, correlating with an increase in the number of women smokers.

No convincing link has been made between this form of cancer and a family's medical history. Only an inconsequential number of people suffering from the disease have a familial history of laryngeal cancer. However, a link has been detected between laryngeal cancer and long-term occupational exposure to certain carcinogens, notably asbestos, nickel, mustard gas, and fumes from sulfuric acid.

Etiology and the disease process: Laryngeal cancer can form in any part of the larynx, although it usually starts in the glottis. Almost all cancers of the larynx start in the squamous cells that line its inner walls, and these cancers are known as squamous cell carcinomas. The cancer can spread (metastasize) to the lymph nodes in the neck, the back of the tongue, and other parts of the throat and neck. It also can reach the lungs, the liver, and other parts of the body.

Incidence: Laryngeal cancer is a relatively rare form of cancer, accounting for about 2 percent of all cancers in the United States. The American Cancer Society has estimated that there would be 2,400 new cases of the cancer, 12,250 people with the disease, and 2,670 deaths from it in 2008. There has been a notable overall decrease in laryngeal cancer since 2000 as increasing restrictions on smoking have been imposed and as heavy and sustained drinking has become less prevalent.

Symptoms: Cancer of the supraglottic larynx may result in a persistent sore throat. Sometimes swallowing is difficult and choking frequent. Changes in the quality of the voice may be detected. Some people suffering from the disease suffer from pain in the ears. If the cancer develops in the glottis, some of these symptoms are present, including significant hoarseness caused by tumors on the vocal cords. Cancer in the subglottis, which involves the true vocal cords and may continue to the first cartilaginous ring that surrounds the trachea, is quite rare, although some cases have been reported. In subglottic laryngeal cancer, besides hoarseness, patients may experience shortness of breath. Their breathing may be labored and noisy.

Symptoms of the disease that cannot be ignored and that require immediate medical attention are hoarseness that persists for two weeks or longer, a sore throat that lingers, difficulty in swallowing accompanied by frequent choking, swelling in the neck, and in some cases, pain in the ears.

Screening and diagnosis: When a small tumor grows in the glottis, it can cause pronounced and prolonged hoarseness, which often will lead patients to their physicians while the cancer is still at in an early stage and is most susceptible to elimination and cure. However, the symptoms often develop gradually and may be ignored until they become quite pronounced.

When symptoms appear, a laryngoscopy is indicated. This procedure can be performed either by using a mirror and light to examine the endangered area or through the use of an endoscope inserted into the affected area for a more extensive examination. Usually tissue is taken from the vocal cord and is biopsied to determine whether it is cancerous. Such techniques work well if the area involved is the supraglottis or glottis. If the subglottis is involved, however, endoscopic examination is essential and even it is not wholly reliable because the vocal cords often obscure the area that requires examination.

Other tests may include computed tomography (CT), magnetic resonance imaging (MRI), and a barium swallow.

The staging system for laryngeal cancer looks at the size of the tumor and whether it has spread to the lymph nodes or distant parts of the body. The stages range from

Stage 0, carcinoma in situ, to Stage IV, with spread of the cancer to distant organs. Stage definitions differ depending on whether the cancer is in the supraglottis, glottis, or subglottis.

Treatment and therapy: If a small cancerous growth is discovered early, it is usually treated with radiation, although in some cases, surgery is indicated. Usually surgery is avoided if possible because it can damage the vocal cords and lead to problems in speaking. Biopsies must be done on any tissue that is removed. If the biopsy indicates a malignancy, further investigation is required to determine whether the malignancy has spread to such sites as the lymph nodes, the throat, the lungs, the throat, the tongue, the liver, and the bones.

Advanced cancers that produce large tumors may require a laryngectomy, the surgical removal of the voice box. This treatment is usually a treatment of last resort because it robs the patient of the ability to speak normally, although extensive speech therapy can teach people to produce speech through an artificial larynx or through such means as esophageal speech. In Stage III and IV laryngeal cancer, surgery is usually followed by both radiation and chemotherapy.

Cancers that develop below the vocal cords are particularly problematic because the vocal cords can prevent these cancers from being seen. Also, subglottal tumors and their lesions do not produce symptoms early in the course of the disease; therefore, by the time symptoms occur, the cancer may be well advanced.

Prognosis, prevention, and outcomes: Most laryngeal cancers are 90 percent curable as long as they are detected early and treated aggressively. The five-year survival rate for Stage I throat cancers is between 75 and 95 percent, whereas the three-year survival rate of those with Stage IV throat cancers sinks to between 15 and 30 percent.

Prevention offers the best hope for controlling laryngeal cancers. The two most identifiable causes of such cancers are smoking and heavy drinking. Although abstinence from tobacco products and alcohol cannot guarantee that someone will not develop laryngeal cancer, it is clear that most of those suffering from this disease have abused tobacco, alcohol, or both. Once symptoms appear, those who smoke or drink should stop doing so immediately.

R. Baird Shuman, Ph.D.

For Further Information

Ko, A., E. H. Rosenbaum, and M. Dollinger. *Everyone's Guide to Cancer Therapy: How Cancer Is Diagnosed, Treated, and Managed Day to Day*. 5th ed. Kansas City, Mo.: Andrews McMeel, 2007.

Litin, Scott C., Jr., ed. *Mayo Clinic Family Health Book*. 3d ed. New York: HarperCollins, 2003.

Lydiatt, William, and Perry Johnson. *Cancers of the Mouth* and Throat: A Patient's Guide to Treatment. Omaha, Nebr.: Addicus Books, 2000.

National Cancer Institute. *What You Need to Know About Cancer of the Larynx*. Bethesda, Md.: National Institutes of Health, 1995.

Silverman, Sol. *Oral Cancer*. Lewiston, N.Y.: BC Decker, 2003.

Stasney, C. Richard. *Atlas of Dynamic Laryngeal Pathology*. San Diego, Calif.: Singular, 1996.

Teeley, Peter, and Philip Bashe. *The Complete Cancer Survival Guide*. New York: Broadway Books, 2005.

Other Resources

American Cancer Society
http://www.cancer.org

Cancer Links
http://www.cancerlinks.com

National Cancer Institute
Throat (Laryngeal and Pharyngeal) Cancer
http://www.cancer.gov/cancertopics/types/throat/

See also: Asbestos; Barium swallow; Bronchography; Chewing tobacco; Cigarettes and cigars; Coal tars and coal tar pitches; Cordectomy; Electrolarynx; Endoscopy; Epidermoid cancers of mucous membranes; Esophageal speech; Head and neck cancers; Laryngeal nerve palsy; Laryngectomy; Laryngoscopy; Mustard gas; Occupational exposures and cancer; Oral and oropharyngeal cancers; Salivary gland cancer; Throat cancer; TNM staging; Tobacco-related cancers; Tracheostomy; Upper Gastrointestinal (GI) series

▶ Laryngeal nerve palsy

Category: Diseases, Symptoms, and Conditions
Also known as: Recurrent laryngeal nerve damage, paralysis of the laryngeal nerve, paralysis of the larnyx

Related conditions: Intrathoracic diseases, neurolaryngological lesion

Definition: Laryngeal nerve palsy is the paralysis of the laryngeal nerve.

Risk factors: Damage to the laryngeal nerve can result from tumors in the neck and chest or from intrathoracic diseases such as tumor or aneurysm of the arch of the aorta or of the left atrium of the heart. Tumors and aneurysms may press on the nerve, causing nerve damage. Damage to the recurrent laryngeal nerve may also occur during surgery on the thyroid gland.

Etiology and the disease process: The vagus nerve is one of twelve cranial nerves. It originates in the brain stem and reaches to the large intestine. In the neck, the vagus nerve branches off a paired nerve called the recurrent laryngeal nerve. When the laryngeal nerve separates from the vagus nerve, it reaches into the chest and loops back up to the voice box (larynx). The recurrent laryngeal nerves extend along either side of the trachea (windpipe) between the trachea and the thyroid gland, and they control movement of the larynx. The larynx is located where the throat divides into the esophagus and the trachea. The larynx is where the voice is produced, and it controls the flow of air into the lungs. It houses the vocal cords and the muscles and ligaments that move the vocal cords. Damage to the laryngeal nerve itself causes laryngeal palsy on the affected side. Less commonly, laryngeal palsy, or paralysis of the larynx, can be the result of damage to the vagus nerve before the recurrent laryngeal nerve branches off. A damaged laryngeal nerve results in reduced movements of the larynx, causing voice weakness, hoarseness, or the complete loss of voice. Although rare, life-threatening cases may occur if the larynx is paralyzed to the extent that air cannot enter the lungs. Damage can occur to either one or both branches of the nerve, and paralysis of the laryngeal nerve may be temporary or permanent.

Incidence: Recurrent laryngeal nerve injury, without injury to the superior laryngeal nerve, is the most common traumatic neurolaryngological lesion. Laryngeal nerve palsy is an uncommon side effect of thyroidectomy. It occurs in 1 to 2 percent of complete thyroidectomies performed to treat cancer, and less often when only part of the thyroid is removed. Most often patients experience only transient laryngeal nerve palsy and within a few weeks spontaneously recover their normal voice.

Symptoms: The effects of laryngeal nerve damage are flaccidity of the ipsilateral vocal fold, loss of adduction (movement of a limb), severe dysphonia or laryngeal dystonia, (involuntary movements of the muscles of the larynx) complete paralytic aphonia (inability to speak), and frequently aspiration of food and drink into the trachea.

Screening and diagnosis: Diagnosis and treatment of the immobile or hypomobile vocal fold are challenging. True paralysis and paresis (impaired movement) result from vocal fold denervation secondary to injury to the laryngeal or vagus nerve. Location of the vocal fold paralysis and paresis may be unilateral or bilateral and central or peripheral. Paralysis may involve the recurrent laryngeal nerve, the superior laryngeal nerve, or both. It is important to confirm that the laryngeal impairment is not caused by arytenoid cartilage subluxation (dislocation of small cartilages in the back of the larynx), cricoarytenoid arthritis or ankylosis (stiffness of a joint), neoplasm, or other mechanical causes. Most common diagnostic tools are strobovideolaryngoscopy, endoscopy, radiologic and laboratory studies, and electromyography (EMG).

Treatment and therapy: Once the recurrent laryngeal nerve is damaged, there is no specific treatment to heal it. Common treatments for laryngeal nerve damage are polytetrafluoroethylene (trademark Teflon) injection, a surgical procedure in which an implant is inserted into the paralyzed vocal cord (medialization thyroplasty); arytenoid adduction procedures; or reinnervation by nerve transfer. With time, most cases of recurrent laryngeal palsy improve spontaneously. In some cases, the larynx may be paralyzed so that air cannot flow past it into the lungs, and an emergency tracheotomy needs to be performed. A tracheotomy is a surgical procedure to make an artificial opening in the trachea, which allows air to bypass the larynx and to enter the lungs. If the paralysis is temporary, the tracheotomy hole can be surgically closed. There are no alternative or complementary therapies to heal laryngeal nerve palsy. When loss of speech is permanent, artificial speech devices exist to produce tone.

Prognosis, prevention, and outcomes: Muscle function can be assessed by observing the movements of the structures or by recording the electrical activity of the muscles via electromyography. Although electromyography is an invasive technique, it may be helpful in patients with voice problems of suspected neurological or neuromuscular etiology. Electromyography recordings are helpful in differentiating vocal fold paralysis from arytenoid dislocation. Electromyography is useful for the diagnosis to establish a reliable prognosis and treatment plan and to monitor muscle denervation and reinnervation. Following acute denervation, the subsequent progression is either chronic denervation or laryngeal nerve regeneration.

Anita Nagypál, Ph.D.

For Further Information

Crumley, R. L. "Unilateral Recurrent Laryngeal Nerve Paralysis." *Journal of Voice* 8, no. 1 (March, 1994): 79-83.

Harti, D. M., and D. F. Brasnu. "Recurrent Laryngeal Nerve Paralysis: Current Concepts and Treatment." *Ear, Nose and Throat Journal* 79, no. 12 (December, 2000): 918.

Rubin, A. D., and R. T. Sataloff. "Vocal Fold Paresis and Paralysis." *Otolaryngolic Clinic of North America* 40, no. 5 (October, 2007): 1109-1231.

Woodson, G. "Evolving Concepts of Laryngeal Paralysis." *The Journal of Laryngology and Otology* 122, no. 5 (May, 2008): 437-441.

Ysunza, A., et al. "The Role of Laryngeal Electromyography in the Diagnosis of Vocal Fold Immobility in Children." *International Journal of Pediatric Otorhinolaryngology* 71, no. 6 (June, 2007): 949-958.

Other Resources

MayoClinic.com
Vocal Cord Paralysis
http://www.mayoclinic.com/health/vocal-cord-paralysis/DS00670

National Cancer Institute
Thyroid Cancer
http://www.cancer.gov/cancertopics/types/Thyroid

See also: Electrolarynx; Esophageal speech; Head and neck cancers; Laryngeal cancer; Laryngectomy; Laryngoscopy; Oral and oropharyngeal cancers; Salivary gland cancer; Throat cancer; Tracheostomy

▶ Leiomyomas

Category: Diseases, Symptoms, and Conditions
Also known as: Myomas, fibroids, uterine fibroids, genital leiomyomas, angioleiomyomas, piloleiomyomas

Related conditions: Leiomyosarcomas

Definition: Leiomyomas are benign tumors that arise from smooth muscle of the digestive tract, piloerector muscle in hair (piloleiomyoma), blood vessels (angioleiomyoma), nipples, and the genital tract (genital leiomyoma). While any organ possessing smooth muscle may become involved, the myometrium (the muscular layer of the uterus) is the most common site. Leiomyomas may arise at any location in the myometrium as a single mass, as a cluster, or as diffuse disease.

Risk factors: One risk factor is a family history of leiomyomas, especially of a tumor involving the skin and uterus called Reed syndrome (familial leiomyomatosis cutis et uteri), which is inherited in an autosomal dominant fashion but expressed variably. The responsible gene, *MCU11*, is located on the long arm of chromosome 1(1q42.3-q43). Women are at risk of developing a uterine leiomyoma during their reproductive years.

Etiology and the disease process: The development of extrauterine leiomyomas is still obscure. The unusual manifestation of pain has been postulated to arise when these tumors stimulate the sympathetic nervous system, causing muscle contraction, but remains poorly understood. Uterine leiomyomas occur only in the presence of estrogen and progesterone stimulation and arise as a result of overproliferation of smooth muscle and connective tissue cells within the myometrium. They have been linked with a specific mutation (G354R) of a tumor-suppressor gene encoding for fumarate hydratase in *MCU11*. Estrogen and progesterone receptor stimulation on these cells accelerate or decrease proliferation, suggesting that leiomyomas depend on estrogen and progesterone.

Incidence: Leiomyomas outside the uterus are rare. In contrast, around 50 percent of women in their reproductive years will develop a uterine leiomyoma in their lifetime, with a peak age of thirty. Leiomyomas account for half of esophageal masses found. Less than 1 percent of uterine leiomyoma cases will experience malignant transformation (leiomyosarcoma).

Symptoms: Patients with most extrauterine tumors experience pain induced by cold, pressure, menses, or pregnancy. On examination, these tumors may appear as flat lesions or skin nodules. A woman of reproductive age who has a leiomyoma proximal to the vascular endometrium will experience bleeding and may exhibit fatigue and pallor. A uterine leiomyoma may be felt through the abdominal wall and mistaken for pregnancy. However, a pregnancy test would be negative. Subtler symptoms may include menometrorrhagia (increased, frequent, and irregular bleeding from the vagina), infertility and pressure symptoms causing difficulty in swallowing, and compression of the bladder and ureter (urine duct from the kidney to the bladder). A blood test may reveal significant anemia when the woman is experiencing frequent and substantial blood loss.

Screening and diagnosis: A diagnosis of an extrauterine leiomyoma may be confirmed by an excisional biopsy, where excision of the entire mass is also therapeutic. A barium contrast study may show a "punched-out" defect in the esophagus. Ultrasound and magnetic resonance imaging (MRI) are not as helpful. A pelvic ultrasound may

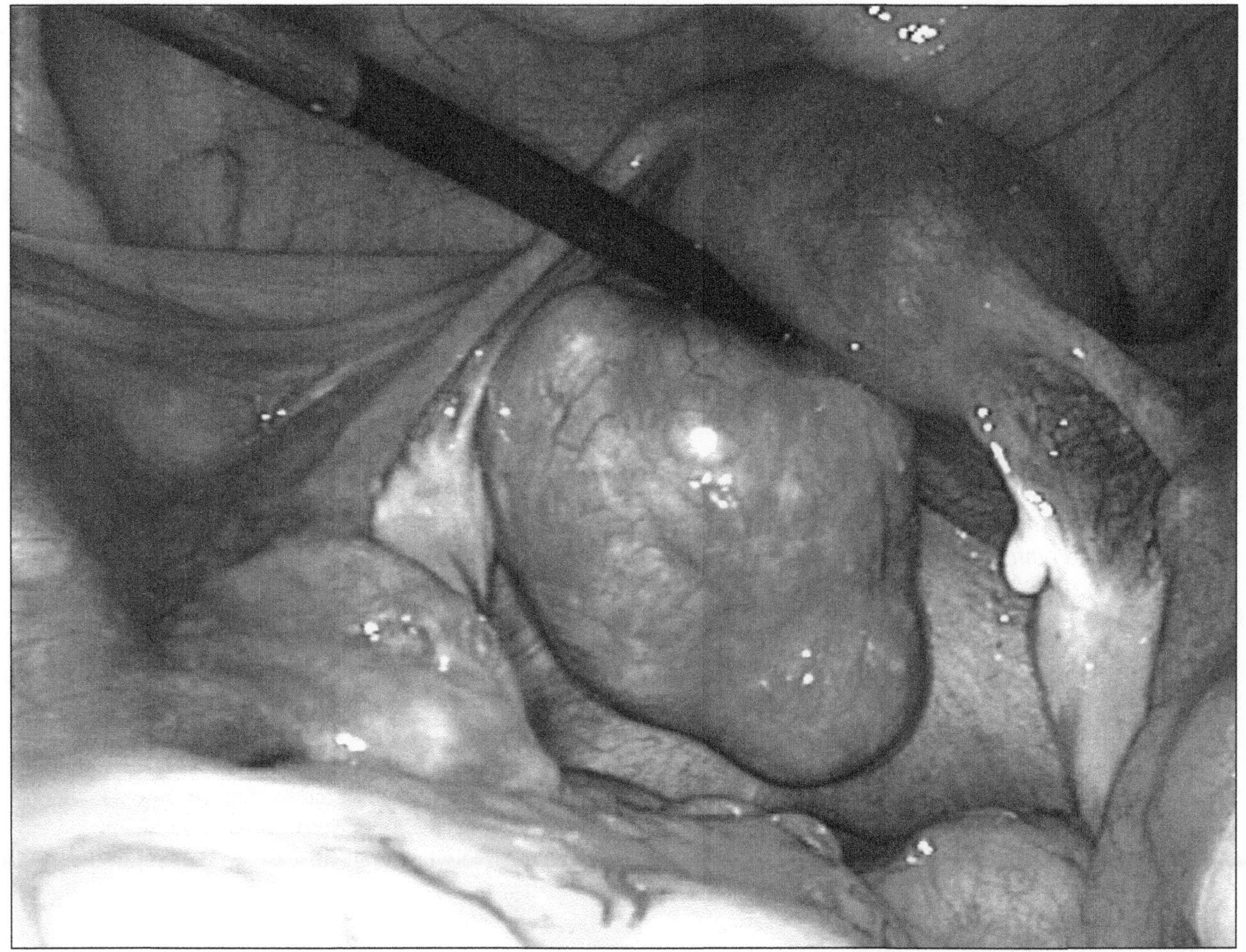

Surgical removal of large subserosal leiomyoma of the uterus. (Wikimedia)

reveal a vague mass darker than the surrounding normal tissue within the myometrium. A distortion in the uterine contour may be the only hint of a leiomyoma. An endometrial biopsy is also performed to rule out endometrial cancer. Specific screening tests other than regular pelvic examinations are not available for leiomyomas.

Treatment and therapy: Apart from excisional biopsy, pain from extrauterine leiomyomas may be alleviated with calcium channel blockers (nifedipine), alpha-receptor blockers (phenoxybenzamine), or gamma-aminobutyric acid (GABA) analogs (gabapentin). Enucleation with repair may be sufficient in esophageal masses.

Treatment of uterine leiomyomas may be conservative or curative. If the patient is symptomatic (for example, anemic from chronic bleeding), no longer desires to bear children, wishes to be pain free, and is amenable to a hysterectomy (surgical removal of the uterus), a curative approach is adapted. If the patient is relatively young and desires to bear children, a conservative approach is preferred.

Conservative treatment consists of options from watchful waiting and myomectomy to newer procedures such as uterine arterial embolization (UAE). UAE involves injecting polyvinyl alcohol foam particles into the uterine arteries, which occludes the leiomyoma's blood supply, inducing tumor involution. As only 10 to 20 percent of patients require definitive treatment, with most leiomyomas shrinking after menopause and pregnancy, monitoring with serial pelvic ultrasound may be done. A myomectomy, in which the leiomyomas are surgically removed, seeks to preserve as much of the muscular integrity of the uterus as possible. Excessive blood loss during an operation may be prevented by chemotherapy with a gonadotropin-releasing hormone (GnRH) analog such as nafarelin or leuprolide acetate. A fertility workup including Fallopian tube patency with a hysterosalpingogram and semen analysis should also be carried out. Curative options include an abdominal or vaginal hysterectomy to remove the uterus along with the mass.

Prognosis, prevention, and outcomes: The overall prognosis of uncomplicated leiomyomas is excellent. As most leiomyomas are benign, patients undergoing surgical excision or a hysterectomy rarely experience recurrence. Postmenopausal women with a history of leiomyoma on hormone replacement may have a recurrence. No preventive measures against developing a leiomyoma are known.

Aldo C. Dumlao, M.D.

For Further Information

Byers, Tim, Susan J. Curry, Maria Elizabeth Hewitt, and National Cancer Policy Board. *Fulfilling the Potential of Cancer Prevention and Early Detection*. Washington, D.C.: National Academies Press, 2003.

Dollinger, Malin, et al. *Everyone's Guide to Cancer Therapy: How Cancer Is Diagnosed, Treated, and Managed Day to Day*. 4th ed. Kansas City, Mo.: Andrews McMeel, 2002.

Parker, James N., and Philip M. Parker, eds. *The Official Patient's Sourcebook on Uterine Fibroids*. San Diego, Calif.: Icon Health, 2002.

Other Resources

American Cancer Society
http://www.cancer.org

LeioMyoSarcoma
http://www.leiomyosarcoma.info

LMSarcoma Direct Research Foundation
http://www.lmsdr.org

The National Leomyosarcoma Foundation
http://www.nlmsf.org

See also: Hereditary Leiomyomatosis and Renal Cell Cancer (HLRCC); Hystero-oophorectomy; Kidney cancer; Leiomyosarcomas; Mitochondrial DNA mutations; Urinary system cancers; Uterine cancer

▶ Leiomyosarcomas

Category: Diseases, Symptoms, and Conditions

Related conditions: Gastrointestinal stromal tumors (GISTs), leiomyomas

Definition: Leiomyosarcomas are rare malignant tumors that arise from smooth muscle, most commonly in between the muscular and mucosal layers of the digestive tract and the myometrium (muscular layer) of the uterus. The stomach and small intestine are the most commonly involved organs. The ileum is the most common region of small bowel affected.

Risk factors: Shared factors implicated in endometrial cancer and leiomyosarcoma include nulliparity (no births), obesity, and diabetes. Pelvic irradiation and chlorophenol exposure were associated specifically with extrauterine leiomyosarcoma in some studies. Concomitant Crohn disease was found in 6 percent of patients in another study.

Etiology and the disease process: The malignant cells are clones of a single, spindle-shaped cell transformed by an external mutagen. Biological etiologies such as Epstein-Barr virus (EBV), as seen in leiomyosarcomas with EBV deoxyribonucleic acid (DNA) from immunosuppressed patients such as transplant recipients and patients infected with the human immunodeficiency virus (HIV), are possible mutagens. One characteristic of a leiomyosarcoma's growth differentiating it from other tumors is its propensity to grow outward into the abdominal cavity instead of inward, causing obstructive symptoms relatively late in the disease. Malignant transformation of a preexisting uterine leiomyoma is possible but has been estimated to occur in only 0.2 percent of cases.

Incidence: While comparatively rare, leiomyosarcomas account for around 2 to 9 percent of all extrauterine sarcomas, with 20 percent of these found within the digestive tract. Uterine leiomyosarcomas make up 4 percent of all uterine cancers. In the United States, the overall occurrence of extrauterine leiomyosarcomas is estimated at 1.4 cases per 100,000.

Symptoms: Most symptoms of a leiomyosarcoma mimic those of other, more common digestive tract cancers such as colorectal cancer. These include overt symptoms such as bleeding or obstruction (constipation) in large tumors. Bleeding may be acute and severe enough to require blood transfusions if a blood vessel has been eroded by a tumor. Patients may complain of vague symptoms such as fatigue, weight loss, malaise (from long-term blood loss), and abdominal pain. Some patients may have no symptoms, delaying diagnosis. In uterine leiomyosarcomas, a mass may be felt through the abdominal wall and mistaken for pregnancy. However, a pregnancy test would be negative. Other symptoms may include menometrorrhagia

Stage at Diagnosis and Five-Year Relative Survival Rates for Adult Leiomyosarcoma, 1988-2001

Stage	*Cases Diagnosed (%)*	*Survival Rate (%)*
Localized[a]	51.0	71.8
Regional[b]	18.6	44.4
Distant[c]	21.9	13.6
Unstaged	8.5	45.4

Source: Data from L. A. G. Ries et al., eds., Cancer Survival Among Adults: U.S. SEER Program, 1988-2001—Patient and Tumor Characteristics, NIH Pub. No. 07-6215 (Bethesda, Md.: National Cancer Institute, 2007)

[a]Cancer still confined to primary site

[b]Cancer has spread to regional lymph nodes or directly beyond the primary site

[c]Cancer has metastasized

(increased, frequent, and irregular bleeding from the vagina), infertility and pressure symptoms causing difficulty in swallowing, and compression or invasion of the bladder and ureter (urine duct from the kidney to the bladder).

Screening and diagnosis: A diagnosis of an extrauterine leiomyosarcoma may be confirmed by ultrasound-guided biopsy. Ultrasound, computed tomography (CT), or magnetic resonance imaging (MRI) are not as helpful. The tumor type is diagnosed by a pathologist, who can determine cancerous changes in cells and the histologic grades (number of cell divisions, defined as five or more in ten microscopic field samples). Immunohistochemical identification may be useful for differentiating leiomyosarcoma from gastrointestinal stromal tumors (GISTs) by identifying GIST markers such as CD34 and tyrosine kinase c-kit (CD117); GIST treatment differs from that for leiomyosarcoma.

Specific screening tests other than regular pelvic examinations are not available for leiomyosarcoma of the uterus. A pelvic ultrasound may reveal a vague mass darker than the surrounding normal tissue within the myometrium. An endometrial biopsy is also performed to rule out endometrial cancer in bleeding women.

The American Joint Committee on Cancer (AJCC) uses the TNM (tumot/lymph node/metastasis) classification for tumor staging of intestinal tumors:

- Stage I: The tumor is less than 5 centimeters (cm), low grade, with no sign of lymph node spread or spread to other parts of the body.
- Stage II: The tumor is greater than 5 cm, localized, low grade, and has not spread to lymph nodes or other parts of the body.
- Stage III: The tumor is either high grade of any size or has spread to regional lymph nodes or the peritoneum.
- Stage IVA: The tumor has metastasized or is deemed unresectable.
- Stage IVB: Tumor rupture has occurred in spite of resection.

For uterine leiomyosarcomas, the staging criteria for uterine cancers developed by the International Federation of Gynecology and Obstetrics (FIGO) is used:

- Stage I: Tumor is limited to the endometrium and myometrium.
- Stage II: Endocervical and cervical stroma are involved.
- Stage III: Invasion of serosa or adjacent reproductive organs has taken place, or malignant cells are found in peritoneal, vaginal, pelvic, or para-aortic lymph nodes.
- Stage IVA: Bladder or bowel mucosa invasion or distant metastases have taken place.

Note that cell grade is not as significant in staging of uterine leiomyosarcomas as in staging intestinal leiomyosarcomas.

Treatment and therapy: Irrespective of location, radical surgical resection of the leiomyosarcoma through abdominal surgery (bowel resection or hysterectomy) is warranted. Although lymph node spread is an ominous sign, it rarely occurs. In such cases, removal of lymph nodes draining the immediate area of the tumor is sufficient. In unresectable tumors, palliative therapy is carried out. This may include intestinal bypass of the tumor followed by radiotherapy. In cases of metastases, palliative resection, radiotherapy, and chemotherapy are carried out.

Prognosis, prevention, and outcomes: Prognosis is based on the cellular grade and size of the tumor upon diagnosis and surgical staging. The five-year survival rate for operable extrauterine leiomyosarcoma is approximately 50 percent. Liver metastasis may occur in as many as 55 percent of patients with recurrence.

Aldo C. Dumlao, M.D.

For Further Information

Byers, Tim, Susan J. Curry, Maria Elizabeth Hewitt, and National Cancer Policy Board. *Fulfilling the Potential of Cancer Prevention and Early Detection*. Washington, D.C.: National Academies Press, 2003.

Dollinger, Malin, et al. *Everyone's Guide to Cancer Therapy: How Cancer Is Diagnosed, Treated and*

Managed Day to Day. 4th ed. Kansas City, Mo.: Andrews McMeel, 2002.

Morra, Marion E., and Eve Potts. *Choices*. 4th ed. New York: HarperCollins, 2003.

Other Resources

American Cancer Society
http://www.cancer.org

LeioMyoSarcoma
http://www.leiomyosarcoma.info

LMSarcoma Direct Research Foundation
http://www.lmsdr.org

The National Leomyosarcoma Foundation
http://www.nlmsf.org

See also: Fibrosarcomas, soft-tissue; Hereditary Leiomyomatosis and Renal Cell Cancer (HLRCC); Leiomyomas; Sarcomas, soft-tissue; Testicular cancer; Uterine cancer; Vaginal cancer

▶ Leptomeningeal carcinomas

Category: Diseases, Symptoms, and Conditions
Also known as: Leptomeningeal carcinomatosis (LC), leptomeningeal metastasis, leptomeningeal seeding, carcinomatous meningitis, neoplastic meningitis

Related conditions: Metastasized cancers most often of the breast, lung, and gastrointestinal tract; malignant melanoma; lymphoma

Definition: Leptomeningeal carcinoma is the growth of cancer in the central nervous system (brain and spinal cord) as a result of the metastasis of a primary cancer.

Risk factors: People develop leptomeningeal carcinoma because they have another type of cancer that spreads (metastasizes) to the central nervous system. Small-cell lung cancers, malignant melanoma, cancers of the gastrointestinal tract, cancers of the blood, and breast cancer are the most likely to metastasize into leptomeningeal carcinoma.

Etiology and the disease process: The central nervous system (CNS) consists of the brain and spinal cord. Three membranes cover the brain. The pia mater is a thin, delicate membrane that lies tightly on top of the cells in the brain and spinal cord. The arachnoid mater is the middle membrane surrounding the central nervous system. It fits loosely, creating space between the pia mater and the arachnoid mater. This space is called the subarachnoid space.

The subarachnoid space is filled with cerebrospinal fluid (CSF). This fluid brings nutrients to the nerve cells, removes wastes, and cushions the central nervous system during movement. Once cancer cells enter the cerebrospinal fluid, they can move freely to any central nervous system location. Leptomeningeal carcinoma develops in the subarachnoid space and usually is found in multiple locations. The outer membrane, or dura mater, does not play a role in this cancer.

Leptomeningeal carcinoma develops secondary to another type of cancer, almost always after the original cancer has been treated and then returned. Blood cancers and cancer cells that have been shed by solid tumors travel through the circulatory system and enter the cerebrospinal fluid, often by burrowing through the wall of a blood vessel. This process is called leptomeningeal seeding. Once in the cerebrospinal fluid, the cancer cells multiply. They are transported through the cerebrospinal fluid and eventually attach to nerve cells in the brain and spinal cord. Here they grow into either flat sheets of tissue (often in the brain) or masses of cells. The cancer cells also tend to spread along nerves emerging from the spinal column.

Incidence: The frequency with which patients develop leptomeningeal carcinoma is not clear, and the disease is probably underdiagnosed. Between 1 and 8 percent of cancer patients are diagnosed with leptomeningeal carcinoma, but on autopsy, about 20 to 25 percent have evidence of the disease. Leptomeningeal carcinoma can occur in adults and children.

Symptoms: Symptoms depend on where the leptomeningeal carcinoma is located. In the brain, masses of cells may interrupt the flow of cerebrospinal fluid and cause an increase in pressure in the brain. Symptoms associated with leptomeningeal carcinoma in the brain include headaches accompanied by nausea and vomiting, disturbances in balance and gait, memory problems, and behavior changes.

Symptoms associated with leptomeningeal carcinoma along the cranial nerves (twelve pairs of nerves that originate in the brain and enervate the head, neck, and upper chest) include double vision or other vision problems, hearing loss, problems swallowing, and dizziness. These are the most common symptoms, occurring in more than 90 percent of patients. More than one cranial nerve is usually involved, so multiple symptoms are present in the same individual.

Symptoms associated with leptomeningeal carcinoma in nerves that originate in the spine include neck and back pain, incontinence, and leg weakness. Most often, patients have a combination of symptoms because multiple sites are affected.

Screening and diagnosis: Diagnosis is made by multiple lumbar punctures. In a lumbar puncture, a small amount of cerebrospinal fluid is withdrawn from the subarachnoid space using a fine needle. Since the physician has little idea where in the central nervous system the leptomeningeal carcinoma is located, the likelihood of correctly diagnosing leptomeningeal carcinoma with a single lumbar puncture is only about 50 percent. When lumbar puncture is repeated three times at different sites, the likelihood of making a positive diagnosis increases to almost 90 percent. Diagnosis also involves contrast-enhanced imaging scans (magnetic resonance imaging, computed tomography, myelography) to identify the location of the leptomeningeal carcinoma for treatment.

Because leptomeningeal carcinoma is the result of metastasis of a primary cancer, it is, by definition, Stage IV cancer.

Treatment and therapy: The goal of treatment is to prevent the development of additional symptoms and prolong the survival of the patient. Treatment options are often limited because leptomeningeal carcinoma is a sign of advanced cancer. Radiation directed to the sites where the cancer is located and chemotherapy drugs injected by lumbar puncture directly into the cerebrospinal fluid are the two main treatments available.

Prognosis, prevention, and outcomes: Leptomeningeal carcinoma is a sign of terminal cancer. If untreated, the average survival time is four to six weeks. When treated, the average survival time is three to seven months, depending on the type of primary cancer. Usually the individual dies from either the primary cancer or complications of cancer treatment rather than directly from leptomeningeal carcinoma.

Martiscia Davidson, A.M.

For Further Information

Bruno, M. K., and J. Raizer. "Leptomeningeal Metastases from Solid Tumors (Meningeal Carcinomatosis)." *Cancer Treatment and Research* 125 (2005): 31-52.

Jaeckle, K. A. "Improving the Outcome of Patients with Leptomeningeal Cancer: New Clinical Trials and Experimental Therapies." *Cancer Treatment and Research* 125 (2005): 181-193.

Kaal, E. C., and C. J. Vecht. "CNS Complications of Breast Cancer: Current and Emerging Treatment Options." *CNS Drugs* 21, no. 7 (2007): 559-579.

Penthoroudiaks, G., and Palvidis, N. "Management of Leptomeningeal Malignancy." *Expert Opinion on Pharmacotherapy* 6, no. 7 (June, 2005): 1115-1125.

Other Resources

eMedicine.com
Leptomeningeal Carcinomatosis
http://www.emedicine.com/RADIO/topic390.htm

National Cancer Institute
http://www.cancer.gov

See also: Brain and central nervous system cancers; Carcinomatous meningitis; Lumbar punctures; Meningeal carcinomatosis

▶ Leukemias

Category: Diseases, Symptoms, and Conditions
Also known as: Hematologic malignancy, liquid tumor

Related conditions: Myelodysplastic syndrome (MDS)

Definition: Leukemias are cancers of the blood that result in abnormally high numbers of white cells, called leukocytes, in the blood and bone marrow. There are some rare forms of leukemia, but the main ones are acute myeloid leukemia (AML), chronic myeloid leukemia (CML), acute lymphoblastic leukemia (ALL), and chronic lymphocytic leukemia (CLL). Leukemias are named for the type of malfunctioning blood cell and the intensity of how the cancer progresses. Acute leukemia occurs suddenly and usually involves large numbers of abnormal cells. Chronic leukemia grows more slowly and may go undetected until the disease progresses. AML is a fast-growing leukemia that involves mature white cells. CML is slow growing, has a disease marker called the Philadelphia chromosome, and affects mature white cells. ALL affects mature lymphocytes and grows rapidly. CLL also affects mature lymphocytes but grows slowly.

Risk factors: Exposure to certain chemicals, such as benzene, is a risk factor for leukemia. Chemicals, solvents, and ionizing radiation can alter deoxyribonucleic acid (DNA), one of the acids found within the nucleus of cells. The damaged DNA causes chromosomal abnormalities linked to cancer. Another risk factor is prior treatment with chemotherapy, or cytotoxic drugs. Leukemia emerging after treatment of another cancer is known as a secondary leukemia.

Etiology and the disease process: The cause of leukemia is unknown, but it is thought that substances that damage DNA lead to the development of leukemia. The proliferation of abnormal white blood cells crowds out red blood cells, platelets, and healthy white cells. The different types of white blood cells are neutrophil, eosinophil, basophil, monocyte, and lymphocyte, and each has a specific role in fighting infection. Red blood cells carry oxygen to the body, and platelets enable blood to clot. Normal white cells, which help the body fight infection by keeping blood and tissues free of contaminants such as bacteria, viruses, and fungi, cannot function properly in the presence of leukemia. White blood cells, as well as red blood cells and platelets, originate from stem cells that mature, or differentiate, into specific types of cells inside the bone marrow. Immature white cells are called blasts, and increased numbers are found in the bone marrow, and sometimes blood, of people with AML and ALL. The presence of leukemic cells leaves less room for the normal white cells, compromising and suppressing the immune system. Myelodysplastic syndrome (MDS) is a disease that affects the normal maturation process of blood cells and may evolve into AML.

Incidence: Leukemia makes up about 3 percent of cancers. New cases of leukemia, estimated by the Leukemia and Lymphoma Society of America, were expected to number 44,240 in 2007. There are 7 percent more cases of chronic versus acute leukemias. The incidence is much higher for the elderly, with half of all cases occurring after the age of sixty-seven. Leukemias account for about 33 percent of all cancers in children up to the age of fourteen. The most common form of leukemia among children under the age of nineteen is ALL. AML is the most common leukemia in adults, with 13,410 new cases projected in 2007. The estimate for CML was 4,570 new cases for 2007. The incidence of all leukemias is about 30 percent higher for men than women. The highest incidence is among whites. Hispanic children of all races under the age of twenty have the highest rates of leukemia

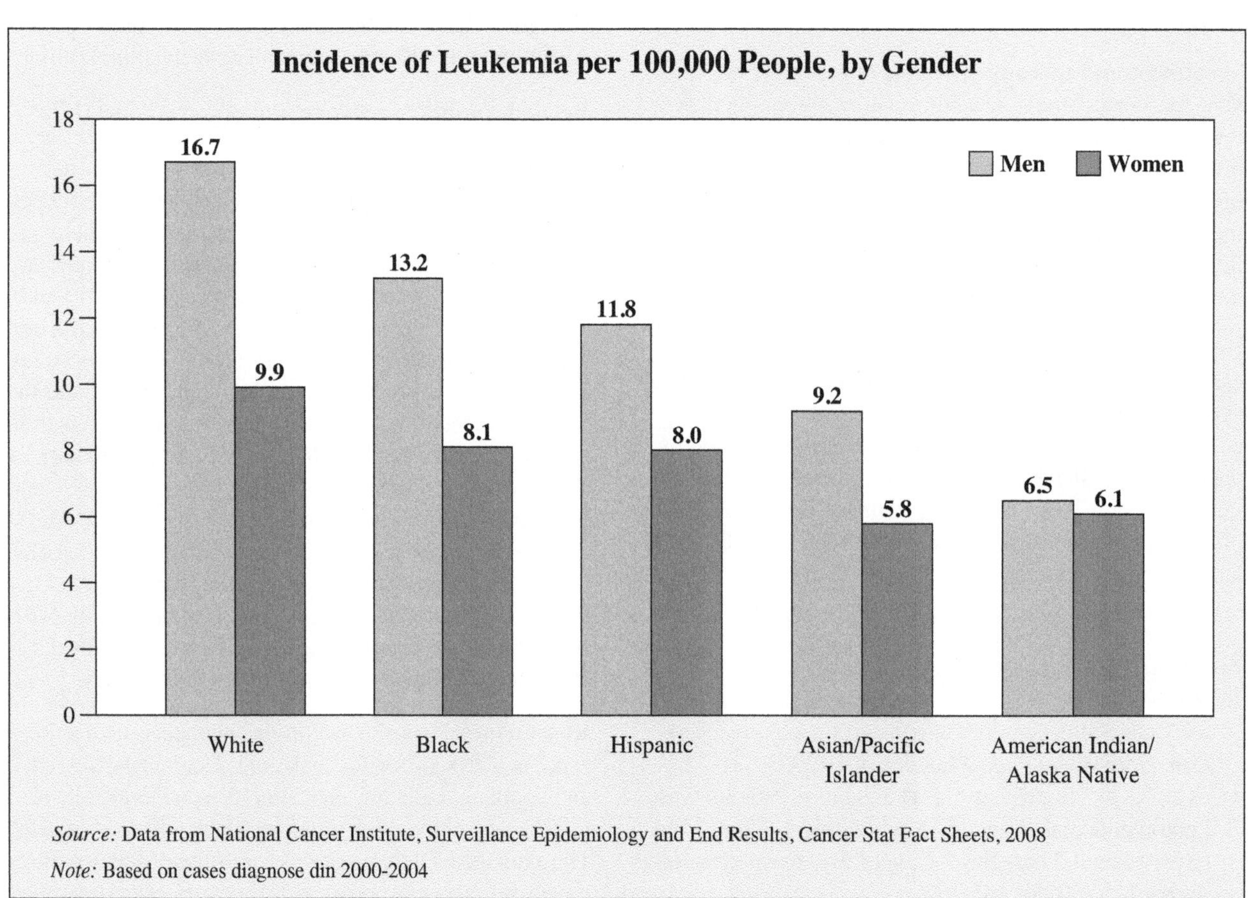

Source: Data from National Cancer Institute, Surveillance Epidemiology and End Results, Cancer Stat Fact Sheets, 2008

Note: Based on cases diagnose din 2000-2004

among children. Leukemia is not a hereditary disease, because most people with leukemia report no family history of the disease.

Symptoms: The early signs of leukemia may manifest as generalized symptoms such as fatigue and shortness of breath that result from a lack of oxygen in the body because of reduced numbers of red blood cells. Pale skin, infection, and wounds that heal slowly are other symptoms. Bruising or bleeding may result when platelets are reduced by the abnormally high white cell counts. Enlarged lymph nodes and joint pain may also be noticed. A complete workup is necessary to determine the cause of the symptoms. There are multiple medical conditions that cause the same symptoms, and therefore these symptoms should not be assumed to be caused by leukemia. However, as leukemia is potentially fatal and early intervention is critical, particularly with acute leukemia, symptoms should be reported promptly to a health care provider.

Screening and diagnosis: Routine blood tests such as a complete blood count (CBC) are used to screen for abnormalities in white and red blood cells and platelets. Diagnosis is made by testing blood and bone marrow in conjunction with a thorough review of medical history and a physical examination. Bone marrow is obtained though a procedure called a biopsy. A small sample of bone marrow is obtained by inserting a needle into bone, typically near the hip. The sample is examined under a microscope to look for malignant cells and through testing called immunophenotyping. White blood cells can be identified by their size and by the way they look when stains are applied. Staining allows visualization of the different cell lines and makes it easier to quantify or estimate the number of each present in the sample. The number of blast cells found in bone marrow or blood is used to diagnosis leukemia versus myelodysplastic syndrome. An increase in the number of blasts may be indicative of conversion from myelodysplastic syndrome to AML.

Genetic testing is the key to diagnosing leukemia because it identifies the cell defect causing the leukemia. Chromosome testing, which reveals important genetic information about type and aggressiveness of the leukemia, is used to guide treatment. Immunophenotyping is a process that enables examination of individual cells in a sample of blood or bone to determine the types of proteins and antigens on their surface. This process helps determine the percentage of abnormal markers on cells, which determines leukemia type. The specific abnormalities found through this testing give a picture of the genetic defect and prognosis for the leukemia.

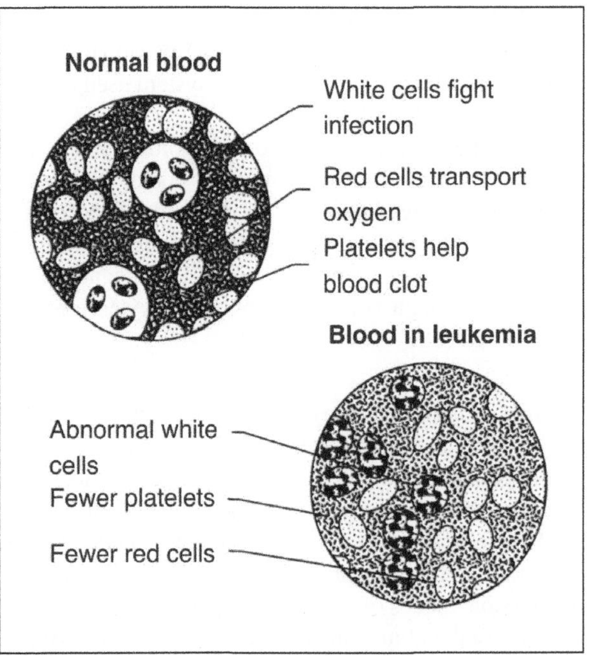

Leukemias are characterized by abnormally high numbers of white cells in the blood.

Karyotyping is done to gain additional information about the genetic features of the chromosomes and thereby confirm a diagnosis of leukemia and identify its subtype. The type of genetic abnormality needs to be determined before treatment begins to ensure utilization of the correct regimen. The abnormality may be a deletion, addition, or translocation of a segment of DNA that controls cell replication and function. The Philadelphia chromosome describes the abnormality of a translocation that confirms the diagnosis of CML. It is the switch of part of chromosome 9 to chromosome 22 and part of chromosome 22 to chromosome 9.

Fluorescence in situ hybridization (FISH) is another genetic test that can confirm or rule out a diagnosis. This test detects abnormalities that may be missed on normal karyotyping. Some abnormalities are more favorable than others in terms of prognosis. The Philadelphia chromosome is also found in approximately a third of the cases of ALL. The information about the leukemia cells gained through cytogenetic testing aids oncologists and hematologists in helping patients weigh the chances of recovery against potential risks inherent in chemotherapy. Radiographs, such as X rays, computed tomography (CT) scans, and magnetic resonance images (MRI), may be needed to rule out other conditions or medical problems.

The staging of leukemia differs for each type. For example, a common staging system for AML is the

French-American-British (FAB) system, which uses eight subtypes labeled MO to M7. The World Health Organization's classification is another system used to identify the extent of disease.

CML may cause few or no symptoms initially and may be discovered during a routine doctor visit when blood samples are obtained. CML is diagnosed according to chronic, accelerated, and aggressive phases based on how far the disease has progressed. CLL is diagnosed and monitored through examination of lymphocytes, a type of white blood cell.

Treatment and therapy: Treatment options depend on the type and aggressiveness of the leukemia as well as the patient's age and other health considerations. Severe symptoms, associated with acute leukemia, require immediate hospitalization and treatment. Chemotherapy, radiation, and bone marrow or stem cell transplantation are possible modes of therapy. Chemotherapy is most frequently used and may involve multiple drugs in different combinations, called regimens. Treatments evolve with ongoing research as more is learned about the mechanisms that cause and arrest the disease. Targeted therapies show promise in the treatment of cancer, including some leukemias. The development of imatinib mesylate (Gleevec) has been important for the treatment of CML. This drug works by depressing an enzyme that causes CML to grow.

In the process of killing leukemia cells, normal cells may be affected, causing side effects that must be closely monitored and treated in a health care setting. In acute leukemia, the white cell count may be dangerously high, requiring treatment with hydroxyurea to reduce the number of white cells before treatment for the leukemia begins.

The initial treatment phase of leukemia is called induction and is designed to put the leukemia into remission. When testing shows improvement in the leukemia but diseased cells remain, it is regarded as a partial remission and the patient may be given a second induction. Consolidation or intensification therapy is another treatment step that increases or improves the chance of a cure. It is given after a remission is achieved with induction therapy. Patients may continue to get other drugs during a maintenance phase of treatment that is given to reinforce remission.

A stem cell or bone marrow transplant is the process of replacing diseased cells with normal or disease-free cells and may be an option after remission to prolong survival. An autologous transplant uses an individual's own cells, and an allogeneic transplant involves cells from another person, called a donor. Chemotherapy and sometimes total body irradiation (TBI) are used to clear as much of the disease as possible prior to the transplant. A person diagnosed with leukemia often needs transfusions of whole blood and platelets and other supportive care while undergoing treatment for the leukemia.

Drugs that have shown promise in the laboratory and in preliminary clinical trials with humans may be an option for the treatment of leukemia. These drugs are considered investigational and are available only through participation in a clinical trial. Oncologists and other physicians who treat leukemia can help patients learn if there is a clinical trial option appropriate for a particular diagnosis.

Prognosis, prevention, and outcomes: Preventive strategies include undergoing routine health screenings to check blood counts and avoiding prolonged exposure to chemicals. Outcomes depend on type of leukemia, availability of treatment options, age, and overall state of health. Survival rates are excellent for children with ALL under the age of fifteen, with almost all cases cured. Treatment for the elderly can be limited by the toxic effects of some chemotherapy regimens that are poorly tolerated by individuals in this age group. The prognosis after treatment for ALL is less favorable in patients who have the Philadelphia chromosome. Acute leukemia that goes into remission after treatment is considered cured after five years.

Linda August Vrooman, R.N., B.S.N., O.C.N.

For Further Information

Ball, Edward D., and Gregory A. Lelek. *One Hundred Questions and Answers About Leukemia*. Sudbury, Mass.: Jones and Bartlett, 2003.

Keene, Nancy. *Childhood Leukemia: A Guide for Families, Friends, and Caregivers*. 3d ed. Sebastopol, Calif.: O'Reilly, 2002.

Lackritz, Barbara. *Adult Leukemia: A Comprehensive Guide for Patients and Families*. Sebastopol, Calif.: O'Reilly, 2001.

Sinclair, Alison. "Genetics 101: Cytogenetics and FISH." *Canadian Medical Association Journal* 167 (2002): 373-374.

Other Resources

American Cancer Society
http://www.cancer.org

American Society of Hematology
http://www.hematology.org

The Leukemia and Lymphoma Society
http://www.leukemia-lymphoma.org

National Cancer Institute
http://www.cancer.gov

National Marrow Donor Program
http://www.marrow.org

See also: Acute Lymphocytic Leukemia (ALL); Acute Myelocytic Leukemia (AML); Aleukemia; Amyloidosis; Anemia; Aplastic anemia; Bone marrow aspiration and biopsy; Bone Marrow Transplantation (BMT); Burkitt lymphoma; Chronic Lymphocytic Leukemia (CLL); Chronic Myeloid Leukemia (CML); Cutaneous T-Cell Lymphoma (CTCL); Disseminated Intravascular Coagulation (DIC); Down syndrome and leukemia; Eosinophilic leukemia; Fanconi anemia; 5Q minus syndrome; Hairy cell leukemia; Hemolytic anemia; Hodgkin disease; Human T-cell Leukemia Virus (HTLV); Hypercalcemia; Leukopenia; Leukoplakia; Lymphocytosis; Lymphomas; Multiple myeloma; Myelodysplastic syndromes; Myelofibrosis; Myeloma; Myeloproliferative disorders; Myelosuppression; Neutropenia; Pheresis; Polycythemia vera; Richter syndrome; Sézary syndrome; Stem cell transplantation; Superior vena cava syndrome; Thrombocytopenia; Thymomas; Thymus cancer; Transfusion therapy; Umbilical cord blood transplantation; Waldenström Macroglobulinemia (WM)

▶ Leukoencephalopathy

Category: Diseases, Symptoms, and Conditions
Also known as: Multifocal demyelinating disease, progressive multifocal leukoencephalopathy (PML)

Related conditions: Acute hemorrhagic leukoencephalopathy, leukoencephalopathy with vanishing white matter, multiple sclerosis

Definition: Leukoencephalopathy is a life-threatening, rapidly progressing disease of the nerves and muscles that affects patients who have a suppressed immune system. It is thought to be caused by a reactivated viral infection that changes form to take advantage of a suppressed immune system. In this disease, the myelin sheath, composed of the fatty tissue that forms a protective covering of the nerve fibers (sometimes called white matter), is destroyed.

Risk factors: This disease occurs only in patients who have had their immune systems suppressed by another disease or for medical procedures that depend on a suppressed immune system, such as organ transplant. It is considered to be an opportunistic infection, or one that takes advantage of a suppressed immune system to damage some part of the body or one of its systems.

This disease is also linked to the JC virus (a polyomavirus named with the initials of the first patient to have been diagnosed with this virus), to which more than 80 percent of the general population has been exposed, most likely in childhood. Some studies show that 85 percent of children have been exposed to this virus before the age of nine. However, in most of the population, this virus stays dormant.

This disease is a rare side effect of some types of cancer treatment that suppress the immune system, which may happen with some types of chemotherapy or with certain types of procedures, such as a bone marrow transplant. Cancer patients—particularly those with Hodgkin disease, leukemia, lymphoma, or sarcoidosis—who have received chemotherapy treatment with methotrexate or radiation therapy are at risk of developing this disease. However, the disease is not limited to cancer patients and may be developed by those who have other immunocompromising diseases or factors such as acquired immunodeficiency syndrom (AIDS) or organ transplants. This disease is, in fact, most common in AIDS patients.

Other factors that are thought to increase risk in combination with a suppressed immune system are exposure to toxic substances, injuries, ischemia (a decrease in blood flow to a body part), and some types of metabolic disorders.

Etiology and the disease process: This disease is thought to be caused by activation of the JC virus. Most of the people exposed to this virus never develop the disease, even if they have a suppressed immune system.

The virus lies dormant, mostly in the kidneys, until the immune system is suppressed somehow. In cancer patients, this suppression is usually through radiation or chemotherapy as part of a treatment strategy, but patients with AIDS or those who have had organ transplants may also get this disease because treatment involves suppressing the immune system. The virus becomes active, taking advantage of the suppressed immune system, and changes into a form that is able to attack the brain. It begins destroying, or perhaps interfering with the formation of, the myelin sheath. The myelin sheath is the fatty substance that covers and protects the nerve fibers in the brain and spinal column. Like other myelin-attacking diseases, such as multiple sclerosis (MS), the process by which the myelin is destroyed is not completely understood.

This loss of the myelin protective sheath keeps nerve signals from traveling to the rest of the body. Other abnormalities or cell growths may also begin to occur in the brain, and these complications further damage healthy brain cells. This eventually leads to progressive loss of muscle coordination and mental dysfunction. These symptoms are extremely varied and depend on the location (where in the brain or spinal column) and the severity (how deep or wide) of the damage to the myelin sheath. Eventually, this disease results in seizures and coma before death. The patient usually dies within a year of diagnosis.

Incidence: This disease occurs only in patients with a suppressed immune system. Even in those patients, only a very small number of people will develop this disease. Only about 5 percent of people living with AIDS will develop this disease; the incidence for cancer patients is even less. However, the incidence of this disease is rising, as more people with cancers that are being treated in ways that suppress the immune system are surviving longer. It is classified as a rare disease by the National Institutes of Health Office of Rare Diseases. This means that this disease affects less than 200,000 people in the entire population of the United States. This number includes patients with AIDS as well as cancer patients.

Symptoms: Symptoms include clumsiness, difficulty walking, facial weakness, fatigue, headaches, loss of muscle coordination, loss of appetite, loss of speech, memory failure, mental dysfunction or deterioration, paralysis on one side of the body, partial or total blindness (sometimes affecting half of the vision in each eye), seizures, slow movements, stammering, stuttering, and weakness. Symptoms may vary greatly because they depend on where in the brain or spinal column the myelin sheath is being destroyed and how much damage has been done.

Screening and diagnosis: There is no screening test or staging developed for this disease. Diagnosis can be uncertain at first. The disease is suspected in patients with compromised immune systems who develop unexplained brain dysfunction. Magnetic resonance imaging (MRI) or computed tomography (CT) scans may suggest this disease by showing lesions or sores on the myelin or white matter in the brain or spinal column. Spinal fluid may be analyzed to determine if the JC virus is present, which can help strengthen a diagnosis. Blood tests are not helpful in diagnosing this disease; there is no effect on the blood, only on the nerves and muscles.

The only sure diagnosis is done by stereotaxic biopsy (a special type of removal of tissue using a computer and a three-dimensional scanning device) of the brain tissue in the affected area. However, this type of biopsy is not generally warranted for this disease because a brain biopsy is a high-risk procedure, especially for those with an already compromised immune system. Generally, the diagnosis of the disease is made by observing by its rapid progression with symptoms becoming more pronounced and widespread.

Treatment and therapy: No treatment or therapy currently exists to reliably cure this disease. Antiviral medications may help by reducing the viral load in the body, increasing the body's T-cell count and generally improving the immune system. However, these medications often have toxic side effects or are not tolerated well by patients, particularly those who already have suppressed immune systems.

Sometimes, other attempts are made to slow the progress of this disease—for example, altering chemotherapy or removing nonvital transplanted organs so that immune-suppressing drug therapy can be stopped—but these treatments have, at best, inconclusive results. Treatment is generally supportive, which means that the treatment attempts to reduce the severity of the symptoms and make a patient as comfortable as possible without truly addressing the main cause of the disease.

Prognosis, prevention, and outcomes: There is no cure for leukoencephalopathy, nor is there any way to prevent the disease other than attempts to keep the immune system healthy and functioning properly.

Prognosis and outcomes are very poor, with most patients (80 percent) dying within six months to a year of diagnosis. Those who survive this disease (about 20 percent) are often left with severe disabilities, both mental and physical.

Marianne M. Madsen, M.S.

For Further Information

Icon Health. *The Official Patient's Sourcebook on Progressive Multifocal Leukoencephalopathy: A Revised and Updated Directory for the Internet Age.* San Diego, Calif.: Author, 2003.

St. Georgiev, Vassel. *Infectious Diseases in Immunocompromised Hosts.* Boca Raton, Fla.: CRC Press, 1998.

Uziel, G., and F. Taroni, eds. *Hereditary Leukoencephalop*athies and Demyelinating Neuropathies in Children. Eastleigh, England: John Libbey Eurotext Ltd, 2004.

Other Resources

Cleveland Clinic Center for Consumer Health Information

Progressive Multifocal Leukoencephalopathy
http://www.clevelandclinic.org/health/health-info/docs/1300/1322.asp?index=6101

Merck Online Medical Library
Progressive Multifocal Leukoencephalopathy
http://www.merck.com/mmpe/sec16/ch217/ch217f.html#sec16-ch217-ch217f-1055

National Institute of Neurological Disorders and Stroke
Progressive Multifocal Leukoencephalopathy
http://www.ninds.nih.gov/disorders/pml/pml.htm

See also: Cognitive effects of cancer and chemotherapy; HIV/AIDS-related cancers; Oligodendrogliomas

▶ Leukopenia

Category: Diseases, Symptoms, and Conditions
Also known as: Neutropenia, low white blood cell count, leucopenia

Related conditions: Neutropenia, which is a subset of leukopenia

Definition: Leukopenia is an abnormally low number of white blood cells, or leukocytes. The laboratory standard measurement of leukocytes ranges from approximately $(4.0 \text{ to } 11.0) \times 10^9$ per liter.

Risk factors: Leukopenia may be related to use of certain drugs (such as barbiturates and chemotherapeutics), radiation therapy, bone marrow or stem cell transplant, severe infections, or bone marrow diseases such as leukemia, myelodysplastic syndromes, acquired immunodeficiency syndrome (AIDS), aplastic anemia, or lupus. Patients older than the age of seventy and those with comorbid diseases, such as diabetes, are at great risk for leukopenia during chemotherapy.

Etiology and the disease process: Chemotherapy and radiation therapy for cancer target the rapidly dividing cancer cells as well as other rapidly dividing cells, that is, hematopoietic stem cells. It takes about ten days for a new leukocyte to differentiate and mature from a hematopoietic stem cell, which means that a patient receiving chemotherapy or radiation therapy can have a low number of leukocytes for days. The role of leukocytes is to safeguard against infection by destroying bacteria. Leukopenia and its associated impaired immunity make a patient more susceptible to infections and may lead to septicemia. Untreated, leukopenia may require hospitalization and use of intravenous anti-infective drugs.

Incidence: Most patients who are receiving chemotherapy, radiation therapy, or a bone marrow transplant experience leukopenia, and very often chemotherapy must be delayed because of it.

Symptoms: Symptoms include recurrent infections, high-grade fever and chills, and diarrhea.

Screening and diagnosis: Leukopenia is defined as a leukocyte count less than approximately 4.0×10^9per liter. Mild leukopenia is defined as a leukocyte count of $(1.0 \text{ to } 2.0) \times 10^9$per liter, and severe as a leukocyte count less than 0.5×10^9per liter. Leukopenia is determined by a blood test.

Treatment and therapy: At this time, white blood cell transfusions are not a treatment option, primarily because of the abbreviated life span of a leukocyte, which is estimated to be between twenty-four and forty-eight hours. Most patients with leukopenia receive hematopoietic growth factors such as filgrastim (Neupoegen), pegfilgrastim (Neulasta), or sargramostim (Leukine) to increase the number of circulating white blood cells.

Prognosis, prevention, and outcomes: Hematopoietic growth factors are the standard for treatment of severe leukopenia at many cancer centers and can rapidly, within hours in some cases, increase leukocyte counts. Left untreated, the patient is at risk for serious and possibly life-threatening infections.

MaryAnn Foote, M.S., Ph.D.

See also: Antineoplastics in chemotherapy; Aplastic anemia; Azathioprine; Candidiasis; Chemotherapy; Colony-stimulating factors (CSFs); Fever; Immunotherapy; Infection and sepsis; Lymphocytosis; Myelosuppression; Neutropenia; Side effects; Thrombocytopenia; Topoisomerase inhibitors; Young adult cancers

▶ Leukoplakia

Category: Diseases, Symptoms, and Conditions
Also known as: Smoker's keratosis

Related conditions: Erythroplakia and hairy leukoplakia

Definition: Leukoplakia is a whitish precancerous lesion found on the mucous membranes of the mouth and tongue that cannot easily be scraped off.

Risk factors: Tobacco use (smoking, chewing, snuff), long-term alcohol use, and chronic irritation of the gums or cheeks from poor dental work increase the risk of developing leukoplakia.

Etiology and the disease process: The grayish-white patches that characterize leukoplakia grow slowly. They begin as smooth plaques, then gradually become rough, wrinkled, and hard. The cells in these plaques often show precancerous changes and may progress to oral cancer.

Hairy leukoplakia is a related, noncancerous condition caused by infection with the Epstein-Barr virus. It is common in people infected with human immunodeficiency virus (HIV) and does not develop into oral cancer. Erythroplakia is a rough, red, precancerous lesion. Sometimes erythroplakia and leukoplakia are found in mixed plaques.

Incidence: Fewer than 1 percent of adults have leukoplakia. It occurs most often in men over the age of forty.

Symptoms: The main symptom is a whitish growth inside the mouth. Lesions are painless but may be sensitive to spicy foods or to touch. Precancerous leukoplakia lesions develop hard surfaces, while hairy leukoplakia growths are fuzzy.

Screening and diagnosis: Most cases of leukoplakia are found during dental visits. When a suspect white patch appears in the mouth, a tissue sample (biopsy) is taken to determine whether the patch shows signs of cancer. A few cells may be collected using a spinning brush, or the entire lesion may be removed. The sample is examined under the microscope for cancer and to rule out other possible causes, such as a fungal infection.

Treatment and therapy: Individuals with leukoplakia should stop using tobacco products. If no cancer cells are found in the biopsy, the lesion may be observed for several months or it may be removed. Many lesions disappear without treatment once tobacco use is stopped. Medications derived from vitamin A and vitamin E have been used to shrink leukoplakia plaques, but these drugs have significant negative side effects.

If abnormal cells are present in the biopsy, the lesion is removed either surgically or by using a laser or very cold probe that freezes and destroys the cells.

Prognosis, prevention, and outcomes: In about 3 to 5 percent of people, leukoplakia progresses to oral cancer. In many cases, leukoplakia disappears spontaneously. Avoiding tobacco, especially smokeless tobacco products, is the most effective way to prevent leukoplakia.

Martiscia Davidson, A.M.

See also: Alcohol, alcoholism, and cancer; Chewing tobacco; Cigarettes and cigars; Epidermoid cancers of mucous membranes; Erythroplakia; Head and neck cancers; Keratosis; Lip cancers; Oral and oropharyngeal cancers; Prevention; Smoking cessation; Tobacco-related cancers

▶ Leydig cell tumors

Category: Diseases, Symptoms, and Conditions
Also known as: Testicular tumors, interstitial cell tumors

Related conditions: Sertoli-Leydig cell tumors

Definition: Leydig cell tumors are a rare type of testicular (or, rarely, ovarian) tumor. They arise from the Leydig cells, which produce testosterone and other male hormones in the testicles. Most often these tumors are benign, but they can sometimes be cancerous.

Risk factors: There are no known risks for this condition; however, it is much more common in men than in women.

Etiology and the disease process: The cause of Leydig cell tumors is unknown, but animal studies have suggested that these tumors may grow following exposure to the female hormone estrogen. Leydig cell tumors secrete testosterone and sometimes estrogen.

Incidence: This condition is most common in men between the ages of thirty and sixty, although it can occur in prepubescent boys and in women (in the ovaries). Only 1 to 3 percent of all testicular tumors are Leydig cell tumors. In about 3 percent of men who develop Leydig cell tumors, the tumors are found in both testicles. Only about 10 percent of Leydig cell tumors are cancerous.

Symptoms: Boys who develop Leydig cell tumors can develop feminine symptoms such as breast tenderness or nipple soreness, and they often go into early puberty. In men, the symptoms more commonly include erectile dysfunction, decreased sexual drive, and infertility. Women with Leydig cell tumors may develop masculine characteristics, such as excessive hair growth and increased muscle mass.

Screening and diagnosis: The doctor will feel the testicles to check for an enlarged mass. An ultrasound can confirm the diagnosis. Blood tests can be used to identify elevated testosterone and estrogen levels. Liver function tests are sometimes performed on patients who have cancerous Leydig cell tumors.

Treatment and therapy: Most Leydig cell tumors can be treated with surgery to remove the tumor. Malignant Leydig cell tumors can be treated with surgery, but they do not tend to respond well to chemotherapy or radiation.

Prognosis, prevention, and outcomes: The prognosis for people with benign Leydig cell tumors is excellent, because surgery can usually treat the problem. However, those with malignant tumors have an average survival rate of only two years.

Stephanie Watson, B.S.

See also: Germ-cell tumors; Infertility and cancer; Orchiectomy; Sertoli cell tumors; Spermatocytomas; Teratocarcinomas; Testicular cancer; Testicular Self-Examination (TSE); Urologic oncology

▶ Li-Fraumeni Syndrome (LFS)

Category: Diseases, Symptoms, and Conditions

Related conditions: Li-Fraumeni-like syndrome (LFL), soft-tissue sarcoma, breast cancer, leukemia, adrenal gland (SBLA) syndrome

Definition: Li-Fraumeni syndrome (LFS) is a genetic abnormality that predisposes individuals to developing cancer at an early age and to developing multiple primary cancers during their lifetime.

Risk factors: About 70 percent of the time, Li-Fraumeni syndrome develops because of a mutation (change) in the deoxyribonucleic acid (DNA) of the *TP53* gene (also called *p53*) on chromosome 17. This gene can be inherited from either parent, and the mutation is present in all cells in the body. Changes in another gene, *CHEK2* (also called *CHK2*), on chromosome 17 and spontaneous (noninherited) changes in these genes account for the remaining 30 percent of individuals with LFS. People who have a mutation causing LFS have a 50 percent chance of passing this mutation to their children whether or not they develop cancer.

Etiology and the disease process: *TP53* is a tumor-suppressor gene. A normal *TP53* controls cell growth and cell death. When it mutates, it loses the ability to regulate cell growth, allowing cells to grow wildly and become malignant. The *CHEK2* gene controls another step in the regulation of cell growth, but when it mutates, the result is the same.

People inherit one copy of *TP53* from each parent. In Li-Fraumeni syndrome, one copy of *TP53* is normal, and the other has mutated. This, in itself, does not cause cancer, because both copies of the gene must be mutated for cancer to occur. However, a mutation in the second copy of the gene is common. Researchers do not understand what triggers this second mutation.

The type of cancer a person gets depends on which type of cell in the body develops the second mutation. The most common types of cancer for people with LFS are breast cancer, soft-tissue sarcomas (cancer arising in cartilage, muscle, fat, or blood vessels), leukemia, osteosarcoma (bone cancer), malignant melanoma, and cancer of the brain, pancreas, esophagus, adrenal cortex, and colon. People with LFS are also at higher risk of developing more than one type of primary cancer during their life, especially if they develop and are cured of a childhood cancer.

Incidence: Li-Fraumeni syndrome appears to be rare. Only about 400 families have been identified as having the mutation. However, the ability to screen for this mutation is relatively new, so the incidence is not well defined. Men and women are equally affected, as are all races and ethnicities.

Although LFS is rare (it is, for example, thought to account for only 1 percent of breast cancer cases), for people who have this condition, the chances of developing cancer are staggeringly high. Various studies have found the following to be true:

- Only about 10 percent of individuals who develop cancer in the general population are diagnosed before age forty-five, while more than 50 percent of people with LFS develop cancer before this age.
- About 85-90 percent of people with LFS develop cancer by age sixty.
- About 40 percent of people with LFS develop cancer before age sixteen.
- About 15 percent of people with LFS whose cancer is cured develop a second primary cancer. Some 4 percent develop a third cancer and 2 percent a fourth cancer.
- People who develop cancer before age sixteen are at highest risk of developing multiple primary cancers.

Symptoms: Li-Fraumeni syndrome has no symptoms. Cancer symptoms depend on the type of cancer the individual develops.

Screening and diagnosis: People are formally diagnosed with Li-Fraumeni syndrome when they meet all three of the following conditions:

- They are diagnosed with sarcoma before age forty-five.
- A biological parent, sibling, or child is diagnosed with any cancer before age forty-five.

• A parent, sibling, child, grandparent, aunt, uncle, niece, or nephew related by blood is diagnosed with any cancer before age forty-five or a sarcoma at any age.

With genetic screening it is possible to detect about 95 percent of *TP53* mutations that cause LFS. Genetic screening is controversial. It is normally offered only when a close blood relative is diagnosed with LFS. Screening should be accompanied by genetic counseling, so that individuals can make informed decisions about their future and the risks of passing this mutation on to any children they might have. Prenatal screening is possible through chorionic villi sampling or amniocentesis. Researchers have found, however, that as many as 60 percent of eligible relatives do not consent to screening for LFS.

Treatment and therapy: No treatment can prevent or reverse this mutation. Cancers are treated as they arise.

Prognosis, prevention, and outcomes: Li-Fraumeni syndrome strongly predisposes individuals to develop cancer at an early age. Individuals who know they come from a family with LFS are encouraged to have complete annual physical examinations and to get prompt medical care for any symptoms that may be an early warning of cancer. Outcomes depend on the type of cancer the individual develops and how soon it is treated.

Martiscia Davidson, A.M.

For Further Information

Field, S. S. Shanley, and J. Kirk. "Inherited Cancer Susceptibility Syndromes in Paediatric Practice." *Journal of Paediatrics and Child Health* 43, no. 4 (April, 2007): 219-229.

Hottinger, A. F., and Y. Khakoo. "Update on the Management of Familial Central Nervous System Tumor Syndromes." *Current Neurology and Neuroscience Reports* 7, no. 3 (May, 2007): 200-207.

Lalloo, Fiona, ed. *Risk Assessment and Management in Cancer Genetics*. New York: Oxford University Press, 2005.

Strahm, B., and D. Malkin. "Hereditary Cancer Predisposition in Children: Genetic Basis and Clinical Implications." *International Journal of Cancer* 119, no. 9 (November 1, 2006): 2001-2006.

Other Resources

Genetics Home Reference
Li-Fraumeni Syndrome
http://ghr.nlm.nih.gov/condition=lifraumenisyndrome

Stanford Cancer Center
Li-Fraumeni Syndrome
http://cancer.stanford.edu/information/geneticsAndCancer/types/lifrmni/

See also: Adrenal gland cancers; Adrenocortical cancer; Astrocytomas; Bone cancers; Brain and central nervous system cancers; Breast cancers; Childhood cancers; Family history and risk assessment; Fibrosarcomas, soft-tissue; Genetic testing; Leukemias; Mediastinal tumors; Mutagenesis and cancer; Neuroectodermal tumors; Rhabdomyosarcomas; Sarcomas, soft-tissue; TP53 protein

▶ Lip cancers

Category: Diseases, Symptoms, and Conditions

Related conditions: Other oral or skin cancers

Definition: Lip cancers are malignant tumors that form in the surface layer cells of the upper or lower lip. Though lip cancers are generally similar to skin cancers, they are often grouped with oral cancers.

Risk factors: Smoking, especially smoking a pipe or cigar, and exposure to sunlight are the two best-documented risk factors for lip cancers. According to some studies, 90 percent of people who have any type of oral cancer smoke.

The aging process itself is also a risk factor; as lip cells age and change, they are more susceptible to cancer cell generation. These factors (smoking, exposure to sunlight, and the aging process) may all work in combination to increase risk. Alcohol consumption is a risk factor for developing other types of oral cancer (about 75 percent of patients with any type of oral cancer drink alcohol frequently) and may contribute to lip cancers as well.

Other risk factors include viral infection (especially with the human papillomavirus, or HPV), poor oral hygiene, a suppressed immune system (often due to organ transplant treatment), or vitamin deficiency.

Etiology and the disease process: Lip cancers almost always (about 90 percent of the time) originate in the flat skin cells (squamous cells) that form the outside covering layer of the lips. These cancers behave like skin cancers. The other 10 percent of lip cancers are basal cell carcinomas or melanomas.

This type of cancer begins with a sore, usually a bleeding sore that does not heal. If not treated, this cancer may move into other portions of the mouth, such as the tongue and the mucous membranes inside the lips. The next spread of the cancer may be into the lymph nodes, and the cancer may spread even farther into other areas of the body. Generally, cancers that begin in the upper lip (about 60 percent of all lip cancers) are more aggressive than those that originate in the bottom lip and may be more likely to spread.

Incidence: Most people (around 90 percent) who develop lip cancers are over the age of forty-five, and as age increases, this type of cancer is even more likely. Men are more likely (up to two to three times) than women to get this cancer. Fair-skinned people are also more likely than those with darker skin to develop lip cancer. About 13 out of 100,000 people in the United States will be diagnosed with lip cancers. The incidence of lip cancers is increasing, especially among women. This is thought to be because people are exposing themselves to the sun more often without using sunscreen, or perhaps because people are less likely to wear a hat as sun protection.

Symptoms: Symptoms include lumps, sores, or white spots on the lips, particularly a bleeding or open sore that does not heal in a reasonable time. Lumps or white spots may or may not be painful. Pain may also be felt in a lymph node near the lip area. Nearly 40 percent of lip cancers begin in the lower lip.

Screening and diagnosis: Dentists often perform a screening for lip and other oral cancers at a regular dental checkup by examining the lips and mouth for suspicious symptoms. X rays may also help spot a lip cancer.

Noncancerous sores, lumps, and white spots often occur on the lips, and lip cancer may resemble these conditions. Because of this, biopsy (removing a small piece of tissue and examining it under a microscope for cancerous cells) is the generally preferred method of diagnosis.

Staging of lip cancer is broken into four parts based on how large the tumor or sore is and how far the cancer has spread.

- Stage I: The tumor is less than 2 centimeters (cm) and has not spread.
- Stage II: The tumor is more than 2 cm but less than 5 cm and has not spread.
- Stage III: The tumor is larger than 4 cm, or the tumor is any size and the cancer has spread to a lymph node in the neck on the side that the cancer is located with the lymph node being no more than 3 cm.
- Stage IV: The cancer has spread to the mouth or other areas around the lip (with or without lymph node involvement); the cancer is any size and has spread to more than one lymph node on the same side of the neck, has spread to lymph nodes on both sides of the neck, or has spread to any lymph node that measures more than 6 cm; or the cancer is any size and has spread to other parts of the body.

Stage at Diagnosis and Five-Year Relative Survival Rates for Lip Cancers, 1988-2001

Stage	*Cases Diagnosed (%)*	*Survival Rate (%)*
Stage I	83.2	96.3
Stage II	5.5	82.7
Stage III	1.5	56.7
Stage IV	2.2	48.1
Unstaged	7.6	88.3

Source: Data from L. A. G. Ries et al., eds., Cancer Survival Among Adults: U.S. SEER Program, 1988-2001—Patient and Tumor Characteristics, NIH Pub. No. 07-6215 (Bethesda, Md.: National Cancer Institute, 2007)

Treatment and therapy: Surgery is generally the first line of treatment for lip cancer, especially in Stages I and II. Chemotherapy (using chemicals in the bloodstream to kill cancer cells) or radiation therapy (using high-energy rays to focus on and kill cancer cells) may also be necessary depending on whether the cancer has spread. Chemotherapy or radiation therapy may also be used before surgery to shrink a tumor. In Stages III and IV, the lymph nodes affected by the cancer are also surgically removed.

Some other types of treatment may be possible depending on the size or extent of the cancer. These types of treatment may involve freezing or burning the cancerous cells on the lips or using chemicals in an acid, cream, solution, or ointment applied to the lips to kill the cancerous cells.

Surgical treatment of this type of cancer always takes into consideration the patient's ability to eat and speak following tissue removal. If treatment of a lip cancer involves surgical removal, reconstructive surgery may be needed. Even with reconstructive surgery, however, there may be significant changes in eating and speaking abilities, especially if muscle tissue is removed. Occupational or speech therapy may improve those functions.

Other treatment may involve counseling for issues dealing with scars or disfigurement from the surgery. Patients may need to work with a nutritionist to ensure proper nutrition and eating habits after surgery or during radiation therapy, when the lips and mouth may be sore, making eating difficult.

A promising treatment for lip cancer therapy is hyperthermia, a process that uses heat to kill cancer cells. In this type of therapy, a special machine heats the body for a certain amount of time. Cancer cells are often more sensitive to heat than healthy cells, so this treatment may kill the cancer while leaving healthy cells intact. This type of therapy may also be combined with other types of therapy, such as freezing or burning the cancer cells.

Prognosis, prevention, and outcomes: Quitting smoking is the most effective prevention for any type of oral cancer. Quitting pipe smoking is helpful for lip cancer in particular, as it is more closely associated with lip cancer. It is thought that the heat of the pipe stem on the lips increases the likelihood of cancer developing on the lips.

Other preventive measures include avoiding sun exposure, using lip balm or lipstick with an sun protection factor (SPF) rating of 15 or more, limiting use of alcohol, and increasing consumption of fruits and vegetables.

Prognosis and outcomes are very good for patients when lip cancer is discovered early, especially in Stage I or II, and the cancer is squamous-cell based, with survival rates of over 90 percent. If the cancer is at Stage III or IV when discovered, survival rates fall to about 50 percent. Survival rates for those with lip cancers that are carcinoma based are about 10 to 20 percent less than the squamous-based survival rates.

Early identification and diagnosis of lip cancer have improved prognosis. Only about 112 individuals die from this cancer each year in the United States.

Marianne M. Madsen, M.S.

For Further Information

Brockstein, Bruce, and Gregory Masters, eds. *Head and Neck Cancer*. Boston: Kluwer Academic, 2003.

"Disorders of the Oral Region: Neoplasms." In *The Merck Manual of Diagnosis and Therapy*, edited by Mark H. Beers and Robert Berkow. 17th ed. Whitehouse Station, N.Y.: Merck Research Laboratories, 1999.

Scully, Crispian, et al. *Dermatology of the Lips*. Oxford, England: Isis Medical Media, 2000.

Other Resources

National Cancer Institute

Lip and Oral Cavity Cancer Treatment

http://www.cancer.gov/cancertopics/pdq/treatment/lip-and-oral-cavity/patient

Support for People with Oral and Head and Neck Cancer

http://www.spohnc.org

See also: Chewing tobacco; Cigarettes and cigars; Epidermoid cancers of mucous membranes; Erythroplakia; Head and neck cancers; Hyperthermia therapy; Leukoplakia; Oral and maxillofacial surgery; Oral and oropharyngeal cancers; Risks for cancer; Skin cancers; Symptoms and cancer; Tobacco-related cancers

▶ Liposarcomas

Category: Diseases, Symptoms, and Conditions
Also known as: Soft-tissue liposarcomas

Related conditions: Soft-tissue sarcomas

Definition: Liposarcomas are the second most common malignant soft-tissue sarcomas in adults after malignant fibrous histiocytoma (MFH). Liposarcoma, a mesenchymal sarcoma, accounts for between 12 and 18 percent of all malignant soft-tissue tumors and usually manifests as a nonspecific soft-tissue mass. Frequently the fat it contains is not radiographically detectable. Liposarcoma demonstrates a wide range of manifestations and prognoses, ranging from a well-differentiated nonmetastasizing neoplasm with good prognosis to a high-grade sarcoma with hematogenous metatastases to the lung and the visceral organs.

Risk factors: A relationship to trauma has been reported. The myxoid and round-cell type of liposarcoma are associated with a reciprocal translocation between chromosomes 12 and 16.

Etiology and the disease process: Liposarcoma is a malignant tumor of mesenchymal origin with the microscopic appearance of adipose tissue, although in some cases it does not contain visible fat. It is made up of several cell types. The well-differentiated type of liposarcoma, which has the best prognosis, has mature lipocytes with varying degrees of nuclear atypia. It is seen in only 15 percent of cases. The most common type, accounting for 40 to 50 percent of all liposarcomas, is the myxoid type, which is composed of proliferating fibroblasts with less than 10 percent fat. This type of tumor often metastasizes to serosal and pleural surfaces, subcutaneous tissue, and bone. The pleomorphic type is seen in approximately 20 percent of cases and

Stage at Diagnosis and Five-Year Relative Survival Rates for Liposarcoma, 1988-2001

Stage	*Cases Diagnosed (%)*	*Survival Rate (%)*
Localized[a]	65.9	90.9
Regional[b]	21.3	74.4
Distant[c]	5.7	30.8
Unstaged	7.1	70.1

Source: Data from L. A. G. Ries et al., eds., Cancer Survival Among Adults: U.S. SEER Program, 1988-2001—Patient and Tumor Characteristics, NIH Pub. No. 07-6215 (Bethesda, Md.: National Cancer Institute, 2007)

[a]Cancer still confined to primary site

[b]Cancer has spread to regional lymph nodes or directly beyond the primary site

[c]Cancer has metastasized

is a highly anaplastic tumor with pleomorphic (many sized and shaped) cells growing in a disorderly fashion. The round-cell type is seen in less than 10 percent of cases, is poorly differentiated, and is often associated with hemorrhage and necrosis. It is highly cellular, composed of primitive small round cells. Retroperitoneal liposarcoma is a slow-growing variant that rarely metastasizes and usually displaces rather than infiltrates or invades surrounding tissues.

Incidence: Liposarcomas represent between 12 and 18 percent of all malignant soft-tissue tumors, and annually 2.5 cases occur per 1 million population.

Symptoms: Liposarcoma usually manifests as a large, painless mass between 2 and 30 centimeters (cm) in size, associated with weight loss in a patient between the ages of fifty and sixty. It is slightly more common in men than in women. Liposarcoma can be painful in 15 percent of patients because of the compression of the adjacent neurovascular bundle or adjacent abdominal organs. Retroperitoneal tumors can weigh several pounds.

Screening and diagnosis: Liposarcomas are best diagnosed by magnetic resonance imaging (MRI) with gadolinium intravenous contrast. The tumor appears as a large hypervascular septated mass containing fat and soft tissue. In contradistinction to a lipoma, liposarcoma enhances with intravenous contrast. Liposarcoma can have large areas of necrosis and hemorrhage and can be located in the trunk or retroperitoneum in approximately 42 percent of cases, in the lower extremities in 41 percent of cases, in the upper extremities 11 percent of the time, and in the head and neck in 6 percent of cases, with predilection for the thigh and retroperitoneum. The more differentiated the tumor, the closer the signal characteristics of the tumor approach that of fat. Myxoid and pleomorphic tumors may demonstrate little or no fat on computed tomography (CT) scans. On nuclear medicine positron emission tomography (PET) scans, the tumor is fluorodeoxyglucose (FDG) avid.

According to the World Health Organization classification, liposarcoma includes well-differentiated, myxoid, pleomorphic, and round-cell types, with the most common type being the myxoid type (50 percent of all liposarcomas). Myxoid liposarcoma can appear benign on MRIs. These gelatinous lesions can demonstrate a cyst-like appearance. High-grade liposarcoma often contains no recognizable fat and as such is indistinguishable from other soft-tissue malignancies.

As with most malignant musculoskeletal tumors, surgical staging depends on pathology, compartmentalization, and presence or absence of metastases:

- Stage Ia: Low grade, intracompartmental
- Stage Ib: Low grade, extracompartmental
- Stage IIa: High grade, intracompartmental
- Stage IIb: High grade, extracompartmental
- Stage IIIa: Low or high grade, intracompartmental, presence of metastases
- Stage IIIb: Low or high grade, extracompartmental, presence of metastases

Treatment and therapy: The treatment depends on the stage at diagnosis. Stage I lesions are handled with surgical resection with wide margins. Stage II lesions are treated with more radical resection, possible amputation, and radiation therapy. Therapy for Stage III lesions includes surgical resection with radiation and chemotherapy.

Prognosis, prevention, and outcomes: The well-differentiated type of liposarcoma has the best prognosis, with overall five-year survival rates exceeding 80 percent. However, even with the well-differentiated type, there can be local recurrence. The well-differentiated type rarely metastasizes, unlike the pleomorphic and round-cell types, which metastasize and have a five-year survival rate of only 50 percent. A size greater than 15 centimeters connotes a poor prognosis. Retroperitoneal liposarcoma is the most radiosensitive of all soft-tissue sarcomas, with an overall five-year survival of 32 percent.

Debra B. Kessler, M.D., Ph.D.

For Further Information

Bergquist, Thomas H. *MRI of the Musculoskeletal System.* 4th ed. Philadelphia: Lippincott Williams & Wilkins, 2001.

Kumar, Vinay, et al., eds. *Robbins and Cotran Pathologic Basis of Disease.* Philadelphia: Elsevier Saunders, 2005.

Stoller, David W. *Magnetic Resonance Imaging in Orthopedics and Sports Medicine.* Philadelphia: J. B. Lippincott, 1993.

Stoller, David W., et al. *Diagnostic Imaging: Orthopedics.* Salt Lake City, Utah: Amirsys, 2006.

Other Resources

The Liddy Shriver Sarcoma Initiative

Liposarcoma
http://liddyshriversarcomainitiative.org/Newsletters/V01N05/Liposarcoma/liposarcoma.htm

Sarcoma Foundation of America

http://www.curesarcoma.org/

See also: Afterloading radiation therapy; Agent Orange; Alveolar soft-part sarcomas; Fibrosarcomas, soft-tissue; Hemangiosarcomas; Hyperthermic perfusion; Magnetic Resonance Imaging (MRI); Malignant Fibrous Histiocytoma (MFH); Malignant tumors; Mesenchymomas, malignant; Sarcomas, soft-tissue; Synovial sarcomas

▶ Liver cancers

Category: Diseases, Symptoms, and Conditions
Also known as: Hepatocellular carcinoma (HCC), malignanat hepatoma, silent disease

Related conditions: Hepatoblastoma, bile duct cancer, angiosarcoma

Definition: Liver cancer is a condition in which the liver develops tumors both internally and externally, with severe disruptions to its normal functioning. When tumors develop as a result of mutations in liver cells (called hepatocytes), the result is primary liver cancer. Liver cancer also occurs as a result of tumors developing in other parts of the body and migrating to the liver through a process called metastasis (secondary liver cancer).

Risk factors: A number of factors are considered potential risks for the development and metastasis of liver cancer.

- Chronic liver infections: Certain types of viruses such as hepatitis B (HBV) and hepatitis C (HCV) invade liver cells and induce chronic liver infections. Of these, HBV infection is more common in South Asia and in Africa, while HCV infection is more prevalent in Japan and the Western countries. HBV infection is acquired at birth and becomes persistent because of exposure to certain substances such as aflatoxins, while HCV infection occurs mainly because of contaminated blood and is spread through intravenous drug usage. People diagnosed with chronic liver infections face the highest risk for developing liver cancers.
- Cirrhosis: When liver cells become heavily damaged, often because of drug or alcohol abuse, a condition called cirrhosis arises. Cirrhosis is the cause of tumor development in 5 percent of liver cancers.
- Aflatoxins: Aflatoxins are produced by some molds and are formed commonly in nuts, corn, and grains. Aflatoxin B^1 is a major environmental factor in inducing hepatocellular carcinoma. Evidence shows that aflatoxins can induce mutations in certain beneficial genes called tumor-suppressor genes and activate the Wnt signaling pathway (a family of cell-signaling molecules) leading to hepatocellular carcinoma.
- Race, gender, and age: The highest prevalence of liver cancer is seen in Southeast Asia (particularly in Vietnam) and sub-Saharan Africa. Men are twice as likely to have the disease as women. In the United States, African Americans are more prone to develop hepatocellular carcinoma. People above the age of sixty also have a higher probability of developing liver cancer.
- Chemicals: Exposure to chemicals such as arsenic and polyvinyl chloride (PVC) poses a risk for development of liver cancer.
- Genetic factors: Certain genetic disorders such as hemochromatosis and Wilson disease predispose individuals to hepatocellular carcinoma.
- Diabetes mellitus: There is increasing evidence to show a correlation between hepatocellular carcinoma and diabetes mellitus.

Etiology and the disease process: Primary liver cancer, like most cancers, commences with a cell that undergoes disruptive mutations affecting normal growth and death processes. These mutations occur primarily through specific interactions between viral infections and chemicals such as aflatoxins. Chronic liver infections with the hepatitis B virus cause inflammation of the liver, resulting in the release of free radicals, chemokines, and cytokines. In high concentrations, these are capable of damaging deoxyribonucleic acid (DNA), resulting in mutations of genes. Viral infections also result in upregulation (an increase in the number of receptors on target cells) of certain proinflammatory cytokines (proteins secreted by the immune system) such as tumor necrosis factor-alpha (TNFα), interferons (IFNs), and interleukins (ILs). Such changes induce DNA damage, rapidly resulting in mutations of specific genes involved in cancer, called tumor-suppressor genes.

A tumor-suppressor gene that has been extensively implicated in many types of cancers, including liver cancers is *TP53*. Mutations in the *TP53* gene result in either prevention of damaged proteins from undergoing apoptosis or blockade of cell-cycle checkpoint controls. These effects result in uncontrolled growth of mutated cells, ultimately leading to tumor formation. Tumors then establish themselves by developing new blood vessels and deriving oxygen and nutrients from their environment.

In patients with cirrhosis, liver cancer starts with the development of small nodules called dysplastic nodules. These are distinct structures and can be easily distinguished from surrounding normal cells by their size, color, or texture. Transforming growth factor-alpha (TGFα) and insulin growth factor 2 (IGF-2) are some of the cytokines that are released during this phase, triggering extensive proliferation of hepatocytes.

Incidence: Liver cancer is the most rapidly growing cancer in the United States and the fifth most common malignancy around the world. It is the third most common cause of cancer-related deaths. According to studies by the National Cancer Institute based on data from 2000 to 2004, the incidence rate for liver cancer in the United States is higher for men than for women. The age-adjusted mortality rate was 7.1 per 100,000 people per year for men and 3.1 per 100,000 for women. The overall five-year survival rate from 1996 to 2003 was 10.8 percent. In 2007, new cases of liver cancer were estimated to reach about 13,650 in men and 5,510 in women, and deaths from liver cancer were estimated at 11,280 men and 5,500 women.

Symptoms: Major symptoms of liver cancer include abdominal pain on the right side that might spread to the back and shoulder, weight loss, loss of appetite, feeling easily satiated, nausea and vomiting, jaundicelike symptoms, and fever.

Screening and diagnosis: Screening of liver cancer involves the following procedures:

- Computed tomography (CT) scans: CT scans are screening techniques by which information about internal organs is computed using X rays.
- Tests for tumor markers: Certain substances are secreted by tumors and thus can be used as tumor markers. Alfa-fetoprotein (AFP) is a typical example of such a marker. Normally the highest amounts of AFP are secreted in fetuses, and the level of the protein gradually decreases in adulthood. Almost a hundredfold increase in levels of AFP can be detected in liver tumor cells. However, some concerns have arisen about false positives and the most appropriate fraction of AFP to use as a tumor marker. Other liver tumor markers include hepatoma-specific gamma-glutamyl transpeptidase (HS-GGT), TGF-α1 and IGF-2.
- Magnetic resonance imaging (MRI): MRI is a technique used to decipher structural details of internal organs using their responses to magnetic fields. MRI has excellent soft-tissue contrast and is ideal for tissues with air spaces and bones. Also, MRI is very flexible with image-plane control, enabling better resolution of details. A tumor can be easily picked up because of its differential responses compared with normal tissue.
- Biopsy: A small amount of tissue removal is called biopsy. Tissue obtained is scrutinized under a microscope to study the cellular architecture. A cancer cell is distinct in its morphology compared with a normal cell and can easily be distinguished. A variety of methods like fine-needle aspirations, cone biopsy, or laparoscopy can be used to excise the sample tissue.

Staging is an important process in cancer testing. Staging determines the extent of cancer formation, and treatment options are decided based on the stage of the cancer at the time of diagnosis. Stages are determined based on the following criteria: size of the tumor, development of tumor in one or both lobes of the liver, growth of tumors in and around major blood vessels, and spread of cancer to lymphatic nodes and other organs of the body. Based on these criteria, liver cancer is divided into four stages, Stages I through IV, some stages having a few subclasses within.

Treatment and therapy: Surgery is still the standard treatment for liver cancers. The choice between the two surgical options, resection and liver transplantation, depends on the stage and extent of spread.

When the tumor is small, has not spread to other regions, and is not complicated by cirrhosis, resection is possible. The process, called partial hepatectomy, removes the portions of the liver beset with the tumor. Liver cells have the remarkable capacity to regenerate following surgery, and surgical methods take advantage of this property.

When resection is not possible because of poor liver function or metastasis, whole-liver transplantation is considered the treatment of choice. Tumors are assessed on the basis of the Milan criteria, which help determine

Stage at Diagnosis and Five-Year Relative Survival Rates for Cancer of the Liver and Intrahepatic Bile Duct, 1996-2004

Stage	Cases Diagnosed (%)	Survival Rate (%)
Localized[a]	33	22.3
Regional[b]	25	7.3
Distant[c]	20	2.8
Unstaged	21	4.4

Source: Data from National Cancer Institute, Surveillance Epidemiology and End Results, Cancer Stat Fact Sheets, 2008

[a]Cancer still confined to primary site

[b]Cancer has spread to regional lymph nodes or directly beyond the primary site

[c]Cancer has metastasized

the suitability for liver transplantation. Typically, patients whose cancers measure up to the following limits—one nodule greater than or equal to 5 centimeters (cm), two to three nodules greater than or equal to 3 cm—are considered to be within limits defined by the Milan criteria and are eligible for liver transplantations. Sometimes these criteria can be expanded, depending on the circumstances.

Liver transplantation requires the availability of either a complete or partial liver, depending on the state of the donor. If the donor is deceased, a whole liver is required, but if the donor is alive, a small portion of the liver is sufficient. Patients slated for whole-liver transplantation have to undergo long periods of waiting (usually close to a year), and this often leads to large numbers of dropouts as well as patients in whom the cancer has spread and who no longer meet the Milan criteria. With liver transplants from living donors, only small portions of the liver are needed, and more patients can benefit from a single donor. However, the acceptable rate of recurrence has not been defined well in cases involving living donors, and there are still lingering concerns about donor safety.

In some cases, nonsurgical options are preferred, and many of these methods have proven to be effective at various stages of liver cancer. Transarterial chemo embolization (TACE) can be used when the tumor is larger than 4 cm and there are multiple lesions. This treatment takes advantage of the fact that the liver receives its blood supply from two main sources—the hepatic artery and the hepatic portal vein—and that the major supplier of blood to the liver is the hepatic artery. In this way, the liver is a unique organ. During TACE, an angiographic catheter is introduced in the branches of the hepatic artery. An anticancer drug (for example, doxorubicin) is injected through the catheter, and the hepatic artery is blocked with occluding agents such as polyvinyl alcohol beads, which get transported to terminal hepatic arteries and occlude the vessels. The liver can still be healthy and functional using a blood supply derived from the alternative route of portal veins.

Percutaneous ethanol injection (PEI) is more effective with a small hepatocellular carcinoma. Cancer cells are susceptible to treatment with ethanol, which is injected directly into the tumor under the guidance of percutaneous ultrasound. Because of the soft nature of the hepatocellular carcinoma within the hardened cirrhotic liver, diffusion of the alcohol is easily attained.

Chemotherapy uses drugs to cure tumors or to alleviate pain. A single class or a combination of a few classes of drugs may be administered in specific cases. Most commonly used drugs are doxorubicin, uracil-tegafur (UFT), or sorafenib.

Tumors that are between 2 and 4 cm are treated with radio frequency ablation. Tumors are exposed to small electrodes emitting radio frequency waves. The energy generated by these waves destroys a specific zone comprising the tumor and a small region surrounding it.

Magnetic resonance-guided microwave coagulation therapy (MR-MCT) makes use of a vertical type, open-configuration magnetic resonance system as opposed to the horizontal type that is typically used.

Immunotherapy involves modifying genes that are part of the body's immune system to combat cancer. The most common immunotherapy strategies are making the tumor more capable of immunogenic responses, modifying the microenvironment surrounding the tumor and making it less immune suppressive, and activation of both specific and nonspecific immune responses. All these methods have selective advantages and have improved chances of cure and survival in liver cancer patients.

Prognosis, prevention, and outcomes: Generally the prognosis for liver cancer is poor, because this particular cancer is difficult to diagnose while in the early stages. Once the symptoms manifest themselves, the cancer generally has already spread to some extent. Therefore, survival rates among people diagnosed with liver cancer are low. Preventive measures include vaccination against known viruses (such as hepatitis B) as well as a healthy diet, avoidance of chemical exposures, and abstinence from alcohol.

The efficacy of various interferons in the treatment of liver cancer is under investigation. Clinical trials involving the targeted drug sorafenib have produced tremendous improvements in patients with advanced liver cancer. Advances in imaging techniques and a better understanding of the molecular mechanisms involving the development of liver cancers have improved the outcomes of this disease.

Geetha Yadav, Ph.D.

For Further Information

Butterfield, L. H. "Recent Advances in Immunotherapy for Hepatocellular Cancer." *Swiss Medical Weekly* 137 (2007): 83-90.

Hanahan, D., and R. A. Weinberg. "Hallmarks of Cancer." *Cell* 100 (2000): 57-70.

Kulik, L. M. "Advancements in Hepatocellular Carcinoma." *Current Opinion in Gastroenterology* 23 (2007): 268-274.

Schwartz, M., et al. "Strategies for the Management of Hepatocellular Carcinoma." *Nature Clinical Practice (Oncology)* 4 (2007): 424-432.

Other Resources

American Cancer Society
http://www.cancer.org

Cancer Backup
Primary Liver Cancer
http://www.cancerbackup.org.uk/Cancertype/Liver/Primarylivercancer

Cancer.Net
http://www.cancer.net/portal/site/patient/

National Cancer Institute
http://www.cancer.gov

See also: Bile duct cancer; Hepatic Arterial Infusion (HAI); Hepatitis B Virus (HBV); Hepatitis C Virus (HCV); Hepatomegaly; Liver biopsy; Percutaneous Transhepatic Cholangiography (PTHC); Virus-related cancers

▶ Lobular Carcinoma In Situ (LCIS)

Category: Diseases, Symptoms, and Conditions
Also known as: Lobular neoplasia

Related conditions: Lobular carcinoma, atypical lobular hyperplasia, ductal carcinoma in situ (DCIS), ductal carcinoma

Definition: Lobular carcinoma in situ (LCIS) is a type of noninfiltrating breast cancer that originates in the breast lobules. It differs from other breast cancers in its propensity to develop in multiple sites in one or both breasts. Unlike other in situ cancers, LCIS is considered a marker rather than a premalignant lesion for subsequent development of invasive breast cancer. Only 25 to 35 percent of patients with lobular carcinoma in situ develop invasive cancer, compared with patients with other in situ lesions, such as ductal carcinoma in situ (DCIS). Between 25 and 70 percent of those with DCIS will develop invasive breast cancer.

Risk factors: Being a woman is a significant risk factor because men do not possess developed lobular breast tissue. Increasing age (forty and above) also contributes to the risk of LCIS. A family history of breast cancer, especially in first-degree relatives, is another significant risk factor, although not specific to any type of breast cancer. White patients have a twelvefold increased risk of LCIS compared with the general population; however, patients of African American origin have a higher rate of recurrence. Other risk factors include obesity, late (or not) first childbirth (older than thirty years), and a prior history of breast cancer.

Etiology and the disease process: The etiology of LCIS has been linked in some studies to loss of heterozygosity in chromosome 16q, 17p, and17q (*BRCA1* tumor-suppressor gene), which predisposes people to unregulated monoclonal proliferation. An alteration in the E-cadherin adhesion complex has also been noted in LCIS. Lobular carcinoma in situ originates from the terminal duct-lobular apparatus, where it is thought that monoclonal cells from the cellular lining (epithelium) of this apparatus undergo uninhibited proliferation within the lobule. Cells do not possess the atypical findings of other cancer cells, such as increased nucleus-to-cytoplasm ratios, increased cellular division, and loss of cellular cohesion or necrosis. However, the cells are enlarged and possess characteristic mucoid globules that help distinguish LCIS from DCIS. An interesting characteristic of LCIS is that invasion of tissue outside the lobule does not ensue, leaving lobular tissue architecture intact. As a result, LCIS can develop in multiple lobules undetected by clinical breast examinations and mammography. In spite of this, development of invasive cancer from LCIS is slow and may take as long as fifteen to twenty years.

Incidence: The overall incidence of LCIS, as documented by breast biopsies with a suspicious mammogram, is estimated at 2 to 5 percent. LCIS accounts for 9.8 percent of all breast malignancies. The diagnosis of LCIS peaks around the mid-forties. It is also interesting to note that more than 90 percent of women diagnosed with lobular carcinoma in situ are premenopausal, which suggests a plausible role of estrogen in LCIS proliferation.

Symptoms: LCIS is often missed due to the lack of overt signs and symptoms like those associated with other breast lesions, such as incidental discovery of a breast mass on self-examination, changes in the skin or nipples, and the presence of pain or nipple discharge. More often than not, LCIS is an incidental finding in otherwise normal breast biopsies. The presence of "neighborhood calcifications" in normal tissue surrounding the lesion on mammography is unique to LCIS and may aid in diagnosis.

Screening and diagnosis: Screening for all breast cancer follows the American Cancer Society (ACS) recommendations. ACS guidelines recommend that breast examinations be conducted every three years as part of a routine checkup beginning at age twenty (annually beginning at age forty) and that screening mammographies be conducted annually starting at age forty. Diagnosis of LCIS depends on the pathologic findings obtained by needle core biopsy. LCIS may accompany invasive cancer in 5 percent of cases. On microscopic examination, cancer cells may be densely packed and occupy the lobular spaces (acini), terminal ducts, or ductules completely without spread to adjacent structures. The cell nucleus, nucleolus, and cytoplasm are dark-staining and large. Immunohistochemical studies may also reveal E-cadherin-negative cells.

Treatment and therapy: Definitive surgical treatment of LCIS is geared toward removal of the multiple sites presumed to be contained in one breast. This is accomplished by surgical removal of the entire breast (total mastectomy) with optional dissection of axillary lymph nodes. The latter is optional because of the rare (less than 1 percent) occurrence of lymph node spread. Prophylactic removal of the opposite breast in the absence of pathological findings is not recommended in spite of the possibility of development of LCIS. Other treatment options include clinical observation and yearly mammography. Tamoxifen, an estrogen-receptor antagonist may be used in reducing the further development of LCIS in the remaining breast. A bilateral total mastectomy is also an option for patients with a familial inheritance of the *BRCA1* gene as demonstrated by genetic studies.

Prognosis, prevention, and outcomes: Prognosis is generally excellent with complete excision. However, progression to multiple or bilateral LCIS is high, approaching 90 percent and 70 percent, respectively. Simultaneous invasive cancer incidence is 5 percent.

Aldo C. Dumlao, M.D.

For Further Information

Harding, Fred. *Breast Cancer: Cause—Prevention—Cure*. Rev. ed. London: Tekline Publishing, 2007.

Knox, Sally M., and Janet K. Grant. *The Breast Cancer Care Book: A Survival Guide for Patients and Loved Ones*. Grand Rapids, Mich.: Zondervan, 2004.

Simone, John. *The LCIS and DCIS Breast Cancer Fact Book*. Raleigh, N.C.: Three Pyramids Publishing, 2002.

Other Resources

American Cancer Society
http://www.cancer.org

Cancer Backup
Lobular Carcinoma in Situ
http://www.cancerbackup.org.uk/Cancertype/Breast/DCISLCIS/LCIS

National Cancer Institute
Lobular Cancer in Situ
http://www.cancer.gov/cancertopics/pdq/treatment/breast/HealthProfessional/page6

See also: Breast cancer in children and adolescents; Breast cancers; Comedo carcinomas; Ductal Carcinoma In Situ (DCIS); Ductal lavage; Invasive ductal carcinomas; Invasive lobular carcinomas; Mastectomy; Medullary carcinoma of the breast; Microcalcifications; Mucinous carcinomas; Tubular carcinomas

▶ Lumps

Category: Diseases, Symptoms, and Conditions
Also known as: Masses

Related conditions: Cysts, fibromas

Definition: Lumps are abnormal masses or swellings on the skin or in the body.

Risk factors: There are many conditions that may cause lumps, such as a cyst, fibroma, injury, or cancer.

Etiology and the disease process: The likely causes of lumps include benign breast diseases, a lipoma (collection of fatty tissue), exostoses (new bone formation), cancer, an injury, an enlarged organ, or a swollen lymph node. Lymph nodes often swell in response to various infections or diseases, including the common cold, infections, viruses, mononucleosis, tonsillitis, lymphoma, Hodgkin disease, and leukemia. A variety of tissues in the body respond to hormonal changes, and as a result, certain lumps are transient. As an example, breast lumps may appear at all ages. Male or female infants may develop breast lumps temporarily in response to receiving estrogen from the mother's milk. Breast-feeding women are prone to benign breast lumps from mastitis (inflammation of the mammary gland). Other underlying conditions for breast lumps include fibrocystic breasts, fibroadenoma, cyst, abscess, fat necrosis, gynecomastia (male breasts), duct papilloma (epithelial tumor growth), sclerosing adenosis (excess growth of breast tissues), and ductal ectasia (dilatation of the subareolar ducts). Fibrocystic breasts and fibroadenomas often occur in women during the reproductive years and are considered a normal variation of breast tissue. Cysts are fluid-filled sacs that can become tender.

Incidence: Lumps commonly occur and often spontaneously resolve.

Symptoms: The signs and symptoma of lumps are swelling or pain, often in the breast, under the skin, and in the groin.

Screening and diagnosis: Lumps are detected by touch, visually, or by the perception of pain. Medical examination can reveal their cause and whether they are benign or malignant. Most common potentially cancer-related lumps develop in the breasts. Although typically lumps in the breast are benign breast cysts, they may be indicators of breast cancer. As a result, lumps found in the breast should be immediately examined to detect potential cases of breast cancer.

Treatment and therapy: The nature and causes of lumps determine how they are treated. Cysts can easily be drained by a physician, but if they do not disappear, surgery may be needed. Generally, if the fluid removed from the cyst is relatively clear and the lump disappears, no further treatment is necessary. However, if the fluid is bloody, the cyst must be inspected for the possible presence of cancer cells.

Prognosis, prevention, and outcomes: Lumps tend to be benign. However, if a malignancy is detected, the survival rate with early diagnosis tends to be higher than after delayed detection.

Anita Nagypál, Ph.D.

See also: Accelerated Partial Breast irradiation (APBI); Biopsy; Breast cancer in children and adolescents; Breast cancer in men; Breast cancers; Breast Self-Examination (BSE); Breast ultrasound; Clinical Breast Exam (CBE); Fibrocystic breast changes; Fibrosarcomas, soft-tissue; Head and neck cancers; Lumpectomy; Mammography; Surgical biopsies; Symptoms and cancer

▶ Lung cancers

Category: Diseases, Symptoms, and Conditions

Also known as: Carcinomas of the lung, small-cell lung cancer (SCLC), oat cell carcinoma, non-small-cell lung cancer (NSCLC)

Related conditions: Mesothelioma

Definition: Lung cancer is an uncontrolled cell growth in lung tissues, which may lead to metastasis and infiltration of other tissues beyond the lungs.

Risk factors: Long-term exposure to tobacco smoke is the main risk factor (90 percent of the cases) for the development of lung cancer. The lifetime risk of developing lung cancer among male smokers is 17.2 percent, and among female smokers the risk is 11.6 percent. This lifetime risk is significantly lower among nonsmokers, accounting for 1.3 percent of cases of lung cancers in men and for 1.4 percent of cases in women. The occurrence of lung cancer in nonsmokers (less than 10 percent of the cases) may be due to genetic factors, secondhand smoke, air pollution, and exposure to occupational respiratory carcinogens such radon gas, chromium, asbestos, and inorganic arsenic. There are more than four thousand chemicals in tobacco smoke, making the identification of the contributing factors to lung carcinogenesis challenging.

Genetic predisposition might also contribute to the risk of lung cancer development. First-degree relatives of patients with lung cancer have an increased risk of lung cancer compared with those of controls. However, familial aggregation of lung cancer might in part be caused by shared exposure to tobacco smoke. A major autosomal susceptibility locus for inherited lung cancer was found at chromosome 6q23-25, which contains numerous potential genes of interest, including *SASH1*, *LATS1*, *IGF2R*, *PARK2*, and *TCF21*. Genetic aberrations associated with lung cancer often encompass multiple genetic aberrations, including deoxyribonucleic acid (DNA) sequence alterations, copy number changes, allele loss, and abnormal promoter methylations.

Etiology and the disease process: The lung is a common place for metastasis of tumors that originate from tissues other than the lung. The site of origin identifies these

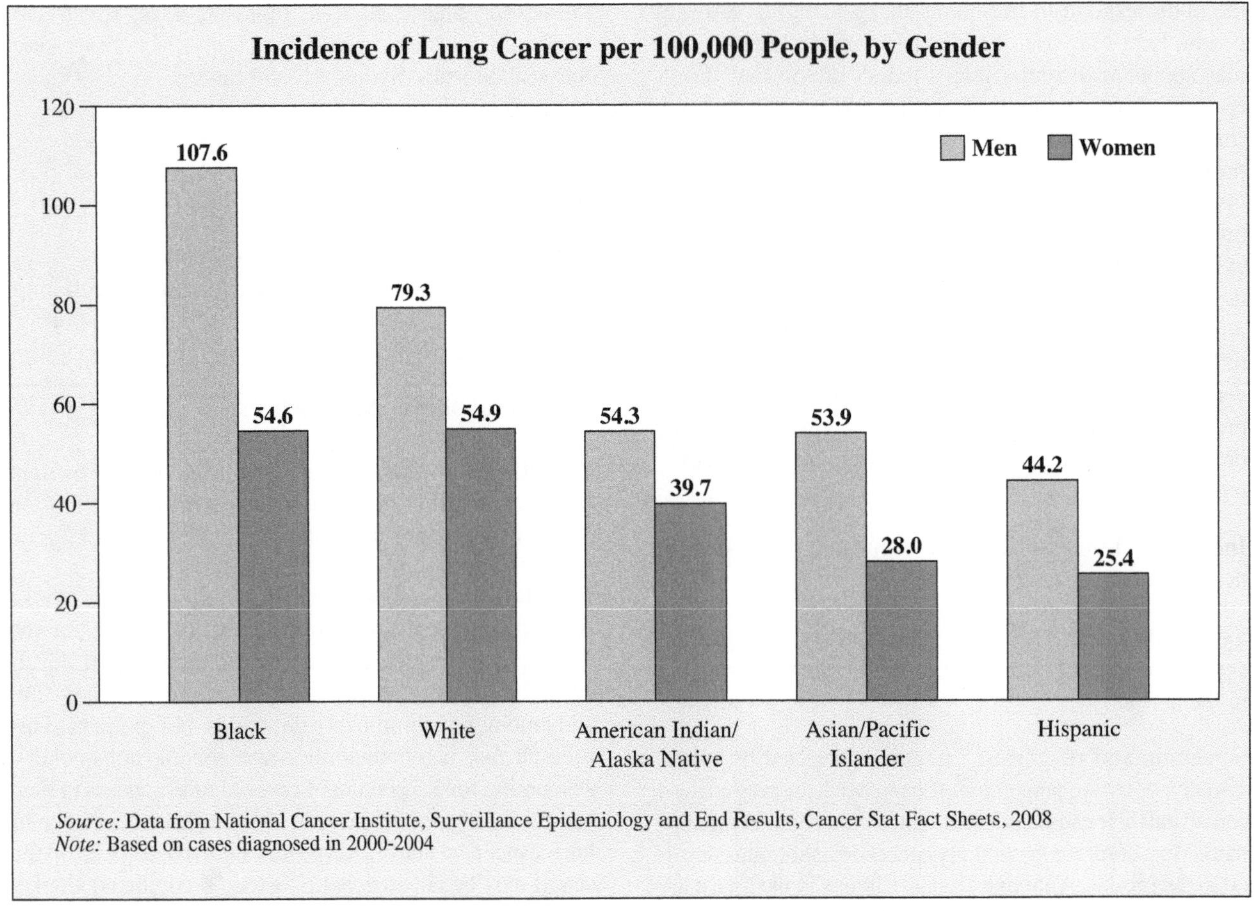

Source: Data from National Cancer Institute, Surveillance Epidemiology and End Results, Cancer Stat Fact Sheets, 2008
Note: Based on cases diagnosed in 2000-2004

nonprimary lung cancers. For example, a breast cancer metastasis to the lung is still called breast cancer. These metastatic lung cancers usually have a distinctive round appearance on chest X ray. Primary lung cancers typically metastasize to the adrenal glands, liver, brain, and bone.

The majority of lung cancers arise from epithelial cells. The two main types of lung carcinomas are histologically defined as SCLC and NSCLC. At diagnosis, it is essential to distinguish which type of lung cancer is present because their treatment varies. SCLC is usually treated with chemotherapy, while NSCLC is often treated with surgery.

There are three main subtypes of NSCLC: squamous cell lung carcinoma, adenocarcinoma, and large-cell lung carcinoma. Squamous cell lung carcinoma, which accounts for 31 percent of lung cancers, usually originates near a central bronchus and often grows more slowly than other cancer types. Adenocarcinoma is associated with smoking, accounts for about 29 percent of lung tumors, and usually arises in peripheral lung tissue. Despite its link to smoking, adenocarcinoma is the most common form of cancer among patients who have never smoked. Variants of adenocarcinoma are adenocarcinoma (not otherwise specified), bronchoalveolar carcinoma, pdenosquamous carcinoma, papillary adenocarcinoma, mucoepidermoid carcinoma, adenoid cystic carcinoma, and other specified adenocarcinomas. Bronchoalveolar carcinoma is more common in women who have never smoked. Large-cell lung carcinoma often develops around the surface of the lung, and it is an aggressive, fast-growing type of NSCLC that tends to metastasize early. This type of malignancy accounts for about 11 percent of lung cancers.

SCLCs are strongly associated with smoking, but they are less common than NSCLCs. SCLCs usually originate in the larger breathing tubes and develop rapidly. Although SCLCs respond well to chemotherapy initially, they often are metastatic at diagnosis and have a worse prognosis than NSCLCs.

Incidence: Lung cancer is the most common cause of cancer-related death in men and the second most common in women worldwide. Lung cancer is responsible for 1.3 million deaths worldwide annually. The incidence of the disease increases with age up to about age seventy. Worldwide, approximately twice as many men as women develop lung cancer. This ratio decreases in areas in which the prevalence of cigarette smoking among women is high. The highest numbers of new lung cancers are found in the United States and Europe. In 2005, the estimated number of new cases in the seven major commercial markets was 393,000, and by 2015 new cases of lung cancer are estimated to reach approximately 561,000. About 80 percent of lung cancers are NSCLC, and 17 percent are SCLC. Over 50 percent of NSCLC patients are diagnosed with an advanced stage of the disease.

Symptoms: Lung cancer symptoms may include dyspnea (shortness of breath), hemoptysis (coughing up blood), chronic coughing or change in regular coughing pattern, wheezing, pain in the chest or abdomen, cachexia (weight loss), fatigue, loss of appetite, dysphonia (hoarse voice), clubbing of the fingernails (uncommon), and dysphagia (difficulty swallowing). At the time of diagnosis, the most common symptom of lung cancer (occurring in more than half of patients) is coughing. Other common symptoms at the time of diagnosis are weight loss and intermittent aching chest pain, which occurs in up to 50 percent of patients. Approximately 60 percent of lung cancer patients develop dyspnea, and up to 35 percent of patients have hemoptysis.

Symptoms and signs of development depend on the organ involved in the spread of disease. With a tumor in the mainstem bronchi, the initial symptom is most often wheezing that may be accompanied by a cough. If the cancer spreads to the left pharyngeal nerve, resulting in left vocal cord paralysis, and hoarseness of the voice occurs, this indicates an unresectable tumor. In addition to laryngeal nerve involvement, the left phrenic nerve is also commonly affected, which could result in paralysis of the left hemidiaphragm. Right paratracheal adenopathy

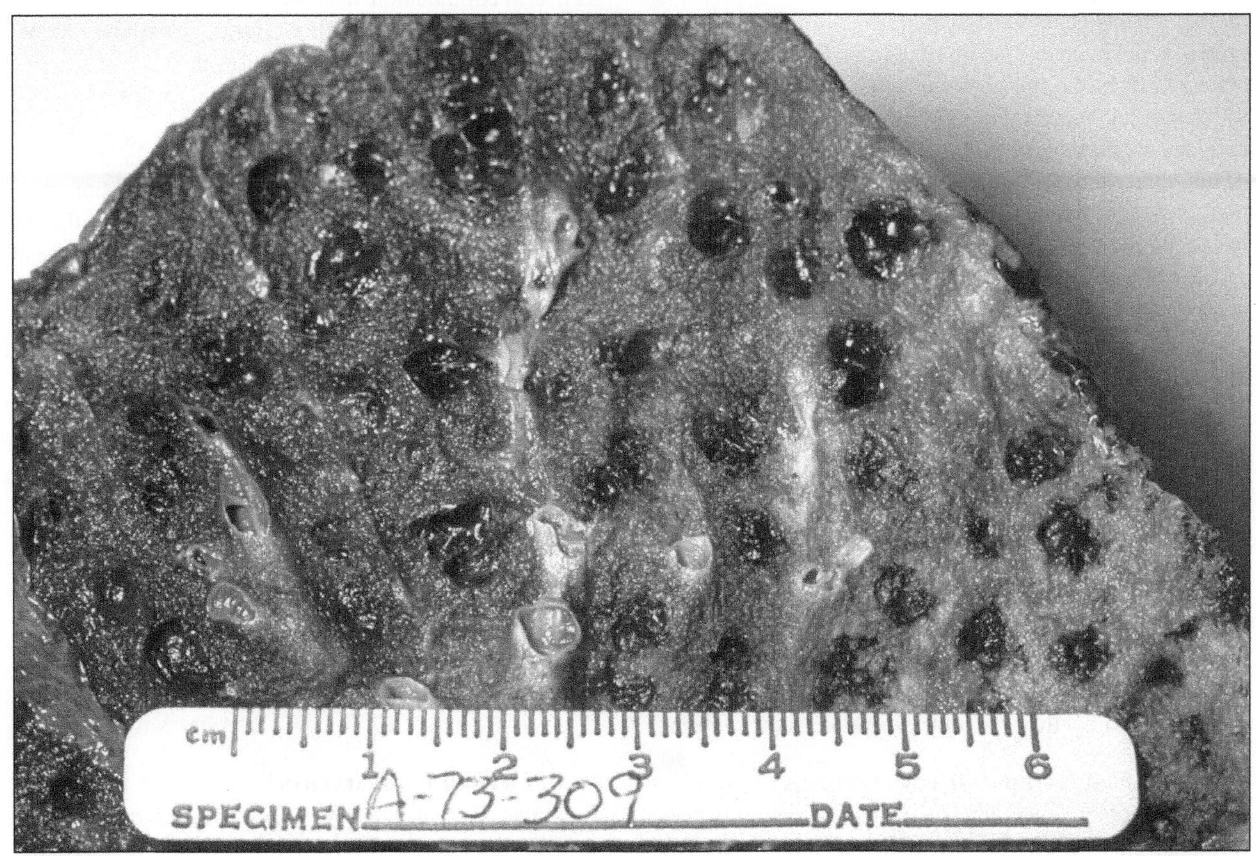

Centrilobular emphysema in a lung, characteristic of smoking, a major risk factor for lung cancer. (Centers for Disease Control and Prevention)

or central enlargement of a tumor in the right upper lobe of the lung often obstructs the superior vena cava. Such a tumor position often causes the patient to have facial or upper extremity swelling, venous swelling in the neck or chest, a cough, and dyspnea. A tumor localized in the apex of the lung usually causes shoulder and upper chest pain. Tumors located in the top of the lung may also cause damage to the brachial plexus and result in Horner syndrome (injury to the sympathetic nerves). Approximately 8 to 15 percent of lung cancer patients have pleural involvement and experience pleuritic chest pain or dyspnea.

Screening and diagnosis: Lung tumors are typically detected by chest radiography done during a general checkup or in response to reported symptoms. When a neoplasm is confirmed, staging of disease is required to develop the appropriate treatment plan and prognosis. Computed tomography (CT) scans and whole-body positron emission tomography (PET) scans are noninvasive staging methods. If clinical symptoms indicate the disease may have spread, other parts of the body may also be scanned.

Invasive staging modalities are used for confirmation of the diagnosis. Pathological diagnosis of neoplastic growth is obtained by sputum (mucus) cytology of tissues extracted from the tumor. Specimen sampling is crucial for diagnostic accuracy of cytology. Typically, transthoracic needle aspiration or endoscopic ultrasound with fine needle aspiration is used for sensitive diagnosis confirmation. For centrally located tumors, flexible bronchoscopy is one of the most common techniques, and it is often accompanied by bronchial washings. Transbronchial needle aspiration with fluoroscopic or CT scan guidance is used for submucosal or peribronchial tumors. In case of peripheral lung lesions, transthoracic lung biopsy offers high sensitivity sampling, and mediastinoscopy is the preferred method to evaluate a tumor in the mediastinal lymph node. Pulmonary function tests are also used.

Lung cancer staging is an assessment of the disease's progression from its original source. Precise staging of lung cancers is essential to develop prognosis and treatment. The most widely used staging system for NSCLC is the International Staging System (ISS), which uses TNM (tumor/lymph node/metastasis) categories that describe four stages of disease. SCLC is classified as limited-stage if it is confined to one half of the chest; otherwise it is extensive-stage.

Treatment and therapy: Treatment depends on the histological type of cancer, the stage, and the patient's performance status (how well the patient is able to perform daily living activities). Treatments include surgery, chemotherapy, and radiotherapy.

Commonly used systemic agents are bevacizumab (Avastin), carboplatin, cisplatin, docetaxel (Taxotere), erlotinib (Tarceva), etoposide, gemcitabine (Gemzar), ifosfamide (Mitoxana), irinotecan (Camptosar), mitomycin (Mutamycin), paclitaxel (Taxol), pemetrexed (Alimta), vinblastine (Velban), and vinorelbine (Navelbine).

The gold-standard therapy for advanced or metastatic disease is platinum-based chemotherapy, a cytotyic theropy that prolongs survival, controls symptoms, and improves quality of life compared with best supportive care (treatment to prevent, control, or relieve side effects or complications and to improve the patient's quality of life). However, patients with poor performance status do not benefit from cytotoxic chemotherapy. Bevacizumab (a monoclonol antibody) plus chemotherapy or chemotherapy alone is beneficial in patients with low performance status, as indicated by the Eastern Cooperative Oncology Group (ECOG) score of 0 to 1. In cases of advanced NSCLC, concurrent chemotherapy with radiation (chemoradiation) is better than sequential chemoradiation, and it is superior to radiation alone. Carboplatin or cisplatin is effective in combination with docetaxel, etoposide, gemcitabine, irinotecan, paclitaxel, vinblastine, and vinorelbine. Erlotinib is often used for nonsmoker patients with active epidermal growth factor receptor mutations or gene amplification. Single agents, such as docetaxel, pemetrexed, tyrosine kinase inhibitor, or erlotinib, are offered for second-line patients. Docetaxel is superior to best supportive care as second-line therapy in terms of quality of life. In addition, erlotinib is also superior to best supportive care in terms of survival as second- and third-line therapy.

Prognosis, prevention, and outcomes: The primary way to prevent lung cancer is to eliminate tobacco smoking. Approximately 42 percent of lung cancer patients survive for at least one year. Worldwide, the five-year survival rate is 14 percent with treatment. In particular, the five-year survival is 16 percent in the United States and 10 percent in Europe. Five-year survival decreases when advanced disease or NSCLC is present at diagnosis. For both men and women, age-standardized lung cancer mortality rates are highest in the United States compared with Japan and many European countries, including France, Germany, Italy, Spain, and the United Kingdom.

Anita Nagypál, Ph.D.

For Further Information

American Cancer Society. *Quick Facts Lung Cancer: What You Need to Know—Now*. Atlanta: Author, 2007.

Desai, Sujal R., ed. *Lung Cancer*. New York: Cambridge University Press, 2007.

Eckardt, John R., and Julia E. Kimmis. *Understanding Lung Cancer: A Guide for Patients and Their Families*. Manhasset, N.Y.: CMP Healthcare Media, 2005.

Gilligan, David, and Robert Rintoul. *Your Guide to Lung Cancer*. London: Hodder Arnold, 2007.

Hunt, Ian, Martin Muers, and Tom Treasure, eds. *ABC of Lung Cancer*. Malden, Mass.: Blackwell, 2008.

Mountain, C. F. "Revisions in the International System for Staging Lung Cancer." *Chest* 111 (1997): 1710-1717.

Roth, Jack A., James D. Cox, and Waun Ki Hong, eds. *Lung Cancer*. 3d ed. Malden, Mass.: Blackwell, 2008.

Other Resources

American Cancer Society
http://www.cancer.org

American Lung Association
Facts About Lung Cancer
Http://www.lungusa.org/site/pp.asp?c=dvLUK9O0E&b=35427

Lung Cancer Online Foundation
http://www.lungcanceronline.org/

LungCancer.org
http://www.lungcancer.org

National Cancer Institute
Lung Cancer
http://www.cancer.gov/cancertopics/types/lung

See also: Air pollution; Bilobectomy; Bronchoalveolar lung cancer; Bronchography; Bronchoscopy; Coughing; Hemoptysis; Klinefelter syndrome and cancer; Lambert-Eaton Myasthenic Syndrome (LEMS); Lobectomy; Mesothelioma; Pleural biopsy; Pleural effusion; Pleurodesis; Pneumonectomy; Pneumonia; Smoking cessation; Soots; Thoracentesis; Thoracoscopy; Thoracotomy; Tobacco-related cancers

▶ Lymphangiosarcomas

Category: Diseases, Symptoms, and Conditions
Also known as: Lymphatic vessel tumors, angiosarcomas, lymphangioendotheliomas, Stewart-Treve syndrome, hemangiosarcomas

Related conditions: Primary or secondary lymphedemas, classical radical mastectomy

Definition: A lymphangiosarcoma is a rare malignant tumor that begins in the cells of the lymph vessels, usually in the upper extremities of individuals who have lymphedema.

Risk factors: Risks factors for lymphangiosarcomas are a history of primary or secondary lymphedema, having had a classical radical mastectomy, or having radiation or chronic infections in a lymphodemous limb.

Etiology and the disease process: Lymphangiosarcoma begins in the cells of the lymphatic vessels. This tumor is seen in the upper arms approximately five to fifteen years after a classical radical mastectomy, specifically in individuals who have long-standing lymphedema. Although the breast cancer may have been cured with the radical mastectomy, a secondary cancer diagnosis of lymphangiosarcoma has a poor prognosis. The radical mastectomy procedure is now outmoded and has been replaced with a more conservative surgical procedure. Lymphangiosarcomas can also arise in individuals with long-standing idiopathic lymphedema of several years. The signs of lymphangiosarcoma are a purple or bruised area on an extremity (usually the upper arm) that becomes a sore that does not heal with necrosis (breakdown) of the skin and underlying tissue. There are often satellite spots from the original site. The tumor metastasizes quickly.

Incidence: Lymphangiosarcoma is rare; the occurrence in patients who had a radical mastectomy for breast cancer is less than 1 percent.

Symptoms: Symptoms of lymphangiosarcoma are purple or bruised areas on the skin of the arms or legs.

Screening and diagnosis: The appearance of purplish, bruised-looking areas on the extremities of an individual with long-standing lymphedema is an indication for further evaluation. A biopsy is taken from the site; diagnosis is made by histologic examination and rules out metastatic disease from a primary tumor or another sarcoma (such as Kaposi sarcoma).

Treatment and therapy: There is not an effective treatment or therapy for lymphangiosarcoma. The lymphangiosarcoma site is removed surgically, and amputation of the affected limb may be necessary. Chemotherapy may also be given after surgical treatment.

Prognosis, prevention, and outcomes: The rate of recurrence is high, and the long-term survival rate is poor, in large part because of the rapid spread of the tumor to the chest wall, the liver, and to bone.

Vicki Miskovsky, B.S., R.D.

See also: Angiosarcomas; Breast cancers; Fibrosarcomas, soft-tissue; Lymphadenectomy; Lymphedema; Mastectomy

▶ Lymphedema

Category: Diseases, Symptoms, and Conditions
Also known as: Lymphatic obstruction

Related conditions: Cancer, malformations of the lymph system

Definition: Lymphedema is a blockage in the lymphatic system that results in swelling, or edema. The lymph system is a network of channels that move lymph, a clear fluid, around cells and through nodes that filter harmful substances such as bacteria.

Risk factors: Surgery and radiation are most often associated with lymphedema. If the patient receives radiation to the underarm or has lymph nodes removed during surgery or as part of a sentinel lymph node biopsy, the lymph channel may be damaged. Lymph node removal for biopsy related to cancer spread is common and may also be done in the chest, groin, pelvic, and neck areas. Tumor growth may also cause lymphedema by compression.

Etiology and the disease process: There are two kinds of lymphedema, primary and secondary. Primary lymphedema is a rare condition inherited at birth, and secondary lymphedema is caused by blockages from infection, surgery, radiation therapy scar tissue, pressure on lymph nodes from a growing tumor, or removal of lymph nodes during surgery. Primary lymphedema is due to a malformation in the lymph system present at birth. Secondary lymphedema is a mechanical interruption in the normal flow of lymph.

When an interruption in the lymph system occurs, the ability to transport fluid is impaired, leading to swelling as the fluid collects in the tissues below the area of blockage. For example, if lymph nodes under the arm or in the groin are removed, the arm or leg may swell. The fluid that collects is interstitial fluid, which causes inflammation. As the fluid collects, the swelling progresses, and the patients note an increase in the size of their arms, legs, or abdomen depending on the site of the blockage. Because the disease is progressive, the swelling continues and may lead to fatigue, the inability to fit clothing over the affected area, and the inability to carry on the activities of daily living. As the disease progresses, the skin in the affected area may become thickened and begin to resemble an orange peel, known as peau d'orange. The skin may break down easily, leading to oozing of fluid through the skin and ultimately infection.

Incidence: Incidence rates for secondary lymphedema vary significantly by site. Some 10 to 40 percent of breast cancer patients with lymph node removal under the arm develop lymphedema. In women with major gynecologic surgery for ovarian and other cancers, the incidence rate ranges from 15 to 44 percent. A limited number of studies of head and neck cancer patients report that up to 5 percent experience lymphedema.

Symptoms: Swelling is the most common and obvious symptom of lymphedema. The patient may also report a feeling of heaviness in the affected body part. Pain and weakness in the limb may be obvious to the patient. Sensations may decrease, including an inability to feel heat or cold. As the disease progresses, the skin becomes hard and loses its elasticity, and the limb may become two to three times its normal size. Lymphedema in the abdominal area may result in bowel and bladder problems. If untreated, fluid oozing from the skin may be noticed, and the skin may seem to disintegrate, leading to open sores.

Screening and diagnosis: Patients at risk for lymphedema should be screened at each doctor's visit and educated to the signs and symptoms of lympedema. Diagnosis of lymphedema is generally made after patients complain of symptoms, such as swelling and fullness. Physical examination, a medical history including medicines taken, and changes since the previous examination are important in diagnosis. There are no specific tests for diagnosing lymphedema. There is no staging of lymphedema, but measurement and recording of the circumference of the affected area are important to monitor progression of the disease.

Treatment and therapy: Treatment of lymphedema is primarily mechanical: elevation of the affected area, manual lymphatic drainage using gentle massage to move fluid toward the center of the body (decongestive therapy), wearing of custom-fitted compression garments on the affected limb, and practicing good skin care and injury protection. Antibiotics may be necessary to prevent or treat infections, but other drugs are not generally effective. Patients are often encouraged to watch their weight, exercise appropriately, and eat protein-rich foods. Bowel and bladder complications such as constipation and urine retention may require treatment. Surgery for lymphedema is not recommended. Because the disease is progressive and treatment is based on symptoms, management and control are the therapies of choice. Patient education is critical to treatment and must be an important part of the therapy for lymphedema.

Prognosis, prevention, and outcomes: There are no clinical studies that support actions to prevent lymphedema. There is no cure for lymphedema so the prognosis depends on the patient's compliance with treatment measures. The use of sentinel lymph node biopsy rather than aggressive lymph node removal may be contributing to a decreasing incidence of the disease. The key to an optimal outcome is early recognition and treatment of the symptoms and compliance with ongoing treatment.

Patricia Stanfill Edens, R.N., Ph.D., FACHE

For Further Information

Fu, M. R. "Breast Cancer Survivors' Intentions of Managing Lymphedema." *Cancer Nursing* 28, no. 6 (2005): 446-457.

Golshan, M., and B. Smith. "Prevention and Management of Arm Lymphedema in the Patient with Breast Cancer." *Journal of Supportive Oncology* 4, no. 8 (2006): 381-386.

Other Resources

American Cancer Society
http://www.cancer.org

National Cancer Institute
Lymphedema
http://www.nci.nih.gov/cancertopics/pdq/supportivecare/lymphedema/patient

National Lymphedema Network
http://www.lymphnet.org

See also: Axillary dissection; Edema; Endotheliomas; Lumpectomy; Lymphadenectomy; Lymphangiosarcomas; Mastectomy; Radiation therapies; Side effects

▶ Lymphocytosis

Category: Diseases, Symptoms, and Conditions
Also known as: Raised lymphocyte count

Related conditions: Lymph symptoms, absolute lymphocytosis, hematological malignancy, lymphoma, leukemia, lymphoproliferative disorders

Definition: Lymphocytosis is an abnormal excess of lymphocytes in the blood. Lymphocytes are a type of white blood cell that help fight infections. A healthy adult has an absolute lymphocyte count (ALC) of 1,300 to 4,000 per microliter of blood. ALC over 4,000 indicates lymphocytosis; however, this number may be higher in children up to six years of age, as their ALC is significantly higher than in adults.

Risk factors: There are more than thirty medical condition that may underlie lymphocytosis. The most common causes include viral and bacterial infections, such as mononucleosis (glandular fever), influenza, pertussis (whooping cough), or tuberculosis. Malignant blood diseases, such as chronic lymphocytic leukemia, follicular lymphoma, hairy cell leukemia, and leukopenia, may also cause lymphocytosis.

Etiology and the disease process: Lymphocytosis indicates an underlying problem, but it is not a disease in itself. The lymph nodes are the most commonly affected organs. Transient stress lymphocytosis may also occur after trauma or extensive psychological or physical stress, and it typically resolves within two days of diagnosis. Transient stress lymphocytosis may be in part mediated by modulation of catecholamine and steroid hormones and cell adhesion molecules.

Incidence: Lymphocytosis is common and occurs in most people throughout life, usually in association with viral infections.

Symptoms: Symptoms of lymphocytosis may include sore throat, fever, and fatigue. However, lymphocytosis typically causes no symptoms and is often discovered incidentally via a routine blood test.

Screening and diagnosis: A complete blood count will identify lymphocytosis. Further investigation is done by assessing the major lymphocyte subsets, such as T cells, B cells, and natural killer cells. The subgroups of T cells are CD4 T cells (helper cells) and CD8 T cells (cytotoxic cells). In a healthy person, approximately 75 percent of lymphocytes are T cells, with a 2:1 ratio of CD4 to CD8, and about equal proportions of the remainder cells are B cells and natural killer cells. A marked increase in lymphocytes may indicate a serious condition, such as the presence of chronic lymphocytic leukemia. Many types of blood cancer are often identified after diagnosing lymphocytosis.

Treatment and therapy: For the best therapy, it is necessary to address the underlying issue that caused lymphocytosis. If a malignant blood disease is detected, cancer treatment may be needed.

Prognosis, prevention, and outcomes: Depending on the cause of lymphocytosis, it may spontaneously resolve or may need medical interaction to relieve its symtoms.

Anita Nagypál, Ph.D.

See also: Acute Lymphocytic Leukemia (ALL); Ataxia tel angiectasia (AT); Biological therapy; Blood cancers; Childhood cancers; Chronic Lymphocytic Leukemia (CLL); Complete Blood Count (CBC); Cutaneous T-Cell Lymphoma (CTCL); Edema; Hairy cell leukemia; Hodgkin disease; Immune response to cancer; Leukemias; Leukopenia; Non-Hodgkin lymphoma; Richter syndrome; Sézary syndrome; Thymomas; Thymus cancer

▶ Lymphomas

Category: Diseases, Symptoms, and Conditions
Also known as: Hodgkin disease, non-Hodgkin lymphoma, Burkitt lymphoma

Related conditions: Cancer of the lymph nodes, cancer of the spleen, leukemia, acquired immunodeficiency syndrome (AIDS)

Definition: Lymphatic cancer is a blood cancer that involves the lymphocytes (white blood cells). Cancerous cells grow and multiply, mostly in the lymph nodes and spleen, where they cause swelling and a suppression of the body's natural immune system. Lymphoma occurs in two forms, Hodgkin disease and non-Hodgkin lymphoma. The presence of abnormal cells known as Reed-Sternberg cells after the scientists who discovered them indicates Hodgkin disease and differentiates this lymphoma from all other types, including Burkitt lymphoma, which are designated non-Hodgkin lymphoma.

Risk factors: As the causes of both Hodgkin disease and non-Hodgkin lymphoma are unknown, the risk factors cannot be definitively determined. However, in non-Hodgkin lymphoma, it is thought that the suppression of the immune system, particularly in high-risk patients such as those who have undergone organic transplantation and are on antirejection medications, is a significant risk factor. A spike in the incidence of non-Hodgkin lymphoma has been detected among people who have had the human immunodeficiency virus (HIV) for four or more years, largely because their immune systems have been compromised.

A link has been detected between the development of lymphoma and exposure to flour in some agricultural jobs. Also, in more advanced cases of the disease, a link has been found to exposure to X rays and to certain forms of chemotherapy.

Heredity appears to have little effect in the development of lymphomas, although physicians who diagnose the disease do record genetic details in their diagnoses.

Etiology and the disease process: The causes of lymphoma are not fully understood. The fact that lymphoma is not a single disease with clear-cut boundaries has made it difficult to understand and assess. Some lymphomas are relatively easy to treat and have good survival rates, whereas other forms of the disease grow very rapidly and aggressively so that successful treatment is more problematic. In the United States, lymphoma has been found most often among the well educated and those in more affluent socioeconomic situations.

The lymphatic system contains two types of cells, the B cells and the T cells. The former manufacture antibodies designed to fight infections. The T cells, on the other hand, regulate the immune system. More than 90 percent of lymphomas in the United States originate in the B cells. Lymphatic cancer cells can be present in the stomach and the intestines, the bones, the skin, the sinuses, and in the lymph nodes.

More than thirty types of non-Hodgkin lymphomas have been identified microscopically, each unique in its morphology. As a result, treatment is most effective if it is directed toward a specific variety of the disease.

Incidence: In 2007, 71,380 were estimated to be diagnosed with lymphoma, and 19,730 were estimated to die of it. The age-adjusted incidence rate was 22 per 100,000 people per year. Both Hodgkin disease and non-Hodgkin lymphoma are found more often in men than in women. Non-Hodgkin lymphoma affects more people in their twenties and in the fifty-five to seventy age group. One variety of non-Hodgkin lymphoma, Burkitt lymphoma, is found largely in the Tropics and in Africa. It is thought to be related in some way to the Epstein-Barr virus. Non-Hodgkin lymphoma is the fifth most frequently occurring cancer in the United States. It is also the third fastest-growing cancer worldwide, with the highest incidence of the disease found in North America, western Europe, and Australia.

Symptoms: The most frequent symptom is a swelling in the lymph nodes in the neck, under the arms, or in the groin, usually referred to as swollen glands. In some cases, particularly in young children, the thymus gland in the upper chest may also be swollen.

The swelling is clearly visible in most cases and usually is not painful. It is sometimes accompanied by other symptoms—loss of appetite, fever, weight loss, and night sweats—that are frequently mistaken for influenza. These symptoms may disappear after a short time, only to reappear.

People suffering from lymphoma often have an overall feeling of illness characterized by lethargy, headaches, and ulceration of the skin accompanied by itching. If the disease has spread to the abdominal area, it may be accompanied by pain and bleeding as well as by swelling. In such cases, the patient may vomit blood or have blackened stools indicating internal bleeding.

Because non-Hodgkin lymphoma usually grows slowly, it may be asymptomatic or may produce only minor symptoms that can easily be ignored in the early stages of the disease. Therefore, this type of lymphoma is frequently diagnosed at Stage III or IV rather than in the earliest stages when the cure rate is greatest. Hodgkin disease, on the other hand, grows and spreads rapidly. Its early symptoms may cause its victims to seek medical intervention in the earlier stages of the disease.

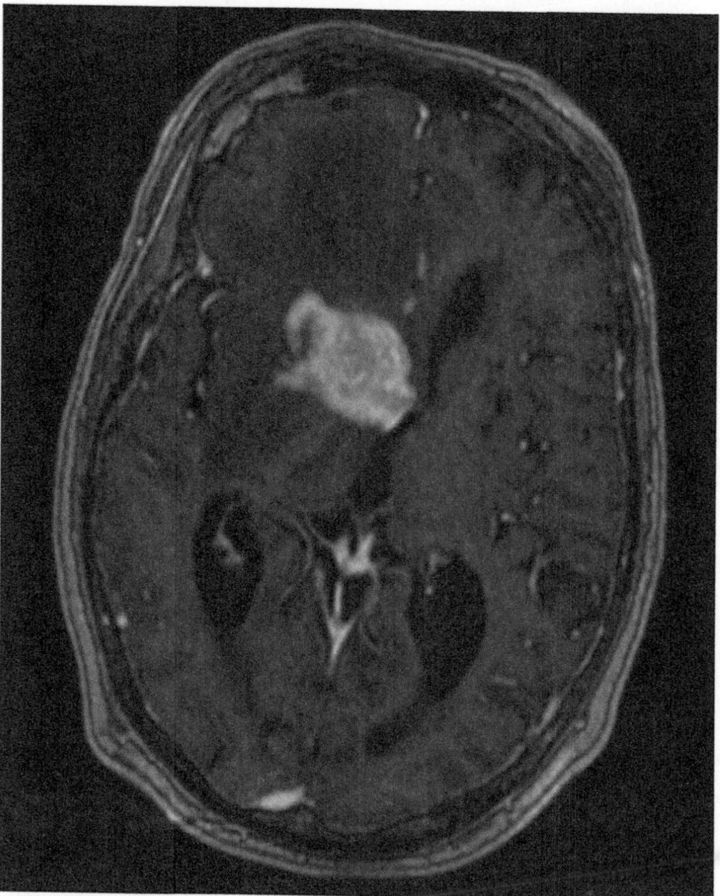

An MRI scan reveals primary central nervous system (CNS) lymphoma in a human brain. (Wikimedia)

Screening and diagnosis: The usual method for diagnosing lymphoma involves the removal and microscopic examination of tissue from the lymph nodes for biopsy. If cancer cells are found, further diagnosis may be indicated and usually will involve X rays of the chest or lymph glands, removal of bone marrow to be biopsied, ultrasound, and scanning by computed tomography (CT), magnetic resonance imaging (MRI), or positron emission tomography (PET).

The Ann Arbor staging system is used for Hodgkin disease and non-Hodgkin lymphoma:

- Stage I: Cancer cells have been found in only one section of the lymph nodes or in just one confined area outside the lymph nodes.
- Stage II: Cancer has been detected in two or more lymph nodes on the same side of the diaphragm.
- Stage III: Cancer cells have been found on both sides of the diaphragm and may have spread to surrounding areas, notably the spleen, the lungs, the liver, or the bone marrow.
- Stage IV: Cancer cells are found in more than one spot within the lymphatic system or in organs located at a significant distance from the lymphatic area.

Treatment and therapy: A biopsy not only determines whether cancer cells are present but also can more specifically identify the kinds of cancer cells that are present. It is important to customize treatment for each individual patient to the greatest degree possible; therefore, identification of the precise kinds of cancerous cells is vital.

For patients with Stage I and Stage II lymphomas, the first avenue of treatment is radiation therapy. If there are signs that the malignancy has spread, radiation may be supplemented by chemotherapy. If the disease has advanced considerably or is likely to, the treatment of choice may be a bone marrow transplant.

When a bone marrow transplant—considered a treatment of last resort—is used, it is also combined with continued radiation therapy and chemotherapy. The patient undergoing such treatment usually has a badly

Age at Death for Lymphoma, 2001-2005

Age Group	*Deaths (%)*
Under 20	0.6
20-34	2.4
35-44	3.4
45-54	7.6
55-64	13.9
65-75	22.9
76-84	32.8
85 and older	16.5

Source: Data from National Cancer Institute, Surveillance Epidemiology and End Results, Cancer Stat Fact Sheets, 2008

Note: The median age at death from 2001 to 2005 was seventyfour, with an age-adjusted death rate of 7.8 per 100,000 men and women per year.

compromised immune system so that the postoperative treatment involves isolation under sterile conditions for an extended period to prevent infection from some of the opportunistic diseases that are found in hospitals.

An alternative treatment is the mini bone marrow transplant. This method involves the use of low-level, minimally toxic chemotherapy or radiation therapy to kill some of the patient's bone marrow, leaving some cancer cells. Cancer-free bone marrow from a donor is then introduced into the patient's bone marrow. In time, this cancer-free bone marrow produces cancer-free cells that attack and destroy the remaining cancerous cells. Stem cell research also appears to have considerable promise in the treatment of lymphoma.

Prognosis, prevention, and outcomes: There is no clear-cut way to prevent lymphoma, although avoiding some occupational and environmental hazards may decrease the likelihood that it will develop. Links have been made between increases in the spread of the disease and such environmental hazards as hydrocarbons and noxious fumes. Avoiding polluted air and water is certainly essential.

Also, diet has profound effects in combating many forms of cancer, including lymphoma. A diet low in fats, limited in animal protein, and containing few refined carbohydrates will strength the immune system and lead to a sense of overall well-being. People should routinely eat at least five servings of fruits and vegetables every day.

The outlook for those suffering from lymphoma depends largely on the stage at which the cancer was detected. Many Stage I patients are cured of the disease. The five-year survival rate among Stage I and Stage II patients approaches 80 percent. Among Stage IV patients, the two-year survival rate is about 50 percent. Each year the statistics are more encouraging as new medications and techniques are developed and employed in treating the disease.

Certainly the key to survival is early diagnosis. Any symptoms should receive the attention of a qualified physician. Particularly dangerous are phantom symptoms, those that disappear after a short time but then return. The interval between their first appearance and their return is crucial because this is the period in which the disease is most susceptible to treatment designed to eliminate it.

R. Baird Shuman, Ph.D.

For Further Information

Adler, Elizabeth M. *Living with Lymphoma: A Patient's Guide*. Baltimore: Johns Hopkins University Press, 2005.

Freedman, Jeri. *Lymphoma: Current and Emerging Trends* in Detection and Treatment. New York: Rosen, 2006.

Holman, Peter, Jodi Garrett, and William Jansen. *One Hundred Questions and Answers About Lymphoma*. Sudbury, Mass.: Jones and Bartlett, 2004.

Litin, Scott C., Jr., ed. *Mayo Clinic Family Health Book*. 3d ed. New York: HarperCollins, 2003.

National Institutes of Health. *What You Need to Know About Hodgkin's Disease*. Bethesda, Md.: National Institutes of Health, 1999.

_______. *What You Need to Know About Non-Hodgkin's Lymphoma*. Bethesda, Md.: National Institutes of Health, 1999.

Park, Alice. "The Cancer Test: Exposing a Growing Tumor's Secrets May Be as Simple as Drawing Blood." *Time*, June 25, 2007, 53.

Teetley, Peter, and Philip Bashe. *Cancer Survival Guide*. Rev. ed. New York: Broadway Books, 2005.

Other Resources

American Cancer Society
http://www.cancer.org

The Leukemia and Lymphoma Society
http://www.leukemia-lymphoma.org

Lymphoma Information Network
http://www.lymphomainfo.net/lymphoma/whatis.html

Lymphoma Research Organization
http://www.lymphoma.org

MedlinePlus
Lymphoma
http://www.nlm.nih.gov/medlineplus/lymphoma.html

See also: Burkitt lymphoma; Castleman disease; Cutaneous T-Cell Lymphoma (CTCL); Epstein-Barr Virus; Hemolytic anemia; Hepatitis C virus (HCV); HIV/AIDS-related cancers; Hodgkin disease; Human T-cell Leukemia Virus (HTLV); Immune response to cancer; Immunocytochemistry and immunohistochemistry; Immunotherapy; Klinefelter syndrome and cancer; Lambert-Eaton Myasthenic Syndrome (LEMS); Leukapharesis; Lymphangiography; Lymphocytosis; Malignant Fibrous Histiocytoma (MFH); Mantle Cell Lymphoma (MCL); Mucosa-Associated Lymphoid Tissue (MALT) lymphomas; Mycosis fungoides; Myeloma; Nijmegen breakage syndrome; Non-Hodgkin lymphoma; Organ transplantation and cancer; Primary central nervous system lymphomas; Richter syndrome; Sézary syndrome; Simian virus 40; Sjögren syndrome; Thymomas; Thymus cancer; Virus-related cancers; Waldenström Macroglobulinemia (WM); Young adult cancers

▶ Malignant Fibrous Histiocytoma (MFH)

Category: Diseases, Symptoms, and Conditions
Also known as: MFH, sarcoma, histiocytoma

Related conditions: Lymphoma, multiple myeloma, hematologic diseases

Definition: Malignant fibrous histiocytoma (MFH) is the most common primary malignant soft-tissue tumor of adulthood. It can also be present in bone. It is usually seen in late adulthood with a peak at age fifty. These are aggressive tumors with a tendency to recur and metastasize.

Risk factors: Malignant fibrous histiocytoma is the most common radiation-induced sarcoma; MFH of bone is more frequent in whites, with a male-to-female ratio of 1.5:1.

Etiology and the disease process: Malignant fibrous histiocytomal cells is thought to derive from primitive mesenchymal cells, with four cell types predominating: storiform/pleomorphic, myxoid, giant cell, and inflammatory.

Incidence: Malignant fibrous histiocytoma accounts for 20 to 30 percent of all soft-tissue sarcomas. It is the most common malignant sarcoma of older adults.

Symptoms: Soft-tissue malignant fibrous histiocytoma usually presents as a painless soft-tissue mass with progressive enlargement over months. Any deep-seated, painless, invasive intramuscular mass in a patient over the age of fifty is most likely MFH. Patients with retroperitoneal MFH have symptoms of fatigue, weight loss, abdominal pressure, fever, and malaise. Osseous MFH usually presents with pain over several months with or without swelling and can be associated with pathologic fracture.

Screening and diagnosis: Soft-tissue malignant fibrous histiocytoma is best diagnosed with magnetic resonance imaging (MRI) with gadolinium contrast. This tumor usually appears as a well-defined hypervascular heterogeneous soft-tissue mass with areas of hemorrhage and necrosis. Osseous MFH usually presents as an aggressive Stage IIb lesion associated with pathologic fracture in approximately 20 percent of cases. Staging depends on pathology, compartmentalization, and presence or absence of metastases:

- Stage Ia: Low grade, intracompartmental
- Stage Ib: Low grade, extracompartmental
- Stage IIa: High grade, intracompartmental
- Stage IIb: High grade, extracompartmental
- Stage III: Presence of metastases

Treatment and therapy: Treatment for Stage I tumors involves surgical resection with wide margins, whereas treatment for Stage II involves surgical resection with adjuvant radiation or chemotherapy.

Prognosis, prevention, and outcomes: Prognosis depends on tumor size, depth, location, histologic subtype, and presence of metastases. Local recurrence is seen in approximately 20 to 31 percent of cases. The five-year survival rate is 80 percent if the tumor is under 5 centimeters (cm) but drops to approximately 40 percent if the tumor is greater than 10 cm at diagnosis (however, for retroperitoneal tumors, the five-year survival is 15 to 20 percent). Metastases can occur to the lung, lymph nodes, bone, and the liver.

Debra B. Kessler, M.D., Ph.D.

See also: Amputation; Fibrosarcomas, soft-tissue; Limb salvage; Liposarcomas; Mesenchymomas, malignant

▶ Malignant rhabdoid tumor of the kidney

Category: Diseases, Symptoms, and Conditions
Also known as: Rhabdoid tumor of the kidney, MRT

Related conditions: Wilms' tumor

Definition: Malignant rhabdoid tumor of the kidney is an extremely aggressive and lethal cancer that occurs only in infants and young children.

Risk factors: Malignant rhabdoid tumor of the kidney is caused by a mutation or deletion of the *INI1* gene. However, there are no known risk factors associated with its development.

Etiology and the disease process: Malignant rhabdoid tumor of the kidney is made up of an overgrowth of rhabdoid (rod-shaped) cells. These cells may appear like epithelial (skin), neural (nerve), muscle, or mesenchymal (rare soft-tissue tumor) cells. A single rhabdoid tumor may include all these types of cells or only one or two. The cells tend to infiltrate the kidney tissue and to metastasize early. A common site of metastasis is the brain.

Incidence: Malignant rhabdoid tumor of the kidney is a rare tumor. According to the National Wilms' Tumor Study (NWTS) group data, only 1.6 percent of cases of childhood renal tumors are malignant rhabdoid tumors. Malignant rhabdoid tumors are equally common in both sexes, and the median age at which it occurs is eleven months.

Symptoms: The most common symptoms observed are fever, hematuria (blood in the urine), fussiness, and hypertension. Other symptoms are those of brain metastasis, such as seizures and loss of previously achieved motor skills.

Screening and diagnosis: There is no routine screening for malignant rhabdoid tumor of the kidney. The most definitive testing includes abdominal ultrasound and abdominal computed tomography (CT) scan. Then the tumor is biopsied.

The staging for malignant rhabdoid tumor of the kidney was devised by the NWTS group and then modified by the Children's Oncology Group (COG). The stages are as follows:

- Stage I: The tumor has not spread beyond the one kidney.
- Stage II: The tumor is localized to the area around the kidney, and there is no evidence of tumor spread.
- Stage III: The tumor has spread into the abdomen.
- Stage IV: There are metastases outside the abdominal or pelvic cavities.
- Stage V: There are bilateral tumors.

Treatment and therapy: The primary treatment is surgical removal of the kidney. It is usually removed through direct incision, to avoid any spillage of cancer cells. At this time, lymph nodes are sampled and the adrenal gland may be removed. Bilateral tumors are not removed. Chemotherapy is performed on all patients with malignant rhabdoid tumor of the kidney.

Prognosis, prevention, and outcomes: The prognosis for malignant rhabdoid tumor of the kidney is poor, with an average survival time of less than one year. There is no way to prevent it.

Christine M. Carroll, R.N., B.S.N., M.B.A.

See also: Childhood cancers; Wilms' tumor

▶ Malignant tumors

Category: Diseases, Symptoms, and Conditions
Also known as: Cancerous tumors

Related conditions: Most cancers

Definition: Malignant tumors are those that invade surrounding tissues. Unlike a benign tumor, which is a self-contained, harmless mass of slow growing cells, malignant tumors are fast growing, fast spreading and harmful. Commonly known as cancer, cells of malignant tumors are abnormal in morphology, tend to be larger than normal, and have odd shapes, and large and irregular nuclei. By entering into the bloodstream or the lymphatic system, these cells spread to surrounding tissue, where they damage the tissues and organs.

Malignant tumors are named using the Latin or Greek root of the organ of origin as a prefix and "sarcoma" or "carcinoma" as the suffix. For example, a malignant tumor of the liver is called hepatocarcinoma; a malignant tumor of the fat cells is called liposarcoma. A sarcoma is a cancer of the connective tissue, and carcinomas originate from epithelial cells.

Risk factors: The most common risk factors for development of malignant tumors include family history, tobacco use, exposure to ultraviolet (UV) radiation, ionizing radiation, certain chemicals, and viruses.

Etiology and the disease process: A mutated cell that continues to divide is a hallmark of cancer. The deoxyribonucleic acid (DNA) repair mechanisms are damaged, and the immune system is compromised such that the tumor cells rapidly multiply undeterred. Additionally, the tumor has an extensive vasculature that provides nutrients and oxygen for its growth.

Symptoms: Unusual bleeding or discharge, a change in the shape or coloration of a wart or mole, a sore throat that does not heal, unexplained weight loss, persistent cough, and anemia are some warning signs. Many symptoms are caused by the fatigue, pain, and stress imposed on the body by malignant tumors.

Screening and diagnosis: X-rays, ultrasound, magnetic resonance imaging (MRI), and computed tomography (CT) scans are used to detect changes in tissues or organs, and blood tests are used to monitor abnormal cell counts. Presence of tumor markers such as prostate specific antigen (PSA), carcinoembryonic antigen (CEA), and human chorionic gonadotropin hormone in the blood are used to screen high-risk individuals.

Treatment and therapy: Malignant tumors can be removed before they metastasize (spread), but frequently they grow back. Besides a person's age, general health, and response to treatment, the outcome depends on the type and location of the cancer, the stage of the disease (the extent to which the cancer has spread), or its grade (how abnormal the cancer cells look and how quickly the cancer is likely to grow and spread). Treatment includes surgery, radiation therapy, chemotherapy, hormone therapy, or biological therapy. However, most often a combination of therapies is required for complete eradication of the malignancy. Choice of a healthy, active, tobacco-free lifestyle with a minimum exposure to harmful UV rays can go a long way in preventing cancer.

Banalata Bono Sen, Ph.D.

For Further Information:

Definition of Tumor, MedicineNet.com
http://www.medicinenet.com/script/main/art.asp?articlekey=14066

The New York Times, Health Guide, Tumor, Feb 2016
http://www.nytimes.com/health/guides/disease/tumor/overview.html

The Truth about Cancer
Benign and Malignant Tumors: What is the Difference? https://thetruthaboutcancer.com/benign-malignant-tumors-difference/

NCI Dictionary of Cancer Terms
http://www.cancer.gov/publications/dictionaries/cancer-terms?cdrid=45771

Nomenclature of Neoplasia
http://library.med.utah.edu/WebPath/NEOHTML/NEOPL103.html

Friberg, S,, & Mattson, S. (1997), On the growth rates of human malignant tumors: Implications for medical decision making. *Journal of Surgical Oncology,* 65(4), 284-97.

See also: Cancer biology; Carcinoma; Invasive cancer; Metastasis; Tumor markers

▶ Mantle Cell Lymphoma (MCL)

Category: Diseases, Symptoms, and Conditions
Also known as: Non-Hodgkin lymphoma, B-cell lymphoma

Related conditions: Hodgkin lymphoma

Definition: Mantle cell lymphoma (MCL), or B-cell lymphoma, is a rare form of non-Hodgkin lymphoma (NHL), with 6 to 8 percent of cases of NHL accounting for MCL. MCL primarily affects the B lymphocytes of the lymphatic system. The lymphatic system is made up of lymph nodes that are linked by lymph vessels responsible for delivering fluid throughout the body, as well as collecting waste from tissues, purifying it, and then returning it to the blood. MCL has two distinct groups: indolent or low-grade lymphoma and aggressive or high-grade lymphoma.

Risk factors: There are no risk factors for MCL.

Etiology and the disease process: Causes for MCL have not been identified; however, it is known that Caucasian males are more susceptible to MCL and that it is most prevalent in adult populations. It has been determined that patients with MCL have an overexpression of cyclin D1, which is a protein that encourages cellular growth. This cyclin D1 overexpression has been traced to a translocation between chromosomes 11 and 14.

Incidence: MCL is found typically in adults in their sixties, affecting males more often than females at a ratio of 3:1. Cases of MCL have been steadily increasing since the 1970's. As the initial symptoms of MCL often go undetected, upon diagnosis the majority of patients already have Stage IV disease.

Symptoms: MCL is often detected because of swelling in the lymph nodes of the neck, groin, or armpit that is painless yet noticeable either visibly or to the touch. Accompanying symptoms often include fatigue, decreased appetite, fever, night sweating, weight loss, itchiness, and breathlessness.

Screening and diagnosis: MCL is diagnosed following surgical removal of a portion of the swollen lymph node. The tissue collected is then sampled to review its cells under a microscope to make the diagnosis. Additional supportive tests may include blood tests, bone scans, marrow biopsies, and X rays to provide information on the extent of the spread of the lymphoma and its type. The information gained from these tests will assist the doctor in determining the appropriate treatment plan for the cancer.

The Ann Arbor staging for non-Hodgkin lymphoma, which is the definitive disease process guide for lymphomas, defines four stages of the disease. Stage I is lymphoma limited to a primary lymph node, organ, or tissue site in one body area. Stage II includes two or more lymph nodes or regions of lymph nodes either on the upper or lower half of the body. Stage III includes two or more lymph nodes or regions of lymph nodes on both the upper and lower parts of the body, and Stage IV includes lymphoma that has spread from the lymph nodes to one or more organs in the body. Each stage also includes a subclassification of either A or B, to identify either the absence of symptoms (A) or the presence of symptoms (B). Additionally, lymphoma that has spread beyond the lymph nodes to the organs can be classified with an E for extranodal.

Relative Survival Rates for Mantle Cell Lymphoma, 1988-2001

Years	*Survival Rate (%)*
1	83.9
2	72.6
3	65.2
5	51.1
8	37.4
10	34.3

Source: Data from L. A. G. Ries et al., eds., *Cancer Survival Among Adults: U.S. SEER Program, 1988-2001—Patient and Tumor Characteristics,* NIH Pub. No. 07-6215 (Bethesda, Md.: National Cancer Institute, 2007)

Treatment and therapy: Treatment for MCL is dependent upon the patient's stage of disease. Patients with indolent MCL who are asymptomatic often manage their disease with a "watch and wait" approach without medication until symptoms appear. As most patients with MCL are diagnosed, however, already at Stage IV, aggressive therapy is often prescribed. Aggressive therapy can consist of chemotherapy alone; however, this is often not enough to treat the cancer. Aggressive therapy typically includes a combination of chemotherapy and radiation. Allogenic stem cell transplantation has also been used to introduce stem cells that are not cancerous into the body to assist the body in its fight against the cancer. Allogenic stem cell transplantation, however, causes side effects which are often deemed intolerable by the patient, is difficult to perform, and is rarely used as a treatment option. Additional therapy, such as treatment with a monoclonal antibody, can also be used in combination with chemotherapy, to target and kill select cancer cells.

The patient may also be given medications to counteract the side effects caused by the first-line therapies, such as steroids to combat nausea, or interferons to allow the body to increase its immune response.

Prognosis, prevention, and outcomes: Prognosis for MCL can be determined by its classification as either indolent or aggressive, and indolent MCL typically has a better prognosis than aggressive MCL. As the majority of cases of MCL are diagnosed as Stage IV, MCL has only a moderate prognosis. Patients diagnosed with MCL most often have an average survival of three to four years. Even in patients with a good or fair prognosis, curing MCL is uncommon.

Anna Perez, M.Sc.

For Further Information

Clarke, C. A., and S. L. Glaser. "Changing Incidence of Non-Hodgkin Lymphomas in the United States." *Cancer* 94 (2002): 2015-2023.

Norton, A. J., J. Matthews, V. Pappa, et al. "Mantle Cell Lymphoma: Natural History Defined in a Serially Biopsied Population over a 20-Year Period." *Annals of Oncology* 6 (1995): 249-256.

Other Resources

American Cancer Society
http://www.cancer.org

Leukemia and Lymphoma Society
http://www.leukemia-lymphoma.org

National Cancer Institute
www.cancer.gov/search/geneticsservices

See also: Angiogenesis inhibitors; Burkitt lymphoma; Non-Hodgkin lymphoma; Proteasome inhibitors; Richter syndrome; Virus-related cancers

▶ Mastocytomas

Category: Diseases, Symptoms, and Conditions
Also known as: Mast cell tumors

Related conditions: Mastocytosis

Definition: Mastocytomas are lesions found in mastocytosis, a disease characterized by an abnormal increase in tissue mast cells. Mastocytomas do not lead to the hematogenous spread of mast cells; there is no known association with mastocytomas and a predilection to develop mast cell leukemia.

Risk factors: Mastocytomas typically develop only in people with mastocytosis.

Etiology and the disease process: Mast cells are ubiquitous throughout the body and are found in almost all body tissues. They release proinflammatory mediators such as histamine on activation. Mastocytosis may be limited to the skin, in which case it is referred to as cutaneous mastocytosis, or may involve systemic organ systems, in which case it is referred to as systemic mastocytosis. Mastocytomas—along with urticaria pigmentosa, diffuse cutaneous mastocytosis, and telangiectasia macularis eruptive perstans—make up the spectrum of cutaneous disease. Accumulations of mast cells in the skin result in these conditions.

Mastocytomas can appear as solitary or multiple lesions and typically affect only children before the age of six months. Mastocytomas more commonly appear as solitary lesions, and if a second lesion or multiple lesions develop, they typically do not occur more than two months after the first lesion. They are rare in adults because they usually resolve early in life. Although mastocytomas most commonly are localized to the skin, other organs, such as the gastrointestinal system, may be affected. They are nodular, usually range in size from three to four centimeters, and frequently occur on an extremity.

Incidence: The incidence of mastocytomas is unknown.

Symptoms: Lesions may be asymptomatic or may intermittently become itchy, red, and swollen if the lesions are stroked. More commonly, lesions are symptomatic.

Screening and diagnosis: The lesions typically demonstrate Darier's sign. Darier's sign occurs when a lesion is stroked and the lesion and the surrounding area become itchy, red, and swollen. On histological examination, mastocytomas show marked tumorlike aggregates of mast cells throughout the dermis.

Treatment and therapy: Mastocytomas that cause mechanical problems or systemic problems can be treated locally with PUVA therapy (psoralen combined with long-wave ultraviolet light). Potent topical steroids under occlusive dressings are also utilized. Surgical excision is also an option but should be considered only as a last option, as the natural course of the lesions is to resolve.

Prognosis, prevention, and outcomes: Mastocytomas usually appear in infancy, and the occurrence of the lesions resolves by adolescence.

Sarah Kasprowicz, M.D.

See also: Benign tumors; Veterinary oncology

▶ Mediastinal tumors

Category: Diseases, Symptoms, and Conditions
Also known as: Mediastinal neoplasias

Related conditions: Pericardial cysts, ectopic thyroid, bronchiogenic cysts

Definition: Mediastinal tumors are benign or malignant growths in the mediastinum, which is the central chest cavity that separates the lungs and contains the heart, aorta, esophagus, thymus, and trachea.

Risk factors: Risk factors include neurofibromatosis (von Recklinghausen disease), Li-Fraumeni syndrome, and a family history of Hodgkin disease.

Etiology and the disease process: The mediastinum is divided into the front, middle, and posterior mediastinum. The anterior mediastinum lies between the heart and the sternum. The middle mediastinum extends from the surface of the heart to the trachea (windpipe), and the posterior mediastinum begins behind the trachea and ends at the front of the vertebral column (backbone). Each mediastinal compartment is subject to specific types of tumors.

Anterior mediastinal tumors include tumors of the thymus (thymomas), lymphomas, teratomas, and thyroid tumors. Thymomas usually occur in adults, but 15 percent of them occur in children. Lymphomas account for 10 to 20 percent of anterior mediastinal tumors. Hodgkin disease causes most adult cases of mediastinal lymphomas. Teratomas (germ-cell tumors) account for 10 to 15 percent of mediastinal tumors. Thyroid tumors grow from goiters and primarily occur in women.

Tumors of the middle mediastinum include lymphomas (most common), mesenchymal tumors, and carcinomas. Mesenchymal tumors account for 6 percent of primary mediastinal tumors and are also called soft-tissue tumors that originate in connective tissue within the chest (about half are malignant).

Neurogenic tumors (derived from nerve cells) are the most common tumors of the posterior mediastinum and include malignant schwannomas and neuroblastomas. Some 19 to 39 percent of mediastinal tumors are neurogenic and are usually benign in adults but malignant in children. Endocrine and mesenchymal tumors are also found in the posterior mediastinum.

Though typically diagnosed in people between the ages of thirty and fifty, mediastinal tumors can occur at any age and in any tissue that passes through the chest.

Incidence: Thymomas occur at a rate of 3 cases per million people per year. Lymphoblastic lymphomas in children occur at a rate of 6 cases per million. There are about 6 cases of mediastinal germ-cell tumors per million in children per year. Some 125 children per year in the United States are diagnosed with mediastinal neuroblastomas.

Symptoms: Half of mediastinal tumors produce no symptoms, but masses in the chest can compress other tissues and prevent proper functioning. The most common symptoms are cough, shortness of breath, and chest pain. Accompanying symptoms include trouble swallowing (dysphagia), chest pain, fever, chills, night sweats, coughing up blood (hemoptysis), hoarseness, unintentional weight loss, wheezing, tender or swollen lymph nodes (lymphadenopathy), and stridor (high-pitched, noisy respiration).

Between 35 and 50 percent of people with thymomas experience myasthenia gravis-like symptoms that include weakness of eye muscles, drooping of one or both eyelids (ptosis), and fatigue. Certain mediastinal tumors can produce neurotransmitters (catecholamines) that significantly raise blood pressure (hypertension). Other types of neurosarcomas can make insulinlike substances that can cause low blood sugar concentrations (hypoglycemia).

Blood work may show abnormally high levels of serum calcium (hypercalcemia) and abnormally low levels of antibodies (hypogammaglobulinemia), circulating blood cells (cytopenia), and normal red blood cells (pernicious anemia).

Screening and staging: Many different types of imaging tests can detect mediastinal tumors. Chest X rays are essential to determine the location of mediastinal tumors. Computed tomography (CT) and magnetic resonance imaging (MRI) scans are common imaging methods for detecting mediastinal masses. CT scans are also used to direct needle biopsies of potentially tumorous masses. Positron emission tomography (PET) scans are used to determine the spread of the tumor to other parts of the body. If the tumor is located in a difficult-to-reach spot, then laparoscopic surgery called mediastinoscopy is used to biopsy the mass.

Most mediastinal tumors are solid tumors, which are graded by TNM (tumor/lymph node/metastasis) staging. T refers to the primary tumor and grades it from 0 to 4. N specifies the spread of the cancer to nearby lymph nodes (ranked 0 to 3). M represents metastasis or spread of the tumor beyond the lymph nodes to other parts of the body (0 or 1).

Treatment and therapy: Thymomas are primarily treated with surgery, followed by radiation or chemotherapy. For lymphomas, chemotherapy followed by radiation is the treatment of choice. For neurogenic tumors, surgery is the treatment of choice. It is possible to surgically resection some mesenchymal tumors and radiation can help in some cases, but some fibrosarcomas are not treatable with surgery or chemotherapy. Malignant schwannomas are very aggressive tumors that require multiagent chemotherapy.

Prognosis, prevention, and outcomes: The outcome is highly dependent on the type of tumor. If untreated, the prognosis is very poor. If properly treated, the prognosis for thymomas, lymphomas, thyroid tumors, teratomas, and some neurogenic tumors is generally quite good. Mesenchymal tumors tend to have a poor prognosis.

Michael A. Buratovich, Ph.D.

For Further Information

Duwe, Beau V., Daniel H. Sterman, and Ali I. Musani. "Tumors of the Mediastinum." *Chest* 128 (2005): 2893-2909.

Huang, Tsai-Wang, et al. "Middle Mediastinal Thymoma." *Respirology* 12, no. 6 (2007): 934-936.

Quint, Leslie E. "Imaging of Anterior Mediastinal Masses." *Cancer Imaging* 7 (2007): S56-S62.

Strollo, Diane C., Melissa L. Rosado de Christenson, and James R. Jett. "Primary Mediastinal Tumors: Part 1, Tumors of the Anterior Mediastinum." *Chest* 112 (1997): 511-522.

_______. "Primary Mediastinal Tumors: Part 2, Tumors of the Middle and Posterior Mediastinum." *Chest* 112 (1997): 1344-1357.

Other Resources

American Cancer Society
http://www.cancer.org

National Cancer Institute
http://www.cancer.gov

See also: Klinefelter syndrome and cancer; Lung cancers; Mediastinoscopy; Stent therapy; Superior vena cava syndrome; Surgical biopsies; Thoracoscopy

▶ Medullary carcinoma of the breast

Category: Diseases, Symptoms, and Conditions
Also known as: Infiltrating breast cancer

Definition: Medullary carcinoma is a rare but invasive breast cancer distinguished microscopically by a well-defined boundary, presence of cells from the immune system at its edges, and large, misshapen cancer cells.

Related conditions: Familial breast cancer

Risk factors: Medullary breast carcinoma is more frequent in women with a genetic predisposition. Mutations in tumor-suppressor genes, whether genetic or unknown in origin, can prevent their normal function of suppressing abnormal growth. This mutation occurs at the *BRCA1* and *BRCA2* genes. In some studies, medullary carcinomas account for up to 19 percent of all cancers in women with a *BRCA1* mutation. In women with a family history of reproductive-system cancers, smoking increases breast cancer risk significantly.

Estrogen can stimulate breast cancers. Changes in deoxyribonucleic acid (DNA), which carries the instructions for all cells, can cause normal cells to become cancerous, and such changes are more likely to occur with age.

Etiology and the disease process: Estrogen exposure tends to encourage breast cancer, and hormones can boost breast cancer growth. Gene mutations can inhibit the body's defenses.

Incidence: These infrequent cancers make up 2 to 7 percent of breast cancer cases.

Symptoms: Most cancers start without symptoms, detectable if at all by only mammography or ultrasound. As the cancer develops, a lump or thickening may begin. An unusual lump in the breast or armpit area, one that feels firm or unlike other breast tissue, or a lump that seems "fixed" and immobile, needs to be investigated.

Screening and diagnosis: Medullary carcinomas are distinguishable by histology (microscopic examination). Monthly self-examination and regular mammography increase early detection. Staging for medullary carcinomas is as follows:

- Stage I: Cancerous cells have invaded nearby tissue.
- Stage II: Cancerous cells are in lymph nodes in the armpit.
- Stage III: Cancerous cells have invaded lymph nodes, breastbone, and other tissues above the waist.

Treatment and therapy: Treatment is the same as for invasive ductal carcinoma: usually a combination of local therapy (affecting only the cancer site, such as surgery and radiation) and systemic therapy using drugs (chemotherapy, hormone therapy, and immunotherapy), either by mouth or intravenously, to kill cancer cells that might have spread elsewhere but are not yet detectable.

Prognosis, prevention, and outcomes: When caught early, medullary breast cancers are curable and prognosis is good, with 70 percent of patients surviving for ten years. Good, balanced nutrition with avoidance of dietary fat and a healthy lifestyle that avoids smoking and includes exercise are among the best strategies for decreasing the chance of developing cancer.

Jackie Dial, Ph.D.

See also: *BRCA1* and *BRCA2* genes; Breast cancer in men; Breast cancer in pregnant women; Breast cancers; Carcinomatosis; Invasive ductal carcinomas; Invasive lobular carcinomas

▶ Medulloblastomas

Category: Diseases, Symptoms, and Conditions

Related conditions: Supratentorial primitive neuroectodermal tumors, neurofibromatosis (von Recklinghausen disease), Gorlin syndrome

Definition: Medulloblastomas are malignant (cancerous) or benign (noncancerous) tumors that form in the cerebellum of the brain. The cerebellum controls balance and movement, posture, and speech. These tumors occur more often in children but may rarely appear in adults.

Risk factors: There is no known cause of medulloblastomas, but, scientists are uncovering changes in genes and chromosomes that may influence the development of these tumors. A small percentage of tumors may tend to occur in families, particularly in families with neurofibromatosis (von Recklinghausen disease), an inherited disease that causes benign tumors to occur on peripheral nerves in the body. A few individuals with Gorlin syndrome, an inherited disease related to basal cell carcinoma and other conditions, also develop medulloblastoma.

Etiology and the disease process: Medulloblastoma is a relatively rare disease, with no known cause other than a familial tendency. The tumor is considered fast growing. Because of the location of the tumor, walking and talking disruptions are common as the disease progresses.

Incidence: The tumor occurs more often in boys than girls, and generally before the age of eight, with a peak incidence between five and ten years of age. In the United States, the incidence of medulloblastoma is 1.5 to 2 cases per 100,000 population (children). Approximately 1,000 cases are diagnosed annually, with 1 in 5 brain tumors in children diagnosed as medulloblastoma.

Symptoms: The classic, initial symptoms of medulloblastoma are morning headaches, nausea, vomiting, and other flulike symptoms. Because the symptoms mimic flu, the tumor may go undiagnosed until symptoms progress to balance problems. Older children may be more easily diagnosed than infants, as infants may initially exhibit an increase in head size and irritability, both common in infants as they grow and develop. Vomiting may make the person feel better, as the intracranial pressure is temporarily relieved. Symptoms increase as the tumor grows.

Screening and diagnosis: There is no screening test for medulloblastoma. Diagnosis begins with a history of symptoms and neurological examination. Radiology studies include magnetic resonance imaging (MRI), including the use of a contrast dye, to identify the presence of a brain tumor, and a positron emission tomography (PET) scan, used to determine if the tumor is active and growing. Other procedures, such as a lumbar puncture to take cerebrospinal fluid (CSF), a bone marrow aspiration and biopsy, and a bone scan, may be done to look for signs of cancer. A confirmed diagnosis is made during surgery, and pathologic examination of the tumor specimen removed determines if the tumor is benign or malignant.

Two risk groups are used in childhood medulloblastoma to determine treatment management, rather than the adult staging process. The average risk group and the poor risk group are differentiated based on the tumor remaining after surgery, spread of cancer cells within the brain and spinal cord, or distant spread of tumor cells to other parts of the body. Adults are staged based on the remaining tumor and whether the tumor has spread using the TNM (tumor/lymph node/metastasis) staging system.

Treatment and therapy: Treatment of medulloblastoma is with surgery, radiation therapy, chemotherapy, and, if necessary, mechanical diversion of cerebrospinal fluid with a shunt to carry blocked fluid out of the brain. Surgery is used to remove as much of the tumor as possible. Imaging studies may show that the tumor is inoperable. A biopsy will still be done to determine the type of tumor and whether it is malignant. If the tumor has grown into the brain stem, removal may not be an option, as the side effects of removal are life-threatening. Steroids are used to decrease swelling in the brain. A shunt, or tube to drain CSF away from the brain, usually to the abdomen, may be placed during surgery. Radiation therapy to the brain and the spinal cord is then used to kill any cells remaining. Radiation may be done with stereotactic radiosurgery, intensity-modulated radiation therapy, or external beam radiation. Chemotherapy may be used in infants to postpone the use of radiation, as cranial radiation side effects may be severe. Chemotherapy may be given either intravenously (into a vein) or intrathecally (into the

Relative Survival Rates for Medulloblastoma, 1988-2001

Years	*Survival Rate (%)*
1	89.2
2	84.6
3	78.4
5	66.4
8	56.8
10	52.5

Source: Data from L. A. G. Ries et al., eds., Cancer Survival Among Adults: U.S. SEER Program, 1988-2001—Patient and Tumor Characteristics, NIH Pub. No. 07-6215 (Bethesda, Md.: National Cancer Institute, 2007)

cerebrospinal fluid) by use of an Ommaya reservoir. In adults, chemotherapy effectiveness is less clear.

Prognosis, prevention, and outcomes: The prognosis for medulloblastoma varies with the patient's age at diagnosis, the size of the tumor, the amount remaining after surgery, and the level of tumor cell spread to other sites in the brain, spinal cord, or elsewhere in the body (metastasis). Approximately 70 percent of adults are alive at five years after diagnosis, and up to 80 percent of children with average-risk classification can be expected to reach five years. With poor risk classification, up to 65 percent of children may survive to five years. The outcome for infants is poor, with a 30 to 50 percent survival. There is no prevention for medulloblastoma. Quality of life may be negatively affected by the side effects of therapy, including learning disabilities, hearing loss from drug therapy, obesity, thyroid deficiency, and other problems depending on treatment and site. Recurrence is always a risk as tumors may be difficult to remove completely.

Patricia Stanfill Edens, R.N., Ph.D., FACHE

For Further Information

Hargrave, D. R., and S. Zacharoulis. "Pediatric CNS Tumors: Current Treatment and Future Directions." *Expert Review of Neurotherapeutics* 7, no. 8 (August, 2007): 1029-1042.

Parker, W., E. Filion, D. Roberge, and C. R. Freeman. "Intensity-Modulated Radiotherapy for Craniospinal Irradiation: Target Volume Considerations, Dose Constraints, and Competing Risks." *International Journal of Radiation Oncology, Biology, Physics* 69, no. 1 (September 1, 2007): 251-257.

Other Resources

American Brain Tumor Association
http://www.abta.org

American Cancer Society
http://www.cancer.org

National Cancer Institute
Childhood Medulloblastoma Treatment
http://www.cancer.gov/cancertopics/pdq/treatment/childmedulloblastoma/patient/

See also: Brain and central nervous system cancers; Craniotomy; Neuroectodermal tumors; Turcot syndrome

▶ Melanomas

Category: Diseases, Symptoms, and Conditions
Also known as: Skin cancer

Related conditions: Basal cell cancer, squamous cell cancer

Definition: Melanomas are malignant tumors of the skin that occur in the melanocytes, the cells that produce melanin (skin pigment).

Risk factors: Melanomas occur most commonly in fair-skinned people, particularly natural blonds and redheads, especially those with a history of sun exposure or multiple serious sunburns. A history of serious sunburns in childhood is a particular risk. Risk for the disease is strongly related to having a family history; which is characteristic of about 1 in 10 of patients with melanoma. Additional risk factors include large or multiple moles and past personal history of melanoma or of less serious skin cancers, known as basal cell or squamous cell cancers. People with diseases that suppress the immune system are at added risk for melanoma. Occupational exposure to coal tar, pitch, creosote, arsenic compounds, or radium increase a person's risk for the disease. Celtic descent, male gender, and older age are also risk factors.

Etiology and the disease process: Repeat exposure to harmful ultraviolet rays from the sun or artificial sources such as sunlamps or tanning booths appears to be the most significant factor contributing to the development of melanoma. This is borne out by the fact that the incidence of melanoma increases in the lower latitudes of the world where the sun is strongest. Additionally, in parts of the world where the ozone layer is thin, the incidence is higher. In Queensland, Australia, for example, where there is a hole in the ozone, between 1979 to 1987, the rate of melanoma doubled to 55.8 per 100,000 men and rose to 42.9 per 100,000 women.

Melanomas can occur on parts of the body not usually exposed to the sun, including the soles of the feet and the genitals. Melanoma starts with an abnormal skin growth, which is generally quite small. When discovered at this early stage, melanomas can be easily removed and the cancer cured. If the growth is not removed, it thickens and invades surrounding tissue and nearby lymph nodes. The cancer can then spread through the lymph nodes to sites distant from the original growth, including vital organs, soft tissues, and other lymph nodes.

Incidence: In the 1970's, the incidence rate of melanoma rose dramatically to about 6 percent a year. Incidence continues to rise but at a slower rate; from 1981 to 2001 the rate of growth was about 3 percent a year.

The American Cancer Society estimated that 59,940 men and women in the United States would be newly diagnosed with melanoma in 2007. Melanoma affects adults of all ages as well as teenagers. Based on statistics for the years 2001 to 2003, the probability of a man in the United States developing melanoma is 1 in 49. For a woman in the United States, the probability is 1 in 73. Rates for whites are ten times higher than for African Americans. However, one type of melanoma, which develops on the palms of the hands, soles of the feet, and nail beds, occurs more frequently in African Americans and Asians.

Symptoms: Melanoma generally first appears as a new mole or a change in the shape, size, or color of an existing mole. The American Cancer Society describes the warning signals in terms of a mnemonic: ABCD. "A" for asymmetry, meaning that the mole is not uniformly round; "B" for border, in that the edges of the mole are irregular; "C" for color, referring to the varied colors (generally in tones of tan, brown, and black) throughout

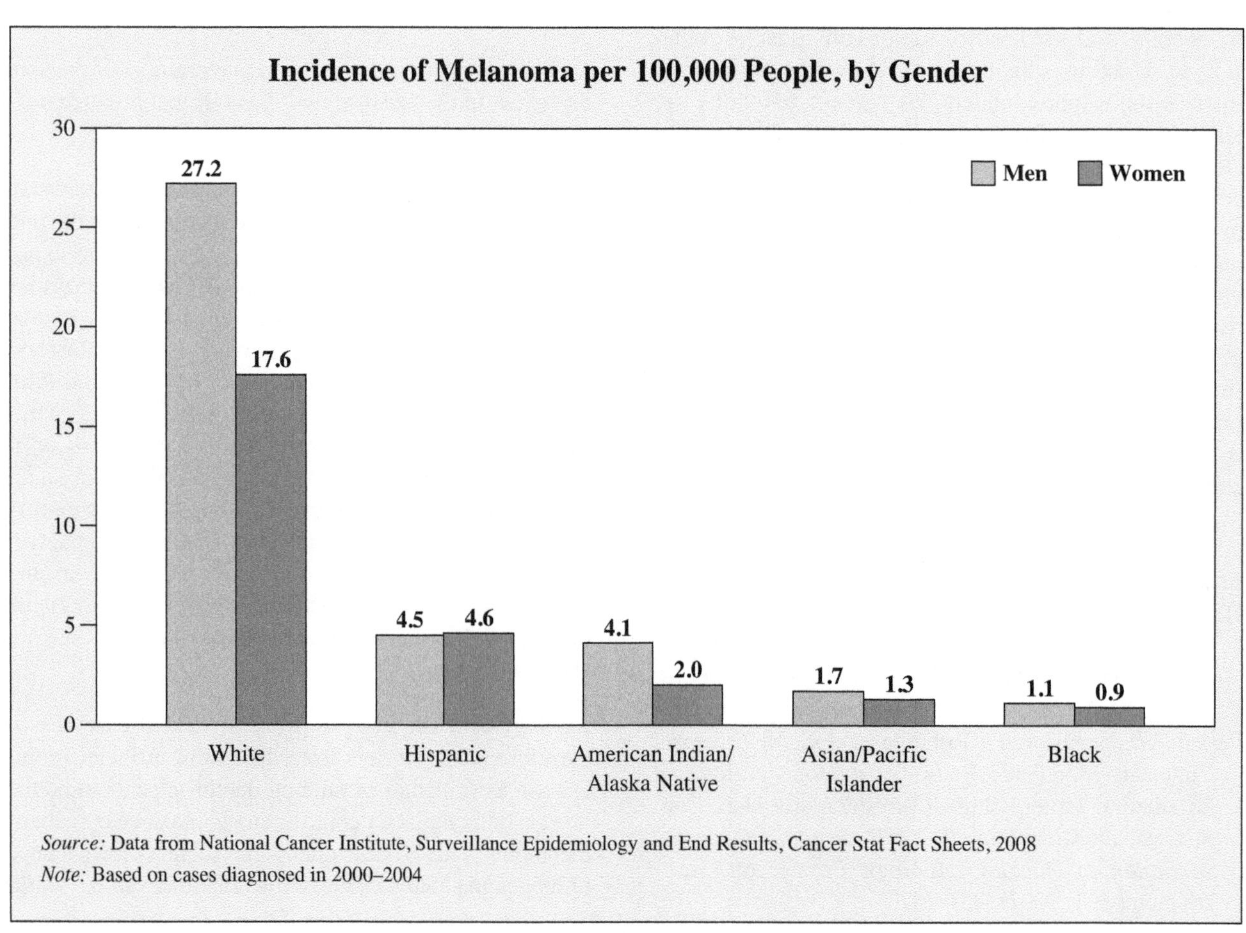

Source: Data from National Cancer Institute, Surveillance Epidemiology and End Results, Cancer Stat Fact Sheets, 2008
Note: Based on cases diagnosed in 2000–2004

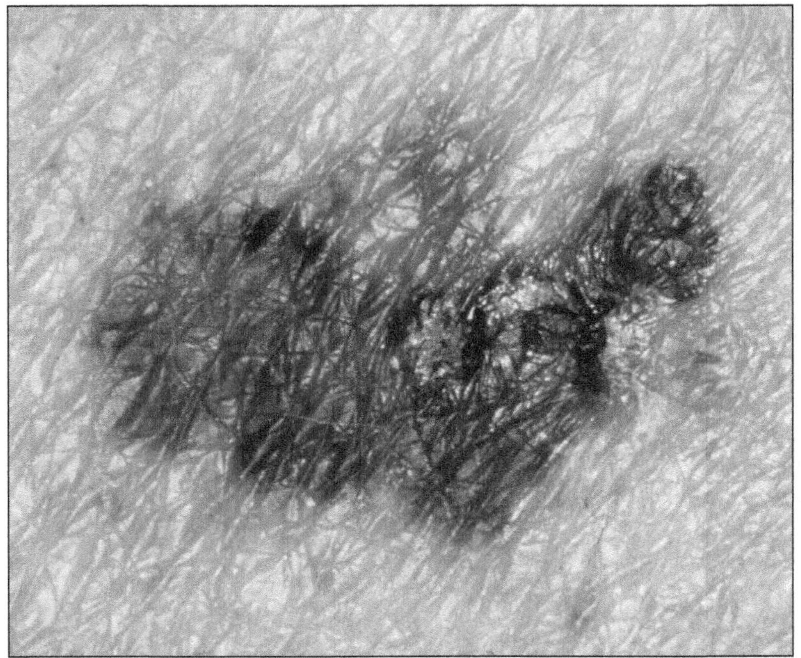

Melanoma. (National Cancer Institute)

the mole; and "D" for diameter, meaning that the mole is larger than 6 millimeters (mm).

Screening and diagnosis: People with serious risk factors or symptoms should have regular full body exams by a dermatologist to identify any skin abnormalities, and baseline photographs should be taken so that any changes can be tracked. Suspect moles or skin abnormalities should be removed and analyzed for cancer cells.

The stages of melanoma are defined as follows:

- Localized, Stage 0: These melanomas involve only the top layer of skin, the epidermis.
- Localized, Stages I and II: These melanomas involve the underlying layer of skin, the dermis, and are rated according to the depth they penetrate the skin (known as the Breslow depth) and their degree of ulceration (how much the epidermis is eroded and exposes the dermis below). Ulceration is determined by a pathologist, using a microscope.
- Regional, Stage III: These melanomas include those in which the cancer has spread to nearby lymph nodes.
- Advanced, Stage IV: These melanomas include those where cancer has spread beyond the region of the skin growth to distant sites in the body, including internal organs and distant lymph nodes.

Treatment and therapy: Significant advances have been made in the early detection of melanoma. All suspect moles or skin growths should be removed and tested for cancerous cells. Removal of localized growths (Stages 0-II) can be done one of three ways: surgically, cutting out the suspect tissue; by electrodessication and curettage, using an electric current to destroy the tissue and then scraping the area with a special tool to remove any possible remaining cancer cells; or by cryosurgery, which freezes the tissue. About 83 percent of melanomas are diagnosed in these early stages while the cancer is still confined to the primary skin growth. Surgery successfully removes the cancer for the majority of patients with early-stage melanoma. In some cases, radiation therapy may be directed at the area following surgery to kill any cancer cells that may remain. Patients with Stages 0 to II melanoma have an excellent prognosis.

If the growth is extensive, the surgeon will remove lymph nodes to determine if the cancer has spread. After their removal, Stage III and IV melanomas may be treated with radiation or immunotherapy (agents that attempt to harness the human body's own disease-fighting properties to kill cancer cells) or chemotherapy (toxic agents targeted to kill cancer cells). Two therapeutic agents approved by the U.S. Food and Drug Administration (FDA) for the treatment of Stage III and IV melanoma are dacarbazine (DTIC, chemotherapy) and interleukin-2 (IL-2, immunotherapy). Some patients with Stage III and IV disease experience a full recovery with chemotherapy; however, positive responses to the drug therapy, when they occur, are most often partial and brief. Much research is being done to explore other possible treatments for melanoma, including combinations of different chemotherapies and new immunotherapies. Some of these agents are not specifically approved by the FDA to treat melanoma. Patients with melanoma may be eligible to become subjects in clinical trials in which these experimental agents or combinations of agents are tested.

Prognosis, prevention, and outcomes: The thickness of a patient's tumor is the best single indicator of the prognosis. After having melanomas of less than 0.76 mm removed, about 96 to 99 percent of patients are cured. About 1 in 10 patients with melanoma is diagnosed after the cancer has already spread to nearby lymph nodes.

For these patients in the regional stage (Stage III), the prognosis is not as good, but survival rates for patients with Stage III disease range widely, depending on how many lymph nodes are affected by the cancer. About 3 of 10 patients with melanoma are diagnosed in an advanced stage (Stage IV), after the cancer has already spread (metastasized) to distant sites. Those with metastases to the skin or soft tissue or to distant lymph nodes appear to fare better than those with lung or other vital organ metastases.

Recommended measures to prevent melanoma include avoiding excessive direct sunshine, especially during the hours when the sun is high in the sky (from about 10 a.m. to 2 p.m.); using sunscreen and protective clothing to prevent sunburn; and not using sunlamps; tanning booths, or other artificial sources of ultraviolet light. People should become familiar with the moles and spots on their bodies and report any changes that could indicate melanoma to their doctors.

Charlotte Crowder, M.P.H., ELS

For Further Information

Kaufman, Howard. *The Melanoma Book: A Complete Guide to Prevention and Treatment.* New York: Gotham Books, 2005.

Poole, Catherine M., and I. V. DuPont Guerry. *Melanoma: Prevention, Detection, and Treatment.* 2d ed. New Haven, Conn.: Yale University Press, 2005.

Schofield, Jill R., and William A. Robinson. *What You Really Need to Know About Moles and Melanoma.* Baltimore: Johns Hopkins University Press, 2000.

Other Resources

Melanoma Center
http://www.melanomacenter.org

Melanoma Research Foundation
http://www.melanoma.org/

National Cancer Institute
Melanoma
http://www.cancer.gov/cancertopics/types/melanoma

Skin Cancer Foundation
Melanoma
http://www.skincancer.org/melanoma/index.php

See also: Breslow's staging; Dermatology oncology; Dysplastic nevus syndrome; Merkel Cell Carcinomas (MCC); Moles; Premalignancies; Risks for cancer; Skin cancers; Squamous cell carcinomas; Sunlamps

▶ Meningeal carcinomatosis

Category: Diseases, Symptoms, and Conditions
Also known as: Carcinomatous meningitis, leptomeningeal carcinomatosis

Related conditions: Almost any type of cancer can be associated with this condition, but it is generally seen with breast, melanoma, and lung cancers.

Definition: Carcinomatous meningitis is the spread of tumor cells from a primary central nervous system (CNS) source, such as a brain tumor, or from a distant source, such as a lung or breast tumor, via the blood to the subarachnoid space, where it spreads via the fluid covering the brain, called the cerebral spinal fluid (CSF) fluid, to involve the coverings of the brain, known as the leptomeninges.

Risk factors: In adults, primary brain tumors such as oligodendroglioma or secondary tumors, also called metastases, from lung, breast, melanoma, lymphoma, ovarian, or gastric cancer can spread to the brain surfaces.

Etiology and the disease process: Unlike other forms of meningitis, where the invading organism is a bacterium, fungus, or virus, the invaders in carcinomatous meningitis are cancer cells. In adults, meningeal carcinomatosis is usually the result of the metastasis of a primary brain tumor or a secondary cancer in a person who has lymphoma, melanoma, or lung, breast, or gastric tumors.

Incidence: The incidence of meningeal carcinomatosis is increasing because cancer patients are surviving longer. It is seen in about 3 to 5 percent of patients who have cancer.

Symptoms: Patients usually complain of nonspecific symptoms of headache, back pain, or weakness in an extremity.

Screening and diagnosis: Meningeal carcinomatosis can be diagnosed by magnetic resonance imaging (MRI) or myelography together with computed tomography (CT). A spinal tap (also called a lumbar puncture), whereby a needle is inserted into the cerebral spinal fluid within the subarachnoid space and the fluid is sampled, is the usual form of diagnosis, although cerebral spinal fluid cytology is negative in 10 percent of cases.

Treatment and therapy: Meningeal carcinomatosis is difficult to cure and the aim of treatment is usually to ameliorate symptoms, usually by chemotherapy injected into the spinal fluid via lumbar puncture (intrathecal methotrexate) or by radiotherapy to the brain.

Prognosis, prevention, and outcomes: Some patients respond to treatment; however, the prognosis is generally poor with death occurring within one month if the disease is untreated.

Debra B. Kessler, M.D., Ph.D.

See also: Carcinomatous meningitis; Leptomeningeal carcinomas; Lumbar puncture

▶ Meningiomas

Category: Diseases, Symptoms, and Conditions
Also known as: Meningeal tumors

Related conditions: Intracranial and spinal tumors, extra-axial brain tumors, neurofibromatosis

Definition: Meningiomas are tumors of the meninges, the thin layers of tissue that surround the brain and spinal cord. This type of neoplasm most likely originates from cells of the arachnoid matter, the middle element of the three meningeal coverings, and occur mainly at the base of the brain and around the cerebral convexities. Meningiomas are visibly demarcated from the brain tissue and thus are classified as extra-axial tumors. They can extend from the surface of the dura matter, the outer meningeal layer, and erode the cranial bones, causing exostosis, or growth of the bone. In general, these are solitary lesions, and more than 80 percent of them are benign. However, multiple lesions are common in patients with neurofibromatosis type 2 (NF2), a genetic disorder that affects the nervous system. Several different histological types have been described, with the meningothelial, fibrous, and transitional forms as the most frequently found.

Risk factors: Although the risk factors for meningiomas are largely unknown, evidence suggests an association of risk with a family or personal history of neurofibromatosis type 2, exposure to ionizing radiation (during full-mouth dental radiographs), and use of sex hormones (oral contraceptives or hormone replacement therapy). Other risks factors that have been explored without conclusive results are head trauma, cell phone use, breast cancer, and allergic diseases.

Etiology and the disease process: The precise origin of the majority of the meningiomas is uncertain. However, several forms of this disease are clearly associated with the loss of a tumor-suppressor gene on chromosome 22, known as merlin and encoded by the *NF2* gene. Merlin belongs to the 4.1 family of proteins, a group of molecules with roles in maintaining cell structure. Genetic defects in merlin account for many sporadic meningioma cases. In addition to merlin, other members of the 4.1 protein family with tumor-suppression activity have been involved in meningioma initiation (for example, 4.1B and 4.1R). However, meningioma progression seems to involve genetic changes in chromosomes other than chromosome 22.

The presence of a high density of progesterone receptors in the vast majority of meningiomas suggests a functional role of progesterone-signaling pathways in the pathogenesis and might explain the twofold and tenfold higher incidence respectively of cranial and spinal meningiomas in women. Other proteins that might participate in the disease process of meningioma include telomerase, transforming growth factor-beta, and somatostatin.

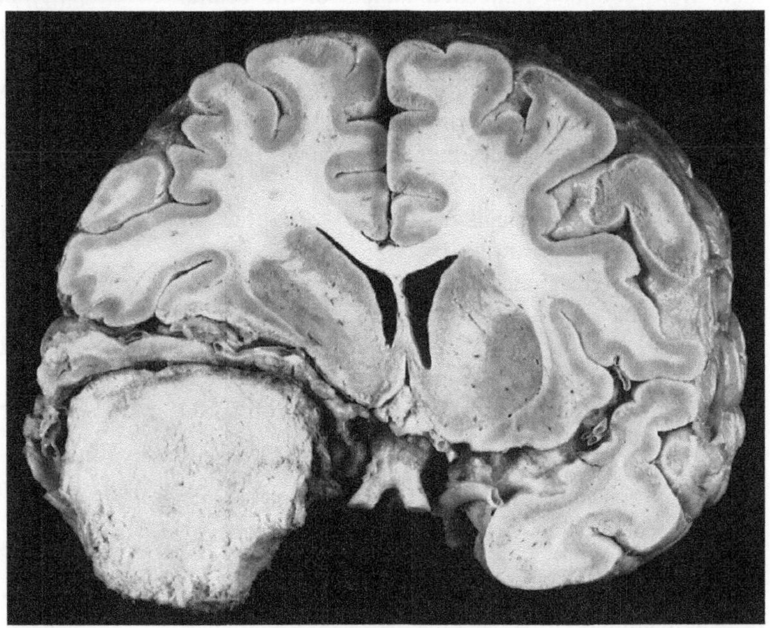

The classic meningioma is a soft, spherical lesion which displaces rather than infiltrates the underlying brain. (The Armed Forces Institute of Pathology (AFIP)/ Wikimedia)

Incidence: Meningiomas are the most common nonglial and most common extra-axial tumors of the brain, with an annual age-adjusted incidence rate of 5 per 100,000 individuals. The relatively frequent autopsy finding of small asymptomatic undiagnosed meningiomas suggests that the actual incidence rate is significantly higher. They are more common in women, and the highest incidence is observed in the sixth and seventh decades of life. Childhood cases of meningioma are rare.

Symptoms: Symptoms of meningiomas depend on the location and size of the lesion and result from increased intracranial pressure and edema of the brain structures adjacent to the tumor. The most common symptoms are headache, unilateral sensory disturbances (for example, hearing or visual loss), vertigo, imbalance, focal seizures, spastic weakness, numbness of the limbs, and painless proptosis or "bulging" eyes, among others.

Screening and diagnosis: No screening tests are available. The tendency of meningiomas to calcify and their abundant blood supply allow their diagnosis by contrast-enhanced computed tomography (CT), magnetic resonance imaging (MRI), and arteriography. On both CT and MRI scans, meningiomas appear as homogeneous, smoothly outlined masses, with attachments to the dura matter. Their extra-axial location differentiates them from common intra-axial tumors of the central nervous system, and their unique image density characteristics differentiate them from Schwannoma, another extra-axial tumor.

The World Health Organization (WHO) classifies meningiomas into three grades based on their histological features and the likelihood of recurrence.

- Grade I: Benign meningiomas, with low risk of recurrence and aggressive growth
- Grade II: Atypical meningiomas, with greater risk of recurrence and aggressive growth
- Grade III: Anaplastic or malignant meningiomas, with the greatest risk of recurrence and aggressive growth

Some 80 percent of all meningiomas are of WHO Grade I on diagnosis.

Treatment and therapy: The primary treatment is complete surgical excision of the tumor. Focused radiation by Gamma Knife or proton beam is used when the lesion is located around vital structures or when it is a high-grade or recurrent tumor. Although effective chemotherapy has not yet been developed, studies on the use of hormonal antagonists and other molecules are ongoing.

Prognosis, prevention, and outcomes: Complete removal of the tumor is achieved in more than 70 percent of the cases, and in most patients, hearing and other functions of the nervous system are preserved. Recurrence depends on the grade of the tumor, ranging from 5 percent for WHO Grade I tumors up to 80 percent for WHO Grade III after five years of treatment. Prevention of meningiomas is difficult since the etiology is poorly understood.

Reyniel Cruz-Aguado, Ph.D.

For Further Information

Claus, E. B., et al. "Epidemiology of Intracranial Meningioma." *Neurosurgery* 57 (2005): 1088-1095.

Lusis, E., and D. H. Gutmann. "Meningioma: An Update." *Current Opinion in Neurology* 17 (2004): 687-692.

Riemenschneider, M. J., A. Perry, and G. Reifenberger. "Histological Classification and Molecular Genetics of Meningiomas." *Lancet Neurology* 5 (2006): 1045-1054.

Other Resources

Brain Tumor Foundation
http://www.braintumorfoundation.org/about.asp

MayoClinic.com
Meningioma
http://www.mayoclinic.com/health/meningioma/DS00901

See also: Acoustic neuromas; Brain and central nervous system cancers; Carcinomatous meningitis; Cell phones; Endotheliomas; Leptomeningeal carcinomas; Meningeal carcinomatosis; Neurofibromatosis type 1 (NF1); Pheochromocytomas; Spinal axis tumors

▶ Merkel Cell Carcinomas (MCC)

Category: Diseases, Symptoms, and Conditions
Also known as: Neuroendocrine carcinoma of the skin

Related conditions: Ectodermal dysplasia

Definition: Merkel cell carcinomas (MCC) are fast-growing cancers in Merkel cells, which are found in the deepest part of the outermost skin layer and are believed to be associated with the sense of touch. The structure of

Merkel cells is characteristic of cells that assist in impulse transmission between an initial stimulus and the nerve impulse that carries messages to the brain. This cancer appears on the face, head, or neck as a firm, painless, shiny bump that can be red, pink, or blue, and it has been found to spread quickly to other parts of the body. Considered rare, MCC has become the second most common cause of non-melanoma skin cancer deaths, with most deaths from the disease occurring within the first three years after diagnosis.

Risk factors: Risk factors include being over the age of sixty-five and having a history of repeated or prolonged sun exposure. People with weakened immune systems, such as those with human immunodeficiency virus (HIV) infection, patients with organ transplants, and those on medications that suppress the immune system, are also at increased risk of developing MCC.

Etiology and the disease process: Although the exact cause of MCC is not known, it is believed that ultraviolet radiation from the sun and other sources plays a significant role in its development. One theory proposes that stem cells in the skin become cancerous and take on the characteristics of Merkel cells. Genetic abnormalities have been found in the cancer cells, leading to speculation that MCC is genetically linked. MCC grows rapidly, typically beginning on the face (especially around the eye), neck, and head. Metastasis to nearby lymph nodes, other areas of skin, liver, bone, and lungs is common and occurs early in the disease. When MCC spreads to other areas of the skin, the lesions grow rapidly and are flesh-colored to red-purple, firm, and deeper in the skin than the primary lesion.

Incidence: Statistics from the National Cancer Institute indicate that about 1,200 new cases of MCC are diagnosed each year in the United States. Although the number of cases is increasing, it still accounts for less than 1 percent of all skin cancers. The average age at diagnosis is sixty-nine. MCC is substantially more common among white people and affects women more often than men.

Relative Survival Rates for Merkel Cell Carcinoma, 1988-2001

Years	*Survival Rate (%)*
1	87.4
3	68.6
5	62.8
10	57.5

Source: Data from L. A. G. Ries et al., eds., Cancer Survival Among Adults: U.S. SEER Program, 1988-2001—Patient and Tumor Characteristics, NIH Pub. No. 07-6215 (Bethesda, Md.: National Cancer Institute, 2007)

Symptoms: The primary skin lesions in MCC usually produce no symptoms. They usually occur as solitary, dome-shaped nodules that are smaller than 2 centimeters (cm) in diameter, but can be larger than 15 cm. The skin surface is typically shiny and the color of the lesions is red, pink, or blue. Although they can develop on any skin surface, they are found on the head or neck in about 50 percent of cases. In 40 percent of the cases, they are found on the arms and legs.

Because metastasis is common with MCC, other symptoms that may be reported include swollen lymph glands and fatigue. New growths, with a different appearance than the primary site, may also be reported.

Screening and diagnosis: Screening for MCC should be performed as part of an annual physical. In addition, people at high risk for MCC should perform routine self-examination. When a nodule is found, a biopsy should be performed to determine its cell type and whether it is benign tissue, MCC or, possibly, another form of cancer. If it is found to be MCC, further testing should follow as soon as possible because of how rapidly it spreads. Additional testing should include sentinel lymph node biopsy, a complete blood count, liver function tests, and a chest X ray. Computed tomography (CT) and positron emission scanning (PET) should also be performed to determine the extent of the cancer's spread.

MCC is divided into three stages depending on the severity of disease.

- Stage I: The disease is localized to the skin at the primary site.
- Stage IA: The primary lesion is less than or equal to 2 cm.
- Stage IB: The primary lesion is greater than 2 cm.
- Stage II: The cancer involves nearby lymph nodes.
- Stage III: The cancer is found beyond the nearby lymph nodes.

The stage at diagnosis is important in determining the possibility of tumor metastasis, the patient's treatment options, and prognosis.

Treatment and therapy: Treatment of MCC is based on the stage of the disease at diagnosis. Most commonly, surgery is performed to remove the primary lesion, along with some normal skin around the lesion's edges. Lymph nodes are also removed to test for cancer cells and spread of the disease. Radiation therapy is usually given to the site of the primary lesion and the lymph nodes. When the cancer has spread beyond the lymph nodes, treatment is mainly palliative to relieve pain. The use of chemotherapy, typically with etoposide and carboplatin, is controversial. Some studies have demonstrated positive results but recommend that it be reserved for metastatic MCC, whereas others have found that, especially with this disease, there was a trend toward decreased survival rates.

Prognosis, prevention, and outcomes: Overall, the two-year survival rate for MCC is 50 to 70 percent. Most recurrences and most deaths from this disease occur within the first three years. The only prevention for MCC is to reduce exposure to ultraviolet light, including the sun.

Dorothy P. Terry, R.N.

For Further Information

Allen, P. J., et al. "Merkel Cell Carcinoma: Prognosis and Treatment of Patients from a Single Institution." *Journal of Clinical Oncology* 23, no. 10 (April 1, 2005): 2300-2309.

Brady, Mary S. "Current Management of Patients with Merkel Cell Carcinoma." *Dermatologic Surgery* 30, no. 2 (February, 2004): 321-325.

Hodgson, N. C. "Merkel Cell Carcinoma: Changing Incidence Trends." *Journal of Surgical Oncology* 89, no. 1 (January, 2005): 1-4.

Other Resources

American Cancer Society

Treating Merkel Cell Carcinoma
http://www.cancer.org/docroot/CRI/content/CRI_2_4_4X_Treatment_of_Merkel_Cell_Carcinoma_51.asp

MayoClinic.com

Merkel Cell Carcinoma
http://www.mayoclinic.com/health/merkel-cell-carcinoma/DS00802

National Cancer Institute

Merkel Cell Carcinoma Treatment
http://www.cancer.gov/cancertopics/pdq/treatment/merkelcell/patient

See also: Skin cancers

▶ Mesenchymomas, malignant

Category: Diseases, Symptoms, and Conditions
Also known as: Mixed-cell sarcomas

Related conditions: Soft-tissue sarcomas

Definition: Malignant mesenchymomas are a type of soft-tissue sarcoma composed of two or more unrelated malignant forms. These rare tumors contain at least two nonepithelial mesenchymal tissues that are neoplastic, with differing histologies are not normally associated together in the same tumor.

Risk factors: There are no readily identifiable risk factors particular to malignant mesenchymoma, although several risk factors associated with soft-tissue sarcomas in general have been identified. These include exposure to chlorophenols in wood preservatives and phenoxyacetic acid in herbicides, exposure to ionizing radiation, and very rare genetic predispositions in some families. Sporadic cases of malignant mesenchymoma in patients previously treated with radiation for breast cancer have been reported.

Etiology and the disease process: Etiology is not at all well understood, and connections with diet, smoking, alcohol, or preexisting conditions have not been established. It is most likely that malignant mesenchymomas arise from a primitive mesenchymal stem cell with the capacity for multipotent differentiation, thus resulting in a soft-tissue sarcoma with mixed neoplastic cell types.

Incidence: Only about 1 percent of newly diagnosed cancers are soft-tissue sarcomas, and malignant mesenchymomas represent only a small fraction of these. These tumors can develop at any age. Reports from the literature indicate ages of onset from one and a half years to eighty-four, with a median age of forty-six years and a slight preponderance of men.

Symptoms: These tumors can arise in any of the connective tissues of the body, although they are most frequently encountered in the arms, legs, hands, feet, and retroperitoneum. Unusual locations such as the neck, fibula, and uterus have also been reported. They are usually first detected as a painless swelling of the soft tissue. Retroperitoneal tumors may become quite massive before detection and may be diagnosed only after the functions of adjacent organs such as the liver or kidneys have been compromised.

Screening and diagnosis: No screening tests exist, although a few mesenchymomas are known to produce excessive amounts of insulin-like growth factor 2 precursor. Diagnosis is always based on direct histological examination of tumor tissue because other sarcomas of single somatic origin can develop in the same locations.

Treatment and therapy: Surgical removal of the tumor, whenever possible, is the treatment of choice. This can be followed by radiation therapy or chemotherapy. Doxorubicin, in combination with several other cytotoxic drugs has proven effective in a few cases, although the benefits of these postsurgical treatments are questionable.

Prognosis, prevention, and outcomes: Malignant mesenchymomas are usually described as high-grade sarcomas with a poor prognosis, although small tumors 5 centimeters or less in diameter have a much better prognosis. None of these tumors are encapsulated, so recurrence following excision is relatively common.

Jeffrey A. Knight, Ph.D.

See also: Fibrosarcomas, soft-tissue

▶ Mesothelioma

Category: Diseases, Symptoms, and Conditions
Also known as: Malignant mesothelioma (MM), pleural mesothelioma, peritoneal mesothelioma, pericardial mesothelioma

Related conditions: Lung cancer, pericardial effusion

Definition: Mesothelioma is a rare cancer of the mesothelium, the collective name for the membranes that surround the body's internal organs. Particular mesothelia—the pleura (which covers the lungs), the peritoneum (which lines the abdominal cavity), and the pericardium (the sac that surrounds the heart)—lend their names to forms of mesothelioma. Pleural mesothelioma and peritoneal mesothelioma are the most common forms. At the cellular level, mesothelioma takes three main forms: epithelioid (50 to 70 percent of cases), in which the cancer cell is typically uniform and cube shaped, with a visible nucleus; sarcomatoid (7 to 20 percent), in which the cells are more irregular and oval shaped, with less visible nuclei; and biphasic (20 to 35 percent), a mixture of the two.

Risk factors: About 80 percent of cases strike those exposed to asbestos, a name that refers to six silicate minerals: the serpentine mineral chrysotile and the amphibole minerals actinolite, amosite, anthophyllite, crocidolite, and tremolite. These minerals were heavily used in many industries and products from the late nineteenth century to the 1980's. Today, although more strictly regulated, they remain components of materials for roofing, thermal and electrical insulation, cement pipe and sheets, flooring, gaskets, friction materials, coatings, plastics, textiles, paper, and other products. Those who work with these materials—in asbestos mining and milling, shipyards, building demolition, heating and insulation, brake repair, and asbestos abatement—as well as family members exposed to their clothing, are at risk.

Etiology and the disease process: Asbestos fibers generally do their damage when inhaled, although ingestion also poses risks. The microscopic fibers pierce the pleural lining and harm its mesothelial cells, resulting in the formation of malignant plaques. These fibers may be transported by the lymphatic system to the abdomen, or the infected person may cough, produce fiber-infested sputum, and re-ingest it into the abdomen, leading to the peritoneal form of mesothelioma. The worst asbestos fibers seem to be the long, thin fibers of the amphibole minerals. The serpentine mineral chrysotile possesses a feathery fiber that may do less damage, although it is more easily suspended in the air and possibly more subject to inhalation.

Researchers do not completely understand the mechanisms whereby the fibers transform normal cells into cancerous ones, but it is believed that the fibers' mechanical action on mesothelial cells, followed by inflammation as macrophages gather during the immune response, sets the stage. Asbestos has also been shown to mediate the entry of foreign deoxyribonucleic (DNA) into cells, resulting in mutations that lead to the activation of oncogenes, the deletion of tumor-suppressor genes, increased production of free radicals, inactivation of natural cell death (hence uncontrolled cell growth), and other errors. This process may be followed by interactions between the fibers and chromosomes that result in abnormalities, particularly of chromosome 22.

Incidence: Although mesothelioma is a rare form of cancer, its incidence increased in the last two decades of the twentieth century, ranging from 7 to 40 per 1 million in Western, industrialized nations, with several thousand cases diagnosed each year in the United States. (Lung cancer from smoking, by way of comparison, typically strikes 1,000 in 1 million.) Perhaps because of the occupational risk factors, mesothelioma strikes men more often than women, and because it takes years to develop, it is diagnosed most often in those aged sixty and older. Cases in younger persons or with shorter onsets have, however, been reported, and the difficulties of diagnosis (mesothelioma is often misdiagnosed as adenocarcinoma) may mask a higher incidence. Pleural mesothelioma accounts for about 75 percent of all cases, peritoneal mesothelioma about 20 percent, and pericardial mesothelioma about 5 percent.

Symptoms: Pleural mesothelioma is marked by fatigue, anemia, shortness of breath, wheezing, hoarseness, cough, sputum containing blood, and chest pain resulting from the accumulation of fluid in the pleural space. Peritoneal mesothelioma is accompanied by weight loss, cachexia (wasting), abdominal swelling, and pain due to ascites (fluid buildup in the abdominal cavity); bowel obstruction, abnormal blood clotting, anemia, and fever may also appear. In advanced cases of mesothelioma, symptoms may include blood clots in the veins and consequent thrombophlebitis, severe bleeding in many body organs resulting from disseminated intravascular coagulation, jaundice, low blood sugar level, pleural effusion, blood clots in the arteries of the lungs (pulmonary emboli), and severe ascites. Other types of pain, problems in swallowing, and swelling of the neck or face may accompany metastatic tumors.

Screening and diagnosis: Because the symptoms of mesothelioma are common to many conditions and because the disease takes so long to cause severe symptoms, it often remains undetected until well advanced. Unfortunately, no screening tests exist, although researchers are investigating blood levels of osteopontin, a protein associated with mesothelioma, as one means of early detection.

For those whose symptoms have prompted a visit to the doctor, a history of exposure to asbestos, along with a physical examination, lung-function tests, and an X ray, are the first diagnostic steps. If the X ray reveals pleural thickening, computed tomography (CT) or magnetic resonance imaging (MRI) scans usually follow. If these scans show an abnormal amount of fluid or a tumor, aspiration will follow, via pleural tap or chest drain, paracentesis or ascitic drain, or pericardiocentesis, depending on the area affected. Cytology performed on the fluid will reveal or rule out cancer; the absence of abnormal cells would suggest another disease, such as tuberculosis or congestive heart failure.

Even these tests, however, are not sufficient to confirm anything more than the presence of cancerous cells. To diagnose mesothelioma, a biopsy must be performed: thoroscopy if the area is located in the chest, laparoscopy if in the abdomen. These procedures involve small incisions that allow both examination of the cavity and retrieval of tissue samples. Bronchoscopy, in which the physician examines the lung's airways by means of a bronchoscope, and mediastinoscopy, a method of examining the lymph nodes, are also used. Open surgery may be required if the samples retrieved are insufficient to confirm the diagnosis.

If pathology confirms the suspicion of mesothelioma, the disease will require staging. The precise TNM (tumor/lymph node/metastasis) system is usually employed:

- Stage I: Mesothelioma is confined to the right or left pleura, perhaps in addition involving the lung, pericardium, and diaphragm.
- Stage II: Mesothelioma extends to the chest wall and esophagus, both sides of the pleura, and perhaps the heart.
- Stage III: Mesothelioma extends through the diaphragm into the abdominal cavity.
- Stage IV: Mesothelioma has spread through the bloodstream to distant organs.

For pleural mesothelioma, the Butchart system is most commonly used:

- Stage I: Malignant melanoma is confined to the right or left pleura, perhaps in addition involving the lung, pericardium, and diaphragm.
- Stage II: Malignant melanoma extends to the chest wall and esophagus, both sides of the pleura, and perhaps the heart.
- Stage III: Malignant melanoma extends through the diaphragm into the abdominal cavity.
- Stage IV: Malignant melanoma has spread through the bloodstream to distant organs.

Relative Survival Rates for Mesothelioma by Area Affected, 1988-2001

	Survival Rate (%)	
Years	*Pleura and Lung*	*Peritoneum and Retroperitoneum*
1	38.2	41.8
3	10.5	25.9
5	6.4	18.4
10	4.3	9.5

Source: Data from L. A. G. Ries et al., eds., Cancer Survival Among Adults: U.S. SEER Program, 1988-2001—Patient and Tumor Characteristics, NIH Pub. No. 07-6215 (Bethesda, Md.: National Cancer Institute, 2007)

Treatment and therapy: Treatment options for advanced mesothelioma include surgery, most often pleurectomy and decortication (removal of the chest lining) and less often extrapleural pneumonectomy (removal of the lung, interior chest lining, hemidiaphragm, and pericardium). These are followed by radiation and chemotherapy. Chemotherapy for pleural mesothelioma includes a combination of pemetrexed, cisplatin, and folic acid to mitigate pemetrexed's side effects. A technique known as "heated intraoperative intraperitoneal chemotherapy," using a heated chemotherapy agent to perfuse affected abdominal and pelvic areas immediately after surgery, has been developed for peritoneal mesothelioma. Investigations into immunotherapies have seen little success, although interferon alpha has shown some promise.

Prognosis, prevention, and outcomes: Because diagnosis generally occurs late and the disease is aggressive, survival rates are low, tending to average between six and nine months following diagnosis, depending on the type of mesothelioma. In the United States, the death rate from mesothelioma increased from 2,000 to 3,000 per year between 1980 and the late 1990's.

Radiation and chemotherapy are offered as palliative treatments in advanced cases. A thin tube or needle may be installed in the affected region (via paracentesis for the abdomen and thoracentesis for the chest cavity) to relieve fluid buildup and consequent pain.

A diagnosis of mesothelioma is not necessarily a death sentence, however: Paleontologist Stephen Jay Gould, who was diagnosed with peritoneal mesothelioma, lived two decades after his diagnosis and succumbed to a different disease. Fortunately, mesothelioma remains a rare and highly preventable disease if asbestos exposure is identified and eliminated.

Christina J. Moose, M.A.

For Further Information

Galateau-Sallé, Françoise, ed. *Pathology of Malignant Mesothelioma*. London: Springer, 2006.

Pass, Harvey I. *One Hundred Questions and Answers About Mesothelioma*. Sudbury, Mass.: Jones and Bartlett, 2004.

Pass, Harvey I., Nicholas J. Vogelzang, and Michele Carbone, eds. *Malignant Mesothelioma: Advances in Pathogenesis, Diagnosis, and Translational Therapies*. New York: Springer, 2005.

Treasure, T., et al. "Radical Surgery for Mesothelioma: The Epidemic Still to Peak and We Need More Research to Manage It." *British Medical Journal* 328 (2004): 237-238.

Other Resources

Mesothelioma Applied Research Foundation
http://www.marf.org

Mesothelioma Center
http://www.mesotheliomacenter.org

See also: Acrylamides; Air pollution; Asbestos; Continuous Hyperthermic Peritoneal Perfusion (CHPP); Erionite; Lung cancers; Mediastinoscopy; Paracentesis; Pericardiocentesis; Pleural biopsy; Pleurodesis; Pneumonectomy; Sarcomas, soft-tissue; Simian virus 40; Surgical biopsies; Thoracoscopy

▶ Metastasis

Category: Diseases, Symptoms, and Conditions
Also known as: Metastatic disease, metastatic cancer

Related conditions: Bone cancer, lung cancer, nodal involvement

Definition: Metastasis is the movement or spreading of cancer cells from their original site to other areas of the body. The capacity to metastasize is a characteristic of all malignant tumors. Cancer cells have the ability to enter the bloodstream and flow to any part of the body, making a new home for themselves. Different cancers have different patterns of spreading. When cancer comes back in a patient at a site distant from the original location although the patient appeared to be free of cancer, this is called metastatic recurrence.

Risk factors: Whether cancer cells will metastasize to other parts of the body depends on many factors, including the type of cancer, the stage of the cancer, and the original location of the cancer. Tumors are usually classified as either benign or malignant. Malignant tumors can spread by invasion and metastasis, while benign tumors just grow locally. Often the term "cancer" is used only in reference to malignant tumors, not benign ones.

Etiology and the disease process: Metastasis can occur through the circulatory system, the lymphatic system, or both routes. Common sites for metastasis are the adrenals, the liver, the brain, and the bones. Different cancer types have different metastatic tendencies; that is, the origin of the cancer can often predict the location of metastatic tumor formation. For example, colon cancer will often metastasize to the liver, while prostate cancer tends to metastasize to the bones. Similarly, in women, stomach cancer will often metastasize to the ovaries. It is believed that the migrating cancer cells attempt to find new organs that resemble the local environment of the primary (original) tumor, where they can engraft and thrive. Breast cancer cells, in a high-calcium environment due to the proximity of calcium-containing breast milk, will often metastasize to the bone marrow (also a site of high calcium content).

Cancer will often spread to neighboring lymph nodes; however, this may be referred to as "nodal involvement" or "regional disease" rather than as metastasis. Cancers that are highly metastatic (and therefore particularly dangerous) have been found to secrete proteins that degrade the extracellular matrix that connects cells and separates the organs. Such cells may have greater ability to leave the primary tumor location, migrate into the blood vessels, and then leave the circulation at a remote site. Once cancer cells engraft at a new location, they must induce the growth and infiltration of new microscopic blood vessels to grow in size. Some treatment approaches have attempted to target and interfere with the ability of metastatic tumors to induce new blood vessel growth.

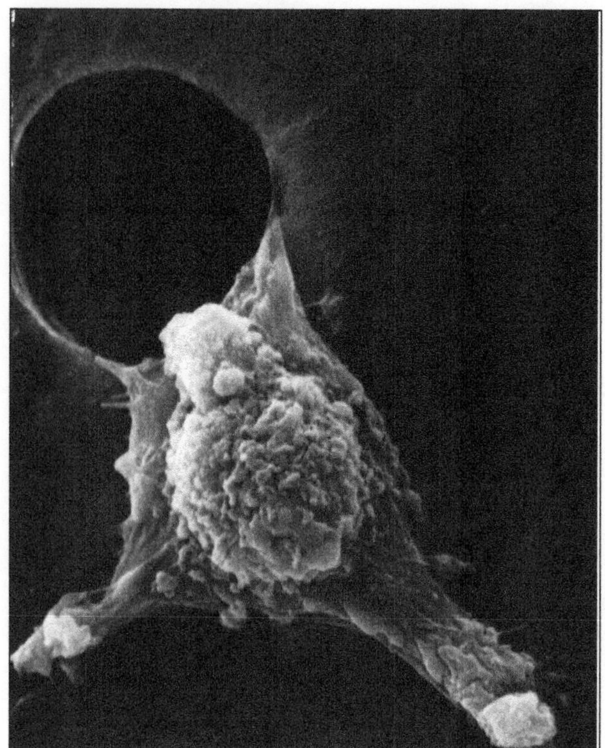

A protein called autocrine motility factor (AMF) *causes cancer cells to grow pseudopodia, which enable them to move to other parts of the body.* (Dr. Raouf Guirgus, Dr. Liotta's Laboratory/ Wikimedia)

Incidence: Metastatic disease is common in many late-stage cancers. Cancers that frequently are the source of metastasis are melanomas and cancers of the lung, breast, colon, kidney, prostate, and pancreas. Therefore, the incidence of metastatic cancer is similar to the incidence of these common cancers after they progress to a metastatic stage.

Symptoms: The exact symptoms experienced by patients with metastatic cancer depend on the type of disease. For instance, lung metastasis can cause coughing or shortness of breath. Brain metastasis can cause symptoms of confusion, seizures, or even coma. Liver metastasis can reveal itself as abdominal pain or jaundice. Bone metastasis is associated with pain in the bones.

Screening and diagnosis: Early metastatic disease may have no signs at all. The more advanced a cancer, the easier it usually is to detect. Each diagnosis of metastasis must be evaluated individually and with care. The extent of each cancer must be determined and all the potential sites of metastasis studied. Metastatic tumors are quite common in the late stages of cancer. Cells collected from a secondary metastatic tumor, when examined under a microscope, can often be identified as cells of the type found in the primary cancer. Therefore, an appropriate treatment regimen may be one that is known to be effective in treating the primary tumor type. The terminology used to describe a metastatic tumor refers to the primary tumor type. For example, breast cancer cells that metastasize to the bone are referred to as "metastatic breast cancer" instead of "bone cancer."

Treatment and therapy: Treatment of metastatic cancer varies widely, depending on the type of cancer and where it has metastasized. Common treatment options include surgery, radiation, and chemotherapy. Biological therapy, radiosurgery, hormone therapy, and laser-immunotherapy can also be treatment options for specific types of metastatic cancer. Treatment must address the symptoms of the metastatic disease along with the primary cancer. Other factors that must be considered in selecting the most appropriate treatment include the size of the metastatic tumor and the patient's age and well-being.

Prognosis, prevention, and outcomes: When a patient is diagnosed with cancer, it is important to determine whether the disease is local or has spread to other locations. The tendency of cancer to spread to secondary organs is what makes the disease potentially life-threatening.

Michael R. King, Ph.D.

For Further Information

Icon Health. *Metastasis: A Medical Dictionary, Bibliography, and Annotated Research Guide to Internet References*. San Diego, Calif.: Author, 2004.

Liotta, L. A., and I. R. Hart, eds. *Tumor Invasion and Metastasis*. Boston: Kluwer, 1982.

Weiss, Leonard. *Principles of Metastasis*. San Diego, Calif.: Academic Press, 1985.

Other Resources

American Cancer Society
What Is Bone Metastasis?
http://www.cancer.org/docroot/CRI/content/CRI_2_4_1X_What_Is_bone_metastasis_66.asp?sitearea=

Children's Hospital Boston
How Cancer Grows and Spreads
http://www.childrenshospital.org/research/Site2029/Documents/CHB_cancer_map.pdf

MetaCancer Foundation
http://www.metacancer.org

See also: Cancer biology; Carcinomatosis; Invasive cancer; Malignant tumors; Tumor markers

▶ Metastatic squamous neck cancer with occult primary

Category: Diseases, Symptoms, and Conditions
Also known as: Metastatic squamous cell carcinoma of the neck from an unknown primary

Related conditions: Head and neck cancers

Definition: Metastastic squamous neck cancer with occult primary is a cancer in which squamous cells (cells from tissues that line the outside of many body organs) metastisize to lymph nodes in the neck or around the collarbone, and the location of the primary tumor is unknown.

Risk factors: The risk factors for metastatic cancer are the same as those for cancer in general. They include tobacco use, unhealthful diet, alcohol abuse, and genetic factors. In addition, the human papillomavirus as a risk factor has been extensively studied in head and neck cancers.

Etiology and the disease process: In the course of the disease, the cancer cells—cells that divide too quickly and without any order—travel from the organ in which they develop (the primary site), through the blood or lymphatic vessels to the lymph nodes in the neck or around the collarbone.

Incidence: Metastastic squamous neck cancer with occult primary is a rare disease that afflicts less than 200,000 individuals in the United States.

Symptoms: Symptoms may include a lump in the neck or throat, pain in the neck or throat, and metastasis.

Screening and diagnosis: Screening tests to diagnose metastatic squamous neck cancer and the primary tumor include physical exams, biopsies, and different imaging procedures. A diagnosis of the disease is made if the primary tumor is not found during testing. Staging is the process used to determine how far the tumor has spread to other body organs, such as the liver or lungs. There is no standard staging process for metastatic squamous neck cancer with occult primary. The tumors are described as untreated or recurrent.

Treatment and therapy: The treatment of the disease depends on how many lymph nodes are affected, on whether the primary tumor has been detected, and on the patient's age and overall health. Surgery is a common treatment, during which the physician cuts out the cancerous lymph nodes and some of the healthy ones around them. Radiation therapy, to kill the cancer cells and to shrink the tumors, may be given alone or before surgery. Chemotherapy is currently administered only in clinical trials, before or at the same time as radiation therapy. Another treatment option is participation in clinical trials of new treatments.

Prognosis, prevention, and outcomes: Prognosis and outcome depend on many factors, for example, the extent of metastasis in the lymph nodes or the response of the cancer to treatment. Avoiding preventable risk factors, such as smoking, may help reduce the disease risk.

Silke Haidekker, Ph.D.

See also: Carcinoma of Unknown Primary origin (CUP); Epidermoid cancers of mucous membranes; Head and neck cancers

▶ Microcalcifications

Category: Diseases, Symptoms, and Conditions
Also known as: Calcifications

Related conditions: Ductal cancer in situ (DCIS)

Definition: Microcalcifications are tiny deposits of calcium phosphate or calcium oxylate found in soft tissues of the body such as the breast. On a mammogram, microcalcifications are seen as fine white flecks with a diameter of less than 1 millimeter. Based on their physical characteristics and location, microcalcifications may be classified as skin, vascular, eggshell, popcornlike, rodlike, punctate (round or oval), milk of calcium, or suture. Although they are very common and most often benign, microcalcifications may be a sign of precancerous changes in the breast.

Risk factors: The incidence of microcalcifications increases with age. However, they are found in women and men of all ages and races.

Etiology and the disease process: Microcalcifications are not associated with dietary calcium. It is thought that they are secreted by the breast cells or are mineralized residue from either normal breast metabolism or abnormal, rapid cell division. They may be related to previous trauma, surgery, infection, or radiation, or they may be an indication of ductal cancer in situ, a noninvasive Stage 0 cancer found in milk ducts of the breast.

Incidence: Microcalcifications and larger macrocalcifications are seen in approximately two-thirds of all mammograms.

Symptoms: The deposits are generally too small to be felt during clinical examinations and do not cause pain.

Screening and diagnosis: Screening mammograms are the standard tool for detecting microcalcifications. Diagnostic mammography, computer-assisted detection software, ultrasound, and comparisons with previous mammograms are used by radiologists to analyze the structure, size, number, shape, and distribution of microcalcifications. The findings are then assigned an assessment category (from 0 to 5), which determines what, if any, follow-up is recommended.

Treatment and therapy: Mammograms classified as categories 1 and 2 are considered negative and require no extraordinary follow-up. Category 3 microcalcifications have a high probability of being benign, but repeat mammograms are typically scheduled to watch for changes in size, number, or shape of deposits. A stereotactic or surgical biopsy of suspicious microcalcifications may be recommended with a category 4 assessment, whereas a category 5 designation indicates a likely malignancy that requires biopsy and surgery or other treatment. Category 0 is used when additional testing is needed before a diagnosis can be made.

Prognosis, prevention, and outcomes: Most microcalcifications are benign. Of those biopsied, more than 80 percent are noncancerous. However, any microcalcifications (especially if they occur in both breasts) are thought to put women at greater risk for breast cancer.

Judy Majewski, M.S.

See also: Breast cancer in children and adolescents; Breast cancer in men; Breast cancers; Breast ultrasound; Calcifications of the breast; Cold nodule; Comedo carcinomas; Ductal Carcinoma In Situ (DCIS); Ductogram; Fibroadenomas; Hormone replacement therapy (HRT); Invasive ductal carcinomas; Mammography; Mastectomy; Medullary carcinoma of the breast; Tubular carcinomas; Wire localization

▶ Moles

Category: Diseases, Symptoms, and Conditions
Also known as: Nevi (singular, nevus or naevus)

Related conditions: Common acquired nevi (acquired in early decades of life), congenital nevi (acquired at birth), freckles, seborrheic keratoses, lentigos (age spots), dysplastic nevi, melanoma, basal cell carcinoma, squamous cell carcinoma

Definition: Moles, or nevi, are clustered melanocytes or nevus cells that appear on the skin, usually brown in color. Melanocytes are cells in the skin that produce the pigment called melanin that protects human skin from the damage of ultraviolet (UV) rays in sunlight.

Risk factors: Although almost everyone has moles, some factors may increase the risk of moles. People with lighter skin and with freckles have a slightly greater risk of developing melanoma. Exposure to ultraviolet rays from the sun can increase the number of moles, and the more moles a person has, the greater the risk of developing melanoma. Damage to the melanocyte deoxyribonucleic acid (DNA) can cause a mole to become cancerous. Lowered immune systems such as those in persons with the human immunodeficiency virus (HIV) or who have had an organ transplant can increase development of moles.

Etiology and the disease process: Nevus cells (melanocytes) are normally localized in the basal layer of the skin (epidermis). A mole of itself is not dangerous and remains a stable part of the skin unless it becomes damaged and then can change into cancer.

Within sunlight are two types of invisible rays: infrared radiation (the sun's heat) and ultraviolet radiation (ultraviolet light). Ultraviolet (UV) light is necessary for plants to live and generate energy. However, UV light can also cause sunburn, aging, and, under the right conditions, skin cancer. UV rays are further differentiated into UVA, UVB, and UVC. Studies are investigating UVA, once thought to be harmless, as a possible cause of skin cancer. Researchers believe that damaged melanocytes may reproduce in an uncontrolled and abnormal way, possibly causing melanoma, one dangerous form of skin cancer. The exact mechanisms by which skin cancer or malignant moles occur is still unclear.

Incidence: Most people have some form of moles, depending on their age, sun exposure, and genetic makeup. Usually people have few moles as an infant or child but may develop moles from puberty to the age of thirty. Often after that time, moles begin to disappear so that older adults may have fewer moles. White adults have an average of twenty-five or fewer moles, but an average person can have ten to forty moles over a lifetime, with a risk of 1:100 turning into a malignant melanoma. With lifestyle changes and more exposure to sunlight, this number can increase.

The number of moles a person has is determined by genetics and exposure to sunlight. Moles are more common on parts of the body that are exposed to sunlight. Some evidence points to a role by the immune system in developing moles because they tend to develop in people with depressed immune systems such those infected with HIV and those who have had organ transplants.

Studies suggest that malignant nevi such as melanoma arise from preexisting moles. If this proves true, the more moles a person has, the higher the incidence of malignant nevi. The percentage of persons with melanoma has increased 100 percent (doubled) in the past thirty years.

Symptoms: Moles come in various colors and shapes. Some are brown and others are pink. Some are yellow, dark blue, or black. Moles can be flat or raised.

Most moles are harmless but people should monitor their moles for changes in color, size, and texture, and for the development of asymmetrical or irregular borders. A benign or noncancerous mole will remain stable in size, color, and shape for years. During pregnancy or puberty, moles may naturally change in color and size, becoming darker and larger.

When a mole bleeds, itches, enlarges, turns multipigmented, or evolves with irregular edges, the patient should see a dermatologist, as this mole may need testing for cancer.

Screening and diagnosis: Health care providers can check their patients' moles during routine physicals or checkups. Also, people can check their own moles periodically. One way to check moles for signs of melanoma

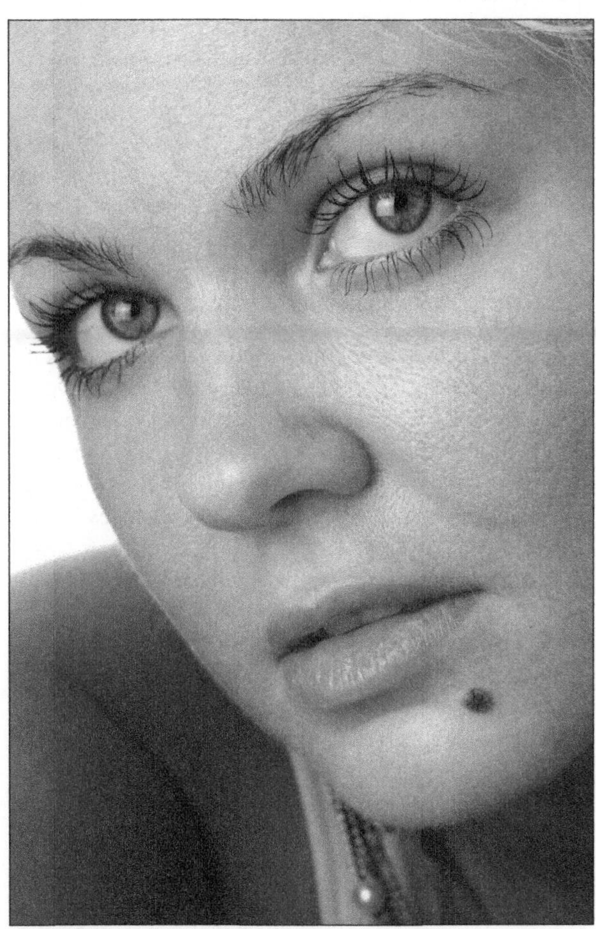

While most moles, like the one on this young woman's face, are harmless, they should be watched for changes in size, color, or shape that could possibly indicate the beginning of cancer. (iStock)

is called the ABCDs of melanomas. "A" stands for asymmetry and indicates that the halves of a single mole should be checked to see if they are different or asymmetrical; a normal mole has identical halves. "B" means to look at the borders or edges of the mole to see if they are irregular; usually a noncancerous mole has regular distinct edges. "C" means that moles should be examined for color that varies within a single mole; ordinary moles are one color, not multipigmented. "D" is a reminder that the diameter of the mole should not exceed the size of a pencil eraser.

If changes appear in the mole, the patient should see a dermatologist who can provide more in-depth testing or removal of the mole. Some symptoms that may need evaluation are bleeding, itching, or an unusual change. The eyes alone cannot diagnosis a malignant mole. The dermatologist will biopsy or excise the mole for the pathologist to inspect. If the mole is malignant, the pathologist can provide a series of tests called staging. These tests may indicate whether the cancer has spread beyond the original site.

Treatment and therapy: Generally nevi require no treatment unless they change into a cancerous mole. However, sometimes they occur in an uncomfortable place and may be surgically removed. Failure to remove such a mole may result in bleeding from irritation.

When a mole is found to be cancerous, the mole, along with some surrounding tissue, is surgically removed.

Prognosis, prevention, and outcomes: Most moles are harmless and are just part of everyday life. However, there are known risk factors that increase the incidence of moles, and some can cause adverse changes in the structure of the moles, leading to malignancies. People at high risk for melanoma should be vigilant for changes in their moles.

Although some exposure to sunlight is healthful because it supplies the body with vitamin D, intense exposure to UV rays—such as tanning—puts people at risk. Sunburn experienced years earlier can still bring about changes in the skin that can precipitate a malignant mole. Young people often will not see the effects of overexposure to the sun's rays until years later, so they may not feel motivated to change their behavior. To decrease the risk of moles as well as the conversion of moles to cancer, people should use sun protection such as sunglasses, sunscreen, long-sleeved garments, and hats.

Robert W. Koch, D.N.S., R.N.

For Further Information

Barnhill, Raymond, Michael Piepkorn, and Klaus Busam. *Pathology of Melanocytic Nevi and Malignant Melanoma.* 2d ed. New York: Springer, 2006.

Hearing, Vincent J., and Stanley P. L. Leong, eds. *From Melanocytes to Melanoma: The Progression to Malignancy.* Totowa, N.J.: Humana Press, 2006.

Poole, Catherine M., and Dupont Guerry IV. *Melanoma: Prevention, Detection, and Treatment.* 2d ed. New Haven, Conn.: Yale University Press, 2005.

Schofield, Jill R., and William A. Robinson. *What You Really Need to Know About Moles and Melanoma.* Baltimore: Johns Hopkins University Press, 2000.

Other Resources

American Academy of Dermatology
Moles
http://www.aad.org/public/publications/pamphlets/common_moles.html

American Cancer Society
http://www.cancer.org

Medline Plus
Moles
http://www.nlm.nih.gov/medlineplus/moles.html

See also: ABCD; Basal cell carcinomas; Carney complex; Chordomas; Choriocarcinomas; Craniosynostosis; Dermatology oncology; Dysplastic nevus syndrome; Gestational Trophoblastic Tumors (GTTs); Hereditary cancer syndromes; Human Chorionic Gonadotropin (HCG); Hydatidiform mole; Melanomas; Premalignancies; Sjögren syndrome; Skin cancers; Squamous cell carcinomas; Ultraviolet radiation and related exposures

▶ Mucinous carcinomas

Category: Diseases, Symptoms, and Conditions
Also known as: Colloid carcinomas, mucinous adenocarcinomas, mucin-producing carcinomas, adenocystic carcinomas, mucoepidermoid carcinomas, gelatinous carcinomas

Related conditions: Breast cancers, ductal carcinoma in situ, colon cancer, pancreatic cancer, eyelid cancer

Definition: Mucinous carcinoma is a type of invasive duct cancer that occurs most frequently in the breast (MCB), although it has also been reported in the colon and pancreas. Primary mucinous carcinoma of the skin (MCS) is recognized as a rare variant of a sweat gland tumor.

Risk factors: Age is the only recognized risk factor. The average age at diagnosis is sixty-seven for mucinous carcinoma of the breast and sixty-three for mucinous carcinoma of the skin.

Etiology and the disease process: In all cases, the distinguishing feature is a type of mucus production called mucin. Poorly differentiated cancer cells are often completely surrounded by mucin in these tumors. The cancer spreads into the normal tissue surrounding it, although the mucin itself does not generally cause major problems.

Incidence: Mucinous carcinoma of the breast is a relatively rare form that accounts for about 1-7 percent of all breast cancer diagnoses. It occurs most frequently in women in their sixties. Mucinous carcinoma of the skin can originate at any location on the body, although the eyelid has been reported as the most commonly affected area (41 percent of cases). There is a slight preponderance of affected males.

Symptoms: Mucinous carcinoma of the breast is usually detected as medium to large size tumors that can be felt. They are usually highly estrogen dependent and a spread to axillary lymph nodes is only found in 10-15% of cases. Mucinous carcinoma of the skin lesions are painless gray or red nodules measuring 0.5 to 7 centimeters in diameter.

Screening and diagnosis: Physical examination, mammograms, ultrasound, and MRI are all important diagnostic tools, and core needle biopsy (of the breast version) and skin biopsy (of the skin version) are essential for accurate tumor classification. Tumor identification is most often straightforward, since the tumor cell morphology and mucin production are so characteristic of this type of cancer. Mucinous carcinomas can be either pure, in which >90% of the cells are mucin-producing, or mixed, which include some cells characteristic of other forms of infiltrating ductal carcinoma. One study reported that 86-92% of pure mucinous breast tumors yield a positive test for estrogen receptors, and almost all test negative for receptors for the HER2/neu protein. Both of these features most commonly correlate with a less aggressive type of cancer.

Treatment and therapy: Since lymph node involvement is rare, surgery can often be conservative (lumpectomy). Surgery is typically followed by radiation therapy, and in more advanced cases (larger tumors) by hormonal therapy. Chemotherapy is generally advised only in cases where the tumors lack estrogen receptors, since hormonal therapy is ineffective in these situations. Standard treatment for mucinous carcinoma of the skin is wide local excision.

Prognosis, prevention, and outcomes: Mucinous carcinoma of the breast has a much better prognosis than other invasive ductal breast carcinomas because it is associated with a low risk of axillary metastases. A ten-year survival rate of more than 90 percent has been reported. Mucinous carcinoma of the skin lesions have a propensity for local recurrence and regional spread, although distant metastases are rare. One study of one hundred cases of primary mucinous carcinoma of the skin reported 29.4 percent local recurrences, 9.6 percent metastases, and an overall mortality rate of 2 percent.

Jeffrey A. Knight, Ph.D.

See also: Adenocarcinomas; Adenoid Cystic Carcinoma (ACC); Breast cancers; Carcinomas; Colorectal cancer; Ductal Carcinoma In Situ (DCIS); Eyelid cancer; Pancreatic cancers

▶ Mucosa-Associated Lymphoid Tissue (MALT) lymphomas

Category: Diseases, Symptoms, and Conditions
Also known as: Extranodal lymphoma, MALT lymphomas, MALTomas

Related conditions: Indolent non-Hodgkin lymphoma (NHL), marginal zone B-cell lymphomas

Definition: Mucosa-associated lymphoid tissue (MALT) lymphomas are a form of non-Hodgkin lymphoma frequently involving the MALT of the stomach and the gastrointestinal tract, usually as a result of *Helicobacter pylori* infection. They are solid tumors that originate from B cells in the marginal zone of the MALT.

Risk factors: Gastric MALT lymphoma is frequently associated (72 to 98 percent) with the presence of *H. pylori.* The causes of MALT lymphoma in other parts of the body are unknown. In general, the incidence of non-Hodgkin lymphoma is two to three times higher among individuals with relatives who developed non-Hodgkin lymphoma, indicating familial clusters. In addition, a compromised immune system is a major risk factor for non-Hodgkin lymphoma development.

Etiology and the disease process: MALT lymphoma starts in mucosa-associated lymphoid tissue, which is lymphatic tissue, such as the stomach, thyroid gland, and lungs. Virtually any mucosal site can be afflicted; however, colorectal involvement of MALT lymphoma is rare.

Disorders Linked to *H. pylori* Infection

- Stomach ulcers
- Duodenal ulcers
- Gastric cancer
- MALT lymphomas
- Possibly pancreatic cancer
- Possibly cardiovascular disease

Source: National Cancer Institute

MALT lymphoma is a cancer of the B-cell lymphocytes. It belongs to the group of marginal zone B-cell lymphomas. Marginal zone lymphoma can be either nodal or extranodal. In particular, MALT lymphoma is an extranodal marginal zone B-cell lymphoma.

Incidence: MALT lymphoma is a relatively rare form of non-Hodgkin lymphoma. Most cases, approximately two out of three, of MALT lymphoma affecting the stomach are caused by infection with *H. pylori*. The disease is more common in people over sixty, but it may occur at any age from early adulthood to old age. MALT lymphoma is slightly more common in women than in men. Ethnicity may play a role in geographic differences among non-Hodgkin lymphoma incidence rates. In particular, gastric lymphomas have the highest recorded incidence in northern Italy.

Symptoms: The most common symptoms experienced by those with MALT lymphomas range from no symptoms to occult or gross gastrointestinal symptoms. Regardless of organ of origin, all MALT lymphomas appear to have similar clinical, pathological, and molecular features.

The symptoms exhibited depend on the site for MALT lymphoma. MALT lymphoma in the stomach may cause indigestion, bleeding into the stomach, weight loss, loss of appetite, and tiredness.

Screening and diagnosis: The initial diagnosis of MALT lymphoma is typically made by esophagogastroduo denos copy (EGD), or upper endoscopy, which is a flexible tube passed down the gullet and into the stomach. Endoscopy is used to obtain photographs of the stomach, and a small sample of cells is extracted for assessment (biopsy). Tests for *H. pylori* are also common when gastrointestinal MALT lymphomas are suspected.

Staging is based on how extensively the cancer has spread throughout and beyond the lymphatic system, which areas are affected, and whether constitutional symptoms, such as fever, night sweats, or weight loss, are present.

The staging of MALT lymphoma is essential for precise prognosis and to develop an effective treatment plan. The Ann Arbor Staging System is the most widely used system for non-Hodgkin lymphoma.

Treatment and therapy: When bacteria are present in the tumor tissue, biological therapy, such as intensive antibiotic treatment, often leads to a complete remission of the lymphoma. Approximately 70 to 80 percent of patients will have a complete regression of malignancy with antibiotic treatment of *H. pylori* when MALT lymphoma is limited to the stomach. If antibiotics do not clear MALT lymphomas or the disease spreads, other treatments are given, including radiotherapy, surgery, or chemotherapy.

Some MALT lymphomas grow very slowly, especially if the site of origin is other than the stomach, and may not cause any problems for many years. In this case, treatment may not be needed immediately, and active monitoring is used instead.

For MALT lymphoma affecting the lung or the bowel, the typical treatment is chemotherapy. Low-grade MALT lymphoma may transform into high-grade lymphoma, in which case it requires more intensive chemotherapy.

MALT lymphoma may be removed during a surgical operation. If the lymphoma is affecting the stomach, total gastrectomy may be needed, which involves the removal of all of the stomach, along with the lower part of the gullet. The gullet is then joined directly to the small intestine. New treatments for MALT lymphoma are being researched.

If patients have been treated for a lymphoma affecting the stomach, typically they will undergo regular follow-up endoscopies and biopsies of the stomach to look for signs of recurrence. Other tests may be used for people whose MALT lymphoma affects areas apart from the stomach.

Side effects of non-Hodgkin lymphoma management may also vary depending on what part of the body is affected and the treatment used. The side effects of biological therapy are most often flulike symptoms, and external radiation to the abdomen may cause nausea, vomiting, and diarrhea.

Prognosis, prevention, and outcomes: The International Prognostic Index is the most widely used prognostic system for non-Hodgkin lymphoma, and it was designed to further clarify lymphoma staging. Paradoxically, in a significant number of cases, aggressive lymphomas can be cured by chemotherapy, while indolent non-Hodgkin lymphomas generally cannot be cured. Approximately 40 percent of indolent malignancies transform into high-grade aggressive lymphomas, and the cure potential of the transformed lymphoma is less favorable than that of aggressive lymphomas without transformation.

Anita Nagypál, Ph.D.

For Further Information

Ferreri, A. J., et al. "Therapeutic Management of Ocular Adnexal MALT Lymphoma." *Expert Opinion on Pharmacotherapy* 8, no. 8 (June, 2007): 1073-1083.

Firat, Y., A. Kizilay, G. Sogutlu, and B. Mizrak. "Primary Mucosa-Associated Lymphoid Tissue Lymphoma of Hypopharynx." *Journal of Craniofacial Surgery* 18, no. 5 (September, 2007): 1189-1193.

Magrath, Ian T., ed. *The Non-Hodgkin's Lymphomas.* New York: Oxford University Press, 1997.

Roh, Jong-Lyel, Jooryung Huh, and Cheolwon. Suh. "Primary Non-Hodgkin's Lymphomas of the Major Salivary Glands." *Journal of Surgical Oncology* 97, no. 1 (October 10, 2007): 35-39.

Troch, M., et al. "Does MALT Lymphoma of the Lung Require Immediate Treatment? An Analysis of Eleven Untreated Cases with Long-Term Follow-Up." *Anticancer Research* 27, no. 5B (September/October, 2007): 3633-3637.

Other Resources

Lymphoma Information Network
Mucosa-Associated Lymphatic Tissue Lymphomas
http://www.lymphomainfo.net/nhl/types/malt.html

Lymphomation.org
MALT Lymphomas
http://www.lymphomation.org/type-malt.htm

See also: *Helicobacter pylori*; Lymphomas; Non-Hodgkin lymphoma

▶ Mucositis

Category: Diseases, Symptoms, and Conditions
Also known as: Oral mucositis, gastrointestinal mucositis

Related conditions: In extreme cases, bacteremia and sepsis

Definition: Mucositis is ulceration in the mouth (oral mucositis) and esophagus, intestines, and anus (gastrointestinal mucositis) as a side effect of radiation or chemotherapy for cancer.

Risk factors: Mucositis is directly related to therapeutic radiation and chemotherapy. There may be genetic factors causing some people to be more sensitive or resistant to cellular damage following therapy.

Etiology and the disease process: Radiation and chemotherapy kill cancer cells but can also damage normal tissue in the gastrointestinal tract. Endothelial cells, which make up the capillaries under the skin, and fibroblast cells, which build connective tissue, are the most sensitive to therapeutic damage. These cells produce important growth factors that maintain the epithelial cells on the surface lining of the gastrointestinal tract. Because of cell death and inflammation, ulcers form along the gastrointestinal tract.

Incidence: Up to 100 percent of patients who receive high-dose radiation treatment will develop some level of mucositis.

Symptoms: Redness of the skin resulting from capiltary congestion (erythema) and swelling are early symptoms. More advanced cases develop ulcers in the mouth and intestines a few days following cancer treatment. Patients may also experience diarrhea, nausea and vomiting, a drop in blood volume (hypovolemia), dry mouth, change of taste, and loss of appetite. Ulcers can become infected, and infection can spread to the blood (bacteremia). Patients often stop eating because of the pain. Severe complications may lead to death due to blood infection (sepsis), electrolyte imbalances, and malnutrition.

Screening and diagnosis: Mucositis is diagnosed by clinical observation of symptoms according to different grades established by the World Health Organization:

- Grade 0: No symptoms
- Grade 1: Erythema
- Grade 2: Erythema, ulcers, can eat solid food
- Grade 3: Ulcers, liquid-only diet
- Grade 4: Ulcers, assisted (parenteral) feeding necessary

Treatment and therapy: After therapy ends, mucositis will resolve without treatment. While mucositis persists, palliative treatment is given, including narcotics for pain, antibiotics for infections, and assisted feeding.

Research on drugs to treat mucositis is ongoing. One drug, palifermin (Kepivance), is approved by the Food and Drug Administration for treating oral mucositis. Palifermin is related to a hormone that stimulates epithelial cells. Given before radiation therapy, palifermin strengthens and protects the oral epithelium, making it much more resistant to developing mucositis.

Prognosis, prevention, and outcomes: Most patients recover from mucositis, though a small percentage of patients die from complications. Cancer therapy is often reduced or stopped because of mucositis, which may compromise cancer care.

Christopher Pung, B.S., C.L.Sp. (CG)

See also: Chemotherapy; External Beam Radiation Therapy (EBRT); Fatigue; Gastrointestinal complications of cancer treatment; Intensity-Modulated Radiation Therapy (IMRT); Radiation therapies; Side effects; Stomatitis

▶ Multiple endocrine neoplasia

Category: Diseases, Symptoms, and Conditions
Also known as: Multiple endocrine neoplasia type 1: Wermer syndrome MEN 1, Multiple endocrine neoplasia type 2): MEN 2, MEN 2A, MEN 2B, Sipple syndrome, mucosal neuroma syndrome, familial medullary thyroid carcinoma

Related conditions: MEN 1: Hyperparathyroidism, pituitary tumor, pancreatic tumor, duodenal tumor MEN 2: Medullary thyroid carcinoma, pheochromocytoma, parathyroid hyperplasia or adenoma, mucosal neuromas of the lips and tongue, gastrointestinal ganglioneuromas

Definition: Multiple endocrine neoplasia type 1 (MEN 1) is a hereditary tumor syndrome characterized by endocrine and nonendocrine tumors, most of which are benign. The characteristic findings include tumors of the parathyroid glands, pituitary gland, pancreas, and duodenum (first part of the small intestine). Neuroendocrine tumors (nerve-cell tumors that may produce hormones) in the pancreas and duodenum are the main cause of tumor-related death. The severity varies within families and between families. Multiple endocrine neoplasia type 2 (MEN 2) is a hereditary cancer syndrome that affects endocrine glands, which produce hormones in the body. MEN 2 is subclassified into three types: MEN 2A, MEN 2B, and familial medullary thyroid carcinoma (FMTC). All three types are associated with medullary thyroid cancer (MTC, a tumor that grows from the C cells in the thyroid gland). MEN 2A and MEN 2B are also associated with pheochromocytoma (an adrenal gland tumor that releases stress hormones). MEN 2A carries an increased risk for parathyroid hyperplasia (in which the parathyroid glands become enlarged and produce too much parathyroid hormone) or parathyroid adenoma (a benign tumor), both of which cause hyperparathyroidism (increased secretion of parathyroid hormone). MEN 2B is associated with mucosal neuromas (tumors growing from a nerve) of the lips and tongue, gastrointestinal ganglioneuromas (benign growths in the intestines), and characteristic facial appearance (a slender face, with prominent, bumpy lips). The disease findings and the severity of the syndrome vary within families and between families.

Risk factors: Because MEN 1 and MEN 2 are hereditary, the main risk factor is having a family history of these disorders. Each child of a person with MEN 1 has a 50 percent chance of inheriting the disorder, as does each child of a person with MEN 2.

Etiology and the disease process: The underlying genetic cause of MEN 1 is a genetic change (mutation) in the MEN1 gene. MEN1 is a tumor-suppressor gene, and the protein it encodes helps stop uncontrolled cell growth and proliferation. The underlying genetic cause of MEN 2 is a mutation in the RET gene. RET is a proto-oncogene,

Relative Survival Rates for Medullary Thyroid Carcinoma, 1988-2001

		Survival Rates (%)					
Stage	*Cases Diagnosed (%)*	*1-Year*	*2-Year*	*3-Year*	*5-Year*	*8-Year*	*10-Year*
Stage II	42.5	97.5	94.5	89.6	89.6	86.3	77.1
Stage III	43.8	100.0	95.4	89.8	82.6	82.3	82.3

Source: Data from L. A. G. Ries et al., eds., *Cancer Survival Among Adults: U.S. SEER Program, 1988-2001—Patient and Tumor Characteristics,* NIH Pub. No. 07-6215 (Bethesda, Md.: National Cancer Institute, 2007)
Note: So few cases were diagnosed at Stages I and IV that percentages and relative survival rates were not meaningful.

which means that it normally functions in cell growth and differentiation. Activating mutations in RET cause it to become an active, unregulated oncogene, turning normal cells into cancer cells.

Usually, each person has two normal copies of the MEN1 gene. A mutation in one copy of the gene is sufficient to cause MEN 1, which is why this condition is referred to as autosomal dominant (autosomal means the MEN1 gene is located on one of the twenty-two pairs of autosomes, which are all the chromosomes except for the X and Y chromosomes). An affected person has a MEN1 gene mutation from the time of conception; however, symptoms of the disease may not manifest until later in life. Most mutations are inherited from a parent, but new mutations do occur.

Usually, each person has two normal copies of the RET gene. An activating mutation in one copy of the gene is sufficient to cause MEN 2, and therefore, this condition is autosomal dominant. A person with MEN 2 may not manifest symptoms until later in life. Most mutations are inherited from a parent, but new, sporadic mutations do occur. The age of onset for medullary thyroid cancer is usually early childhood in MEN 2B, early adulthood in MEN 2A, and middle age in familial medullary thyroid carcinoma.

Incidence: MEN 2 has a higher incidence than MEN 1. Approximately 0.2 to 2 per 100,000 people have MEN 1. Approximately 1 in 30,000 people has MEN 2.

Symptoms: In MEN 1, parathyroid tumors can cause high calcium levels in the blood, nausea, fatigue, muscle pains, constipation, abdominal pain, kidney stones, and bone fractures. Symptoms of pituitary tumors vary depending on the type of hormone being made by the tumor. Tumors of the pancreas and duodenum cause many different symptoms depending on the tumor type.

In MEN 2, symptoms of medullary thyroid cancer may include a thyroid nodule (lump on the throat) and enlarged lymph nodes in the neck. Pheochromocytomas release catecholamines (stress hormones) that can cause dangerously high blood pressure levels. Hyperparathyroidism can cause high calcium levels in the blood, nausea, fatigue, muscle pains, constipation, abdominal pain, kidney stones, and bone fractures. In MEN 2B, gastrointestinal ganglioneuromas can cause constipation or megacolon (abnormally large colon).

Screening and diagnosis: Physicians diagnose MEN 1 in a person with an endocrine tumor in two of the three tissue systems usually affected in this syndrome: parathyroid glands, pancreas, and pituitary gland. Genetic testing can be used to confirm a suspected diagnosis or to test a family member who is at risk for the disease but has no symptoms.

The criteria to diagnose MEN 2 are different depending on the subtype. MEN 2A is diagnosed by the presence of two or more endocrine tumors (in one person or in close blood relatives). MEN 2B is diagnosed in a person with mucosal neuromas on the lips and tongue, medullary thyroid cancer, and, in some cases, pheochromocytoma. Familial medullary thyroid carcinoma is diagnosed in families with four or more cases of medullary thyroid cancer without any other findings of MEN 2. Tools used to check for disease include a blood test to measure levels of calcitonin (a hormone produced by medullary thyroid cancer) and urine testing to check for catecholamines and metanephrines (breakdown products of epinephrine) released by pheochromocytomas. Blood and urine testing may also be done to assess for hyperparathyroidism.

Treatment and therapy: A combination of surgery and medication may be used to treat MEN 1 tumors.

In MEN 2, the only way to cure medullary thyroid cancer is to remove the thyroid gland (thyroidectomy) at a young age. A patient who has had a thyroidectomy must take thyroid hormone replacement therapy. Because the risk for cancer is so high, removing the thyroid gland is recommended for people who have a RET mutation, even if they do not yet have cancer. Surgery to remove the adrenal gland is necessary to treat patients with pheochromocytoma. Sometimes pheochromocytomas occur in both adrenal glands. All or some of the four parathyroid glands may be removed to treat hyperparathyroidism.

Prognosis, prevention, and outcomes: Because MEN 1 and MEN 2 are genetic conditions, their manifestations cannot currently be prevented. However, in MEN 1, physicians recommend monitoring that includes blood testing for hormone levels and imaging of the head and abdomen.

In MEN 2, monitoring individuals who have a family history of the disease or have a RET gene mutation can detect problems early and lead to more effective treatment and better outcomes. Such monitoring includes yearly blood testing for calcitonin levels, blood pressure checks, and urine testing for catecholamines and metanephrines. The medical team caring for patients decides the age at which monitoring should start.

Abbie L. Abboud, M.S., C.G.C.
Updated by: Richard P. Capriccioso, M.D.

For Further Information

Giusti, F., Marini, F., & Luisa Brandi, M. (2015). Multiple endocrine neoplasia I. In R. A. Pagon, M. P. Adam, H. H. Ardinger, S. E. Wallace, A. Amemiya, L. J. H. Bean, T. D. Bird, C-T. Fong, H. C. Mefford, R. J. H. Smith, & K. Stephens (Eds.), *Gene reviews*. Seattle,

WA: University of Washington. Available from: http://www.ncbi.nlm.nih.gov/books/NBK1538/

Marquard, J., & Eng, C., (2015). Multiple Endocrine Neoplasia Type 2. In R. A. Pagon, M. P. Adam, H. H. Ardinger, S. E. Wallace, A. Amemiya, L. J. H. Bean, T. D. Bird, C-T. Fong, H. C. Mefford, R. J. H. Smith, & K. Stephens (Eds.), *Gene reviews*. Seattle, WA: University of Washington. Available from: http://www.ncbi.nlm.nih.gov/books/NBK1257/

Marx, S. J. & Wells, S. A. Jr. (2012). Multiple endocrine neoplasia. In S. Melmed, K. S. Polonsky, P. R. Larsen, & M. Kronenberg (Eds.), *Williams textbook of endocrinology* (12th ed.) (pp. 1728–1767). Philadelphia, PA: Elsevier.

Moline J, & Eng C. (2011). Multiple endocrine neoplasia type 2: An overview. *Genetics in Medicine,* 13(9), 755–764. http://www.ncbi.nlm.nih.gov/pubmed/21552134

Other Resources

AMEND

Association for Multiple Endocrine Neoplasia Disorders
http://www.amend.org.uk/

Genetics Home Reference

Your Guide to Understanding

Multiple Endocrine Neoplasia

http://ghr.nlm.nih.gov/condition=multipleendocrineneoplasia

See also: Duodenal carcinomas; Endocrine cancers; Endocrinology oncology; Family history and risk assessment; Gastrinomas; Histamine 2 antagonists; Human growth factors and tumor growth; Islet cell tumors; Neuroendocrine tumors; Pancreatic cancers; Parathyroid cancer; Pheochromocytomas; Pituitary tumors; Thyroid cancer; Zollinger-Ellison syndrome

▶ Multiple myeloma

Category: Diseases, Symptoms, and Conditions
Also known as: MM, myeloma, plasma cell myeloma, cancer of the bone marrow

Related conditions: Multiple gammopathy of undetermined significance (MGUS), smoldering myeloma, indolent myeloma

Definition: Multiple myeloma is a cancer involving several clusters of cancerous plasma cells (a type of white blood cell found in the bone marrow that produces immunoglobulins to fight infection) in various bones of the body.

Risk factors: No one is sure what causes multiple myeloma. People who have been exposed to agricultural and other chemicals such as Agent Orange, some types of radiation, and some viruses appear to be more susceptible to multiple myeloma. People with multiple myeloma are usually diagnosed in their fifties and sixties. The disease is identified more often in men than in women and more often in African Americans than in members of other ethnic groups. Scientists have not been able to associate multiple myeloma with a genetic trait, but research suggests that chromosome 13 may be incomplete or entirely missing in myeloma cells.

Patients with a condition known as multiple gammopathy of undetermined significance (MGUS) have a relatively large amount of immunoglobulin protein (the M-protein) present in their blood. MGUS itself is benign, but about 16 percent of individuals with the condition eventually exhibit symptoms of multiple myeloma. Patients with smoldering or indolent myeloma, often a precursor disease, exhibit higher levels of calcium and kidney dysfunction, anemia, and bone disease.

Etiology and the disease process: Multiple myeloma occurs when abnormal plasma cells in the bone marrow multiply, accumulate, and overtake the healthy plasma cells. As the plasma cells circulate in the bloodstream, they often settle in other bones and interfere with the body's ability to produce normal antibodies, which leads to difficulty fighting infections.

Incidence: Approximately 53,000 Americans have multiple myeloma. Slightly fewer than 20,000 Americans were expected to be diagnosed with multiple myeloma in 2007. Using statistics gathered from 2002 to 2004, the National Cancer Institute estimates that 0.61 percent (1 in 165) of men and women born today will be diagnosed with multiple myeloma at some time during their lifetime.

Symptoms: The early stages of multiple myeloma may be uneventful and indistinct from other maladies. Multiple myeloma is often marked by successive infections, weight loss, fatigue or weakness, broken bones, or bone pain, most commonly in the ribs or back.

Screening and diagnosis: Kidney problems are often the first indication that something is wrong. High levels of protein in the blood can cause kidney damage, and high

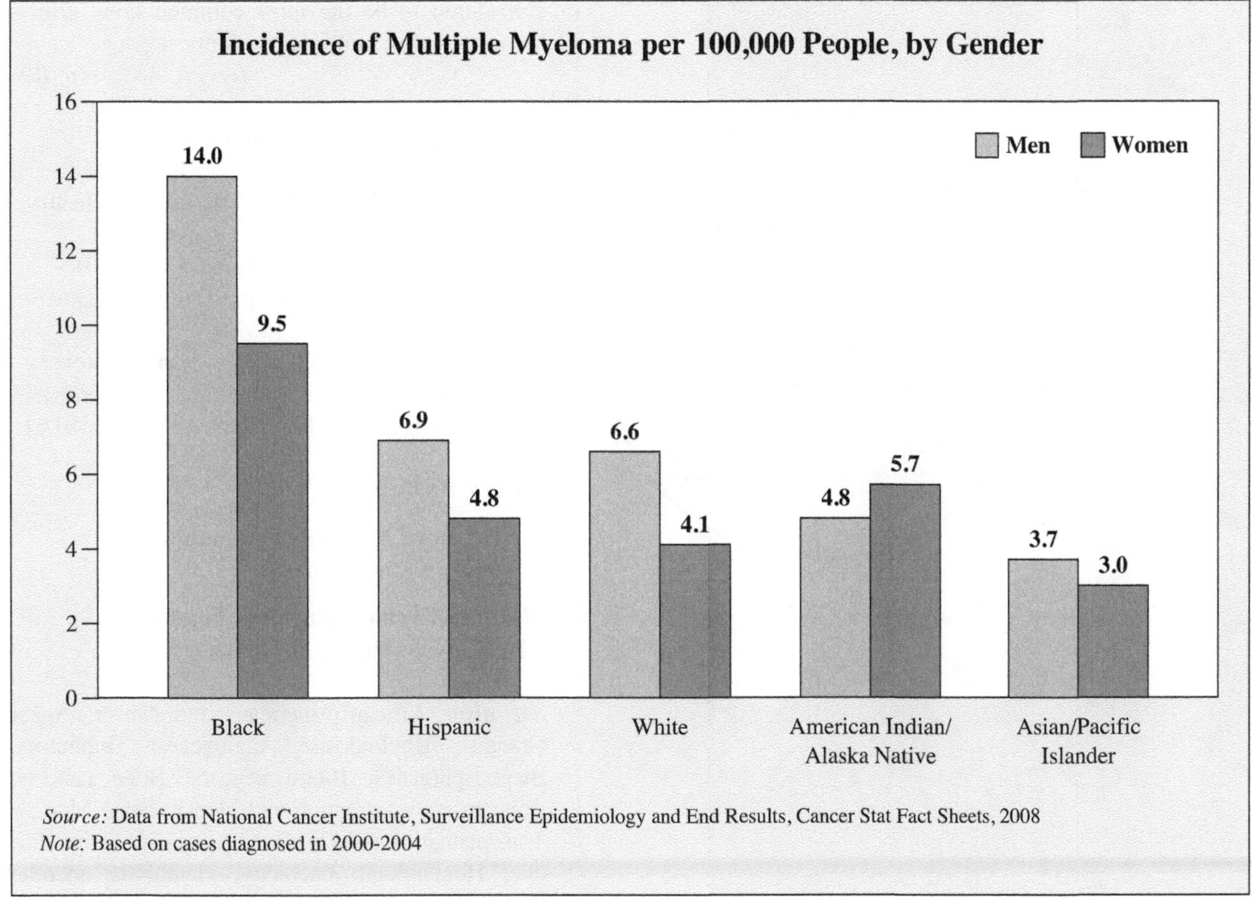

Source: Data from National Cancer Institute, Surveillance Epidemiology and End Results, Cancer Stat Fact Sheets, 2008
Note: Based on cases diagnosed in 2000-2004

levels of calcium may indicate the beginning or presence of kidney problems. Symptoms of kidney problems include greater thirst and urine production, a loss of appetite, fatigue, muscle weakness, restlessness, confusion or an inability to concentrate, constipation, and nausea and vomiting. An accurate diagnosis requires consideration of the patient's history and symptoms, a complete physical, and an evaluation of laboratory results.

A diagnosis of multiple myeloma requires blood tests to determine the amount of calcium and plasma cells in the blood and the patient's degree of anemia. Technologists will look for the presence of M-protein, beta-2 microglobulin (β2M), and other proteins in a blood sample and for the presence of the Bence-Jones protein (a type of M-protein) in the urine. Additional testing will include imaging studies—X rays, computed tomography (CT) scans, or magnetic resonance imaging (MRI) studies—to examine whether bone cavities exist and whether they might be caused by a tumor. This is followed by taking a tissue sample from a large bone to examine whether myeloma cells are present in the marrow.

Most clinicians use the International Staging System to categorize multiple myeloma using the following criteria:

- Stage I: Serum β2M less than 3.5 milligrams/deciliter (mg/dl) and serum albumin greater than or equal to 3.5 grams/deciliter (g/dl)
- Stage II: Serum β2M less than 3.5 mg/dl and albumin less than 3.5 g/dl or serum β2M 3.5 to 5.5 mg/dl
- Stage III: Serum β2M greater than 5.5 mg/dl

Higher serum β2M levels and lower serum albumin levels usually indicate active or advanced disease. Increased values of C-reactive protein and serum lactate dehydrogenase also may indicate active disease.

Treatment and therapy: There is no cure for multiple myeloma, but several treatment options exist and new options are being developed. The aim of most therapy is to ease a patient's symptoms and slow the progression of disease, relieve pain and discomfort, and stabilize the immune system and metabolic functions. Various combination therapies are being used to combat multiple

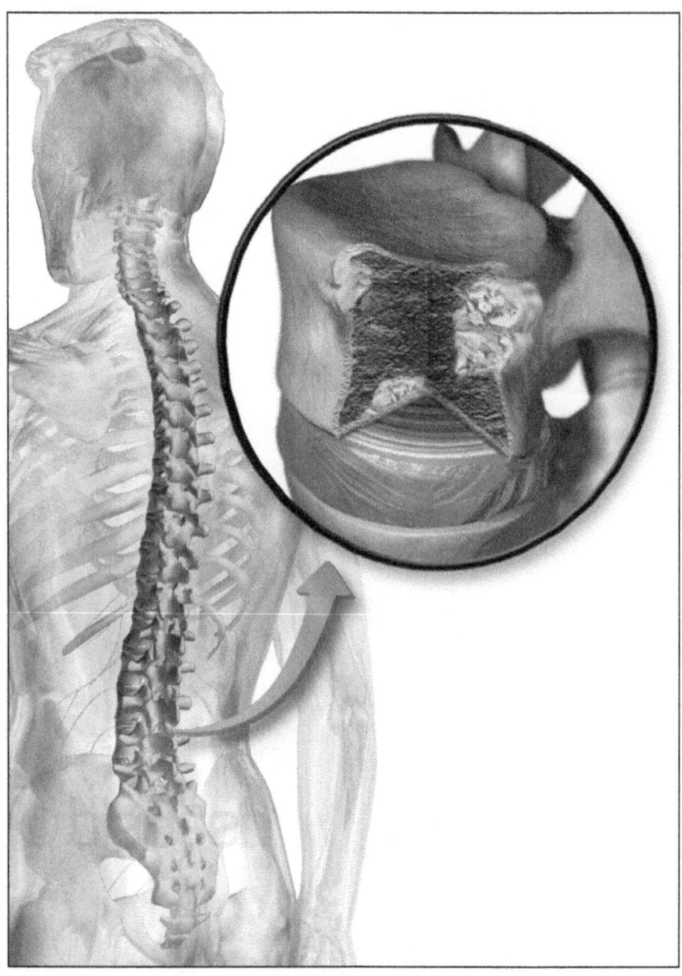

Illustrating multiple myeloma. (Blausen Medical Communications, Inc./ Wikimedia)

myeloma. These include dexamethasone, either alone or in combination with thalidomide or melphalan; melphalan plus prednisone; a combination drug known as VAD (vincristine/doxorubicin/dexamethasone); and bortezomib, either alone or in combination with other drugs such as dexamethasone, lenalidomide, or doxorubicin liposomal (Doxil). Additional therapies include the use of cyclophosphamide or etoposide. Each drug combination has advantages and disadvantages, and not all drug combinations work well in all patients. Some patients have had extremely good results using these drugs, and many have experienced disease remission.

Prognosis, prevention, and outcomes: Most patients live many years after a diagnosis of multiple myeloma. Physicians may offer treatments for bone pain, infections, anemia, and fatigue or weakness, which are considered to be the most common body effects associated with multiple myeloma.

Terry A. Anderson, B.S.

For Further Information

Anderson, Kenneth C., and Irene Ghobrial, eds. *Multiple Myeloma*. New York: Informa Healthcare, 2007.

Brian, G., M., et al. "International Uniform Response Criteria for Multiple Myeloma." *Leukemia* 20, no. 9 (2006): 1467.

Dominik, D., et al. "Multiple Myeloma: A Review of the Epidemiologic Literature." *International Journal of Cancer* 120, suppl. 12 (2007): 40-61.

Other Resources

International Myeloma Foundation
http://www.myeloma.org

Multiple Myeloma Research Foundation
http://www.multiplemyeloma.org

See also: African Americans and cancer; Agent Orange; Amyloidosis; Angiogenesis inhibitors; Bisphosphonates; Blood cancers; Bone cancers; Bone marrow aspiration and biopsy; Bone Marrow Transplantation (BMT); Bone pain; Curcumin; Hair dye; Hematologic oncology; Hemolytic anemia; Hepatitis C Virus (HCV); Hypercalcemia; Immunoelectrophoresis (IEP); Interferon; Malignant Fibrous Histiocytoma (MFH); Melphalan; Motion sickness devices; Myeloma; Myelosuppression; Proteasome inhibitors; Protein electrophoresis; Spinal axis tumors; Waldenström Macroglobulinemia (WM)

▶ Myasthenia gravis

Category: Diseases, Symptoms, and Conditions
Also known as: Familial myasthenia gravis, neonatal myasthenia gravis, congenital myasthenia gravis, juvenile myasthenia gravis

Related conditions: Autoimmune disorders, thymomas

Definition: The term "myasthenia gravis" comes from Latin and Greek meaning grave (severe) muscle weakness; this describes the condition very well. Although there are several forms of myasthenia gravis, the most common is a chronic autoimmune neuromuscular condition in which there is sporadic, severe weakness of the voluntary muscles of the body, especially those of the face and throat.

Risk factors: Most cases of myasthenia gravis appear to be sporadic (caused by unknown factors). An elevated risk has been noted for women between the ages of twenty and forty with family history of the disease, drug ingestion, or other autoimmune disorders. Myasthenia gravis is inherited in about 5 percent of all cases, associated with specific immune system alleles (HLA-B8 and DR3).

Etiology and the disease process: In myasthenia gravis, the body produces antibodies that attack its own proteins (an autoimmune response). With the exception of drug-induced myasthenia gravis (D-penicillamine ingestion, for example), there is no known causative agent or pathogen that accounts for onset of the disease, which can be quite sudden. As with other cancers, the body's regulatory mechanisms are not operating properly, in this case allowing antibody-producing cells that should be screened out to continue being produced.

In most cases of myasthenia gravis, the antibodies produced are directed against the acetylcholine (ACh) receptor. Receptors are proteins on the cell membrane that bind to a particular class of compounds, thus triggering the cell to perform some function or action. Acetylcholine receptors are present in the motor end plate of voluntary muscles, where they are stimulated by nerves. An electrical impulse in a nerve causes acetylcholine to be released; it binds with the receptor on the muscle cell, allowing sodium and calcium to move into the cell and stimulating it to contract. The acetylcholine is then broken down by the enzyme cholinesterase (so hyperstimulation does not occur) and recycled within the nerve cell. If antibodies to the receptor are present, they bind to the receptor first, so that very little acetylcholine can bind. Thus, sodium and calcium influx is limited, and muscle contraction is limited or nonexistent. In some cases, antibodies may actually destroy the receptors on the muscle cell membranes altogether, leaving muscles unable to contract even in the presence of a strong nerve signal.

The antibodies against acetylcholine receptors are produced by B cells, circulating white blood cells (leukocytes). B cells are activated by T-helper cells, which develop within the thymus. Therefore, myasthenia gravis is often associated with thymoma (tumor of the thymus), although the exact mechanism of this association is not clearly understood.

A second form of antibody in some patients develops against the receptor protein muscle-specific kinase (MuSK), required for formation of the nerve-muscle junction during early development. The result is an incomplete junction, making it harder for acetylcholine to span the gap and stimulate the muscle.

Drugs to Be Avoided by People with Myasthenia Gravis

MG-Causing Drugs

- Alpha-interferon
- Botulinum toxin
- D-Penicillamine

Drugs That Increase Muscle Weakness

- Antibiotics: particularly aminoglycosides, ciprofloxacin, telithromycin
- Beta-blockers: propranolo, timolol maleate eyedrops
- Calcium channel blockers
- Iodinated contrast agents (for X rays)
- Neuromuscular blocking agents: succinylcholine and vecuronium; only anaesthesiologists familiar withMG should use these
- Quinine, quinidine, procainamide

Source: Myasthenia Gravis Foundation of America

Incidence: The overall U.S. incidence is listed at 20 cases per 100,000 population, although many authors report it to be much higher. The discrepancy comes from the difficulty of diagnosis from initial symptoms. All ethnic groups and genders are susceptible, but there is a difference in age distribution. Generally this disease is seen in women under the age of forty, and in men and women between the ages of fifty and seventy. However, it can strike at any age including at birth (neonatal myasthenia gravis, congenital myasthenia gravis) or in children (juvenile myasthenia gravis). About 15 percent of those who contract myasthenia gravis have a thymoma.

Symptoms: The primary symptom of myasthenia gravis is muscle weakness, especially those muscles that control eye and eyelid movement, chewing, talking, facial expression, and swallowing. This weakness usually increases during periods of muscle activity and decreases with periods of rest.

Screening and diagnosis: Myasthenia gravis can be difficult to diagnose. The symptoms can be subtle and hard to distinguish from other neurological disorders. A thorough physical exam is the first step in diagnosis, including various tests aimed at muscle fatigability (keeping arms stretched forward for sixty seconds or looking at the feet for sixty seconds while lying on the back). Blood tests can help to identify specific acetylcholine antibodies but may be negative (due to sensitivity of the assay) in up to 50 percent of cases, especially in the early stages. Repetitive nerve stimulation (with electrical impulses) can be used to measure fatigability, as can single fiber electromyography, a sensitive test that records the electrical impulse in muscle fibers.

Classification (staging) of myasthenia gravis is as follows:

- Stage I: Eye muscle weakness or ptosis of any severity; no other evidence of muscle weakness
- Stage II: Eye muscle weakness of any severity; mild weakness of other muscles
- Stage III: Eye muscle weakness of any severity: moderate weakness of other muscles
- Stage IV: Eye muscle weakness of any severity: severe weakness of other muscles
- Stage V: Severe weakness leading to intubation of the airway

Treatment and therapy: Myasthenia gravis is generally controlled through medication. The medications have two purposes: lessening muscle weakness and reducing the autoimmune response. Cholinesterase inhibitors (such as neostigmine and pyridostigmine) allow the acetylcholine to remain near the receptor for a longer period of time, thus increasing the chance that it will bind. Immunosuppresive drugs (such as prednisone, cyclosporine, or azathioprine) help reduce the antibody formation but may take weeks or months to show effects. For patients in a critical state, plasmapheresis may also be used to remove circulating antibodies from the bloodstream.

Patients experiencing myasthenia gravis caused by a thymoma may have the thymoma surgically removed (thymomectomy) to prevent possible spread of cancer in the event the thymoma is cancerous; most thymomas, however, are benign.

Prognosis, prevention, and outcomes: With proper treatment, patients have a normal life expectancy. However, those with malignant thymoma may experience rapid decline. Quality of life varies quite markedly, but myasthenia gravis is not a progressive disease, and therefore, some lifestyle changes can lessen the symptoms in some individuals. In some patients, symptoms come and go; for some the symptoms decrease after three to five years of treatment.

Kerry L. Cheesman, Ph.D.

For Further Information

Baron-Faust, Rita, and Jill P Buyon. *The Autoimmune Connection: Essential Information for Women on Diagnosis, Treatment, and Getting on with Life*. Chicago: Contemporary Books, 2003.

Keesey, John Carl. *Myasthenia Gravis: An Illustrated History*. Roseville, Calif.: Publishers Design Group, 2002.

National Institutes of Health. *Understanding Autoimmune Diseases*. NIH Publication 98-4273. Bethesda, Md.: Author, 1998.

_______. *Understanding the Immune System: How It Works*. NIH Publication 03-5423. Bethesda, Md.: Author, 2003.

_______. *Questions and Answers About Autoimmunity*. NIH Publication 02-4858. Bethesda, Md.: Author, 2002.

Shannon, Joyce Brennfleck, ed. *Movement Disorders Sourcebook: Basic Consumer Health Information About* Neurological Movement Disorders. Detroit: Omnigraphics, 2003.

Vincent, Angela, and Camilla Buckley. "Myasthenia Gravis and Other Antibody-Associated Neurological Diseases." In *The Autoimmune Diseases*, edited by Noel R. Rose and Ian R. Mackay. Boston: Elsevier/Academic Press, 2006.

Other Resources

American Cancer Society
http://www.cancer.org

Myasthenia Gravis Foundation of America
http://www.myasthenia.org

National Institute of Neurological Disorders and Stroke
NINDS Myasthenia Gravis Information Page
http://www.ninds.nih.gov/disorders/myasthenia_gravis/myasthenia_gravis.htm

See also: Lambert-Eaton Myasthenic Syndrome (LEMS); Mediastinal tumors; Mediastinoscopy; Surgical biopsies; Thymomas; Thymus cancer

▶ Mycosis fungoides

Category: Diseases, Symptoms, and Conditions
Also known as: Cutaneous T-Cell Lymphoma (CTCL), cutaneous lymphoma, MF

Related conditions: Sézary syndrome (SS), lymphomatoid papulosis, cutaneous anaplastic large-cell lymphoma, adult T-cell leukemia/lymphoma, peripheral T-cell lymphoma, lymphomatoid granulomatosis, granulomatous slack skin disease, pagetoid reticulosis

Definition: Mycosis fungoides (MF) is the most common type of cutaneous T-cell lymphoma (CTCL). Mycosis fungoides was named after the mushroom-like skin tumors that were noted in the first patient diagnosed with the condition. A low-grade lymphoma that primarily affects the skin, it generally has a slow course and often remains confined to the skin. Over time, in only about 10 percent of the cases, it does slowly progress to the lymph nodes and internal organs such as the liver, lungs, and bone marrow.

The cutaneous T-cell lymphomas are a group of rare skin cancers that includes Sézary syndrome, lymphomatoid papulosis, cutaneous anaplastic large-cell lymphoma, adult T-cell leukemia/lymphoma, peripheral T-cell lymphoma, lymphomatoid granulomatosis, granulomatous slack skin disease, and pagetoid reticulosis.

Risk factors: The cause of mycosis fungoides is unknown. There is no supportive research indicating that this is a hereditary disease. Exposure to Agent Orange may be a risk factor for developing mycosis fungoides for veterans of the Vietnam War, but no direct cause-effect relationship has been established.

Etiology and the disease process: Mycosis fungoides is a special variant of lymphoma with major involvement of the skin as well as hilar and mediastinal lymphadenopathy. It is associated with reticular nodular pulmonary lesions and is often complicated by pneumonias, primarily caused by *Staphlococcus aureus* or *Pseudomonas aeruginosa*. The condition is not contagious. It is not an infection, and there are no infectious agents known to cause the disease. There has been research investigating the role of viruses, but the results are inconclusive.

Incidence: In the United states, approximately 1,000 new cases of mycosis fungoides occur per year. It affects men twice as often as women and is more common in blacks than in whites. Mycosis fungoides can begin at any age, but the most common age is fifty years old.

Symptoms: Mycosis fungoides progresses through four stages, which are defined by the skin symptoms, including the patch phase, skin tumors phase, skin redness stage, and lymph node stage, where mycosis fungoides begins to spread or metastasize, usually first to the lymph nodes, then to the liver, lungs, or bone marrow.

Screening and diagnosis: Typically there are about six years from the onset of symptoms to the diagnosis of mycosis fungoides. Confusion with other conditions is common. A sample of the skin known as a skin biopsy is usually performed. Other laboratory tests can be done to determine the progression of the cancer. There is no cure for mycosis fungoides, so long-term survival depends on early diagnosis and treatment.

Treatment and therapy: Treatments are directed at either the skin or the entire body (systemic therapy). Skin-directed treatments include ultraviolet light (psoralen and ultraviolet A, or PUVA, UVB, narrow-band UVB), topical steroids, topical chemotherapies (nitrogen mustard, carmustine), topical retinoids, local radiation to single lesions, or total skin electron beam (TSEB). Systemic treatments include oral retinoids, photopheresis, photochemotherapy (also known as PUVA), fusion proteins, interferon, systemic chemotherapy (most commonly cyclophosphamide, doxorubicin, vincristine, and prednisone), and orphan drugs such as bexarotene (Targretin). These treatments may be prescribed alone or in combination.

Prognosis, prevention, and outcomes: The course of mycosis fungoides is unpredictable, as some patients will progress slowly, some will progess rapidly, and some will not progress at all. Most patients will experience only skin symptoms, without serious complications. About 10 percent will experience progressive disease with lymph node involvement or spread to the liver, lungs, or bone marrow.

Many patients live normal lives while they treat their disease, and some are able to remain in remission for long periods of time. Although there is no known cure for mycosis fungoides, research has indicated that patients diagnosed with early-stage mycosis fungoides (which is 70 to 80 percent of patients) will have a normal life expectancy.

Debra B. Kessler, M.D., Ph.D.

For Further Information

Dummer, R. "Future Perspectives in the Treatment of Cutaneous T-cell Lymphoma (CTCL)." *Seminars in Oncology* 33, no. 1 (2006): S33-S36.

Girardi, M., P. W. Heald, and L. D. Wilson. "The Pathogenesis of Mycosis Fungoides." *The New England Journal of Medicine* 350, no. 19 (2004): 1978-1988.

Kumar, Vinay, et al., eds. *Robbins and Cotran Pathologic Basis of Disease*. Philadelphia: Elsevier Saunders, 2005.

Other Resources

Cutaneous Lymphoma Foundation
http://www.clfoundation.org/

The Skin Site
Mycosis fungoides
http://www.skinsite.com/info_mycosis_fungoides.htm

See also: Agent Orange; Cutaneous T-Cell Lymphoma (CTCL); Lymphomas; Sézary syndrome; Skin cancers

▶ Myelodysplastic syndromes

Category: Diseases, Symptoms, and Conditions
Also known as: Myelodysplasia

Related conditions: Acute myeloid leukemia

Definition: Myelodysplastic syndromes characterize a range of hematological disorders in which the bone marrow stem cells either do not mature into red or white blood cells or do not function properly. This lack of healthy blood cells can lead to life-threatening conditions.

Risk factors: No one is certain what causes myelodysplastic syndromes. Most researchers believe that a variety of factors will lead to different myelodysplastic syndrome subtypes, but no one has been able to pinpoint what causes their onset. Scientists believe that prior therapy for cancer and exposure to environmental toxins places individuals at great risk for myelodysplastic syndromes. The cancer-treatment drugs chlorambucil, mechlorethamine, and procarbazine are all toxic to the bone marrow and seem to lead to the onset of myelodysplastic syndromes later in life. This is particularly true when these drugs are used in combination with certain forms of radiation therapy.

People who have been exposed to benzene and ionizing radiation appear to be susceptible to myelodysplastic syndromes. Benzene is found in gasoline, detergents, furniture polish, and cigarette smoke. Some researchers believe that a connection can be made between myelodysplastic syndromes and people who have had long-term exposure to certain agricultural chemicals and heavy metals.

Other risk factors for myelodysplastic syndromes include the congenital disorders Fanconi anemia and Down syndrome. People who smoke cigarettes, which contain benzene and other cancer-causing substances, are also more likely to be at risk for myelodysplastic syndromes.

Etiology and the disease process: Myelodysplastic syndromes rarely occur in people younger than the age of sixty, although they are appearing more often in children and adults who survive chemotherapy regimens for cancer treatment. Myelodysplasia is diagnosed more often in men than women, but there appears to be no association with ethnicity. Scientists have not been able to associate myelodysplastic syndromes with a genetic trait.

Secondary myelodysplastic syndromes most often appear after treatment for acute lymphocytic leukemia, Hodgkin disease, and non-Hodgkin lymphoma, but they can also arise after chemotherapy for cancer of the breast, lung, testis, or intestinal tract, and after treatment for some autoimmune diseases.

Incidence: Approximately 10,000 to 15,000 Americans are diagnosed with myelodysplastic syndromes each year. This number may be rising as the number of those who survive cancer treatment increases. Approximately 80 to 90 percent of those who receive a myelodysplastic syndrome diagnosis are the age of sixty and older.

Symptoms: The early stages of myelodysplastic syndromes may be uneventful and indistinct from other diseases. Myelodysplastic syndromes are often marked by anemia, which leads to shortness of breath and fatigue during light exertion. Other symptoms may include unusually pale skin, easy bleeding or bruising, tiny red spots (petechiae) just beneath the skin, weight loss, and frequent infections. About 20 percent of patients with myelodysplastic syndromes exhibit infections or bleeding, and about 20 percent of patients have no symptoms and are diagnosed during routine blood tests.

Screening and diagnosis: A complete blood count will help determine the number of platelets, red and white blood cells, and hemoglobin levels in red cells. A peripheral blood smear may help determine the shape, size, and appearance of blood cells. Myelodysplastic syndromes are usually diagnosed after other diseases, such as leukemia, have been excluded. Bone marrow tests will help confirm a diagnosis of myelodysplastic syndrome. These include aspiration and biopsy to obtain bone and marrow tissues, which are then analyzed using cytochemistry, flow cytometry, immunocytochemistry, and cytogenetic profiles.

Some physicians use the French-American-British (FAB) system to classify myelodysplastic syndromes into five subtypes. In the 1990's, the World Health Organization expanded the FAB into seven subtypes on the basis of circulating blood counts or changes in the bone marrow. These subtypes are refractory anemia, refractory anemia with ringed sideroblasts, refractory cytopenia with multilineage dysplasia, refractory cytopenia with multilineage dysplasia and ringed sideroblasts, refractory anemia with excess blasts (types 1 and 2), unclassified myelodysplastic syndromes, and myelodysplastic syndromes associated with isolated del(5q) chromosome abnormality.

Physicians use the International Prognostic Scoring System to assess a patient's health. Although the system is not a precise science, it uses three factors—the percentage of blasts in the bone marrow, an assessment of the number of cell types in the circulating blood (cytopenia), and an assessment of cellular chromosomal abnormalities—each of which is assigned a score to determine a patient's degree of health.

Treatment and therapy: Most patients require a transfusion of red blood cells to help relieve anemia. Drugs such as darbepoetin and erythropoietin may help the body produce more red blood cells and thus reduce the need for transfusions.

The U.S. Food and Drug Administration has approved two drugs specifically for the treatment of myelodysplastic syndromes. Azacitidine (approved May 19, 2004) and decitabine (approved May 2, 2006) are administered to stimulate blast cells to mature into healthy blood cells, but the pharmaceuticals are ineffective in some people and may cause additional problems.

The only potential cure for myelodysplastic syndromes is allogeneic (donor) stem cell transplantation, but few patients are eligible for the procedure because it poses high risks.

Prognosis, prevention, and outcomes: Patients with fewer bone marrow blasts and a greater number of cells in the blood and better cytogenetic profiles may demonstrate a longer median survival time, whereas patients with more blasts, fewer blood cells, and chromosome 7 abnormalities have a shorter survival time.

Terry A. Anderson, B.S.

For Further Information

Deeg, H. J., et al. *Hematologic Malignancies: Myelodysplastic Syndromes*. New York: Springer, 2006.

Hellstr-Lindberg, E., and L. Malcovati. "Supportive Care, Growth Factors, and New Therapies in Myelodysplastic Syndromes." *Blood Reviews* 22, no. 2 (March, 2008): 75-91.

Other Resources

Aplastic Anemia & MDS International Foundation
http://www.aamds.org/aplastic

Myelodysplastic Syndromes Foundation
http://www.mds-foundation.org

See also: Acute Myelocytic Leukemia (AML); Anemia; Benzene; Blood cancers; Cigarettes and cigars; Down syndrome and leukemia; Fanconi anemia; 5Q minus syndrome; Ionizing radiation; Leukemias; Leukopenia; Myelosuppression; Neutropenia; Premalignancies

▶ Myelofibrosis

Category: Diseases, Symptoms, and Conditions
Also known as: Agnogenic myeloid metaplasia, idiopathic myelofibrosis, aleukemic megakaryocytic myelosis, leukoerythroblastosis

Related conditions: Myeloproliferative disorders, including polycythemia rubra vera (increased numbers of red blood cells) and essential thrombocytosis (overproduction of platelets in the bone marrow)

Definition: Myelofibrosis is a disorder that disrupts the normal production of blood cells, leading to scarring of the bone marrow.

Risk factors: Myelofibrosis is most common in patients over fifty years old. Exposure to radiation, benzene, or radioactive thorium dioxide (a chemical used during some radiology procedures) also increases one's risk. There may also be an association between myelofibrosis and certain autoimmune diseases (in which the body attacks its own cells), leukemias and lymphomas, and other myeloproliferative disorders.

Etiology and the disease process: Hematopoiesis is the process of making blood cells. It begins in the bone marrow with a hematopoietic stem cell that can develop into specialized blood cells, including red blood cells (which transport oxygen), white blood cells (which are involved in the immune system), and platelets (which form clots).

Myelofibrosis develops when the genetic material in a single hematopoietic stem cell changes or acquires a mutation, and then begins to replicate and affect normal blood cell production. Approximately 50 percent of patients with myelofibrosis have stem cells with mutations in the *JAK* kinase gene; mutations in the *GATA-1* and *MPL* genes are less common. Mutated stem cells may affect cellular proliferation, survival, and immune responses. They may also stimulate fibroblast cells, causing them to secrete collagen that can build up scar tissue in the bone marrow. Cytokines (signals secreted from cells to affect activity of other cells), including transforming growth factor-beta (TGF-β), basic fibroblast growth factor, and platelet-derived growth factor (PDGF), may also induce bone marrow scarring.

The accumulation of scar tissue may displace normal blood cells being produced within the marrow. Therefore, blood cell production may begin to occur in other parts of the body, most often the spleen and liver. However, blood cell production in those tissues is not as efficient and increases organ size. Severe anemia (a lack of red blood cells) can also occur, leading to weakness and fatigue. The abnormal hematopoietic stem cells can also spread to other organs in the body and form tumors (primarily in the adrenals, kidneys, lymph nodes, breasts, and lungs).

Incidence: Myelofibrosis is rare, with an incidence rate ranging from 0.3 to 1.5 cases per 100,000 people. Among clonal hematologic disorders, myelofibrosis is the least prevalent.

Symptoms: In the early stages, myelofibrosis does not cause any symptoms. However, as normal blood cell production becomes more affected, multiple signs may arise, including tiredness, weakness, shortness of breath, an enlarged liver or spleen, easy bruising and bleeding, fever, frequent infections, and bone pain.

Screening and diagnosis: Screening for myelofibrosis includes blood tests to determine the number of red blood cells and their shape, because low numbers and teardrop-shaped cells indicate myelofibrosis. To examine enlargement of the liver and spleen, physical exams, as well as imaging tests (ultrasounds, magnetic resonance imaging, and computed tomography scans) may be performed.

A bone marrow biopsy, in which a needle is used to withdraw the bone marrow from the hip bone, may be done to confirm a diagnosis. The harvested bone marrow cells can be viewed under a microscope to examine signs of scarring and the types and number of cells within the marrow.

The following criteria for staging have been accepted by the World Health Organization:

- A1: No other myeloproliferative disorders
- A2: Early clinical stage, with slight anemia and slight enlargement of the spleen
- A3: Intermediate clinical stage, with moderate anemia, teardrop-shaped red blood cells, enlargement of the spleen, and no other symptoms
- A4: Advanced clinical stage, severe anemia, and one or more other symptoms

Treatment and therapy: There are many treatment options for myelofibrosis symptoms. Blood transfusions may improve anemia. Androgen (a hormone) or thalidomide (a drug) in combination with corticosterioids may increase red blood cell production. Hydroxyurea, a chemotherapeutic agent, can shrink enlarged spleens and may reduce bone marrow scarring. Radiation and interferon-alpha not only reduce spleen size but also may alleviate bone pain. When other treatments do not work, the spleen may be surgically removed in a process known as a splenectomy.

The only way to cure myelofibrosis is through a stem cell transplant in which the patient, after being treated with high-dose chemotherapy to kill the diseased cells, is provided with healthy blood stem cells from a donor. Because this is an intensive procedure, patients must be healthy enough to undergo the process and numerous side effects may occur.

Prognosis, prevention, and outcomes: The mean survival time from diagnosis ranges from 3.5 to 5.5 years. Patients with severe anemia, certain symptoms (weight loss, fatigue, night sweats, and fever), and those older than the age of sixty-five tend to have poorer mean survival rates. In approximately 15 percent of patients, myelofibrosis can progress to acute lymphocytic leukemia or lymphoma, which can be fatal.

There are no known ways to prevent myelofibrosis. To alleviate or prevent symptoms of anemia, the diet should include nutrients that promote blood formation, such as iron, folic acid, and vitamin B12.

Elizabeth A. Manning, Ph.D.

For Further Information

Hennessy, B. T., et al. "New Approaches in the Treatment of Myelofibrosis." *Cancer* 103, no. 1 (January 1, 2005): 32-43.

Spivak, J. L., et al. "Chronic Myeloproliferative Disorders." *Hematology/The Education Program of the American Society of Hematology* (2003): 200-224.

Tefferi, A. "The Forgotten Myeloproliferative Disorder: Myeloid Metaplasia." *Oncologist* 8, no. 3 (2003): 225-231.

Tefferi, A., and D. G. Gilliland. "Oncogenes in Myeloproliferative Disorders." *Cell Cycle* 6, no. 5 (March 1, 2007): 550-566.

Other Resources

MayoClinic.com
Myelofibrosis
http://www.mayoclinic.com/health/myelofibrosis/DS00886

MedlinePlus
Primary Myelofibrosis
http://www.nlm.nih.gov/medlineplus/ency/article/000531.htm

See also: Anemia; Chronic Myeloid Leukemia (CML); Myeloproliferative disorders; Polycythemia vera

▶ Myeloma

Category: Diseases, Symptoms, and Conditions
Also known as: Multiple myeloma, plasma cell myeloma

Related conditions: Non-Hodgkin lymphoma, other blood cancers

Definition: Myeloma is a cancer of the plasma cells found in the bone marrow. Plasma cells produce antibodies, which fight infection. In myeloma, abnormal plasma cells in the bone marrow overproduce monoclonal immunoglobulins. Multiple myeloma occurs when there are multiple bones affected.

Risk factors: As nearly all cases of multiple myeloma are diagnosed in adults over the age of forty, age is considered the most significant risk factor. It is thought, however, that myeloma is the result of several unknown factors working together.

Etiology and the disease process: The definitive cause of myeloma has not been determined. However, as age is its primary risk factor, potential causes include age-related factors such as long-term exposure to carcinogens, toxins, genetic variations, and decreased immune response.

Incidence: Myeloma is most commonly found in African Americans and occurs more frequently in women. Multiple myeloma is the second most common type of blood cancer (non-Hodgkin lymphoma is the first). Approximately 16,000 new cases are diagnosed each year. The average age of diagnosis is sixty-eight, and very few cases are diagnosed in people under the age of forty.

Symptoms: A common symptom is back pain, often accompanied by bone pain of the pelvis, ribs, and neck. Patients with myeloma have also reported excessive fatigue, iron deficiency, decreased immunity (frequent colds or sickness), a decrease in appetite, constipation, "pins and needles" in the feet and legs, and abnormal bleeding of the nose or gums.

Screening and diagnosis: There is no standard screening for myeloma; however, patients considered at risk and exhibiting symptoms should see a hematologist (a doctor who specializes in blood disorders) and have a series of tests performed to determine a diagnosis. Blood tests, urinalysis, X rays, bone scans, and bone marrow biopsy are typically performed.

There are two systems for staging myeloma: the Durie-Salmon Staging System and the International Staging System.

Treatment and therapy: Treatment for myeloma, like that for most cancers, depends on the stage of disease. Patients are often treated with chemotherapy and radiation, as well as additional therapies to target plasma cells.

Prognosis, prevention, and outcomes: Prognosis for myeloma depends on the stage at which the patient is diagnosed and the patient's overall health. While myeloma is not curable, it can be treated and managed. Most patients survive for at least one year following diagnosis, while at least half survive an additional five years and twenty out of every hundred patients diagnosed live an additional ten years.

Anna Perez, M.Sc.

See also: African Americans and cancer; Aging and cancer; Blood cancers; Bone cancers; Immunotherapy; Lactate Dehydrogenase (LDH) test; Leukapharesis; Multiple myeloma; Non-Hodgkin lymphoma; Stem cell transplantation; Thrombocytopenia; Umbilical cord blood transplantation

▶ Myeloproliferative disorders

Category: Diseases, Symptoms, and Conditions
Also known as: Blood cancers, chronic granulocytic leukemia, chronic myeloid leukemia, agnogenic myeloid metaplasia, primary myelofibrosis, myelosclerosis with myeloid metaplasia, idiopathic myelofibrosis, essential thrombocytosis

Related conditions: Leukemia

Definition: Myeloproliferative disorders are a group of slow-growing blood cancers, in which the bone marrow produces too many red blood cells, white blood cells, or platelets. All myeloproliferative disorders arise from an overproduction of one or more types of blood cells.

Risk factors: The reason for the abnormal increase in blood cells is not well understood. Genetics and environmental factors such as overexposure to radiation may be risk factors for some of these malignancies. Some types of myeloproliferative disorders have been associated with familial clusters; one such case is marked by a mutation of the erythropoeitin receptor.

Etiology and the disease process: No obvious etiology exists for myeloproliferative disorders. These malignancies begin in the bone marrow when a greater than normal number of stem cells develop into one or more types of blood cells. Normally, the bone marrow makes stem cells that develop into mature blood cells. There are three types of mature blood cells. Red blood cells are mature blood cells that carry oxygen and other materials to all tissues of the body. White blood cells are mature blood cells that fight infection and disease. Platelets are mature blood cells that help prevent bleeding by causing blood to clot. The type of myeloproliferative disorder is based on which kind of mature blood cells are overproduced. Usually one type of blood cell is affected more than the others. The disorders get worse as the number of blood cells increase. There are six types of chronic myeloproliferative disorders:

- Chronic myelogenous leukemia (CML) is a slowly progressing disease of overproduction of white blood cells, but not lymphocytes, in the bone marrow. CML is also called chronic granulocytic leukemia and chronic myeloid leukemia.
- Polycythemia vera is a disease in which too many red blood cells (and occasionally, white blood cells and platelets) are produced in the bone marrow and blood, causing the blood to thicken. The spleen is often enlarged as the extra blood cells may collect in it. Patients with polycythemia vera may also have bleeding problems and are at high risk for blood clotting.
- Chronic idiopathic myelofibrosis is a progressive, chronic disease in which the bone marrow is replaced by fibrous tissue, and blood is made in the liver and the spleen instead of in the bone marrow. The hallmark of this disease is an enlarged spleen. Chronic idiopathic myelofibrosis causes progressive anemia and is also called agnogenic myeloid metaplasia, primary myelofibrosis, myelosclerosis with myeloid metaplasia, and idiopathic myelofibrosis.
- Essential thrombocythemia is an increased number of thrombocytes (platelets) in the blood. The cause of this malignancy is not known. It is also called essential thrombocytosis.
- Chronic neutrophilic leukemia is a disease in which neutrophils, a type of white blood cell, are found in excess in the blood. The excess neutrophils in chronic neutrophilic leukemia may cause the spleen and liver to become enlarged. This disorder may not progress for years, or it may develop quickly into acute leukemia.
- Chronic eosinophilic leukemia is a disease in which eosinophils, a type of white blood cell, are found in the tissues, bone marrow, and blood. Similar to chronic neutrophilic leukemia, chronic eosinophilic leukemia may stay the same for years, or it may develop quickly into acute leukemia.

Incidence: Myeloproliferative disorders typically occur later in life. The prevalence of these diseases is low (approximately 5 per 1 million people), and they occur more commonly in men and women of East European Jewish ancestry compared with other populations. Men are more likely than women to develop polycythemia vera, primary myelofibrosis, and CML. However, women are 1.5 times more likely than men to develop essential thrombocytosis.

Symptoms: Many individuals with myeloproliferative disorders have no symptoms when their physicians first make the diagnosis. However, as the hematocrit or platelet count increases, most patients develop symptoms including headache, blurred vision, plethora (excess of body fluid), elevated white blood cell count, and hematocrit. A sign that is common to all myeloproliferative disorders, except of essential thrombocytosis, is an enlarged spleen, which may cause abdominal pain. Other signs of myeloproliferative disorders often include fatigue, difficulty breathing, intense itching (pruritus) after bathing in warm water, stomach aches, purple spots or patches on the skin, nosebleeds, gum or stomach bleeding, blood in the urine, throbbing and burning pain in the skin, high blood pressure, and blockage of blood vessels. Blockage of blood vessels may cause heart disease, stroke, or tissue death of the extremities.

As the disorders progress, patients may also develop cerebrovascular events, such as thrombosis. Thrombosis in small blood vessels may lead to serious events, such as cyanosis, erythromelalgia (painful vessel dilation in the extremities), ulceration, or gangrene (tissue death) in the fingers or toes. Thrombosis in larger vessels may lead to myocardial infarction, deep-vein thrombosis, transient ischemic attacks, and stroke.

Screening and diagnosis: Many of the myeloproliferative disorders are discovered by primary care physicians on routine blood tests. There is no standard staging system for chronic myeloproliferative disorders. Complete blood count is necessary for proper diagnosis, which includes the number of red blood cells and platelets, the number and type of white blood cells, the amount of hemoglobin (the protein that carries oxygen) in the red blood cells, and what portion of the blood sample is made up of red blood cells. Bone marrow aspiration and biopsy is used to look for signs of blood cancer. In addition, cytogenetic analysis or NextGen sequencing is often done to detect certain changes in the chromosomes or specific mutations.

Treatment and therapy: Treatment is based on the type of myeloproliferative disorder. Ten types of standard treatment are used: watchful waiting (monitoring a patient's condition), phlebotomy (removal of blood), platelet apheresis (removal of platelets from the blood), transfusion therapy, chemotherapy, radiation therapy, other drug therapy, surgery, splenectomy (removal of the spleen), and biological therapy.

Unfortunately, there are no known cures for most myeloproliferative disorders. However, there are treatments available that help alleviate symptoms and prevent complications associated with the disorders. The method used to alleviate symptoms depends on the type of myeloproliferative disorder. For polycythemia vera, phlebotomy is used to lower red blood cell count. In essential thrombocytosis and primary myelofibrosis, symptoms are treated with medications. Medications such as interferon may also improve survival rates of patients with certain myeloproliferative disorders.

When enlargement of the spleen becomes painful, a surgeon may perform a splenectomy to alleviate pain. Replacing the abnormal stem cells in the bone marrow with healthy stem cells may also help control the disorder. Bone marrow transplant is ideal for most patients with CML.

Prognosis, prevention, and outcomes: Though myeloproliferative disorders are serious, they are most often slow to develop; therefore, patients with these conditions often live for many years after diagnosis. Some complications of myeloproliferative disorders include enlargement of the spleen and liver, gout, anemia, bleeding, kidney or liver failure, heart attacks or stroke, and infection. In particular, CML can transform into acute leukemia.

The survival rates of those with myeloproliferative disorders depend on the type of disorder and symptoms. For example, the median survival rate for those with polycythemia vera is more than ten years with treatment. The major causes of death in untreated polycythemia vera patients are thrombosis and hemorrhage. Primary myelofibrosis and CML may be fatal within three to six years after diagnosis. However, if CML transforms into acute leukemia, the median survival rate may be only three months. Patients with other types of myeloproliferative disorders can live longer, especially when diagnosed early. Specifically, patients with primary thrombocythemia may have a normal life expectancy, and patients with polycythemia vera have a survival rate of between ten and twenty years.

Anita Nagypál, Ph.D.
Updated by: Catherine J. Walsh

For Further Information

Hoffman, R., Benz, E. J., Silberstain, L. E., Heslop, H., Weitz, J., & Anastasi, J. (2013). Hematology: Basic principles and practice (6th ed.). New York: Churchill Livingstone.

Michiels, J. J., De Raeve, H., Berneman, Z., & Schrovens, W. (2006). The 2001 World Health Organization and updated European clinical and pathological criteria for the diagnosis, classification, and staging of the Philadelphia chromosome-negative chronic myeloproliferative disorders. *Seminars in Thrombosis and Hemostasis,* 32: 307-340.

Talarico, L. D. (1998). Myeloproliferative disorders: A practical review. *Patient Care,* 30: 37-57.

Yavorkovsky, L. L., & Cook, P.(2001). Classifying chronic myelomonocytic leukemia. *Journal of Clinical Oncology,* 19: 3790-3792.

Barbui T, Thiele, J., Vannucchi, A. M., & Tefferi, A. (2015). Rationale for revision and proposed changes of the WHO diagnostic criteria for polycythemia vera, essential thrombocythemia and primarily myelofibrosis. *Blood Cancer Journal,* 5(8):e337. This article reviews proposed 215 changes to WHO classification of myeloproliferative neoplasms to accommodate newer information on disease-specific mutations and distinguishing morphologic features.

Barbui, T., & Tefferi, A. (Eds.). (2012). *Myeloproliferative neoplasms: Critical concepts and management (Hematologic Malignances).* New York: Springer. This book discusses myeloproliferative neoplasms including polycythemia vera, essential thrombycythemia, and primary myelofibrosis. This book includes recent advances and practical issues for physicians, including contemporary diagnostic approaches.

National Cancer Institute. (2011). 21st Century Adult Cancer Sourcebook: Chronic Myeloproliferative Disorders – Chronic Myelogenous Leukemia, Polycythemia Vera, Myelofibrosis, Thrombocythemia, Neutrophilic Leukemia. Progressive Management. This sourcebook includes information from cancer experts and includes information on signs, symptoms, treatment options, diagnostic testing, prognosis and survival.

Brady L. Stein, Brandon J McMahon. *Contemptorary management of myeloproliferative neoplasms.* 1st Edition. This book is a comprehensive guide to diagnosis and management of MPN. Jaypee Brothers Meidcal Pub, 2015.

Other Resources

Leukemia and Lymphoma Society
Myeloproliferative Disorders.
http://www.leukemia-lymphoma.org/all_page.adp?item_id=311829

Myeloproliferative Neoplasms
www.lls.org This website provides general information on MPNs and includes resources for patients and caregivers and also information on current research.

National Institutes of Health/National Cancer Institute
Myeloproliferative Neoplasms
http://www.cancer.gov/cancertopics/types/myeloproliferative

Provides review of disease and current treatment information for patients and caregivers.

MPN Research Foundation
mpnresearchfoundation.org

A website that shares information for MPN patients and their families about their disease, research, and new treatments and also provides support material.

See also: Acute Myelocytic Leukemia (AML); Blood cancers; Chronic Myeloid Leukemia (CML); Cyclophosphamide; Hypercoagulation disorders; Leukemias; Melphalan; Myelofibrosis; Polycythemia vera

▶ Myelosuppression

Category: Diseases, Symptoms, and Conditions
Also known as: Bone-marrow suppression, pancytopenia

Related conditions: Anemia, neutropenia, leukopenia, thrombocytopenia

Definition: Myelosuppression is a condition in which bone marrow function is decreased, with fewer than normal numbers of red blood cells, white blood cells, and platelets. Complete loss of bone-marrow function is called myeloablation.

Risk factors: Risk factors include having had chemotherapy, radiation therapy, or bone marrow or stem cell transplants, and having myelodysplastic syndromes.

Etiology and the disease process: Chemotherapy and radiation therapy for cancer destroy the rapidly dividing cancer cells as well as other rapidly dividing cells, or hematopoietic stem cells. As with anemia, leukopenia, and thrombocytopenia, hematopoietic stem cells are damaged by drugs used in chemotherapy or by radiation therapy. Cell counts often return to baseline values when treatment is stopped, reduced, or delayed.

Incidence: Nearly all patients who are being treated for cancer experience myelosuppression at some point and to some degree.

Symptoms: Depending on which cell line is involved, patients may feel weak, short of breath, and tired (anemia); may be susceptible to infections and have fevers (leukopenia); or may bruise and bleed easily (thrombocytopenia).

Screening and diagnosis: For routine monitoring during cancer therapy, myelosuppression is generally measured through blood tests. Anemia would be suspected with a red blood cell count less than 3.5×10^9 per liter in women and less than 4.3×10^9 per liter in men; leukopenia would be suspected with a white blood cell count less than 1.0 to 2.0×10^9 per liter; and thrombocytopenia would be suspected with a platelet count less than 200×10^9 per liter. Sometimes aspiration or core needle biopsy of the bone marrow is done to aid in the diagnosis of leukemia, lymphomas, and multiple myelomas, diseases associated with severe myelosuppression.

Treatment and therapy: Treatment for myelosuppression depends on which cell line is involved. Simply stopping or reducing the amount of chemotherapeutic drugs or radiation therapy given may relieve the myelosuppression. Anemia may be treated with red blood cell transfusions, steroids, supplements, or erythropoiesis-stimulating proteins such as epoetin alfa (Procrit, Epogen) or darbepoetin alfa (Aranesp). Leukopenia may be treated with hematopoietic growth factors such as filgrastim (Neupogen), pegfilgrastim (Neulasta), and sargramostim

(Leukine). Thrombocytopenia may be treated with platelet transfusions or with a recombinant form of interleukin (oprelvekin, or Neumega).

Prognosis, prevention, and outcomes: Left untreated, myelosuppression can impair a patient's quality of life, increase the need for hospitalization and transfusions of red blood cells or platelets or both, increase the need for intravenous anti-infectives, and increase risk of bleeding and infections. Use of hematopoietic, erythropoietic, and thrombocyte growth factors and transfusions is routine in supportive cancer treatment.

MaryAnn Foote, M.S., Ph.D.

See also: Anemia; Chemotherapy; External Beam Radiation Therapy (EBRT); Leukopenia; Neutropenia; Radiation therapies; Thrombocytopenia

▶ Nasal cavity and paranasal sinus cancers

Category: Diseases, Symptoms, and Conditions
Also known as: Nose cancers, sinus cancers

Related conditions: Lymphoma, melanoma, hemangiopericytoma, osteosarcoma, chondrosarcoma, adenosarcoma, squamous cell carcinoma

Definition: Nasal cavity and paranasal sinus cancers are cancers that arise in the paranasal sinuses or the nose. Many types of cancer can originate in the paranasal sinuses and nose. These include squamous cell carcinoma, adenocarcinoma, adenoid cystic carcinoma, lymphomas, chondrosarcoma, osteosarcoma, hemangiopericytoma, malignant melanoma, and esthesioneuroblastoma, as well as metastatic lesions from cancers of the kidney, lung, and breast.

Squamous cell carcinomas arise from the epithelial (skin) cells of the sinuses and are the most common type of paranasal sinus tumor. Adenocarcinoma tends to arise in the mucus-producing glands of the upper nasal cavity. This type of nasal cavity cancer is most common in woodworkers and people working with toxic chemicals and substances. Adenoid cystic carcinomas arise out of the salivary gland tissue and have a tendency to migrate to nearby nerve tissue. These tumors are slow growing but often metastasize to distant organs. Lymphomas arise from the cells of the lymph nodes and exhibit ulceration and necrosis (tissue death) of the lymph tissue in the nasal cavity or paranasal sinuses. Chondrosarcomas are rare in the nose and sinuses and arise out of the connective tissue. Osteosarcomas are cancers of the facial bones. Hemangiopericytomas are tumors of blood vessels. They are quite rare in the nose and sinuses. Malignant melanomas arise out of the epithelial tissue of the nasal septum and the lateral nasal wall. They appear to be more common in smokers and metastasize early. Esthesioneuroblastomas arise out of the sensory epithelial cells that control olfaction (smelling) and are quite rare.

Risk factors: The primary risk factor for nasal and paranasal sinus cancer is smoking. Occupational exposure to inhaled toxic substances can also put a person at risk for developing sinus cancer. These substances include dusts from wood, textiles, and leather; glues; formaldehyde; solvents; nickel and chromium dust; mustard gas; isopropyl alcohol; and radium. It is thought that heavy air pollution could lead to nasal and paranasal sinus cancers. These types of cancers do not appear to be hereditary.

Etiology and the disease process: Nasal cavity and paranasal sinus cancers develop in the walls of the nose or the walls of the six sinuses. Each side of the face has a maxillary, ethmoid, and sphenoid sinus. The paranasal sinuses are actually spaces that exist within the nasal and facial bones. Cancer occurs when a single cell mutates and grows uncontrollably. This tumor tends to invade nearby structures, which causes the symptoms of this type of cancer.

Incidence: Cancers of the nasal and paranasal sinuses are considered rare. Each year, only about 2,000 people in the United States develop one of these cancers. They are more common in men than in women. These cancers occur more frequently in countries other than the United States, such as Japan and South Africa.

Symptoms: The symptoms of nasal and paranasal sinus cancers are much like those of chronic sinus disease. They include blocked sinuses, decreased sense of smell, frequent sinus headaches, purulent drainage from the nose, facial swelling, epistaxis (bleeding from the nose), and frequent infections. Some patients will experience more definitive symptoms, such as a growth or mass on the nose, face, or soft palate; a lump inside the nose; numbness in areas of the face or head; loosening, pain, or numbness of the teeth; continuous tearing of the eyes; trouble opening the mouth; and swelling of the eyes.

Screening and diagnosis: No routine screening is performed for nasal or paranasal sinus cancers, because of their rarity. Diagnosis is achieved by physical examination, nasal endoscopy, computed tomography (CT) scan of the nose and sinuses, or magnetic resonance imaging (MRI) of the sinuses and orbits. If there is a visible mass, it is biopsied (a slice of tissue is removed for microscopic examination) to determine whether it is cancer, and if so, what type of cancer.

Only esthesioneuroblastomas and cancers of the maxillary sinuses, nasal cavity, and ethmoid sinuses are staged. The sinus cancers are staged using the American Joint Committee on Cancer (AJCC) staging system. This system uses the TNM (tumor/lymph node/metastasis) groupings. For esthesioneuroblastomas, the staging can be performed using one of two systems: the Kadish system or the UCLA system. Since esthesioneuroblastomas are extremely rare, these staging systems will not be discussed.

For cancers of the maxillary sinus, the stages are as follows:

- Stage 0 (T0, N0, M0): The cancer is confined to the epithelium and still resembles normal tissue.
- Stage I (T1, N0, M0): The cancer is confined to the nasal mucosa and has not spread to other sinuses or invaded the bones of the nose.
- Stage II (T2, N0, M0): The cancer has invaded the bones of the maxillary sinus, excluding the posterior wall. These bones include the hard palate and the opening into the maxillary sinus. The cancer has not spread beyond the maxillary sinus.
- Stage III (T1-3, N0-1, M0): The cancer has invaded the posterior wall of the maxillary sinus or has grown through the other bones of the sinus into the skin, the eye socket, or the ethmoid sinus. It may have metastasized to a single lymph node on the same side as the tumor. The involved node is a maximum of 3 centimeters (cm) in width.
- Stage IV (T1-4, any N, M0-1): The cancer has spread to the eye, the skull, the nasopharynx, or the sphenoid and frontal sinuses. There may be lymph node involvement. For a tumor to be Stage IV, there must be more than one node involved, nodes of greater than 3 cm, or involvement of nodes on the side opposite the tumor. Any maxillary cancer that has metastasized to other organs is Stage IV.

The stages for nasal cavity and ethmoid cancers are as follows:

- Stage 0 (T0, N0, M0): The cancer is confined to the epithelium and is very early stage.
- Stage 1 (T1, N0, M0): The cancer is localized to either the nasal cavity or the ethmoid sinus and its bones. There is no presence of lymph node involvement or metastases.
- Stage II (T2, N0, M0): The cancer has invaded another cavity close to the tumor, but there is no lymph node involvement or metastases.
- Stage III (T1-3, N0-1, M0): Either the cancer has invaded other structures, such as the eye socket, the palate, or the maxillary sinus, and there is no lymph node involvement or metastases, or it has invaded those structures, and one lymph node is involved. This node is a maximum of 3 cm.
- Stage IV (any T, any N, M0-1): The cancer has invaded other structures, such as the eye, skull, or the sphenoid or frontal sinuses, or the cancer has spread to two or more lymph nodes and these nodes are larger than 3 cm, or the cancer has spread to distant organs.

Treatment and therapy: Nasal cavity and paranasal cancers are treated with a combination of surgical resection of the tumor, radiation therapy, and chemotherapy. The actual surgical procedure performed will depend on the location of the tumor, the stage of the tumor, and whether it can be removed en block (as one piece of tissue). Cancer cells can be left in the surgical site if the tumor is incised (cut into).

Stage I and II cancers can be treated with computer-aided transnasal endoscopic surgery, which is performed using an endoscope that is inserted into the nostrils and then into the sinuses. Other surgical procedures used for tumors that remain within the nasal cavity are sublabial (under the upper lip) or lateral rhinotomy (incision along one side of the nose) approaches. Surgical procedures for Stage III and IV tumors may include midfacial degloving (separating the skin, subcutaneous tissue, nerves and tendons from the facial bones), orbital exenteration (removal of the eye and orbital bones), or craniofacial resections. After the latter surgical procedures, it may be necessary to perform grafts of skin or fascia (fibrous connective tissue that separates body structures) and to insert dental, orbital, or other prostheses to reconstruct the face. Tumors that have metastasized to the brain, the spinal column, and the optic nerve, and into the cavernous sinus (bilateral large venous blood vessels that drain blood from the dura mater that covers the brain) are generally considered inoperable.

Radiation therapy may be performed before or after surgery, and it may be applied internally or externally. Radiation therapy before surgery can decrease the size of the tumor and simplify tumor resection. If radiation therapy is performed after surgery, it is used to destroy any tumor cells that remain. Radiation therapy may be applied by an external beam or by radioactive objects placed within the nasal cavity, such as seeds, wires, or catheters. For radiation administered by an external beam, a mask is created to position the head precisely. Radiation beams must be carefully aimed to prevent radiation exposure of the thyroid and pituitary glands. Research is being performed on developing medications that can sensitize tumors to radiation.

Nasal cavity and paranasal sinus cancers can be treated with chemotherapy either before or after surgery. Chemotherapy before surgery is performed to decrease the size of the tumor so that surgical removal is easier. Chemotherapy administered after surgery is intended to destroy any remaining cancer cells. Traditional chemotherapy drugs include cisplatin and 5-fluorouracil for paranasal sinus cancers. Vincristine (Oncovin), cyclophosphamide (Cytoxan), doxorubicin (Adriamycin), and cisplatin are used to treat esthesioneuroblastomas. Epidermal growth factor receptor (EGFR) inhibitor drugs are also being used to treat nasal cavity and paranasal sinus cancers. These drugs interfere with the growth and division of tumor cells by inhibiting a hormone that encourages their growth. Some EGFR drugs being used are cetuximab (Erbitux), gefitinib (Iressa), and erlotinib (Tarceva). Genetic therapy is being explored and drugs tested against tumors with mutations of the *TP53* (also known as *p53*) tumor-suppressor gene.

Prognosis, prevention, and outcomes: Prognosis depends on the stage and location of the tumor and the age and condition of the patient. People with Stage I and II cancers of the nasal cavity and the paranasal sinuses often have full recovery after their treatments. For people with Stage III and IV cancers, full recovery is less likely. These patients, if they are cured, may be left with disfiguring facial changes due to surgery and radiation therapy. People who are elderly or in poor general health are less likely to survive Stage III and IV cancers.

Nasal cavity and paranasal sinus cancers cannot be prevented. There are many cases with no known cause. However, avoiding risk factors can decrease the likelihood of developing one of these cancers.

The outcome of a nasal cavity or paranasal sinus cancer depends on the type of tumor and the tissue from which it arises, the size of the tumor, and whether it has metastasized. Some types, like melanoma, are rapidly fatal. Other types grow slowly and may be resected successfully. The more extensive the tumor, the more likely it is that it will affect the cranial nerves and the sense of smell. More advanced tumors are quite likely to cause facial deformity as well as interference with tasting, smelling, and vision. Damage to the cranial nerves by surgery can affect the ability to open, close, and move the eyes; chew and swallow; and to change facial expressions.

Christine M. Carroll, R.N., B.S.N., M.B.A.

For Further Information

Carper, Elise, Kenneth Hu, and Elena Kuzin. *One Hundred Questions and Answers About Head and Neck Cancer*. Sudbury, Mass.: Jones and Barlett, 2008.

Genden, Eric M., and Mark A. Varvares, eds. *Head and Neck Cancer: An Evidence-Based Team Approach*. New York: Thieme, 2008.

Petruzelli, Guy, ed. *Practical Head and Neck Oncology*. San Diego: Plural, 2008.

Other Resources

American Cancer Society

Detailed Guide: Nasal Cavity and Paranasal Cancer
http://www.cancer.org/docroot/CRI/content/CRI_2_4_1X_What_is_nasal_cavity_and_paranasal_cancer.asp?sitearea=

American Rhinologic Society

An Introduction to Nasal Endoscopy
http://american-rhinologic.org/patientinfo.introendoscopy.phtml

National Cancer Institute

Paranasal Sinus and Nasal Cavity Cancer Treatment
http://www.cancer.gov/cancertopics/pdq/treatment/paranasalsinus

See also: Air pollution; Bone cancers; Cigarettes and cigars; Head and neck cancers; Lymphomas; Melanomas; Occupational exposures and cancer; Sarcomas, soft-tissue; Squamous cell carcinomas; Tobacco-related cancers

▶ Nausea and vomiting

Category: Diseases, Symptoms, and Conditions
Also known as: Emesis, retching, heaving, gagging, being sick to the stomach, seasickness, throwing up, butterflies in the stomach, dry heaves

Related conditions: Chemotherapy, radiation therapy, food poisoning, morning sickness during pregnancy, inner ear syndrome, infections

Definition: Nausea is the uneasy sensation that one is about to vomit, expelling stomach contents or undigested food through the mouth. Nausea can sometimes result in dry heaves when the stomach is empty.

Risk factors: Because nausea and vomiting are symptoms of many disorders as well as cancer therapies, the risk depends on the individual patient's medical condition and circumstances.

Etiology and the disease process: Nausea and vomiting are not diseases but symptoms—a sign that something is wrong within the body. Nausea and vomiting are complex body functions coordinated by the vomiting center in the brain stem of the body's central nervous system. Retching usually occurs after nausea and before vomiting as the body prepares to expel the stomach contents.

Nausea and vomiting can occur as a reaction to many prompts, including overeating, ingesting too much alcohol or sugar, infection, viruses, inner ear disorders, irritation of the throat or stomach lining, food poisoning from contaminated food or fluids, migraine headaches, unpleasant smells or sights, stress, severe anxiety or emotional circumstances, medications, or treatments for cancer. A person experiencing a heart attack, appendicitis, or head injury with increased pressure on the brain may have nausea and vomiting. Determining the cause is critical to finding the appropriate treatment and correcting the problem.

Cancer patients may experience nausea and vomiting for several reasons. Cancer treatments such as chemotherapy can affect patients by causing side effects of nausea and vomiting. Not all chemotherapy causes nausea and vomiting. The level of nausea that chemotherapy induces can range from low to severe. Factors such as the amount of the drug used or the route of administration can affect the incidence of nausea and vomiting. The characteristics of the person receiving chemotherapy—age, gender, or history of motion sickness—can influence the occurrence of nausea and vomiting. Sometimes nausea and vomiting will happen when patients enter an environment in which they have received chemotherapy because of odors or a mental association with the setting (anticipatory nausea and vomiting).

Cancer patients may have nausea and vomiting as an extension of their disease. The tumor may have spread to the gastrointestinal tract, the liver, or the brain. Also, high-dose radiation treatments given for certain types of cancer can cause nausea and vomiting in the hours following therapy. Other causes for nausea and vomiting in cancer patients include bowel obstructions, infections, anxiety, and certain medicines.

Usually the side effects of treatment can be controlled with medication, but if they are uncontrolled, they can result in serious metabolic dysfunction or anxiety and depression for the cancer patient and family.

Medicines Used to Treat Nausea in Cancer Patients

Drug	*Use*
Aprepitant	Used for acute and delayed nausea and vomiting
Aexamethasone	Corticosteroid, given orally and intravenously; used alone or in combination
Aiphenhydramine	Antihistamine, used for low-risk chemotherapy or when other antiemetics have failed; used in combination and also to reduce side effects from other antiemetics
Aolasetron, granisetron, ondansetron	New antiemetics, given orally or intravenously
Aronabinol, nabilone	Tetrahydrocannabinol (THC) is main ingredient; used when other antiemetics have failed
Haloperidol	Tranquilizer, used when other antiemetics have failed; used in combination
Lorazepam, alprazolam	Anxiety drugs; generally used in combination
Metoclopramide	Used for low-risk chemotherapy or when other antiemetics have failed; used alone or in combination
Olanzapine	Used when other antiemetics fail
Palonosetron	Used for acute and delayed nausea and vomiting; given intravenously
Prochlorperazine	Used for low-risk chemotherapy or when other antiemetics have failed; used alone or in combination
Promethazine	Used when other antiemetics have failed

Source: National Comprehensive Cancer Network

Incidence: Almost every person will experience nausea and vomiting at some stage of life for various reasons. Approximately 50 percent of all cancer patients have nausea and vomiting during their treatment or as their disease progresses. Some sources estimate that as many as 7 or 8 out of 10 (70 to 80 percent) cancer patients have some nausea and vomiting.

Symptoms: Nausea produces a queasy feeling in the stomach and increased salivation in the mouth. Sometimes a stomachache or headache will occur before the nausea occurs. The person may experience dizziness, a fast heart rate, skin temperature changes (either feeling chilled or hot and flushed), and difficulty swallowing with nausea. Retching usually precedes vomiting as the body prepares to push out the stomach contents. However, sometimes vomiting occurs without nausea. Loss of fluids and electrolytes can leave the patient feeling drained and fatigued.

Screening and diagnosis: The severity, duration, and frequency of nausea and vomiting will determine the need for further assessment and intervention by the health care provider. The key to screening and diagnosing nausea and vomiting is finding the underlying cause. Patients should review any health conditions they have that might contribute to nausea and vomiting such as migraine headaches or pregnancy (morning sickness).

Health care providers can prepare cancer patients for the likely possibility of nausea and vomiting during their treatment process. The degree to which nausea and vomiting affects the patient depends on many factors. Extension of cancer with metastatic disease to vital organs can increase the incidence of nausea and vomiting.

Treatment and therapy: Nausea and vomiting do not necessarily need treatment unless they continue for extended periods of time, as can occur with several types of radiation and chemotherapy. The first approach to treatment is to determine the cause. If the cause can be defined and treated successfully, the nausea and vomiting will subside.

Sometimes a simple breath of fresh air can resolve the problem. Some people successfully use ginger ale, cola, or crackers to decrease the nausea. Vomiting will immediately relieve nausea but nausea may return. Simple nausea and vomiting usually respond to limiting the intake of food and fluids. Gradually patients may take clear liquids, then small amounts of dry toast or crackers. If this is well tolerated without more nausea and vomiting, patients can return to a regular diet.

If the nausea and vomiting continue uncontrolled, further examination is necessary to remove or treat the cause. Over time, patients with uncontrolled nausea and vomiting will become dehydrated and may suffer an electrolyte imbalance. Patients with continuous nausea and vomiting may need antiemetics, medications that suppress these symptoms. If severe dehydration has occurred, patients may need to be given intravenous fluids by a health care provider. Dehydration and electrolyte imbalance can be serious and can even be life-threatening.

Alternative or complementary therapies may help control or minimize nausea and vomiting. Nonpharmacologic therapies include biofeedback, guided imagery, attentional distraction, massage, and hypnosis. Behavior therapy such as desensitization may be useful for anticipatory nausea and vomiting. Ginger, an herb used to decrease nausea and vomiting, can be used in food or taken in capsules. Acupressure may help some patients. Dietary approaches such as eating food with minimal smell (either cold or at room temperature) while having chemotherapy may decrease nausea and vomiting. Avoiding certain types of foods, such as high-fat, spicy, or salty foods, helps some patients.

Prognosis, prevention, and outcomes: Most people experience uncomplicated nausea and vomiting at some time in their lives but can regain their health through addressing the cause and allowing the body time to heal. However, a health care provider should be notified if people have nausea and vomiting that continue for longer than forty-eight hours, experience extreme dizziness, vomit blood, or are unable to retain fluids within twenty-four hours.

If people have begun taking a new medication before the onset of nausea and vomiting, they should notify their health care provider to possibly change the drug. People should consult a health care provider when they have yellowing of the skin or eyes, difficulty swallowing, mental confusion, dehydration and extreme thirst, trouble with urination, or constant or sharp pain in the chest or lower abdomen. Certain conditions when accompanied by nausea and vomiting may indicate a medical emergency, such as diabetic shock, severe headache, consistent chest pain, difficulty breathing, profuse sweating, or exposure to a known allergen.

At least half of all cancer patients will experience some nausea and vomiting at some point in their disease process. Using antiemetics or complementary therapies such as relaxation, massage, or meditation can sometimes produce a better outcome to the nausea and vomiting resulting from chemotherapy or radiation therapy. Education and knowledge can go a long way in helping patients help themselves.

Robert W. Koch, D.N.S., R.N.

For Further Information

Anderson, Greg. *Cancer: Fifty Essential Things to Do.* New York: Penguin Books, 1999.

Donnerer, Josef, ed. *Antiemetic Therapy.* New York: Karger, 2003.

Lyss, Alan P., and Humberto M. Fagundes. *Chemotherapy and Radiation for Dummies.* Hoboken, N.J.: Wiley, 2005.

Tonato, M., ed. *Antiemetics in the Supportive Care of Cancer Patients.* New York: Springer, 1996.

Other Resources

American Cancer Society

What Can I Do About Nausea and Vomiting?
http://www.cancer.org/docroot/MBC/content/MBC_2_2X_What_Can_I_Do_About_Nausea_and_Vomiting.asp?sitearea=MBC

National Cancer Institute

Nausea and Vomiting
http://www.cancer.gov/cancertopics/pdq/supportivecare/nausea/patient

National Comprehensive Cancer Network

Nausea and Vomiting Treatment Guidelines for Patients with Cancer
http://www.nccn.org/patients/patient_gls/_english/_nausea_and_vomiting/contents.asp

See also: Acupuncture and acupressure for cancer patients; Adjuvant therapy; Antinausea medications; Cachexia; Chemotherapy; Complementary and alternative therapies; External Beam Radiation Therapy (EBRT); Gastrointestinal complications of cancer treatment; Ginseng, panax; Living with cancer; Medical marijuana; Motion sickness devices; Nutrition and cancer treatment; Radiation therapies; Side effects; Taste alteration; Weight loss

▶ Nephroblastomas

Category: Diseases, Symptoms, and Conditions
Also known as: Wilms' tumors

Related conditions: Beckwith-Wiedemann syndrome, WAGR complex (Wilms' tumor aniridia-genitourinary anomalies-mental retardation), Denys-Drash syndrome

Definition: Nephroblastomas are the most common malignant kidney tumors of early childhood.

Risk factors: Nephroblastomas may arise sporadically (in otherwise healthy children) or can be inherited. A nephroblastoma is sometimes linked to birth defects such as aniridia (absence of the iris), hemihypertrophy (enlargement of one side of the body), and genitourinary abnormalities. Birth defect syndromes associated with nephroblastoma include Beckwith-Wiedemann syndrome (tongue and internal organ enlargement and omphalocele), WAGR syndrome (Wilms' tumor aniridia-genitourinary anomalies-mental retardation), and Denys-Drash syndrome (Wilms' tumor, kidney disease, and pseudohermaphroditism). Children aged seven and younger are at highest risk, although older children and adults are occasionally affected. No gender or racial predilection exists.

Etiology and the disease process: There is compelling evidence that genetic factors (two mutational events involving the inactivation of tumor-suppressor genes) may be responsible for tumor development. As a result, primitive embryonic cells of the kidney fail to develop and instead multiply to form a tumor.

Incidence: Annually, 450 to 500 children in the United States are diagnosed with a nephroblastoma, with 24 percent of these cases forming part of a developmental defect syndrome.

Symptoms: Most patients have a painless abdominal mass, usually an incidental finding by the doctor or the parent. Some complain of abdominal pain, bloody urine, nausea and vomiting, anorexia, weight loss, and constipation.

Screening and diagnosis: Lab tests, a thorough family medical history, and diagnostic imaging—ultrasound, chest X ray, computed tomography (CT) scan, and magnetic resonance imaging (MRI)—will help determine the extent of tumor spread. Surgical tumor removal and tissue sampling will confirm the diagnosis. Tumor staging helps establish the treatment plan:

- Stage I: Tumor confined to the kidney, completely resectable
- Stage II: Tumor metastasis to local surrounding area, completely resectable
- Stage III: Tumor metastasis to surrounding area, not completely resectable
- Stage IV: Tumor metastasis to distant organs (lungs, liver, and brain)
- Stage V: Tumor present in both kidneys

Treatment and therapy: Treatment consists of a combination of surgery, chemotherapy, and radiotherapy. Surgery can be partial, complete, or radical nephrectomy (surgical removal of the kidney). The drugs dactinomycin, doxorubicin, vincristine, and cyclophosphamide are used for chemotherapy. Radiotherapy is usually confined to Stage III and IV nephroblastoma.

Prognosis, prevention, and outcomes: The prognosis is good, with an overall survival rate of 90 percent. Outcomes for nephroblastoma patients have vastly improved since the 1970's, thanks to concerted efforts by the National Wilms' Tumor Study Group (NWTSG) and the International Society of Pediatric Oncology (SIOP).

Ophelia Panganiban, B.S.

See also: Beckwith-Wiedemann Syndrome (BWS); Denys-Drash syndrome and cancer; Pediatric oncology and hematology; Wilms' tumor; Wilms' tumor Aniridia-Genitourinary anomalies-mental Retardation (WAGR) syndrome and cancer

▶ Neuroblastomas

Category: Diseases, Symptoms, and Conditions
Also known as: Childhood autonomic nervous system tumors

Related conditions: Ganglioneuroblastomas, ganglioneuromas

Definition: Neuroblastomas are cancers, most often found in infants and young children, that grow from primitive, embryonic nerve cells. Two-thirds of tumors begin in the adrenal glands or the sympathetic nervous system ganglia, with growth in the abdomen. The remaining third of neuroblastomas grow in the chest, neck, or pelvis, but all evolve from sympathetic nervous system ganglia.

Risk factors: Heredity may play a role in some neuroblastomas and is the only known risk factor. Infants with the familial form of neuroblastoma usually have a parent or someone in the family who had a neuroblastoma as an infant, and familial cases are usually diagnosed before one year of age. When familial neuroblastoma develops, there may be two or more tumors in various organs in the body. It is necessary to differentiate metastasis from multiorgan familial neuroblastoma.

Etiology and the disease process: There is no known cause of neuroblastoma other than heredity, which is involved in only 1 to 2 percent of cases. Neuroblastoma may form before birth and is occasionally found by fetal ultrasound. Most tumors develop before five years of age. Tumors are generally found only as the cancer grows and causes symptoms by pressing on organs. The tumor has usually metastasized by the time of diagnosis, and metastasis to the bone is common. Most tumors are fast growing, but in rare cases, the tumor cells may die spontaneously (apoptosis), and the tumor disappears. Occasionally, the tumor cells may quit dividing and become normal ganglia. This causes the tumor to become a ganglioneuroma, which is benign.

Incidence: The incidence rate of neuroblastoma in children under one year of age is 35 per million, decreasing to 1 per million between ten and fifteen years of age. Neuroblastoma is slightly more common in boys than in girls, with a ratio of 5:4. Neuroblastoma accounts for 25 percent of cancers in children under one year of age and 7 percent of cancers in children under the age of fifteen.

Symptoms: Common symptoms of neuroblastoma include fatigue; diarrhea; a swollen abdomen; difficulty breathing as the tumor gets larger or spreads to the chest area; dark circles under the eyes; pale or flushed, red skin; excessive sweating; bone pain or tenderness; rapid pulse;

Possible Causative Factors for Neuroblastoma

Studies have looked at these factors as possible causes for neuroblastoma, but so far the results have been inconclusive or contradictory.

Pregnancy-Related Factors
- Previous miscarriage (higher risk per one study, lower per another)
- Fertility drug use before pregnancy
- Alcohol use during pregnancy
- Smoking during pregnancy (higher risk per one study, lower per another)
- Taking certain medications during pregnancy: amphetamines, diuretics, tranquilizers, muscle relaxants, vaginal anti-infection drugs

Paternal Factors
- Father's exposure to electromagnetic fields, pesticides, dust, rubber, paint, radiation

Birth-Related Factors
- Birth defects
- Low birth weight

Source: L. A. G. Ries et al., eds., Cancer Incidence and Survival Among Children and Adolescents: United States SEER Program, 1975-1995, NIH Pub. No. 99-4649 *(Bethesda, Md.: National Cancer Institute, SEER Program, 1999)*

high blood pressure; poorly controlled movement of the extremities; or paralysis. Symptoms depend on the site of the tumor, and parents may notice or feel a mass in the abdomen, chest, or neck.

Screening and diagnosis: There is no screening test for neuroblastoma. If a family has a history of neuroblastoma, it is important to tell the pediatrician at the first visit. Parents should take note of any unusual lumps, swellings, or changes in bowel or bladder patterns, as the symptoms ofneuroblastoma often manifest in this manner. The diagnosis of neuroblastoma begins with a careful physical examination, as masses may be palpated (felt) in the abdomen, chest, or neck. A twenty-four-hour urine test, blood work, and cytogenetic analysis to look for changes in chromosomes are done. A bone marrow aspiration or biopsy specimen may also undergo cytogenetic analysis and pathology review. Imaging (X-ray) studies may include ordinary X rays, computed tomography (CT) scans, ultrasound, a magnetic resonance imaging (MRI) scan, and a positron emission tomography (PET) scan.

Once a diagnosis is made, staging neuroblastoma is important to determine the treatment needed. The first step is to determine if the tumor has spread to other parts of the body. Additional tests may be indicated, including lymph node biopsy or fine needle aspiration of fluid from a lymph node as well as imaging studies with dye injection or injection of a small amount of radioactive tracer material. Four stages are used to classify neuroblastoma: Stages I, IIA and IIB, III, and IV and IVS. The higher the stage, the more extensive the disease and its spread. Neuroblastomas are categorized as low risk, intermediate risk, and high risk based on stage, with treatment determined by risk group.

Treatment and therapy: Because neuroblastoma is rare, treatment in a clinical research trial is recommended by the National Cancer Institute. Treatment for neuroblastoma is multimodal, which means that surgery, radiation therapy, chemotherapy, and in rare instances watchful waiting may be used. The higher the risk group, the more aggressive the therapy. Surgery is the initial treatment of choice to remove as much of the tumor as possible and to biopsy lymph nodes. Radiation therapy may be used, especially if part of the tumor has been left behind after surgery or if distant metastases exist. Chemotherapy is used to kill any cells remaining after surgery or to attack cells that may have spread elsewhere in the body. Patients may be watched carefully until a change in their condition indicates the method of therapy. A team will make the best treatment decisions for the child based on staging, location of the tumor, and other factors.

Prognosis, prevention, and outcomes: The prognosis for neuroblastoma depends on the age of the child at diagnosis, the stage of the disease, the site of the tumor, the size of the tumor, and the type of tumor cells. Infants do better than older children. Low-risk group survival at five years is 95 percent, intermediate group survival is 85 to 90 percent, and high-risk group survival is approximately 30 percent. Neuroblastoma cannot be prevented.

Patricia Stanfill Edens, R.N., Ph.D., FACHE

For Further Information

Maris, J. M., M. D. Hogarty, R. Bagatell, and S. I. Cohn. "Neuroblastoma." *Lancet* 369, no. 9579 (June 23, 2007): 2106-2120.

Nishimura, H., et al. "Proton-Beam Therapy for Olfactory Neuroblastoma." *International Journal of Radiation Oncology, Biology, Physics* 68, no. 3 (July 1, 2007): 758-762.

Other Resources

American Cancer Society
http://www.cancer.org

National Cancer Institute
Neuroblastoma Treatment
http://www.cancer.gov/cancertopics/pdq/treatment/neuroblastoma/patient

See also: Adrenal gland cancers; Beckwith-Wiedemann Syndrome (BWS); Bone Marrow Transplantation (BMT); Brain and central nervous system cancers; Breast cancer in children and adolescents; Childhood cancers; Horner syndrome; *HRAS* gene testing; Mediastinal tumors; *MYC* oncogene; Nasal cavity and paranasal sinus cancers; Pediatric oncology and hematology; Stem cell transplantation; Syndrome of Inappropriate Antidiuretic Hormone production (SIADH); Tumor markers; Umbilical cord blood transplantation

▶ Neuroectodermal tumors

Category: Diseases, Symptoms, and Conditions
Also known as: Primitive neuroectodermal tumors (PNETs)

Related conditions: Medulloblastomas, peripheral neuroepitheliomas, central neuroblastomas, ependymoblastomas, Gorlin syndrome, nevoid basal cell carcinoma syndrome, Askin tumor (thoracopulmonary PNET), peripheral PNET/Ewing sarcoma family tumor (pPNET/ESFT), extraosseous Ewing sarcoma

Definition: Neuroectodermal tumors refer to a group of cancers that were formerly thought to have a common origin from the neuroectodermal tissue layer cell line (neural crest) in the embryo. Presently, they are classified according to cell differentiation. They possess embryonic cell characteristics of brain (neuronal), neuronal support (glial), or mesenchymal cells depending on the degree of differentiation assumed. Neuroectodermal tumors may arise from bone or soft tissue (peripheral Ewing sarcoma family tumor, pPNET/ESFT), or neurons in the peripheral or central nervous system (medulloblastomas; infratentorial PNET, or iPNET; supratentorial PNET, or sPNET). Medulloblastomas represent the prototype neuroectodermal tumor.

Risk factors: Neuroectodermal tumors have risk factors associated with alterations in the patient's genome as a sporadic mutation, as part of a syndrome, or as a result of environmental exposure to a mutagen. Syndromes associated with the risk of developing iPNET include multiple-tumor, autosomal dominant diseases such as Gorlin syndrome, Turcot syndrome, and Li-Fraumeni syndrome. Exposure of children to pesticides, particularly organophosphates, has been implicated in several studies as an environmental risk factor for the subsequent development of PNET. Organophosphates have been associated in at least one study with a mutation in the PON1(-108T) allele, which is responsible for expression of the organophosphate detoxification pathway (cytochrome P450/paraoxonase) in the liver.

Etiology and the disease process: The genesis of neuroectodermal tumors is associated with chromosomal changes. The most common chromosomal aberration seen in medulloblastomas is deletion of the short arm of chromosome 17 (17p13.3), seen in as many as 30 to 40 percent of medulloblastoma cases. Other gene aberrations associated with medulloblastomas may involve the *TP53*, *PAX*, and sonic hedgehog (*SHH*) genes and the tumor-suppression region *RASSF1A*, among others. The Ewing sarcoma family tumor (ESFT) is associated with the translocation t(11;22)(q24;q12), expressing the *EWS-FLI1* fusion protein modulator.

Incidence: The Swedish Cancer Registry reported that medulloblastomas represented 21 percent of all primary pediatric brain malignancies. The incidence of all neuroectodermal tumors is highest in children, with 0.5 medulloblastoma cases per 100,000 per year reported in the United States. Medulloblastomas represent the most common solid malignant brain tumor found in children (30 percent), with the incidence decreasing to only 1 percent of brain tumors found during adulthood. The majority of medulloblastomas occur in the cerebellum, below the tentorium (extension of the protective tissue covering the brain); only 4 percent of neuroectodermal tumors occur above the tentorium (midbrain, cerebral cortex). Neuroectodermal tumors outside the central nervous system occur in 1 percent of all sarcomas found.

Symptoms: More often than not, the more common signs and symptoms relate to obstruction of cerebrospinal fluid (CSF) flow and subsequent pressure buildup and tissue compression. Symptoms of increased pressure include nausea, vomiting, morning headache, and vision changes. Brain stem compression or encroachment can manifest as irritability, lethargy, and decreased social interaction. Cerebellar signs of involvement include frequent loss of balance. Physical examination findings may include papilledema (swelling of both optic nerves); abnormal eye movements; gaze, gait, and limb incoordination; deficits in affected cranial nerves, especially those going to the throat, mouth, shoulders, and tongue; and an increase in head circumference in babies less than two years old. In other sites, neuroectodermal tumors such as pPNET/ESFT can manifest as localized bone pain, a soft-tissue mass located along the middle of long bones with fever and weight loss.

Screening and diagnosis: The final diagnosis of a neuroectodermal tumor is mainly pathological, when a tissue sample is examined microscopically and with immunohistochemistry (tests determining cell markers). However, the neuroanatomical location of the tumor as suggested by clinical history, physical examination, and neuroimaging tests such as magnetic resonance imaging (MRI) can suggest a medulloblastoma. Alternatively, a computed tomography (CT) scan may reveal the tumor but has significantly less resolution than an MRI. There are no screening tests available for neuroectodermal tumors. X rays and CT of the affected limb may reveal signs of simultaneous bone destruction and remodeling ("sunburst sign") and a periosteal reaction (disruption in the continuity of the outer bone) as well as bone infiltration. X rays and CT of the chest should also be done to find metastases.

Treatment and therapy: Treatment of a neuroectodermal tumor irrespective of location includes surgical removal, radiation therapy, and chemotherapy. Surgical removal must be able to extract the entire primary tumor and probable areas of spread, and restore normal cerebral spinal fluid circulation. The latter may be achieved with the addition of a device diverting excess cerebral spinal fluid to the abdominal cavity (ventriculoperitoneal shunt). For other neuroectodermal tumors outside the nervous system, the same therapeutic principles apply. In children with limb involvement, amputation may be done because of the stunting effect of therapeutic radiation levels on growth plates.

Prognosis, prevention, and outcomes: The prognosis of neuroectodermal tumors after therapy completion is good. Five-year survival rates for central nervous system tumors approach 75 percent with aggressive surgical removal, radiotherapy, and chemotherapy. pPNET/ESFT exhibits similar survival rates with the same treatment, as opposed to radiotherapy and chemotherapy alone (50 percent). Prevention of recurrence includes interval imaging and "second look" surgeries when residual disease is present.

Aldo C. Dumlao, M.D.

For Further Information

Eiser, Christine. *Children with Cancer: The Quality of Life*. Mahwah, N.J.: Lawrence Erlbaum Associates, 2004.

Pagé, Michel. *Tumor Targeting in Cancer Therapy*. Totowa, N.J.: Humana Press, 2004.

Parker, James N., and Philip M. Parker, eds. *The Official Parent's Sourcebook of Ewing's Family of Tumors*. San Diego, Calif.: Icon Health, 2002.

Other Resources

National Cancer Institute

Childhood Supratentorial Primative Neuroectodermal Tumors and Pineoblastoma
http://www.cancer.gov/cancertopics/pdq/treatment/childSPNET

WebMd

Primitive Neuroectodermal Tumors of the Central Nervous System
http://www.emedicine.com/NEURO/topic326.htm

See also: Brain and central nervous system cancers; Ewing sarcoma; Medulloblastomas; Pineoblastomas

▶ Neuroendocrine tumors

Category: Diseases, Symptoms, and Conditions
Also known as: NET

Related conditions: Multiple endocrine neoplasia (MEN) type 1 (Wermer syndrome), MEN type 2A (Sipple syndrome), MEN type 2B, carcinoid tumors, islet cell tumors, pheochromocytomas, thyroid carcinomas (medullary), parathyroid carcinomas, Zollinger-Ellison syndrome (gastrinoma), prolactinomas, Cushing syndrome, small-cell lung carcinomas

Definition: Neuroendocrine tumors are a group of rare tumors affecting organs that originate embryologically from the neural crest, the layer that gives rise to the brain, spinal cord, peripheral nerves, and endocrine glands (organs that secrete hormones). These tumors mostly arise from hormone-secreting tissues; however, some tumors may not secrete hormones at all.

Neuroendocrine tumors may be classified as functional or nonfunctional, or hereditary or nonhereditary. The hereditary MEN syndromes consist of two main variants, MEN 1 and MEN 2. MEN 1 has pituitary, parathyroid, and pancreas involvement. MEN 2A manifests as medullary thyroid cancer (MTC), pheochromocytoma (adrenal medulla tumor), and parathyroid hyperplasia. MEN 2B is essentially type 2A without parathyroid involvement and with the addition of mucosal neuromas and gut ganglioneuromas with a Marfanoid body habitus. Isolated medullary thyroid cancer may also be familial but less aggressive compared to MEN-associated variants of the disease. The nonhereditary tumors include pheochromocytoma, carcinoid tumors, islet cell, small-cell, and nonfamilial medullary thyroid carcinomas.

Risk factors: Although most cases involving a single organ are more sporadic, the most prominent risk factor for the development of neuroendocrine tumors is a genetic predisposition. The MEN syndromes are autosomal dominant, implying that every generation has an afflicted individual, with a 50 percent probability of offspring inheriting the disease. Exposure to leuprolide acetate and medroxyprogesterone acetate in female rats was associated with a higher incidence of pancreatic islet cell tumors.

Etiology and the disease process: The genetic etiology of the heritable as well as most sporadic cases of somatic (mature, differentiated cells) cell mutations in parathyroid adenomas, gastrinomas, insulinomas, and bronchial carcinoids most commonly originates from *MEN1* tumor-suppressor gene mutations, with the *RET* proto-oncogene implicated in sporadic medullary thyroid carcinoma cases. MEN 1 originates from one of two etiologies: a mutation within the embryonic crest cell or inactivation of the tumor-suppressor gene *MEN 1*, located on the long arm of chromosome 11 (11q13). In MEN 2A, MEN 2B, and familial medullary thyroid carcinoma, the origin is believed to be a mutation in the *RET* proto-oncogene, located on the long arm of chromosome 10 (10q11.2). Gastrinomas originate from HER2/neu (human epidermal growth factor receptor 2/neu) proto-oncogene.

Incidence: The overall occurrence of neuroendocrine tumors is extremely rare, accounting for only 0.5 percent of all malignant cancers. However, an increase in the number of cases of these tumors has been observed. The gastrointestinal tract has the highest incidence of neuroendocrine tumors, accounting for 62 to 67 percent of all primary tumors, followed by the lungs (22 to 27 percent) in one study conducted in the Netherlands.

Symptoms: The symptoms associated with neuroendocrine tumors vary widely and are often insidious in onset. Tumors may be found during the course of an unrelated imaging study. Some neuroendocrine tumors are related to location rather than the disease entities they mimic. For example, pancreatic tumors may manifest as poorly controlled diabetes in glucagonoma and somatostatinoma; pituitary tumors as amenorrhea in prolactinomas, unintentional skin darkening, high blood pressure, and psychosis in Cushing disease; sudden episodes of high blood pressure, cold sweats, and palpitations in pheochromocytomas; or as a plethora of unrelated signs and symptoms such as flushing, abdominal cramps, diarrhea, or new-onset heart murmur in carcinoid tumors.

Both nonfunctioning tumors and bulky functioning tumors can compress or infiltrate surrounding tissue or structures and cause obstructive symptoms.

Screening and diagnosis: Diagnosis of neuroendocrine tumors is often difficult and missed because of misleading disease symptoms. Medullary thyroid cancer, especially when a family history is present, should initiate a comprehensive search for high calcitonin, blood and urine calcium (medullary thyroid, parathyroid), adrenocorticotropic hormone (ACTH), growth hormone, thyroid-stimulating hormone (TSH), prolactin levels (pituitary), and twenty-four-hour urine metanephrine (adrenal medulla) levels as well as computed tomography (CT) or magnetic resonance imaging (MRI) of the head, neck, chest, and abdomen, as appropriate, to look for primary as well as metastatic sites. Insulin-to-glucose ratios, chromogranin A, gastrin levels, octreoscans, endoscopy, and CT and MRI imaging studies are useful for aiding in pancreatic tumor diagnosis.

Although neuroendocrine tumors have a clear genetic etiology, genetic testing for *RET* is reserved for patients presenting with medullary thyroid cancer.

Treatment and therapy: Treatment of neuroendocrine tumors includes surgical removal, radiation therapy, and chemotherapy and is highly dependent on the tumor location and type. Precautions should be taken to stabilize the patient preoperatively for many functioning tumors. Control of blood pressure, high glucose levels, electrolyte imbalances, and gastrin excess are essential. Surgery must be able to remove the entire primary tumor and, if needed, structures susceptible to infiltration. For islet cell tumors, chemotherapy with streptozocin, doxorubicin, and 5-fluorouracil (5-FU) alone or in combination have proved beneficial (54 to 69 percent response rate).

Prognosis, prevention, and outcomes: Most cases of neuroendocrine tumors have a good prognosis with radical surgery, chemotherapy, or radiotherapy. Metastatic disease at the time of diagnosis implies a poor prognosis. Gastrinomas in particular have poorer prognosis, as 60 percent are malignant; associated with MEN 1 syndrome, they have a better prognosis than gastrinoma alone. Medullary thyroid cancer and MEN 2 have a five-year survival rate of 90 percent, attributable to early treatment of medullary thyroid cancer. Observation for recurrence is needed, through periodic clinical examinations, laboratory tests for tumor markers, and CT and MRI. Genetic counseling and testing are helpful in individuals with a strong family history of neuroendocrine tumors.

Aldo C. Dumlao, M.D.

For Further Information

Clark, Orlo H. *Endocrine Tumors*. Hamilton, Ont.: BC Decker, 2003.

Fossel, Michael B. *Cells, Aging, and Human Disease*. New York: Oxford University Press, 2004.

Kelloff, Gary, Ernest T. Hawk, and Caroline C. Sigman. *Cancer Chemoprevention*. Totowa, N.J.: Humana Press, 2005.

Other Resources

American Cancer Society

Detailed Guide: Gastrointestinal Carcinoid Tumors

http://www.cancer.org/docroot/CRI/content/CRI_2_4_1X_What_are_gastrointestinal_carcinoid_tumors_14.asp

Dana-Farber Cancer Institute
Neuroendocrine Tumors
http://research.dfci.harvard.edu/neuroendocrine/

See also: Cushing syndrome and cancer; Endocrine cancers; Lung cancers; Multiple endocrine neoplasia type 1 (MEN 1); Multiple endocrine neoplasia type 2 (MEN 2); Parathyroid cancer; Pheochromocytomas; Thyroid cancer; Von Hippel-Lindau (VHL) disease; Zollinger-Ellison syndrome

▶ Neurofibromatosis type 1 (NF1)

Category: Diseases, Symptoms, and Conditions
Also known as: von Recklinghausen's neurofibromatosis, von Recklinghausen disease

Related conditions: Neurofibromas, iris Lisch nodules, optic gliomas, café-au-lait spots, freckling, learning disabilities, bone complications such as scoliosis or bone overgrowth

Definition: Neurofibromatosis type 1 (NF1) is a hereditary disorder of the nervous system that affects growth and development of nerve cell tissues. This disorder is associated with neurofibromas (bumplike tumors under the skin or elsewhere in the body that develop anywhere along a nerve), café-au-lait spots (flat spots on the skin that are darker than the surrounding area), freckling in places not exposed to the sun (such as the armpit and groin), eye developments such as optic glioma (a tumor growing on the nerve to the eye) and Lisch nodules (harmless growths on the colored part of the eye), and bone problems such as scoliosis (curvature of the spine) or bone overgrowth. Up to 10 percent of affected individuals have malignant peripheral nerve sheath tumors (tumors that form along the protective covering around nerves located outside the brain and spinal cord), which are the most common malignant tumors associated with NF1. Although rare, malignant brain tumors do occur. Fewer than 1 percent of people with NF1 have pheochromocytomas (adrenal gland tumors that release stress hormones) that cause dangerously high blood pressure. Approximately half of individuals with NF1 have a learning disability, although it is usually mild. The severity of the disorder varies within families, between families, and even within an individual at different times during life.

Risk factors: Because NF1 is hereditary, the main risk factor is having a family history of this disorder. Each child of a person with NF1 has a 50 percent chance of inheriting the disorder.

Etiology and the disease process: The underlying genetic cause of NF1 is a mutation, or a genetic change, in the *NF1* gene. The purpose of the protein made by the *NF1* gene is not fully understood, but it most likely helps stop uncontrolled cell growth and proliferation. Mutations in the *NF1* gene either prevent the protein from being made or cause the protein to be made incorrectly, and the multistep process of tumorigenesis (formation or production of tumors) is left unchecked.

Usually, each person has two normal copies of the *NF1* gene. A mutation in one copy of the gene is sufficient to cause NF1, which is why this condition is referred to as autosomal dominant (autosomal means the *NF1* gene is located on one of the twenty-two pairs of autosomes, which are the nonsex chromosomes). An affected person has an *NF1* gene mutation from the time of conception; however, symptoms of the disease may be present at birth or not manifest until later in life. Nearly all individuals with NF1 have signs and symptoms of the disorder by the end of childhood. The average life expectancy of affected individuals is reduced about fifteen years.

Incidence: Approximately 1 in 3,000 people has NF1, which makes it one of the most common dominantly inherited genetic disorders. Nearly half of people with NF1 inherit the disorder from a parent. The other 50 percent have a new gene mutation, meaning the mutation occurred for the first time in those individuals.

Symptoms: Symptoms vary and are usually mild to moderate and not life-threatening. Adults with NF1 may have anywhere from a few neurofibromas to hundreds or thousands, and these tumors—which continue to develop throughout life—can affect any organ in the body. Neurofibromas can cause pain and disfigurement and, more rarely, cause problems with organ function. Malignant peripheral nerve sheath tumors can cause pain, numbness, or paralysis. Optic gliomas can lead to blindness. Of the learning disabilities observed in more than half of people with NF1, visual-spatial performance and attention deficits are the most common.

Screening and diagnosis: Doctors diagnose NF1 based on certain criteria, which include having two or more of the following: six or more café-au-lait spots, two or more neurofibromas or one plexiform neurofibroma (weblike neurofibroma that entwines surrounding tissues), freckling in the armpit or groin, optic glioma, two or more Lisch nodules, an unusual bone complication, or a first-degree relative (parent, sibling, or child) with NF1.

Because NF1 is caused by mutations in the *NF1* gene, genetic testing can be used to confirm a suspected diagnosis. However, diagnostic genetic testing is rarely needed because doctors can easily diagnose the disease based on clinical findings. Genetic testing detects more than 95 percent of *NF1* gene mutations in individuals who have been clinically diagnosed by a physician.

Treatment and therapy: The main focus of treatment for NF1 is controlling symptoms. Surgery can be performed to treat bone malformations or to remove tumors that cause pain or disfigurement. In the case of malignancy, the tumor is surgically removed if possible, and the patient may also have adjuvant chemotherapy and radiotherapy.

Prognosis, prevention, and outcomes: The way neurofibromatosis affects a person over a lifetime varies widely. Because NF1 is a genetic condition, its manifestations cannot be prevented. However, physicians recommend that individuals with NF1 have monitoring that includes a yearly physical examination, a yearly ophthalmologic examination (eye exam) for children (less frequently for adults), regular blood pressure checks, and regular assessment of development for children.

Abbie L. Abboud, M.S., C.G.C.

For Further Information

Ferner, R. E. "Neurofibromatosis 1." *European Journal of Human Genetics*. 15 (2007): 131-138.

Korf, Bruce R., and Allan E. Rubenstein. *Neurofibromatosis: A Handbook for Patients, Families, and Health Care Professionals*. New York: Thieme Medical, 2005.

Tonsgard, J. H. "Clinical Manifestations and Management of Neurofibromatosis Type 1." *Seminars in Pediatric Neurology* 13 (2006): 2-7.

Other Resources

Children's Tumor Foundation: Ending Neurofibromatosis Through Research
http://www.ctf.org

Neurofibromatosis, Inc
http://www.nfinc.org

See also: Acoustic neuromas; Astrocytomas; Ependymomas; Fibrosarcomas, soft-tissue; Gastrointestinal Stromal Tumors (GISTs); Gliomas; Mediastinal tumors; Medulloblastomas; Meningiomas; Pheochromocytomas; Sarcomas, soft-tissue; Schwannoma tumors; Spinal axis tumors

▶ Neutropenia

Category: Diseases, Symptoms, and Conditions
Also known as: Agranulocytosis, granulocytopenia

Related conditions: Leukopenia, aplastic anemia, myelodysplastic syndromes

Definition: Neutropenia is a decreased number of circulating neutrophils, which are the most abundant type of white blood cell and are an essential component of the immune response to infections, especially bacterial or fungal infections. Neutrophils are the first to respond to an infection, ingesting the microorganisms and killing them, thus preventing an infection or lessening its severity. A patient who has a significantly reduced number of neutrophils is at increased risk for infection.

Normal total white blood cell counts range from 5,000 to 10,000 cells per cubic millimeter (mm3) of blood, with neutrophils making up 50 to 70 percent of the circulating white blood cells. Therefore, the normal absolute number of neutrophils is about 2,500 to 7,000 neutrophils/mm3 of blood. People are considered to have neutropenia when levels drop below 500 neutrophils/mm3 of blood.

Risk factors: Because most chemotherapeutic agents work to kill fast-growing cells, including neutrophils, almost all cancer patients are at risk for neutropenia. Radiation therapy for cancer treatment can also cause neutropenia. Other factors, including age, nutritional status, and previous exposure to chemotherapy or radiation, increase the risk of neutropenia in someone undergoing chemotherapy or radiation therapy. Patients with hematologic cancers, such as leukemias or lymphomas, are also at increased risk for neutropenia.

Etiology and the disease process: Four main circumstances lead to neutropenia: prolonged, severe infection; decreased survival of neutrophils; abnormal distribution of neutrophils to a body site; and decreased production of neutrophils. In the case of cancer patients, the problem is decreased production. Most anticancer drugs work to disrupt the growth of cancer cells, which tend to grow very quickly. These drugs target cell components involved in cell division and deoxyribonucleic acid (DNA) synthesis. As a result, other fast-growing cells in the body may also be affected by the drugs. This includes the cells of the bone marrow that are precursors to blood cells. Neutrophils are short-lived (surviving two to three days) in the body, with millions of new neutrophils released every minute from the bone marrow. Therefore, the bone marrow cells that are rapidly dividing to make new neutrophils are at high risk for damage from anticancer agents.

Radiation therapy can cause neutropenia if the targeted treatment area includes bones that contain productive marrow (not all marrow actively produces blood cells). Additionally, patients who need a bone marrow transplant must have the diseased bone marrow completely destroyed before the transplant.

Incidence: Chemotherapy is the most common cause of neutropenia, but its incidence among patients varies. Each drug and drug combination has been shown to cause neutropenia at a different rate. For example, the cisplatin/fluorouracil combination used to treat head and neck cancers has been shown to cause neutropenia in only 9 percent of patients. Cisplatin combined with gemcitabine to treat bladder cancer causes neutropenia in 71 percent of patients. The other risk factors, such as age, also contribute to the different incidence rates.

Symptoms: Because low neutrophil counts predispose patients to infection, the first symptom is usually fever, followed by symptoms specific to the infection, including a cough, a sore throat, bronchitis, sinusitis, pneumonia, gingivitis, sores around the mouth and anus, fatigue, and frequent or unusual infections.

Screening and diagnosis: A complete blood count (CBC) with differential tests for levels of the different types of cells in the blood can screen for neutropenia. The differential portion of the test tells the percentage of each type of white blood cell, including the percentage of neutrophils. From this, the absolute number of neutrophils/mm3 can be calculated to determine if a patient is neutropenic and at risk for infection. Patients with borderline levels at 500 to 1,500 cells/mm3 have a slight-to-moderate risk of infection, while patients with counts below 500 cells/mm3 (neutropenic) have a severe risk of infection.

Treatment and therapy: The first priority of treatment is to address fever and underlying infection. Antibiotics or antifungals are necessary to treat the infection. The patient may also require granulocyte-macrophage colony-stimulating factor (GM-CSF) or granulocyte colony-stimulating factor (G-CSF). These drugs stimulate the bone marrow to increase production of neutrophils and are used following chemotherapy and following bone marrow transplantation. Additionally, changes in the chemotherapy regimen may be necessary. The physician may choose to lower the dose of medication, remove a drug from the regimen, or change the most harmful drug to a less toxic drug.

Prognosis, prevention, and outcomes: A neutropenic cancer patient who acquires an infection has a mortality rate of 4 to 30 percent. To prevent neutropenia in cancer patients receiving treatment, doctors can lower the dose of chemotherapy for patients who have a documented history of neutropenia. Doctors can also use colony-stimulating factors in patients at higher risk for neutropenia, such as when a treatment regimen is known to cause neutropenia in a high percentage (greater than 40 percent) of patients. Most cases of chemotherapy-induced neutropenia resolve within two weeks of discontinuing drug treatment.

Michelle L. Herdman, Ph.D.

For Further Information

Beers, Mark H., ed. *The Merck Manual of Diagnosis and Therapy*. 18th ed. Whitehouse Station, N.J.: Merck, 2006.

Mosby's Drug Consult 2007. St. Louis: Mosby Elsevier, 2007.

Tisdale, James E., and Douglas A. Miller. *Drug-Induced Diseases: Prevention, Detection, and Management*. Bethesda, Md.: American Society of Health-System Pharmacists, 2005.

Other Resources

American Cancer Society
http://www.cancer.org

Cancer Symptoms.org
Neutropenia
http://www.cancersymptoms.org/neutropenia/index.shtml

Neutropenia Support Association
http://www.neutropenia.ca/index.html

See also: Aplastic anemia; Chemotherapy; Leukopenia; Myelodysplastic syndromes; Side effects

▶ Night sweats

Category: Diseases, Symptoms, and Conditions
Also known as: Sleep hyperhydrosis

Related conditions: Menopause, obstructive sleep apnea, infection, low blood sugar, lymphoma and other cancers, certain medications

Definition: Night sweats are excessive nighttime sweating that causes the individual to wake up and may require the individual to bathe or change nightclothes.

Risk factors: There are some diseases and conditions that may be associated with an increased incidence of night sweats. Individuals who have obstructive sleep apnea, a disorder in which breathing is interrupted during sleep, are more likely to experience night sweats. Risk factors for sleep apnea, such as obesity, therefore may also be risk factors for night sweats. Women experiencing menopause are also more likely to experience night sweats.

Etiology and the disease process: Night sweats can be caused by a number of underlying diseases and conditions as well as by a simple excess of bedding or an overly warm room. Some of the most common medical causes of night sweats include the changing hormone balance that occurs during menopause, obstructive sleep apnea, infection, low blood sugar, cancer (especially lymphoma), and certain medications. Other causes can include infection with the human immunodeficiency virus (HIV), tuberculosis, hyperthyroidism, epilepsy, and head injury.

Incidence: There are very few significant scientific studies on the incidence of night sweats; however, they are believed to be very common. One study of night sweats found that 41 percent of the 2,267 patients who were studied reported night sweats. Many physicians report a significant percentage of individuals they see in their general practice complaining of night sweats.

Symptoms: The symptoms of night sweats are waking up in the night because of excessive sweating. Night sweats are considered mild if they wake sleepers, who then remove some or all bed coverings and may turn over the pillow to use the dry side. Night sweats that make sleepers feel the need to wash the sweat off their hands or faces are considered moderate. Night sweats are considered severe when the sweating is so excessive as to cause sleepers to change their clothes or to take a shower. Some people who experience night sweats also experience excessive sweating during the day.

Screening and diagnosis: The physician will typically take a history of the patient's night sweat experiences and perform a physical exam to see if any common causes of night sweats seem to be a likely cause. The physician may also ask a series of questions, which may involve travel history, to determine if the patient has been in any areas that increase the likelihood of becoming infected with a disease such as tuberculosis, or if there is a risk of infection with HIV. The doctor may also ask the patient's sleeping partner about symptoms of which the individual may be unaware, such as the loud snoring that often accompanies obstructive sleep apnea.

If these steps fail to determine why the night sweats are occurring, the doctor may order blood tests or additional screening procedures to test for other causes. The doctor will also ask the patient about other unusual symptoms, even those that do not seem to be related. Many diseases and conditions that can cause night sweats usually cause other symptoms as well. Types of cancer that cause night sweats are usually associated with unintentional weight loss and fever. Tuberculosis is also usually accompanied by weight loss, a cough, and a low-grade fever.

Treatment and therapy: Most night sweats are treated by trying to assess the underlying cause of the night sweats and treating that disease or condition, including a possible lymphoma. Resolving the underlying problem will usually eliminate the night sweats. However, while the underlying problem is being diagnosed and treated, or if no treatable underlying cause can be found, there are some techniques that may help relieve the symptoms.

Reducing the quantity of bedclothes or switching from heavy blankets made of insulating materials such as wool to lighter blankets made of fabrics such as cotton may help reduce the occurrence of night sweats or reduce their severity. Sleeping with a window open or a fan pointed toward the bed may also help to relieve the problem. Avoiding spicy food, excessive exercise before bedtime, alcohol, and tobacco may help to reduce the severity of night sweats.

Prognosis, prevention, and outcomes: Sleeping in a cool room without an excess of bedding may be able to help prevent some episodes of night sweats. The prognosis for most cases of night sweats is good. Treating the underlying cause if one can be found is usually effective at eliminating the night sweats. Night sweats can be extremely frustrating as they can lead to poor quality of sleep and increased drowsiness during the day. Treating night sweats successfully can lead to a better quality of sleep, as well as an increased quantity of sleep, which can improve mood and lead to a better quality of life overall.

Robert Bockstiegel, B.S.

For Further Information

Freedman, Jeri. *Lymphoma: Current and Emerging Trends in Detection and Treatment.* New York: Rosen, 2006.

Souhami, Robert, and Jeffrey Tobias. *Cancer and Its Management.* 5th Edition. Malden, Mass.: Blackwell, 2005.

Yarbro, Connie Henke, Margaret Hansen Frogge, and Michelle Goodman, eds. *Cancer Symptom Management.* Sudbury, Mass.: Jones and Bartlett, 2004.

Other Resources

MedicineNet.com

Eight Causes of Night Sweats
http://www.medicinenet.com/script/main/art.asp?articlekey=57394

Sleep Disorders Guide

Sleep Hyperhydrosis
http://www.sleepdisordersguide.com/topics/sleep-hyperhidrosis.html

See also: Hormonal therapies; Hormone replacement therapy (HRT); Hot flashes; Hysterectomy; Lymphomas; Symptoms and cancer

▶ Nijmegen breakage syndrome

Category: Diseases, Symptoms, and Conditions

Also known as: Berlin breakage syndrome, Seemanova syndrome II, ataxia telangiectasia variant V1

Related conditions: Bloom syndrome, Fanconi anemia, ataxia telangiectasia

Definition: Nijmegen breakage syndrome is a rare autosomal recessive condition that causes chromosomal instability, sensitivity to radiation, and increased incidence of malignant lymphomas.

Risk factors: A risk factor for Nijmegen breakage syndrome is the inheritance of a mutation in both copies of the *NBS1* gene.

Etiology and the disease process: The *NBS1* gene encodes the nibrin protein, which helps heal double-stranded breaks (DSBs) in deoxyribonucleic acid (DNA) molecules. Sometimes double-stranded breaks occur as a result of DNA-severing agents or as a normal physiological process during gamete and antibody production. Without the capacity to repair double-stranded breaks, cells are unable to repair damage to DNA, make antibodies to fight infections, or produce viable gametes.

Incidence: As of 2007, there were only 200 estimated cases of Nijmegen breakage syndrome worldwide.

Symptoms: Children born with Nijmegen breakage syndrome show microcephaly (small head), growth retardation, progressive mental retardation, and characteristic facial features (birdlike face, sloping forehead, and receding jaw). The immune system is unable to fight infections, and recurrent sinus, pulmonary, and ear infections are common. More than half of Nijmegen breakage syndrome patients also show skin pigmentation irregularities. At puberty, female Nijmegen breakage syndrome patients fail to experience sexual maturation. Their ovaries are small and poorly developed (premature ovarian failure). Finally Nijmegen breakage syndrome patients show increased tendencies to develop lymphomas.

Screening and diagnosis: Cytogenetic analyses, which isolate and view chromosomes from individual cells, show chromosomal instabilities that typically involve chromosomes 7 and 14. Immunologic testing shows an inability of immune cells to divide rapidly or properly synthesize antibodies in response to infections. Nijmegen breakage syndrome patients are also extremely sensitive to ionizing radiation or clastogens (substances that cause chromosome breaks). DNA sequencing of the *NBS1* gene should reveal loss-of-function mutations in this gene.

Treatment and therapy: Antibiotic treatments and intravenous administration of antibodies are used to treat recurrent infections that accompany immune system deficiency. Bone marrow transplants can permanently treat the immune system defects in children with Nijmegen breakage syndrome. Prepuberty female patients are treated with hormone replacement therapy to allow the development of secondary sexual characteristics and prevent osteoporosis. Cancer treatments in patients with Nijmegen breakage syndrome patients must avoid radiation and chemotherapeutic agents that damage DNA, since they can cause toxic complications.

Prognosis, prevention, and outcomes: Prophylactic antibiotics are prescribed to prevent recurring infections, and vitamin E supplements are recommended to ameliorate chromosome instability. The long-term prognosis for Nijmegen breakage syndrome patients is typically quite poor. Most patients die from aggressive malignancy or complications from infections.

Michael A. Buratovich, Ph.D.

See also: Ataxia Telangiectasia (AT); Childhood cancers; Chromosomes and cancer; Fanconi anemia

▶ Nipple discharge

Category: Diseases, Symptoms, and Conditions
Also known as: Breast discharge

Related conditions: Galactorrhea, mastitis, papilloma, Paget disease of breast intraductal breast carcinoma

Definition: Nipple discharge refers to secretions from either one (unilateral) or both (bilateral) breasts. Discharge can be spontaneous or appear only when expressed through squeezing and "milking" the nipple, and it can be occasional or constant. It can be clear, milky, brown, green, yellow, pink, or deeply bloody.

Risk factors: Nipple discharge is more likely to be the result of underlying malignancy when it is a unilateral discharge, occurs in a woman past reproductive age, is associated with a mass, or contains blood. Older women with nipple discharge are much more likely to have a malignancy than younger women.

Etiology and the disease process: High levels of the hormone prolactin can cause galactorrhea, which is a milky discharge. Galactorrhea is the most common nipple discharge. Medications that commonly cause galactorrhea include psychotropics, oral contraceptives, and antiemetics.

Incidence: Nipple discharge is very common and usually benign. As many as 80 percent of women are able to express fluid with manual manipulation. Although it is far more common in women, men may occasionally exhibit nipple discharge.

Symptoms: Discharge may be spontaneous or occur only with manual expression, or "milking," of the nipple. It may be a few drops of fluid or a continual leakage.

Screening and diagnosis: A clinical breast exam includes taking a history of breast nipple discharge and examination of the nipples with gentle squeezing to see if fluid is expressed. Milky fluid in breast-feeding women is of no concern as long as the woman does not have symptoms of infection (breast is painful to the touch, redness is present, milk has a foul odor or has changed color), and many women continue to express milk long after they stop breast-feeding. Other testing includes cytologic examination of the discharge, mammography, and ductoscopy.

Treatment and therapy: Often discharge will resolve if all stimulation of the breast is ceased; this means the woman must avoid the urge to check to see if the discharge is still occurring. Sometimes drugs that cause increased prolactin need to be adjusted, and any nipple discharge that is suspicious in terms of malignancy must be evaluated. Nipple discharge can also be a symptom of disorders in other hormone-producing glands, and those conditions may need to be treated.

Prognosis, prevention, and outcomes: Prognosis and outcomes depend on the type of discharge. Prevention

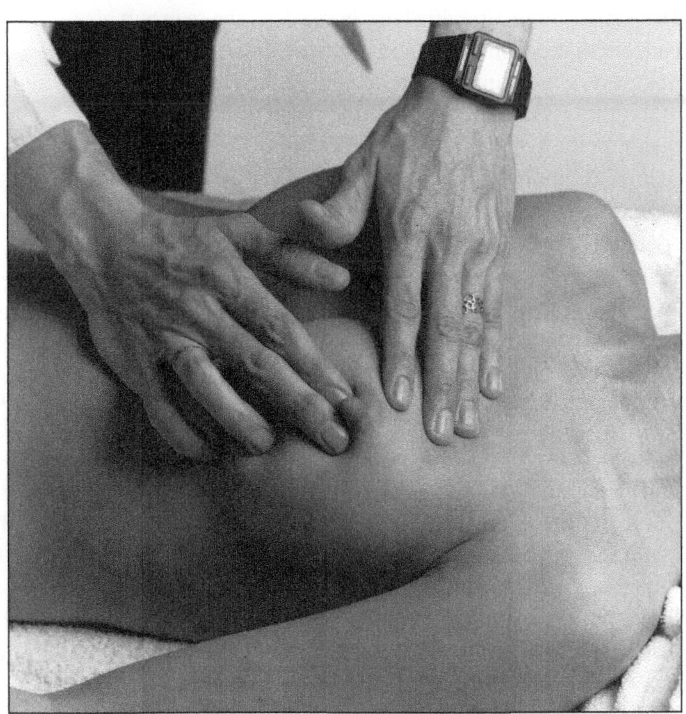

A doctor examines a woman's breasts, checking for possible signs of cancer, such as nipple secretions. (National Cancer Institute/Wikimedia)

can often be managed by decreasing medications that increase prolactin and avoiding a cycle of stimulation of the nipple.

Clair Kaplan, R.N., M.S.N., A.P.R.N. (WHNP), M.H.S., M.T. (ASCP)

See also: Breast cancer in men; Breast cancer in pregnant women; Breast cancers; Clinical Breast exam (CBE); Comedo carcinomas; Duct ectasia; Ductal Carcinoma In Situ (DCIS); Ductogram; Estrogen-receptor-sensitive breast cancer; HER2/neu protein; Invasive ductal carcinomas; Invasive lobular carcinomas; Lobular Carcinoma In Situ (LCIS); Mammography

▶ Non-Hodgkin lymphoma

Category: Diseases, Symptoms, and Conditions
Also known as: Lymphoma, non-Hodgkin's lymphoma, NHL

Related conditions: Hodgkin disease, autoimmune disorders

Definition: Non-Hodgkin lymphoma describes a group of cancers that originate in the lymphatic system. The lymphatic system drains lymph (interstitial fluid) from tissues and returns it to the blood. A wide range of immune cells reside in the lymphatic system that fights disease and infection. Lymphatic tissue consists of the lymph nodes, spleen, liver bone marrow, and other types of lymphatic tissue distributed throughout several other organs in the body (e.g., Peyer's patches in the gastrointestinal tract). Non-Hodgkin lymphoma develops in white blood cells called lymphocytes, of which there are two main types: B-cells and T-cells. Most lymphomas (85 to 90 percent) originate in B-cells.

Risk factors: Some known and potential risk factors for non-Hodgkin lymphoma include age (over sixty); gender (more common in men); a compromised immune system (such as from drugs and other treatments or acquired immunodeficiency syndrome, AIDS); autoimmune disorders, such as rheumatoid arthritis and Sjögren syndrome; history of certain infections, such as with Epstein-Barr virus (increases risk of Burkitt lymphoma), Helicobacter pylori, and possibly hepatitis C virus; radiation exposure; and chemical exposure (such as pesticides and fertilizers).

Despite the list of known and suspected risk factors for non-Hodgkin lymphoma, most people diagnosed have no known risk factors, and many who have risk factors never develop the disease.

Etiology and the disease process: For most patients, the exact cause of non-Hodgkin lymphoma is unknown. One suspected cause is the activation of certain abnormal genes that allow uncontrollable lymphocyte division and growth. This uncontrolled growth causes lymph nodes and other lymphatic tissues to swell. Because lymphatic tissue is in various locations throughout the body, non-Hodgkin lymphoma can start almost anywhere and tends to be widespread, although slower growing types may be confined to one place. Typically, non-Hodgkin lymphoma begins in the lymph nodes and spreads to other parts of the lymphatic system. Occasionally, non-Hodgkin lymphoma invades organs outside the lymphatic system, including the stomach, brain, and lungs.

Incidence: Non-Hodgkin lymphoma is the seventh most common type of cancer in the US, and its rapidly increasing incidence in the United States is primarily unexplained (rates have nearly doubled since the 1970s). According to the National Cancer Institute, in 2015, an estimated 71,850 non-Hodgkin lymphoma cases were diagnosed and 19,790 deaths were attributed to the disease. A person's risk of contracting non-Hodgkin lymphoma is 1 in 50. The disease is more common among Caucasians than African-Americans or Asian-Americans.

Non-Hodgkin lymphoma occurs in all age groups, but the risk of developing the disease increases with age (95 percent of cases occur in adults age forty and older). Some subtypes are more common in certain age groups. In children, non-Hodgkin lymphoma is most commonly diagnosed between the ages of seven and eleven, and some types of non-Hodgkin lymphoma are among the most common childhood cancers.

Symptoms: Symptoms vary depending on the area of the body in which the tumor originated and the areas to which the cancer has spread. Swollen, painless lymph nodes in the neck, underarms, stomach, or groin are commonly the only sign of non-Hodgkin lymphoma in early stages.

Generalized symptoms include fever, unexplained weight loss, fatigue, excessive sweating, night sweats, chills, easy bruising, itchiness, and unusual opportunistic infections.

Tumors in the stomach can cause pain and swelling, which can lead to loss of appetite, constipation, nausea, and vomiting. Tumors in the thymus or chest lymph nodes can cause coughing and shortness of breath. Lymphoma of the brain can cause headaches, personality changes, and seizures.

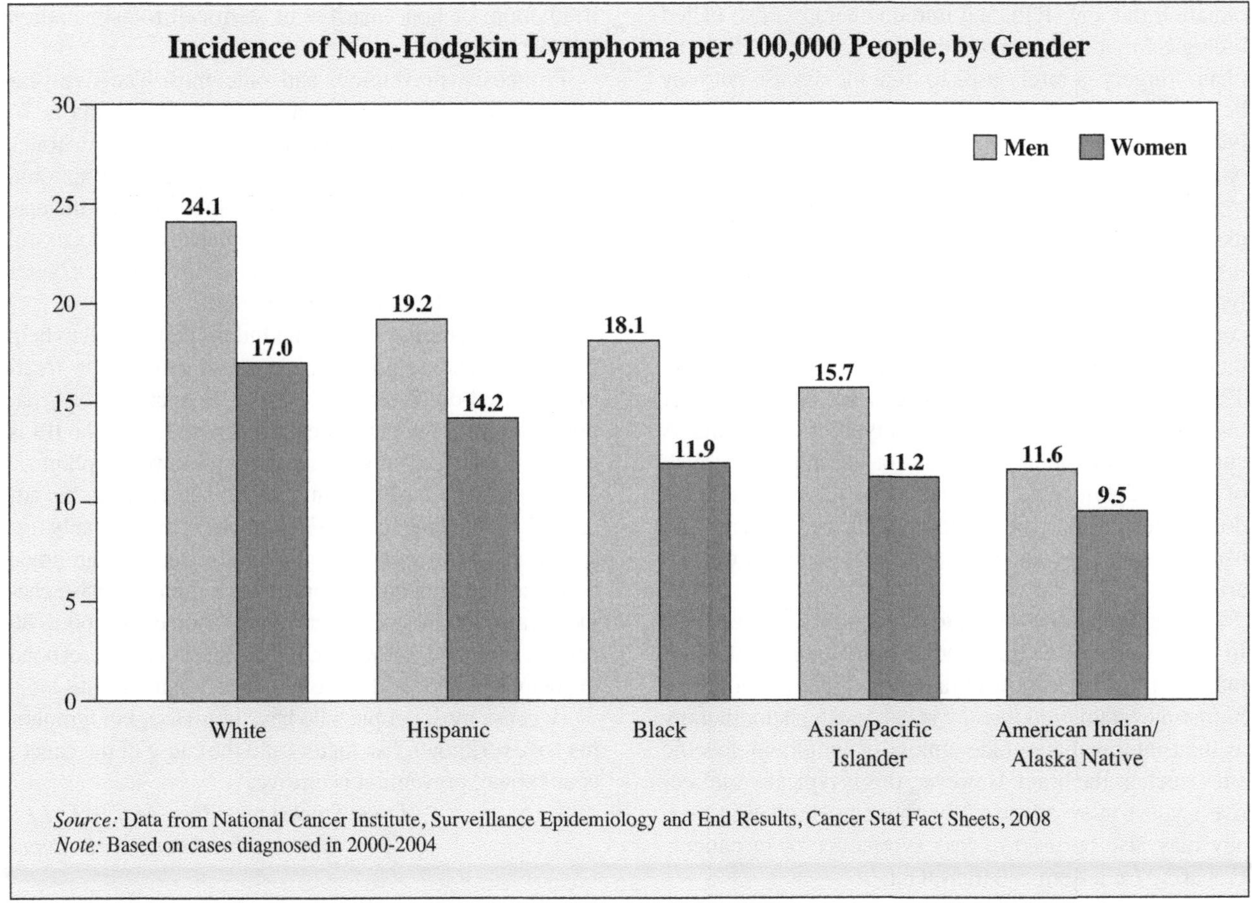

Source: Data from National Cancer Institute, Surveillance Epidemiology and End Results, Cancer Stat Fact Sheets, 2008
Note: Based on cases diagnosed in 2000-2004

Screening and diagnosis: Many tests are used to diagnose non-Hodgkin lymphoma and assess the spread of the disease. Diagnosis begins with a medical history and physical examination, which commonly focuses on the lymph nodes, liver, and spleen. Blood and urine tests may be performed to help rule out infections and other diseases that cause swollen nodes.

A biopsy is the best way to definitively diagnose lymphoma and determine the subtype.

Lymph node biopsy from the neck, armpits, or groin is most common. Bone marrow biopsy may be performed to establish whether the disease has spread.

Imaging tests such as X-rays, magnetic resonance imaging (MRI), and computed tomography (CT) scanning may be used to detect the presence of non-Hodgkin lymphoma, determine the size of tumors, and determine the extent to which the cancer has spread.

Staging helps to determine treatment. A system commonly used to stage non-Hodgkin lymphoma is the Ann Arbor staging system. This system classifies lymphoma into four stages:

- Stage I: Lymphoma is limited to a single region, usually one lymph node or one lymph node region in the body.
- Stage II: Lymphoma involves two or more regions, usually an affected lymph node or lymphatic organ and a second affected area, that are next to each other and on the same side of the diaphragm.
- Stage III: Lymphoma has spread to both sides of the diaphragm.
- Stage IV: Widespread disease has affected nonlymphatic organs.

A lettering system is commonly used in combination with the stage to indicate the presence of symptoms. An "E" indicates involvement of organs outside the lymph system; a "B" indicates the presence of weight loss, night sweats, or unexplained fever; and an "A" indicates the absence of symptoms.

Treatment and therapy: Treatment of non-Hodgkin lymphoma depends on the type and stage of the disease, symptoms, and the patient's age and overall medical condition. The main treatments used are chemotherapy, radiation therapy (RT), and immunotherapy (also called biological therapy), targeted therapy, and stem cell transplant. Surgery is rarely used to treat the disease but may be used to relieve problems caused by non-Hodgkin lymphoma, such as bowel obstruction and spinal cord compression.

Chemotherapy is the primary treatment for non-Hodgkin lymphoma. It may be used alone or in combination with other treatments. Intermediate- and high-grade lymphomas and advanced low-grade lymphomas are commonly treated with multiple agents; single-drug therapy may be used for early-stage, low-grade disease. The exact medications, routes, doses, and duration of treatment depend on the stage and type of lymphoma. A common chemotherapy regimen for the initial treatment of non-Hodgkin lymphoma includes cyclophosphamide, doxorubicin, vincristine, and prednisone. Patients are usually treated on an outpatient basis unless problems arise.

Radiation therapy is used to kill or shrink cancer cells. In some cases of Stage I and II non-Hodgkin lymphoma, curative treatment with radiation therapy is possible. Sometimes, radiation therapy is used with chemotherapy to treat intermediate-grade tumors or tumors in specific sites, such as the brain. However, this is typically ineffective against more advanced lymphomas. Radiation therapy may also be used to ease symptoms, or in patients preparing for a stem cell transplant.

Immunotherapy is an evolving treatment in which man-made substances mimic substances produced by the immune system and are used to either kill lymphoma cells or slow their growth. Immunotherapies for non-Hodgkin lymphoma include monoclonal antibodies (mAbs) and interferons. For example, rituximab is a mAb approved by the Food and Drug Administration for the treatment of B-cell non-Hodgkin lymphoma; it is frequently used in combination with chemotherapy. Some forms of radioimmunotherapy, in which mAbs are attached to radioactive substances, are also used to treat non-Hodgkin lymphoma (e.g., ibritumomab and tositumomab). Other monoclonal antibodies used to treat non-Hodgkin lymphoma include alemtuzumab, obinutuzumab, and brentuximab vedotin, which are attached to chemotherapy drugs.

Targeted therapies work by blocking the processes inside of cells that turn them into cancer cells, such processes of cell growth, maturation, gene expression, and cell death. This type of therapy may have fewer side effects than conventional chemotherapy treatments. Some examples of drugs include bortezomib and ibrutinib.

If non-Hodgkin lymphoma recurs, treatment with high-dose chemotherapy, total-body or total-lymph node irradiation, or bone marrow or stem cell transplantation may be necessary.

Prognosis, prevention, and outcomes: The five-year relative survival rate for non-Hodgkin lymphoma is 70 percent while ten-year survival rate is 59 percent. Rates vary depending on the patient, type of lymphoma, and stage of the disease. As with most other cancers, the earlier the diagnosis, the greater the chances for successful treatment. Typically, the type of tissue involved is a better prognostic predictor than cancer stage.

The International Prognostic Index (IPI) is used to help predict lymphoma growth and patient response to treatment. Based on patient age, cancer stage and spread, patient function, and lactate dehydrogenase levels, the IPI is mainly used in patients with more aggressive lymphomas.

Low-grade non-Hodgkin lymphomas tend to be advanced when diagnosed. Even though they usually respond well to treatment, they may also recur. High-grade non-Hodgkin lymphomas sometimes require intensive chemotherapy, but they are often curable (some have 60 to 80 percent cure rates). However, if the cancer does not respond to chemotherapy, the disease can rapidly cause death.

Because most people who have non-Hodgkin lymphoma have no known risk factors and the cause of the cancer is unknown, prevention is elusive.

Jaime Stockslager Buss, M.S.P.H., ELS
Updated by: Michelle Herdman

For Further Information

Adler, E. M. (2015). *Living with lymphoma: A patient's guide*. Baltimore: Johns Hopkins University Press.

Baker, T. (2012). *Non-Hodgkin lymphoma. Seattle*, WA: Amazon Digital Services LLC.

Rossi, Carla. (2014). *The living end of cancer: One woman's faith-based journey through Non-Hodgkin lymphoma.* Seattle, WA: Amazon Digital Services LLC.

Other Resources

Leukemia and Lymphoma Society
www.lls.org/

Lymphoma Research Foundation
http://www.lymphoma.org

National Cancer Institute
http://www.cancer.gov

American Cancer Society
http://www.cancer.org

See also: Agent Orange; Anthraquinones; Antimetabolites in chemotherapy; Azathioprine; Biological therapy;

Blood cancers; Burkitt lymphoma; Childhood cancers; Cutaneous T-Cell Lymphoma (CTCL); Dioxins; Elderly and cancer; Epstein-Barr Virus; Hair dye; Helicobacter pylori; Hepatitis C virus (HCV); HIV/AIDS-related cancers; Hodgkin disease; Immune response to cancer; Klinefelter syndrome and cancer; Lambert-Eaton Myasthenic Syndrome (LEMS); Lymphomas; Mantle cell Lymphoma (MCL); Mucosa-Associated Lymphoid tissue (MALT) lymphomas; Myeloma; Oncogenic viruses; Pediatric oncology and hematology; Pesticides and the food chain; Primary central nervous system lymphomas; Radiopharmaceuticals; Richter syndrome; Simian virus 40; Splenectomy; Veterinary oncology; Virus-related cancers; Waldenström Macroglobulinemia (WM)

▶ Obesity-associated cancers

Category: Diseases, Symptoms, and Conditions
Related conditions: Various cancers of the blood, bone and body organ(s).

Definition: According to the National Institutes of Health (NIH), the terms "overweight" and "obesity" refer to body weight that is greater than what is considered healthy for a certain height. Body mass index (BMI) is used to classify body weight. For adults, a *normal* BMI range is 18.5 to 24.9 and *overweight* is a range of 25.0 to 29.9. The *obese* category is stratified into three classes (see Table 1), with a range of 30.0 to 39.9 and *extreme obesity* is a BMI of 40 and above (see table labeled Classification of Overweight and Obesity by BMI).

Obesity is characterized by an excessive amount, or abnormal distribution, of body fat or adipose tissue. Central obesity is an abnormal distribution of body fat around the waist and abdomen. In 2013, obesity was designated as a disease by the American Medical Association (AMA).

Risk factors: Obesity is a known risk factor for cancers of the breast (post-menopausal), esophagus, colon, rectum, kidney, pancreas, gallbladder, thyroid and endometrium. Preliminary research shows a possible link with other cancers, including liver, cervical, ovarian, testicular and prostate, as well as multiple myeloma and non-Hodgkin's lymphoma. Obesity has also been shown to affect the prognosis of cancer treatment.

Obesity is generally caused by poor diet, through an excessive intake of calories, in conjunction with physical inactivity. Other influences on weight gain are readily available high-calorie food choices, psychological factors such as stress or depression, health conditions such as hypothyroidism, and certain medications, like those used to treat depression (e.g., citalopram, paroxetine, fluoxetine, sertraline) and migraine headaches (e.g., valproic acid).

Etiology and the disease process: A variety of mechanisms have been identified to elucidate the relationship between obesity and certain cancers. Adipocytes, or fat cells, are a source of hormones and other substances that affect cell growth and cellular death, and potentially enable damaged cells to survive and grow. Levels of these chemicals may be elevated or decreased in the obese, increasing the risk for cancer and tumor growth. Obesity also affects factors that regulate cell growth and proteins that orchestrate how the body utilizes certain hormones, like sex hormone-binding globulin (SHBG).

Excess body fat affects the endocrine system by interfering with insulin, a hormone made by the pancreas, and insulin-like growth factor-1 (IGF-1), which contributes to insulin resistance or high levels of insulin in the blood (hyperinsulinemia); this condition may promote the development of certain tumors. Stress and food contaminants can also disrupt hormonal function by affecting insulin signaling and energy homeostasis. The immune system may be compromised by reduced levels of natural killer (NK) cells in obese patients.

Fat cells produce proteins called adipokines, which play a role in glucose and fatty acid catabolism by altering metabolic signaling pathways. The ratio of certain adipokines may influence the aggressiveness of tumor cells. For example, leptin, a more abundant adipokine in the obese, promotes cell proliferation while adiponectin, a less abundant protein in the obese, down regulates cell growth. Adipocytes also drive changes in energy

Classification of Overweight and Obesity by BMI (guideline excludes pregnant women)

	Obesity Class	*BMI (kg/m^2*
Underweight		<18.5
Normal		18.5 – 24.9
Overweight		25.0 – 29.9
Obese	I	30.0 – 34.9
	II	35.0 – 39.9
Extreme Obesity	III	≥ 40

Body Mass Index

Category	BMI	58	59	60	61	62	63	64	65	66	67	68	69	70	71	72	73	74	75	76
Height (inches)		58	59	60	61	62	63	64	65	66	67	68	69	70	71	72	73	74	75	76
		Weight (pounds)																		
Normal	19	91	94	97	100	104	107	110	114	118	121	125	128	132	136	140	144	148	152	156
Normal	20	96	99	102	106	109	113	116	120	124	127	131	135	139	143	147	151	155	160	164
Normal	21	100	104	107	111	115	118	122	126	130	134	138	142	146	150	154	159	163	168	172
Normal	22	105	109	112	116	120	124	128	132	136	140	144	149	153	157	162	166	171	176	180
Normal	23	110	114	118	122	126	130	134	138	142	146	151	155	160	165	169	174	179	184	189
Normal	24	115	119	123	127	131	135	140	144	148	153	158	162	167	172	177	182	186	192	197
Overweight	25	119	124	128	132	136	141	145	150	155	159	164	169	174	179	184	189	194	200	205
Overweight	26	124	128	133	137	142	146	151	156	161	166	171	176	181	186	191	197	202	208	213
Overweight	27	129	133	138	143	147	152	157	162	167	172	177	182	188	193	199	204	210	216	221
Overweight	28	134	138	143	148	153	158	163	168	173	178	184	189	195	200	206	212	218	224	230
Overweight	29	138	143	148	153	158	163	169	174	179	185	190	196	202	208	213	219	225	232	238
Obese	30	142	148	153	158	164	169	174	180	186	191	197	203	209	215	221	227	233	240	246
Obese	31	148	153	158	164	169	175	180	186	192	198	203	209	216	222	228	235	241	248	254
Obese	32	153	158	163	169	175	180	186	192	198	204	210	216	222	229	235	242	249	256	263
Obese	33	158	163	168	174	180	186	192	198	204	211	216	223	229	236	242	250	256	264	271
Obese	34	162	168	174	180	186	191	197	204	210	217	223	230	236	243	250	257	264	272	279
Obese	35	167	173	179	185	191	197	204	210	216	223	230	236	243	250	258	265	272	279	287
Obese	36	172	178	184	190	196	203	209	216	223	230	236	243	250	257	265	272	280	287	295
Obese	37	177	183	189	195	202	208	215	222	229	236	243	250	257	265	272	280	287	295	304
Obese	38	181	188	194	201	207	214	221	228	235	242	249	257	264	272	279	288	295	303	312
Obese	39	186	193	199	206	213	220	227	234	241	249	256	263	271	279	287	295	303	311	320
Extremely Obese	40	191	198	204	211	218	225	232	240	247	255	262	270	278	286	294	302	311	319	328
Extremely Obese	41	196	203	209	217	224	231	238	246	253	261	269	277	285	293	302	310	319	327	336
Extremely Obese	42	201	208	215	222	229	237	244	252	260	268	276	284	292	301	309	318	326	335	344
Extremely Obese	43	205	212	220	227	235	242	250	258	266	274	282	291	299	308	316	325	334	343	353
Extremely Obese	44	210	217	225	232	240	248	256	264	272	280	289	297	306	315	324	333	342	351	361
Extremely Obese	45	215	222	230	238	246	254	252	270	278	287	295	304	313	322	331	340	350	359	369
Extremely Obese	46	220	227	235	243	251	259	267	276	284	293	302	311	320	329	338	348	358	367	377
Extremely Obese	47	224	232	240	248	256	265	273	282	291	299	308	318	327	338	346	355	365	375	385
Extremely Obese	48	229	237	245	254	262	270	279	288	297	306	315	324	334	343	353	363	373	383	394
Extremely Obese	49	234	242	250	259	267	278	285	294	303	312	322	331	341	351	361	371	381	391	402

Source: National Heart, Lung, and Blood Institute

homeostasis with effects on other tumor growth regulators, such as mTOR and AMP-activated protein kinase.

Biologic mechanisms thought to promote prostate cancer and/or prostate cancer progression include low testosterone levels; increased levels of estrogen, leptin, insulin growth factor-one (IGF-1); consumption of dietary saturated fats; decreased levels of adiponectin; and co-existing diabetes or metabolic syndrome.

Substances secreted in adipose tissues, like Tumor Necrosis Factor (TNF-α) and Interleukin-6 (IL-6), initiate inflammatory responses that can lead to insulin resistance and other pathological effects, including dyslipidemia and non-alcoholic fatty liver disease (NAFLD).

Obesity-induced hypoxia increases the expression of MMPs, a specialized group of enzymes, and vascular endothelial growth factor (VEGF), which suggests that hypoxia may modulate the angiogenic process that potentiates tumor growth. Increases in BMI are correlated with increased levels of VEGF and could contribute to a poorer prognosis for cancer in obese patients.

Other proposed mechanisms include: oxidative stress, shared genetic susceptibility, chronic inflammation, crosstalk between tumor cells and surrounding adipocytes and, migrating adipose stromal cells.

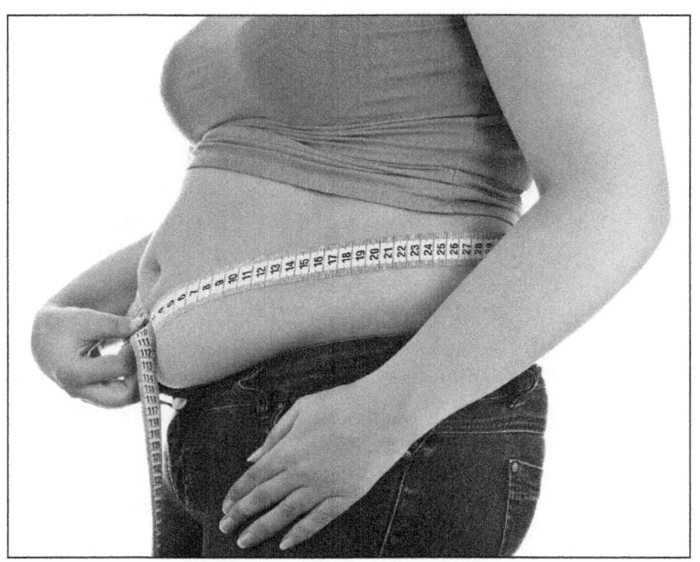

(iStock)

Incidence: As many as 84,000 cancer diagnoses, annually, are attributed to obesity and overweight, and obesity is implicated in 15 to 20 percent of total cancer-related mortality. Obesity is overtaking tobacco as the leading preventable cause of cancer.

Obesity is estimated to be the cause of cancer in 20 percent of cases, with an increased risk of malignancies associated with diet, weight change, body fat distribution and lack of physical activity. Results from the 2007-2008 National Health and Nutrition Examination Survey (NHANES) show that 68 percent of U.S. adults, age 20 years and older, are overweight or obese. In 1988-1994, by contrast, only 56 percent of adults age 20 and older were overweight or obese. In addition, the percentage of children who are overweight or obese has also increased. Among children and teens ages 2 to 19, 17 percent are estimated to be obese, based on the 2007–2008 survey; in 1988–1994, that same figure was only 10 percent.

An estimated 1 out of every 3 cancer deaths in the United States is linked to excess body weight, poor nutrition and/or physical inactivity. Of these, the strongest evidence points to the association of body weight and cancer; excess body weight contributes to 1 out of 5 cancer-related deaths.

Symptoms: There are no specific symptoms for obesity-associated cancers.

Screening and Diagnosis: Screening for obesity begins with a comprehensive review of medical, social and nutritional history to identify health conditions, genetic factors and medications that may influence weight. Physical examination, anthropometric measurements and laboratory studies; such as serum lipid panel, fasting glucose and a thyroid function test are also part of the screening process.

Anthropometric measurements are used to assess the size, shape and composition of the human body. These measurements include BMI, waist circumference, waist-to-hip ratio and skin-fold test. BMI is one of the most common screening tools for obesity but it has limitations.

Limitations to using BMI, as the sole indicator of cardiometabolic health that encompasses blood pressure, triglyceride, cholesterol, glucose, insulin resistance and C-reactive protein, are found in data covering the years 2005 to 2012 that was collected from the National Health and Nutrition Examination Survey (NHANES). Nearly half of overweight individuals (BMI 25.0 to 30.0), 29 percent of obese individuals (30.0 to 35.0) and 16 percent of obesity type II/III individuals (BMI 35.0 to 40.0 and above) were cardiometabolically healthy. It is noteworthy that greater than 30 percent of normal weight individuals (BMI 18.5 to 25.0) were found to be cardiometabolically unhealthy.

Cancer risk increases with a waist measurement of more than 35 inches in females and greater than 40 inches in males. A research study conducted to learn more about the effects of central obesity found that participants with normal-weight central obesity had double the mortality risk compared to those with BMI-defined obesity.

Testing for obesity-related cancers is utilized when symptoms develop and is specific to cancer type.

Treatment and therapy: Resources and support for obesity management are accessible through healthcare providers, community and commercial programs and over the Internet. Programs should include diets that meet the United States recommended daily allowance, as well as exercise counseling and behavior modification.

The NIH guidelines suggest nonpharmacologic treatment, i.e. lifestyle changes, for six months, and then consideration of medication if weight loss is unsatisfactory in those with a BMI greater than 30 or a BMI greater than 27, with other risk factors. Patients with extreme obesity (BMI > 40) may be considered for gastric bypass or other gastroplasty procedures.

Smaller portion sizes and limited between-meal snacks help reduce caloric intake. Foods high in calories, fat and added sugars provide limited nutrients and should be eliminated. Consumption of sugary beverages also increases body fat. In a clinical trial, individuals who consumed at least one serving of a sugar-sweetened beverage, over a six-year period, had a 27 percent increase in visceral adipose tissue than those who did not. Alcohol consumption should be avoided or limited.

Sedentary behaviors, such as sitting, lying down and watching TV and other forms of screen-based entertainment should be limited. The American Cancer Society (ACS) recommends that adults get at least 150 minutes of moderate-intensity or 75 minutes of vigorous-intensity activity each week (or a combination of these), preferably spread throughout the week. Children and teens should get at least one hour of moderate to vigorous activity at least three days a week.

Treatment for obesity-associated cancers is specific to cancer type, staging and consideration of new onset or progression. For patients with a cancer history, striving for a healthy weight during and following cancer treatment may lower risk of recurrence.

Prognosis, Prevention and Outcomes: Lifestyle factors, such as physical activity and diet, are known modifiable risks for obesity, making early childhood education crucial to prevention. Prognosis and outcomes for obesity-associated cancers depend upon how well the incidence of obesity is controlled and the extent to which it is managed. Sufficient weight reduction must be achieved early enough to avoid the irreversible effects of obesity. Unchecked obesity has grave implications for long-term health because of its association with arthritis, diabetes, heart disease, stroke and respiratory disorders, as well as cancer. As little as a 5 to 10 percent weight reduction can have a dramatic impact on health and may mitigate the risk of obesity-associated cancers.

According to a projection of future health and economic burden of obesity, there will be an estimated 500,000 additional cases of cancer in the United States by 2030, if current obesity trends continue. Based on the same analysis, if every adult reduced their BMI by 1 percent (roughly the equivalent of losing 1 kg or 2.2 pounds for an adult of average weight), it would prevent an increase in the number of cancer cases and eliminate about 100,000 new cases.

Dorothy P. Terry
Updated by: Linda August Vrooman, RN, MSN, OCN, CCRC, FNP-BC, NP-C

For Further Information

American Cancer Society (2012). Cancer Facts & Figures 2012: American Cancer Society. http://www.cancer.org/research/cancerfactsfigures/cancerfactsfigures/cancer-facts-figures-2012

Bullwinkle, E. (2015). Abstract 3203: Multiple myeloma microenvironment and obesity. *Cancer Research*, 75(15 Supplement), 3203-3203. doi:10.1158/1538-7445.AM2015-3203

De Pergola, G., & Silvestris, F. (2013). Obesity as a Major Risk Factor for Cancer. *Journal of Obesity*, 2013, 291546. doi:10.1155/2013/291546

Jung, U. J., & Choi, M.-S. (2014). Obesity and Its Metabolic Complications: The Role of Adipokines and the Relationship between Obesity, Inflammation, Insulin Resistance, Dyslipidemia and Nonalcoholic Fatty Liver Disease. *International Journal of Molecular Sciences,* 15(4), 6184-6223. doi:10.3390/ijms15046184

Kwon, H., & Pessin, J. E. (2013). Adipokines Mediate Inflammation and Insulin Resistance. *Frontiers in Endocrinology,* 4, 71. doi:10.3389/fendo.2013.00071

Ligibel, J. A., Alfano, C. M., Courneya, K. S., Demark-Wahnefried, W., Burger, R. A., Chlebowski, R. T., . . . Hudis, C. A. (2014). American Society of Clinical Oncology position statement on obesity and cancer. *J Clin Oncol,* 32(31), 3568-3574. doi:10.1200/jco.2014.58.4680

Ma, J., McKeown, N. M., Hwang, S.-J., Hoffman, U., Jacques, P. F., & Fox, C. S. (2016). Sugar-Sweetened Beverage Consumption is Associated With Change of Visceral Adipose Tissue Over 6 Years of Follow-Up. *Circulation.* doi:10.1161/CIRCULATIONAHA.115.018704

National Cancer Institute (n.d). *Obesity and Cancer Risk.* Retrieved 15 February 2016, from http://www.cancer.gov/about-cancer/causes-prevention/risk/obesity/obesity-fact-sheet#q3

Sahakyan, K. R., Somers, V. K., Rodriguez-Escudero, J. P., Hodge, D. O., Carter, R. E., Sochor, O., . . . Lopez-Jimenez, F. (2015). Normal-Weight Central Obesity: Implications for Total and Cardiovascular Mortality. *Ann Intern Med,* 163(11), 827-835. doi:10.7326/m14-2525

Tomiyama, A. J., Hunger, J. M., Nguyen-Cuu, J., & Wells, C. (2016). Misclassification of cardiometabolic health when using body mass index categories in NHANES 2005-2012. *Int J Obes.* doi:10.1038/ijo.2016.17

van Kruijsdijk, R. C. M., van der Wall, E., & Visseren, F. L. J. (2009). Obesity and Cancer: The Role of Dysfunctional Adipose Tissue. *Cancer Epidemiology Biomarkers & Prevention,* 18(10), 2569-2578. doi:10.1158/1055-9965.EPI-09-0372

Other Resources

Agency for Healthcare Research and Quality (AHRQ)
http://www.ahrq.gov/

American Association for Cancer Research (AACR)
http://www.aacr.org/Pages/Home.aspx

American Cancer Society (ACS)
http://www.cancer.org/

American Institute for Cancer Research (AICR)
http://www.aicr.org/

American Society of Clinical Oncology (ASCO)
www.asco.org

American Urological Association (AUA)
https://www.auanet.org/

Centers for Disease Control and Prevention (CDC)
http://www.cdc.gov/

Clinical Trials.gov
https://clinicaltrials.gov/

Leukemia and Lymphoma Society (LLS)
http://www.lls.org/

National Cancer Institute (NCI)
http://www.cancer.gov/

National Center for Biotechnology Information (NCBI)
http://www.ncbi.nlm.nih.gov

National Health and Nutrition Examination Survey (NHANES)
http://www.cdc.gov/nchs/nhanes.htm

National Institutes of Health (NIH)
http://www.nih.gov/

North American Association of Central Cancer Registries (NAACCR)
http://www.naaccr.org/Home.aspx

The Obesity Society
http://www.obesity.org/

USDA.gov
http://www.usda.gov/wps/portal/usda/usdahome

U. S. National Library of Medicine National Institutes of Health
https://www.nlm.nih.gov/

World Cancer Research Fund International (WCRF)
http://www.wcrf.org/

See also: Appendix cancer; Bile duct cancer; Breast cancers; Cervical cancer; Comedo carcinomas; Craniopharyngiomas; Endometrial cancer; Gallbladder cancer; Gynecologic cancers; Hepatomegaly; Klinefelter syndrome and cancer; Leiomyosarcomas; Medulloblastomas; Nutrition and cancer prevention; Pancreatic cancers; Paraneoplastic syndromes; Rectal cancer; Risks for cancer; Stomach cancers; Urinary system cancers; Uterine cancer

▶ Oligodendrogliomas

Category: Diseases, Symptoms, and Conditions
Also known as: Glial brain tumors, OD

Related conditions: Elevated intracranial pressure, personality changes, neurological deficits

Definition: Oligodendrogliomas are a type of glial tumor arising in the brain in which the oligodendroglial cell is the predominant cell type. There are several kinds of glial cells in the central nervous system, but each functions in support of the nerve cells (neurons). The oligodendrocytes are glial cells that coat the axons in the central nervous system with an insulating membrane called myelin. Without myelin, the nerve impulses flowing down the axon lose efficiency.

The third most common of the glial neoplasms, oligodendrogliomas usually originate in the cerebral hemispheres (predominantly the frontal lobe) but on rare occasions can arise in the cerebellum, brain stem, and spinal cord. Although they are typically considered a rare

Relative Survival Rates of Adults with Oligodendroglioma by Race, 1988-2001

	Survival Rates (%)	
Years	*Whites*	*Blacks*
1	89.1	79.6
2	81.7	71.9
3	77.9	63.1
5	68.8	50.2
8	58.7	37.6
10	52.2	28.5

Source: Data from L. A. G. Ries et al., eds., *Cancer Survival Among Adults: U.S. SEER Program, 1988-2001—Patient and Tumor Characteristics, NIH Pub. No. 07-6215 (Bethesda, Md.: National* Cancer Institute, 2007)

neoplasm, newer diagnostic techniques such as genotyping indicate that the condition is more common than once thought.

Oligodendroglioma neoplasms often contain anaplastic cells, primitive, undifferentiated cells that are a distinguishing feature of emerging embryonic cells and are often seen in malignant neoplasms. Tumors with anaplastic cells are called anaplastic oligodendrogliomas.

Risk factors: There are no known causes or risk factors for oligodendroglioma. The problem occasionally clusters in some families, but this is unrelated to any mechanisms of inheritance. The disease strikes men about twice as often as women, with the risk equally distributed among the races. Although the median age of diagnosis is between forty and fifty years, oligodendroglioma can occur at any age. The anaplastic variant usually occurs between the ages of sixty and seventy. Children are less frequently affected, accounting for 6 percent of oligodendroglioma cases.

Etiology and the disease process: Oligodendrogliomas evolve from primitive precursor glioma cells. The tumor begins as a slow-growing, mixed tumor, combining elements of astrocytes (another type of glial cell), neurons, and oligodendroglial cells. The tumor consists of poorly defined anaplastic components, mature oligodendroglial cells, or a mixture of the two. It is impossible to predict how long it will take for patients to experience symptoms because although oligodendrogliomas usually grow quite slowly, they can quickly evolve into an aggressive malignancy and shorten the crisis point from upwards of thirty years to only a few months. When the neoplasm exhibits features of oligodendroglioma cells with astrocytic components, it is called oligoastrocytoma, but this is less common.

Incidence: Intracranial tumors are second only to stroke as the most common neurological cause of death. In the United States, the incidence of oligodendrogliomas compared with all intracranial tumors may be as high as 19 percent, and they may represent 20 to 54 percent of all gliomas. Oligodendrogliomas may account for 4 percent of all brain tumors, with an annual incidence in the United States of 0.3 per 100,000 people.

Symptoms: Symptoms depend on the size, location, invasiveness, and rate of growth of the tumor. Warning signs will vary but may include seizures, vomiting, fatigue, headache, numbness, pain, ataxia, paralysis, sensations of tingling or burning, hearing or vision deficits, and changes in temperature and taste sensitivity. The most common first symptom is a seizure, representing half of all patients.

Screening and diagnosis: Imaging studies and biopsy examination are central to a diagnosis of oligodendroglioma. Laboratory tests are useful only in excluding other causes and determining overall health. Magnetic resonance imaging (MRI) is performed with and without the radiocontrast medium gadolinium. Computed tomography (CT) scans are helpful in revealing some details missed in MRI studies, and sometimes immunohistochemical markers further help in establishing the diagnosis. However, ultimately, only biopsy will result in a definitive diagnosis. Following biopsy, most pathologists will simply grade oligodendrogliomas according to the presence or absence of anaplastic features.

Treatment and therapy: Treatment depends on the patient's symptoms and the location and nature of the tumor. As with most cancers, the three mainstays of treatment are chemotherapy, radiation, and surgery. Chemotherapy using a combination of procarbarazine, lomustine, and vincristine has been used in the earliest diagnosed stage of the tumor, but typically relapses occur between eighteen months and two years. Newer treatments in combination with radiation may prolong the time until relapse, but the classic treatment for oligodendroglioma remains surgical resection. Often, however, the tumor is poorly defined, making complete resection impossible. In the past, when surgery completely removed the tumor, further treatment was believed unnecessary. However, several years following total resection, almost all patients suffer recurrence of the tumor at the surgical site. Regardless of whether resection is complete or incomplete, typically no further treatment is given until relapse occurs. In the event of relapse, chemotherapy is the treatment of choice; radiation is reserved for patients not responding to chemotherapy.

Prognosis, prevention, and outcomes: The prognosis depends on the growth rate of the tumor, its location, and its pressure effects inside the cranium. Some specific prognostic indicators have been noted: Older age at the time of diagnosis, the presence of a neurological deficit, or a central location in a child's brain usually results in a shorter survival time. From the time of diagnosis, the median survival time ranges between three and seventeen years. Five-year survival rates range from 39 to 75 percent and ten-year rates from 19 to 59 percent, but ultimately all patients will die of the disease.

Richard S. Spira, D.V.M.

For Further Information

Baumann, Nicole, and Danielle Pham-Dinh. "Biology of Oligodendrocyte and Myelin in the Mammalian Central Nervous System." *Physiological Reviews* 18, no. 2 (2001): 871-927.

Central Brain Tumor Registry of the United States. *Primary Brain Tumors in the United States: Statistical Report, 1992-1997.* Chicago: Author, 2000.

Ellis, T. L., V. W. Stieber, and R. C. Austin. "Oligodendroglioma." *Current Treatment Options in Oncology* 4, no. 6 (2003): 479-490.

Kleihus, P., and W. K. Cavenee. *Pathology and Genetics of Tumours of the Nervous System.* New York: Oxford University Press, 2000.

Mason, W. P. "Oligodendroglioma." *Current Treatment Options in Neurology* 7, no. 4 (July, 2005): 305-314.

Ohgaki, H., and P. Kleihues. "Population-Based Studies on Incidence, Survival Rates, and Genetic Alterations in Astrocytic and Oligodendroglial Gliomas." *Journal of Neuropatholy and Experimental Neurology* 64, no. 6 (June, 2005): 479-489.

Van den Bent, M. J. "Advances in the Biology and Treatment of Oligodendrogliomas." *Current Opinion in Neurology* 17, no. 6 (December, 2004): 675-680.

Other Resources

The Brain Tumor Foundation

Tumor Types: Oligodendrogliomas
http://www.braintumorfoundation.org/Oligodendrogliomas.php

National Cancer Institute

Adult Brain Tumors Treatment
http://www.cancer.gov/cancertopics/pdq/treatment/adultbrain/Patient

See also: Brain and central nervous system cancers; Carcinomatous meningitis; Gliomas; Meningeal carcinomatosis

▶ Oral and oropharyngeal cancers

Category: Diseases, Symptoms, and Conditions

Also known as: Mouth cancer, tongue cancer, salivary gland cancer, gum cancer, throat (instead of oropharyngeal) cancer

Related conditions: Neck cancer, esophageal cancer

Definition: Oral cancer is a collective term that encompasses cancers of the lips, mouth, tongue, gums, and salivary glands. Oral cancers mostly occur on the lips, tongue, or floor of the mouth but may also occur inside the cheeks, in the gums, or on the roof of the mouth. The oropharynx or throat is situated between the soft palate and the hyoid bone. The top of the oropharynx connects with the oral cavity and, further up, with the nasopharynx. The bottom of the oropharynx connects with the supraglottic larynx and the hypopharynx. The oropharynx consists of the base of the tongue (including the pharyngoepiglottic folds and the glossoepiglottic folds), the tonsillar region, the soft palate (including the uvula), and the pharyngeal walls. Practically all oral and oropharyngeal cancers are squamous cell carcinomas (SCCs), which refer to cancers that originate in squamous cells.

Because the lymphatic system is one of the major ways that tumors spread or metastasize to other organs, knowledge of the location of lymph nodes in this area is crucial for understanding oral and oropharyngeal cancer. The lymph nodes that supply the head and neck run parallel to the jugular veins and can be classified into five levels: Level I, which refers to the submental and submandibular lymph nodes; Level II, which includes the upper jugular lymph nodes; Level III, which refers to the mid-jugular lymph nodes; Level IV, containing the lower jugular lymph nodes; and Level V, which refers to the lymph nodes of the posterior triangle.

Risk factors: Risk factors include cigarette smoking, chewing tobacco, excessive alcohol intake, extensive exposure to ultraviolet light, denture irritation, leukoplakia (white spots on the tongue or inside the cheeks), erythroplakia (red patches inside the mouth that bleed readily when bruised), and infection with human papillomavirus (HPV). Infection with HPV has been linked to one in five oral cancers. One study conducted at the Johns Hopkins University concluded that HPV infection is a stronger risk factor for oropharyngeal squamous cell carcinoma than tobacco and alcohol use. Gastroesophageal reflux disease (GERD), in which stomach acids enter the esophagus and destroy the esophageal lining, also contributes to the risk of throat cancer.

Etiology and the disease process: Oral and oropharyngeal cancers appear to be caused by deoxyribonucleic acid (DNA) damage in the cells in the mouth and throat. This DNA damage can occur from exposure to too much ultraviolet light from the sun, or from cigarette smoking, tobacco chewing, or excessive alcohol intake. Most oral and oropharyngeal cancers are carcinomas of

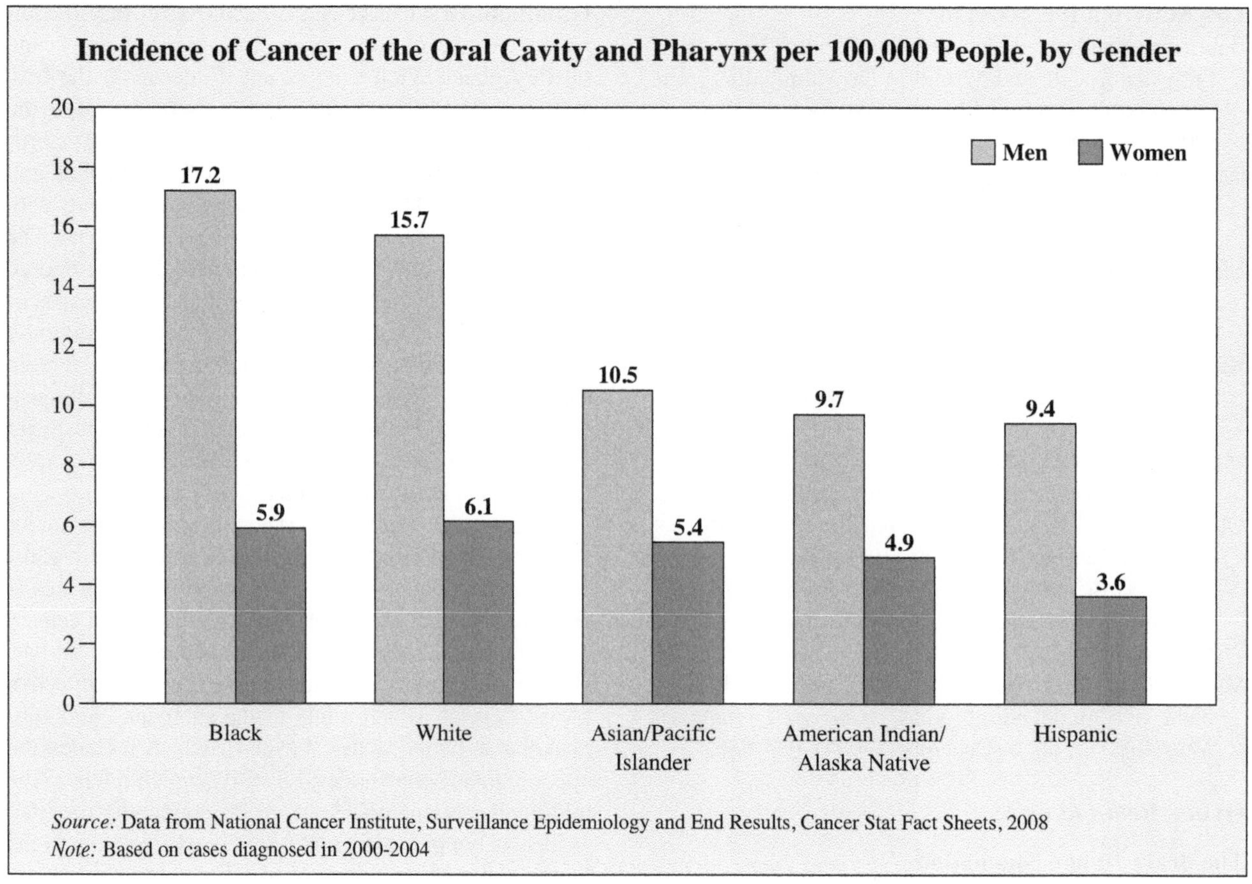

the squamous cells, the flat cells that make up the mucosal epithelium, the layer of cells lining the inside of the mouth, nose, larynx, and throat. Less common are lymphomas, lymphoepitheliomas, and minor salivary gland carcinomas. A rare type of oral cancer is verrucous carcinoma, which usually does not metastasize but can penetrate deeply into nearby tissue.

Incidence: According to the American Cancer Society, there are approximately 30,990 new cases of oral and oropharyngeal cancer annually in the United States, with an estimated 7,430 deaths from oral and oropharyngeal cancer each year. The incidence is higher in men than in women. Oropharyngeal cancer is still a relatively rare type of cancer, and both oral and oropharyngeal cancer rates have been decreasing since 1975 in the United States.

Symptoms: Symptoms of oral and oropharyngeal cancer include lumps of white, red, or dark patches inside the mouth that do not recede with time, mouth sores that do not heal or that enlarge over time, lumps in the neck, persistent pain in the mouth, thickening of the cheek, swelling or pain in the jaw, soreness in the throat or a feeling that something is caught in the throat, difficulty chewing or moving the tongue (late-stage symptom), difficulty moving the jaw (late-stage symptom), pain around the teeth, loosening of the teeth, numbness of the tongue or mouth, and changes in the voice.

Screening and diagnosis: Frequent oral examinations are the best way to detect signs of oral and throat cancer. When a tumor is detected, it is graded or staged to determine how benign or aggressive it is. The TNM (tumor/lymph node/metastasis) staging system is a standard way of classifying tumors. T stands for the size of the primary tumor and which tissues of the oral cavity or oropharynx the tumor has spread to, if any. N refers to the extent of spread to regional lymph nodes. M is used to denote whether the tumor has metastasized to other organs. The most common metastatic site is the lungs, followed by the liver and the bones. Within each of these designations, there are several subcategories.

Following TNM staging, the tumor is classified as Stage 0, I, II, III, or IV. Stage 0 refers to a tumor that is confined to the outer layer of oral or oropharyngeal tissue and has not penetrated deeper or metastasized. Stage I tumors are 2 centimeters (cm) or smaller in diameter and have not metastasized. Stage II tumors are between 2 cm and 4 cm in diameter and have not metastasized. Stage III tumors are larger than 4 cm in diameter and have not metastasized, although they may have invaded one of the nearby lymph nodes. Stage IV is further divided into three substages: Stage IVA, in which tumors have spread to nearby sites and may or may not have invaded one or more nearby lymph nodes, Stage IVB, in which tumors may or may not have spread to nearby sites but have spread to one or more lymph nodes, and Stage IVC, in which tumors have metastasized to distant organs.

Treatment and therapy: Primary care physicians will often refer patients to specialists, including oral and maxillofacial surgeons, otolaryngologists (ear, nose, and throat doctors), medical oncologists, radiation oncologists, and plastic surgeons. At specialized cancer treatment facilities, several of these specialists often work together to provide tailored care for patients. Treatment options include radiation therapy, oral chemotherapy, and surgery, as well as combinations of these treatments. The most commonly used treatment is a combination of radiation therapy and chemotherapy with the drug cisplatin. In some cases, surgery may be necessary to remove the cancer cells from a localized region. The surgery is often followed by radiation therapy to destroy any remaining cancer cells. Chemotherapy is sometimes given before other treatments to potentially enhance effectiveness of the follow-up treatment. In addition, treatments for symptoms and the side effects of therapies are often administered concomitantly.

Radiation therapy can take the form of external radiation from specialized equipment or internal radiation, when radioactive substances are placed in seeds, needles, or plastic tubes and inserted in the tissue. A newer form of radiation therapy, intensity-modulated radiotherapy, focuses radiation to more selectively kill the tumor instead of the surrounding healthy tissue. Surgery can be performed to remove tumors in the mouth or throat, or lymph nodes in the neck.

In addition to radiation, chemotherapy, and surgery, targeted therapies are also available. These include cetuximab (Erbitux), docetaxel (Taxotere), and angiogenesis inhibitors. Cetuximab is a monoclonal antibody directed at a protein that is abundant on cancer cells in this region. In a phase III clinical trial conducted at multiple locations in the United States and Europe (lead author James A. Bonner, of the University of Alabama at Birmingham), treatment with cetuximab combined with radiation therapy was shown almost to double the median survival of patients with nonmetastatic head and neck cancer. Another phase III study showed that patients with inoperable head and neck cancer who were administered multidrug chemotherapy that included docetaxel, followed by radiation therapy, survived four months longer with fewer side effects compared with patients on standard therapy. Another study involved 358 patients with inoperable head and neck cancer that had metastasized to lymph nodes in the neck. These patients were randomly selected to receive either standard chemotherapy with cisplastin and 5-fluorouracil, or cisplastin, 5-fluorouracil, and docetaxel. Both groups received radiation therapy after chemotherapy. The group treated with docetaxel had a longer median survival time and progression-free survival (time during which the cancer does not progress)—18.6 months and 12.7 months, respectively—compared with the group that was treated with standard chemotherapy—14.5 months and 8.4 months, respectively. Docetaxel was also associated with fewer side effects such as vomiting, nausea, and mouth sores. This provides support for the rationale of targeted therapy, which is expected to affect normal healthy tissues less than more nonspecific chemotherapy drugs.

Before starting any treatment, it is important for patients to ask their physicians about the treatment length and procedure, risks, side effects, and the results that may be expected.

Prognosis, prevention, and outcomes: The prognosis is good if detected and treated early. However, oral and throat cancers are often not diagnosed until they are late stage, often because they may be painless at early stages or cause minor pains similar to a toothache. The stage of cancer will also determine the type of treatment to use. After treatment, the cancer may reappear (recur or relapse). The recurrence can occur in the mouth or throat (local recurrence), in the lymph nodes (regional relapse), or in a distant site in the body, often the lungs (distant recurrence). A relapse is associated with a poorer prognosis. The five-year relative survival rate is a statistic that calculates the survival of cancer patients relative to the expected survival for people without cancer. This statistic can be used as a guide, but other factors, such as age, health, and tumor properties, must be considered before arriving at a complete prognosis. By studying patients treated between 1985 and 1991, the five-year relative survival rate for oral cavity cancer was calculated to range from 83 percent for Stage I cancer to 47 percent for Stage IV tumors. The one-year survival rate for all stages was 84 percent. The five-year relative survival rate for oropharyngeal cancer ranges from 57 percent for Stage I cancer to 30 percent for Stage IV cancer.

Ing-Wei Khor, Ph.D.

For Further Information

Bonner, J. A., et al. "Radiotherapy plus Cetuximab for Squamous-Cell Carcinoma of the Head and Neck." *New England Journal of Medicine* 354 (2006): 567-578.

D'Souza, G., et al. "Case-Control Study of Human Papillomavirus and Oropharyngeal Cancer." *New Enland Journal of Medicine* 357 (2007): 1944-1956.

Genden, Eric M., and Mark A. Varvares, eds. *Head and Neck Cancer: An Evidence-Based Team Approach.* New York: Thieme, 2008.

Lydiatt, William M., and Perry J. Johnson. *Cancers of the Mouth and Throat: A Patient's Guide to Treatment.* Omaha, Neb.: Addicus Books, 2001.

Nikolakakos, Alexios P., ed. *Oral Cancer Research Advances.* New York: Nova Biomedical Books, 2007.

Vermorken, J. B., et al. "Cisplatin, Fluorouracil, and Docetaxel in Unresectable Head and Neck Cancer." *New England Journal of Medicine* 357 (2007): 1695-1704.

Other Resources

American Cancer Society

Detailed Guide: Oral Cavity and Oropharyngeal Cancer
Http://www.cancer.org/docroot/CRI/CRI_2_3x.asp?rnav=cridg&dt=60.

Cancer Research UK

Types of Mouth and Oropharyngeal Cancer.
Http://www.cancerhelp.org.uk/help/default.asp?page=13033

MayoClinic.com

Oral and Throat Cancer
Http://www.mayoclinic.com/health/oral-and-throat-cancer/DS00349

National Cancer Institute

Oral Cancer
http://www.cancer.gov/cancertopics/types/oral

See also: Candidiasis; Chewing tobacco; Cigarettes and cigars; Coal tars and coal tar pitches; Cordectomy; Electrolarynx; Endoscopy; Epidemiology of cancer; Epidermoid cancers of mucous membranes; Epstein-Barr Virus; Erythroplakia; Esophageal speech; Glossectomy; Head and neck cancers; Hypopharyngeal cancer; Laryngeal cancer; Laryngeal nerve palsy; Laryngectomy; Laryngoscopy; Leukoplakia; Lip cancers; Oral and maxillofacial surgery; Salivary gland cancer; Throat cancer; Tobacco-related cancers

▶ Orbit tumors

Category: Diseases, Symptoms, and Conditions
Also known as: Eye socket tumors, rhabdomyosarcomas, dermoid cysts, capillary hemangiomas, lymphoid tumors, cavernous hemangiomas, neurofibromas, schwannomas, optic gliomas, skin cancers of the eyelids, osteomas

Related conditions: Arteriovenous malformations, gene mutations, trauma, systemic diseases, congenital anatomic defects, chronic inflammation or infection, metastasis from adjacent or distant primary tumors

Definition: Orbit tumors are tumors found in the orbit, also known as the eye socket, which encases the eyeball, optic nerve, extraocular muscles, blood vessels, and soft tissue. Orbit tumors can be primary, in which the tumor originates from the orbit, or metastatic, in which the tumor develops from adjacent or distant tissue and invades the orbit. Most orbit tumors are benign but, because of their space-occupying nature, are readily conspicuous.

Risk factors: The presence of an invasive tumor in adjacent tissue may increase the risk of developing an orbit tumor. There are no other clearly identifiable risk factors for developing orbit tumors.

Etiology and the disease process: The etiology of orbit tumors varies and encompasses the etiologies of arteriovenous malformations, gene mutations, trauma, systemic diseases (such as amyloidosis or lymphoma), congenital anatomic defects, chronic inflammation or infection, and metastasis from adjacent or distant primary tumors.

Incidence: Orbit tumors can develop in children and adults, with different incidence rates depending on tumor type. In children, rhabdomyosarcoma is the most common malignant orbit tumor and accounts for 3 percent of orbit tumors; capillary hemangioma, which occurs in 1 to 4 percent of infants, is the most common benign pediatric tumor. The most common orbit tumors in adults are lymphoid tumors, cavernous hemangioma, and metastatic tumors, which respectively make up 4 to 13 percent, 4 percent, and 8 percent of all orbital neoplasms. Other orbit tumors include dermoid cysts, neurofibromas, schwannomas, optic gliomas, skin cancer of the eyelid, and osteomas.

Symptoms: The most common symptom is proptosis (forward displacement of the eye). Eye pain, visual abnormalities such as double vision or even visual loss, orbital edema, and eye redness are other symptoms of orbit tumors.

Screening and diagnosis: The diagnosis of orbit tumors relies on a meticulous patient history, thorough physical exam, and magnetic resonance imaging (MRI) or computed tomography (CT) scans. The diagnosis is confirmed by performing a tissue biopsy, either by fine-needle aspiration biopsy (FNAB) or by open biopsy of the orbit (orbitotomy). Histological analysis will determine the type of orbit tumor and lay the groundwork for a treatment plan.

Treatment and therapy: Treatment depends on the tumor type. Surgical removal is usually the best option, especially with disfiguring, massive lesions. Some tumors require external beam radiotherapy or adjuvant chemotherapy. In pediatric patients, dermoid tumors are best treated by surgical excision, while capillary hemangiomas spontaneously regress, therefore not requiring any intervention. In adults, radiotherapy is the treatment of choice for lymphoid tumors, while surgery effectively treats cavernous hemangioma.

Prognosis, prevention, and outcomes: The prognosis and outcomes depend on the type of tumor. Most primary orbit tumors are benign and therefore have a good prognosis. Metastatic orbit tumors (with a primary source of cancer elsewhere in the body) usually signify a poor prognosis.

Ophelia Panganiban, B.S.

See also: Eyelid cancer; Gonioscopy; Lacrimal gland tumors; Neurofibromatosis type 1 (NF1); Ophthalmic oncology; Retinoblastomas; Rhabdomyosarcomas; Rothmund-Thomson syndrome; Sjögren syndrome

▶ Organ transplantation and cancer

Category: Diseases, Symptoms, and Conditions
Related conditions: Immune suppression, Kaposi sarcoma, nonmelanoma skin cancer, lymphoma

Definition: Transplantation of organ

When organs are transplanted, there is a potential to mechanically transmit diseases from the donor to the patient. Infections, malignant conditions, and autoimmune diseases are examples of easily transmittable conditions. Patients who receive transplanted organs must use long-term immunosuppressive therapy, drugs used to prevent organ rejection by suppressing the immune function of the body. If the immune system is weakened, the chance of developing cancer increases. Cancer risk is high for patients on dialysis for end-stage renal disease, often a precursor to kidney transplant.

Risk factors: Those having undergone organ transplantation are at risk for developing cancers.

Etiology and the disease process: An organ such as a liver, lung, or kidney, and less often a heart, can contain malignant cells or a tumor at the time of transplantation into a patient. Coupled with immunosuppressive therapy, which weakens the immune system, a cancer transplanted with an organ is generally aggressive and difficult to manage. There are approximately 125,000 people waiting for organ transplants. If a donor has been cancer free for a long period of time, donation may be an acceptable risk according to the United Network for Organ Sharing and a study of the UK Transplant Registry. As organs are more difficult to locate for transplant, older donors and donors with health issues may be used, which increases the risk for cancer transmission from a transplanted organ to the patient.

Although the immune system is most effective at fighting infection, it protects against cancer to a lesser degree by recognizing abnormal cells and attempting to control them. When the immune system is suppressed by drugs to prevent organ rejection, the body loses its ability to fight infection and abnormal cells. Cancers with a viral etiology are most encouraged by immunosuppressive therapy.

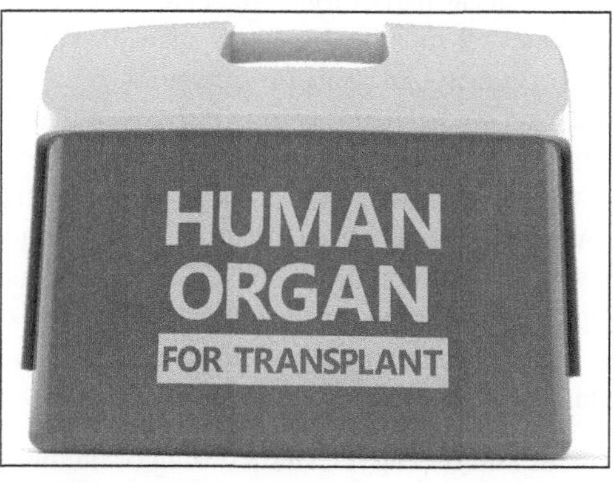

(iStock)

Kaposi sarcoma, tumors just under the skin, may be transmitted by organ donation from donors infected with human herpesvirus 8 (HHV-8) but also may develop in patients with a preexisting infection when the immune system cannot help the body fight the infection. Lymphoma is most likely to occur in the first year after transplant or when treatment for organ rejection is started. The most common cancer in transplant patients is skin cancer. Cancer usually occurs in the first few years following a transplant.

Incidence: The incidence of developing cancer after transplant is 1 to 2 percent higher than it is in the normal population, and there is a fifteen- twentyfold higher incidence of some cancers. Patients on immunosuppressive therapy have a much greater risk of developing cancer than the normal population. The cumulative probability for cancer after transplant is approximately 15 percent. Nonmelanoma skin cancers account for 90 percent of skin cancers in transplant patients, and skin cancer in the transplant group has a rate 100 times higher than that of the normal population. In a study by the United Network for Organ Sharing, malignancies caused 26 percent of deaths in kidney patients surviving at least ten years. Liver recipients had a 24 percent death rate from cancer at one year after transplant, and 21 percent of deaths in cardiac recipients in the first two years were from cancer. Kaposi sarcoma develops in organ recipients at a rate 500 times that of the normal population. Breast, colorectal, and cervical cancer risks are also increased after transplant.

Symptoms: Symptoms depend on the cancer type that develops after transplantation. Skin cancers may be visible on the surface of the skin.

Screening and diagnosis: Transplant patients need to receive routine screenings for cancer according to recommended cancer screening guidelines and have routine physician visits as part of follow-up care. Patients should inspect their skin monthly for any changes that could indicate skin cancer. An annual examination by a dermatologist is recommended. There is discussion that better screening of donors before organ donation should be a priority to prevent cancer transmission from affected organs. When symptoms present, diagnosis may include radiology tests, laboratory tests, and physical examination. Staging depends on the cancer diagnosed and the status of the tumor, lymph nodes, and presence or absence of metastasis at diagnosis.

Treatment and therapy: Careful dosing of immunosuppressive therapy to prevent organ rejection without totally depressing the immune system is critical. Some cancers may respond to changing the drugs and doses used in immunosuppressive therapy. If cancer is diagnosed, the treatments depend on the disease but generally include chemotherapy, radiation, and surgery.

Prognosis, prevention, and outcomes: The prognosis for patients developing cancer after transplant varies by the type of cancer. Patients should avoid sun exposure because of the high risk of skin cancer. Screening patients and donors carefully before transplant may prevent some cancers. Lower doses of immunosuppressive therapy may contribute to preventing cancer. There are newer types of immunosuppressive drugs that may decrease the incidence of cancer, including one that reverses the presence of skin cancers. Approximately one-third of all organ transplant patients die from cancer.

Patricia Stanfill Edens, R.N., Ph.D., LFACHE

For Further Information

Desai R, Collett D, Watson CJ, Johnson P, Evans T, Neuberger J. "Estimated risk of cancer transmission from organ donor to graft recipient in a national transplantation registry." *Br J Surg* 101, no. 7 (June 2014):768-774.

Green M, Covington S, Taranto S, Wolfe C, Bell W, Biggins SW, Conti D, DeStefano GD, Dominguez E, Ennis D, Gross T, Klassen-Fischer M, Kotton C, LaPointe-Rudow D, Law Y, Ludrosky K, Menegus M, Morris MI, Nalesnik MA, Pavlakis M, Pruett T, Sifri C, Kaul D. "Donor-derived transmission events in 2013: a report of the Organ Procurement Transplant Network Ad Hoc Disease Transmission Advisory Committee." *Transplantation* 99, no. 2 (February 2015): 282-287.

Kauffman, H. M., et al. "Deceased Donors with a Past History of Malignancy: An Organ Procurement and Transplantation Network/United Network for Organ Sharing Update." *Transplantation* 84, no. 2 (July 27, 2007): 272-274.

Serraino, D., et al. "Risk of Cancer Following Immunosuppression in Organ Transplant Recipients and in HIV-Positive Individuals in Southern Europe." *European Journal of Cancer* 43, no. 14 (September, 2007): 2117-2123.

Other Resources

American Cancer Society
http://www.cancer.org

National Cancer Institute
http://www.cancer.gov

National Marrow Donor Program
http://www.marrow.org

United Network for Organ Sharing
http://www.unos.org/qa.asp

See also: Azathioprine; Blood cancers; Bone Marrow Transplantation (BMT); Childhood cancers; Colony-Stimulating Factors (CSFs); Cyclosporin A; Denys-Drash syndrome and cancer; Graft-Versus-Host Disease (GVHD); Stem cell transplantation; Umbilical cord blood transplantation

▶ Ovarian cancers

Category: Diseases, Symptoms, and Conditions
Also known as: Cancer of the ovaries

Related conditions: Abdominal cancer, colon cancer, cancer of the diaphragm, lymphatic cancer, peritoneal cancer, stomach cancer

Definition: Ovarian cancers result from the development of a malignant tumor in the ovaries and can be divided into three main types. The most common is epithelial ovarian cancer, which originates in the surface cells of an ovary. The second type, germ-cell ovarian cancer, starts in the interior cells of an ovary, where eggs are produced. A third main type, stomal ovarian cancer, begins in the connective tissue cells that hold an ovary together and generate the female hormones estrogen and progesterone.

Risk factors: One of the most important risk factors involved in the development of ovarian cancers is inherited gene mutations. Inheritance of mutated breast cancer genes, *BRCA1* and *BRCA2*, is responsible for up to 10 percent of all ovarian cancers. Other factors include having had breast or colon cancer, having a family history of ovarian cancer, not having given birth, taking fertility drugs, and using hormone replacement therapy after menopause. Age is an important risk factor. More than half of the deaths caused by ovarian cancer occur in women between the ages of fifty-five and seventy-four.

Etiology and the disease process: The exact cause of ovarian cancers is still unknown. Some specialists have suggested that ovarian cancer in younger women is related to the tissue-repair process subsequent to ovulation. The formation and division of new cells at the site where an egg is released through a small tear in the ovarian follicle may produce genetic errors. Other specialists believe that the origin of ovarian cancers in younger women is related to the production of abnormal cells associated with the increased hormone levels that occur before and after ovulation.

Ovarian cancers are classified according to the histology of the tumor. Between 85 and 90 percent of ovarian cancers are epithelial ovarian cancers, which are classified by cell type and graded from 1 to 3. About 5 percent of ovarian cancers are germ-cell tumors, which develop in the egg-producing cells of the ovary and generally occur in younger women. Another type of ovarian cancer develops in the stomal cells, the tissue that holds the ovary together.

Ovarian cancer cells metastasize by spreading into the naturally occurring fluids in the abdominal cavity. These cells frequently become implanted in other peritoneal structures, particularly the uterus, the intestines, the omentum, and the urinary bladder. New tumor growths often occur in these areas. In rare instances, ovarian cancer cells spread through the bloodstream or lymphatic system to other parts of the body.

Incidence: Ovarian cancer is the fifth leading cause of cancer-related death in women. Each year, more than 20,000 women in the United States are diagnosed with ovarian cancers and about 15,000 succumb to the disease. Ovarian cancers are most common in industrialized nations. In the United States, a woman has a 1.4 to 2.5 percent chance of developing ovarian cancer in her lifetime.

Symptoms: In the majority of cases, ovarian cancer produces no symptoms or only mild symptoms until it progresses to an advanced stage. Symptoms include general

Stage at Diagnosis and Five-Year Relative Survival Rates for Ovarian Cancer, 1996-2004

Stage	*Cases Diagnosed (%)*	*Survival Rate (%)*
Localized[a]	19	92.4
Regional[b]	7	71.4
Distant[c]	68	29.8
Unstaged	7	24.8

Source: Data from National Cancer Institute, Surveillance Epidemiology and End Results, Cancer Stat Fact Sheets, 2008
[a]Cancer still confined to primary site
[b]Cancer has spread to regional lymph nodes or directly beyond the primary site
[c]Cancer has metastasized

abdominal discomfort, such as bloating, cramps, pressure, and swelling; nausea, diarrhea, or constipation; frequent urination; loss of appetite or feeling bloated after a light meal; and the loss or gain of weight for no apparent reason. Other symptoms can include fatigue, back pain, pain during sexual intercourse, abnormal bleeding from the vagina, menstrual irregularities, shortness of breath, and fluid around the lungs.

Screening and diagnosis: A medical doctor first evaluates a patient's medical and family history, then performs, a thorough physical examination of the pelvic region. The presence of any abnormal growths should be further investigated using ultrasound imaging and computed tomography (CT) scans. Ultrasound can detect the difference between healthy tissues, fluid-filled cysts, and tumors. CT scans produce detailed cross-sectional images of regions within the body. In some cases, X rays of the colon and rectum following a barium enema help identify the presence of ovarian cancers. The level of cancer antigen 125 (CA 125) should be assessed with a blood test; however, this marker identifies only about 10 percent of early ovarian cancers. The amount of four other cancer-related proteins in the blood shows some promise for diagnosing ovarian cancers.

A biopsy must be performed for a definitive diagnosis of ovarian cancer. Biopsies are usually done on tumors removed during surgery, although sometimes they are done during a laparoscopy or using a needle guided by ultrasound or CT scans. If ovarian cancer is present, the stage of the disease is assessed. Staging for ovarian cancer is as follows:

- Stage I: The cancer is limited to one or both ovaries.
- Stage II: The cancer has extended into the pelvic region, such as the uterus or Fallopian tubes.
- Stage III: The cancer has spread outside the pelvis or is limited to the pelvic region but is present in the small intestine, lymph nodes, or omentum.
- Stage IV: The cancer has metastasized to the liver or tissues outside of the peritoneal cavity.

These stages are further broken down into levels of seriousness from A to C.

Treatment and therapy: Depending on the stage of ovarian cancer, surgery is often performed to remove the ovaries, uterine tubes, uterus, omentum, and associated lymph nodes. This process is referred to as surgical debulking. The stage of the disease determines whether additional therapy is needed. Typically, chemotherapy is employed, and if the cancer is localized, radiation therapy is sometimes used. The most effective chemotherapy drugs used in treating ovarian cancers are carboplatin and paclitaxel (Taxol), administered intravenously. The combination reduces cell division in ovarian tumors.

Intraperitoneal therapy, or pumping chemotherapy drugs directly into a patient's abdomen, extends the lives of ovarian cancer victims by an additional year or more; however, it can cause side effects such as stomach pain, numbness in the extremities, and possible infection. In January, 2006, the National Cancer Institute recommended an individualized combination of intravenous and intraperitoneal therapy for ovarian cancer patients. New chemotherapy drugs, vaccines, gene therapy, and immunotherapy treatments are being explored as options for treating ovarian cancers.

Prognosis, prevention, and outcomes: More than 60 percent of ovarian cancer patients are in Stage III or IV at the time of diagnosis, so the prognosis is not promising. The five-year survival rate for all stages of epithelial ovarian cancer is only 35 to 38 percent. With early diagnosis, aggressive surgery, and chemotherapy, the five-year survival rate is above 90 percent and the long-term survival rate approaches 70 percent. For germ-cell ovarian cancer, the prognosis is better than for epithelial ovarian cancer.

Eating well, exercising, and properly managing stress help produce good overall health and reduce the risk of developing ovarian cancers. Measures that help prevent ovarian cancer include having children and breast-feeding them, using oral contraceptives (30 percent reduction), and having a tubal ligation. For women who have a high risk of developing ovarian cancers, removal of the ovaries may be the best prevention.

Alvin K. Benson, Ph.D.

For Further Information

Bardos, A. P., ed. *Trends in Ovarian Cancer Research.* Hauppauge, N.Y.: Nova Science, 2004.

Bartlett, John M. S. *Ovarian Cancer: Methods and Protocols.* Totowa, N.J.: Humana Press, 2000.

Conner, Kristine, and Lauren Langford. *Ovarian Cancer: Your Guide to Taking Control.* Sebastopol, Calif.: O'Reilly, 2003.

Dizon, Don S. *One Hundred Questions and Answers About* Ovarian Cancer. 2d ed. Sudbury, Mass.: Jones and Bartlett, 2006.

Icon Health. *Ovarian Cancer: A Medical Dictionary, Bibliography, and Annotated Research Guide to Internet References.* San Diego, Calif.: Author, 2004.

Nathan, David G. *The Cancer Treatment Revolution: How Smart Drugs and Other New Therapies Are Renewing Our Hope and Changing the Face of Medicine.* New York: Wiley, 2007.

Other Resources

American Cancer Society
Detailed Guide: Ovarian Cancer
http://www.cancer.org/docroot/CRI/CRI_2_3x.asp?dt=33

MayoClinic.com
Ovarian Cancer
http://www.mayoclinic.com/health/ovarian-cancer/DS00293

National Institutes of Health
http://www.cancer.gov/cancertopics/types/ovarian/

Ovarian Cancer National Alliance
http://www.ovariancancer.org/

See also: Cervical cancer; Endometrial cancer; Fallopian tube cancer; Fertility drugs and cancer; Gynecologic cancers; Ovarian cysts; Ovarian epithelial cancer; Uterine cancer; Vaginal cancer; Vulvar cancer

▶ Ovarian cysts

Category: Diseases, Symptoms, and Conditions
Also known as: Functional ovarian cysts, physiologic ovarian cysts

Related conditions: Ovarian cancer, uterine cancer, lymphatic cancer, peritoneal cancer

Definition: Ovarian cysts are growths that develop within or on the surface of an ovary. They may consist of fluid-filled sacs, semisolid material, or solid material. Fluid-filled cysts are not likely to be cancerous. Most cysts that develop during a woman's childbearing years are not cancerous.

Risk factors: No specific risk factors have been identified. Most ovarian cysts develop as part of the ovulation process. The likelihood of an ovarian cyst causing cancer increases with the size of the growth and the age of the woman. Women over the age of fifty with ovarian cysts have a higher risk of developing ovarian cancer.

Etiology and the disease process: Functional ovarian cysts, which are not disease related, commonly occur during a woman's normal menstrual cycle. Tiny cysts develop to hold the eggs. When an egg matures, the cyst breaks open to allow the egg to move through the Fallopian tube. Typically, the cyst then dissolves. When the cyst continues to grow and does not break open to release the egg, it is termed a follicular cyst. Follicular cysts usually disappear within sixty days. If follicular cysts continue to grow inside an ovary during repeated menstrual cycles, the patient is said to have polycystic ovaries. If a cyst continues to grow after the egg is released, it is called a corpus luteum cyst. This type of cyst can grow as large as four inches in diameter and will sometimes twist the ovary, causing pelvic or abdominal pain. These cysts can also fill with blood and rupture, causing internal bleeding and intense pain. Corpus luteum cysts typically disappear within a few weeks.

Other types of ovarian cysts include endometriomas, cystadenomas, and dermoid cysts. If tissue from the uterine lining grows outside the uterus, a condition known as endometriosis, it sometimes attaches to an ovary and forms a cystic growth known as an endometrioma. These growths can be very painful during menstruation or sexual intercourse. Growths that develop from the outer epithelial cells of an ovary, known as cystadenomas, typically fill with a fluid, can become twelve inches in diameter or larger, and generate much pain by twisting the ovary. Dermoid cysts form from the germ cells that produce human eggs. They can grow rather large and produce painful twisting of an ovary. They are seldom cancerous.

Incidence: Virtually all women who have menstrual periods will develop ovarian cysts of one type or another. About 20 percent of women have polycystic ovaries. Up to 60 percent of women with endometriosis have endometriomas. The vast majority of ovarian cysts are not cancerous.

Symptoms: Although many women experience no symptoms associated with ovarian cysts, some signs may include abdominal pressure or pain, backache, incomplete urination, unexplained weight gain, painful menstrual periods and abnormal bleeding, pelvic pain during sexual intercourse, tender breasts, and nausea and vomiting. If sudden, severe abdominal or pelvic pain occurs, or pain accompanied by fever and vomiting develops, medical attention should be sought immediately.

Screening and diagnosis: Ovarian cysts are usually found during routine pelvic exams. If a cyst is found, ultrasonic imaging is used to determine its shape, size, location, and content. To determine whether the cyst is malignant, a cancer antigen 125 (CA 125) blood test is sometimes done. For some women with ovarian cancer, this protein occurs in increased levels. Functional uterine fibroids and endometriosis can also increase the CA 125 level. CA 125 tests are recommended for patients over the age of thirty-five who have a high risk for ovarian cancer.

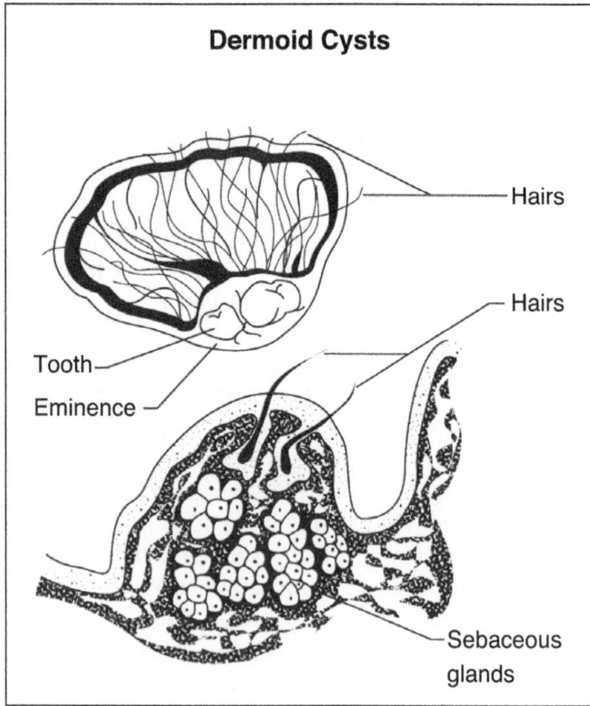

Treatment and therapy: For women still in their childbearing years who have fluid-filled cysts, the most common approach is to wait and watch. If a cyst persists, gets larger, looks unusual, causes too much pain, or the patient goes through menopause, surgical removal may be the best option. For smaller cysts that do not look abnormal in ultrasound images, a laparoscopy may be performed. Using a small incision near the navel, a scope is used to further investigate the cyst. If nothing unusual is found, the cyst is removed. For larger, suspicious-looking cysts, a laparotomy is done. Through larger openings in the stomach, the cyst is removed and tested for cancer by the pathologist. If the cyst is malignant, the doctor will proceed to remove the affected ovary and associated uterine tissues and lymph nodes.

Prognosis, prevention, and outcomes: Although ovarian cysts cannot be prevented, regular pelvic examinations are important to diagnose any problems as early as possible. Any mentrual cycle changes that are abnormal or persist should be discussed with a medical doctor. For women who frequently develop ovarian cysts, a doctor may prescribe birth control pills to reduce the risk of their formation by preventing follicle formation. In most cases, fluid-filled cysts are benign.

Alvin K. Benson, Ph.D.

For Further Information

Bartlett, John M. S. *Ovarian Cancer: Methods and Protocols*. Totowa, N.J.: Humana Press, 2000.

Conner, Kristine, and Lauren Langford. *Ovarian Cancer: Your Guide to Taking Control*. Sebastopol, Calif.: O'Reilly, 2003.

Hammerly, Milton, and Cheryl Kimball. *When the Doctor Says It's PCOS (Polycystic Ovarian Syndrome)*. Beverly, Mass.: Fair Winds Press, 2003.

Icon Health. *Ovarian Cysts: A Medical Dictionary, Bibliography, and Annotated Research Guide to Internet References*. San Diego, Calif.: Author, 2004.

Reznek, Rodney, ed. *Cancer of the Ovary*. Cambridge, England: Cambridge University Press, 2007.

Vliet, Elizabeth Lee. *It's My Ovaries, Stupid!* 2d ed. Tucson, Ariz.: Her Place Press, 2007.

Other Resources

American Cancer Society
Detailed Guide: Ovarian Cancer
http://www.cancer.org/docroot/CRI/CRI_2_3x.asp?dt=33

MayoClinic.com
Ovarian Cancer
http://www.mayoclinic.com/health/ovarian-cancer/DS00293

National Institutes of Health
http://www.cancer.gov/cancertopics/types/ovarian/

Ovarian Cancer National Alliance
http://www.ovariancancer.org/

See also: Amenorrhea; Antiestrogens; CA 27-29 test; CA 125 test; Cervical cancer; Endometrial cancer; Fallopian tube cancer; Fertility drugs and cancer; Gynecologic cancers; Hysterectomy; Ovarian epithelial cancer; Peutz-Jeghers Syndrome (PJS); Uterine cancer; Vaginal cancer; Vulvar cancer

▶ Ovarian epithelial cancer

Category: Diseases, Symptoms, and Conditions
Also known as: Epithelial carcinoma

Related conditions: Abdominal cancer, colon cancer, lymphatic cancer, peritoneal cancer

Definition: Epithelial ovarian cancer results from the development of a malignant tumor that originates in the cells on the outer surface of an ovary. Between 85 and 90 percent of all ovarian cancers are epithelial ovarian cancers.

Risk factors: A history of ovarian cancer within a family—particularly in a woman's mother, sister, or daughter—increases the risk that a woman will develop epithelial ovarian cancer. Inherited gene mutations, specifically the mutated breast cancer genes *BRCA1* and *BRCA2*, are responsible for 5 to 10 percent of all epithelial ovarian cancer. The risk of developing epithelial ovarian cancer is higher in women who have had breast or colon cancer and is highest among women aged fifty and older.

Etiology and the disease process: The exact cause of ovarian epithelial cancer is unknown but it originates in the cells of tissue that cover an ovary. Epithelial ovarian cancer cells can be readily distinguished under a microscope. These cells are differentiated and classified as serous, mucinous, endometrioid, or clear cell types. Serous epithelial cancer cells are the most common. Undifferentiated epithelial ovarian cancer cells tend to grow and spread more rapidly than the four differentiated types. Epithelial ovarian cancers are classified by cell type and graded from 1 to 3. Grade 1 cells look similar to normal tissue and are less dangerous to the patient. Grade 3 cells look quite different from normal tissue and have the worst prognosis.

Epithelial ovarian cancer cells often metastasize by spreading into the abdominal cavity, where they can become implanted in the uterus, the intestines, the omentum, or the bladder. Sometimes they will metastasize to the lungs. On rare occasions, epithelial ovarian cancer cells spread into the bloodstream or lymphatic system and move to many other parts of the body.

Incidence: Epithelial ovarian cancer is one of the leading causes of cancer-related deaths in women. Each year, more than 18,000 women in the United States are diagnosed with ovarian epithelial cancer and about 14,000 succumb to the disease.

Symptoms: Epithelial ovarian cancer is often not detected until it has progressed to an advanced stage. Symptoms include bloating, swelling, or pain in the abdominal area and gastrointestinal problems involving nausea, diarrhea, or constipation.

Screening and diagnosis: If epithelial ovarian cancer is suspected, a doctor will conduct a thorough physical examination of the pelvic region. The shape, size, and position of the uterus and ovaries are assessed. If any growths or abnormal areas are found, they will be further investigated with ultrasonic imaging and computed tomography (CT) scans. The level of cancer antigen 125 (CA 125), which is raised with ovarian cancer, is measured with a blood test. Levels of other cancer-related proteins in the blood are being evaluated for diagnosing ovarian epithelial cancer.

Definitive diagnosis of epithelial ovarian cancer is made through biopsy. Usually when the tumor is removed, a sample of the tissue is analyzed and the stage of the disease is assessed. The staging of epithelial ovarian cancer is as follows:

- Stage I: The cancer is limited to one or both ovaries.
- Stage II: The cancer has metastasized into other parts of the pelvic region.
- Stage III: The cancer has spread to areas outside of the pelvis or has extended into the small intestine or omentum.
- Stage IV: The cancer has metastasized outside the peritoneal cavity.

Depending on the degree of seriousness, these stagings are further broken down into categories ranging from A to C.

Treatment and therapy: Depending on the stage of epithelial ovarian cancer, surgery is often performed to remove the ovaries, uterus, omentum, and associated lymph nodes. After recovery, the patient typically undergoes a regimen of chemotherapy. The most effective chemotherapy drugs used in treating ovarian epithelial cancers are carboplatin and paclitaxel (Taxol), adminstered intravenously. A combination of intravenous chemotherapy and intraperitoneal therapy, the pumping of chemotherapy drugs directly into a patient's abdomen, is recommended by the National Cancer Institute in the treatment of epithelial ovarian cancer patients.

Prognosis, prevention, and outcomes: Because epithelial ovarian cancer is not usually detected until it is in an advanced stage, the prognosis is not promising. The five-year survival rate for all stages of epithelial ovarian cancer is 35 to 38 percent. With early diagnosis, aggressive surgery, and chemotherapy, the five-year survival rate is above 90 percent, and the long-term survival rate approaches 70 percent.

The risk of developing ovarian epithelial cancer can be reduced with a good diet, exercise, and proper management of stress. Other factors that reduce the risk are bearing children and breast-feeding them if possible. Women with a high risk of developing ovarian epithelial cancer may consider removal of the ovaries as a preventive measure.

Alvin K. Benson, Ph.D.

For Further Information

Parker, James N., and Philip M. Parker, eds. *The Official Patient's Sourcebook on Ovarian Epithelial Cancer*. San Diego, Calif.: Icon Health, 2002.

Pfragner, Roswitha, and R. Ian Freshney, eds. *Culture of Human Cancer Cells*. Hoboken, N.J.: Wiley-Liss, 2004.

Reznek, Rodney, ed. *Cancer of the Ovary*. New York: Cambridge University Press, 2007.

Other Resources

American Cancer Society
Detailed Guide: Ovarian Cancer
Http://www.cancer.org/docroot/CRI/CRI_2_3x .asp?dt=33

MayoClinic.com
Ovarian Cancer
http://www.mayoclinic.com/health/ovarian-cancer/ DS00293

National Institutes of Health
http://www.cancer.gov/cancertopics/types/ovarian/

Ovarian Cancer National Alliance
http://www.ovariancancer.org/

See also: Cervical cancer; Endometrial cancer; Fallopian tube cancer; Fertility drugs and cancer; Gynecologic cancers; Ovarian cancers; Ovarian cysts; Uterine cancer; Vaginal cancer; Vulvar cancer